Advances in Neuroscience: Neural Developments in Humans

Advances in Neuroscience: Neural Developments in Humans

Edited by Adam Atkinson

STATES
ACADEMIC PRESS
www.statesacademicpress.com

States Academic Press,
109 South 5th Street,
Brooklyn, NY 11249, USA

Visit us on the World Wide Web at:
www.statesacademicpress.com

ISBN: 978-1-63989-023-1

Cataloging-in-Publication Data

Advances in neuroscience : neural developments in humans / edited by Adam Atkinson.
p. cm.
Includes bibliographical references and index.
ISBN 978-1-63989-023-1
1. Neurosciences. 2. Nervous system. 3. Human beings. 4. Brain. I. Atkinson, Adam.
RC341 .A28 2022
616.8--dc23

Table of Contents

Preface

The scientific study of the nervous system is referred to as neuroscience. It is a multidisciplinary field that combines anatomy, physiology, developmental biology, molecular biology, cytology, mathematical modeling and computer science to understand the fundamentals of neurons and neural circuits. Neurons are the specialized cells that play a significant role in communication. Neuroscience studies the brain and its impact on behavior and cognitive functions. It also covers the study of functional, cellular, behavioral, computational, evolutionary, medical and molecular aspects of the nervous system. There are several branches of neuroscience such as affective neuroscience, clinical neuroscience, behavioral neuroscience, cognitive neuroscience, cultural neuroscience, computational neuroscience, developmental neuroscience, etc. The topics covered in this extensive book deal with the core subjects of neuroscience. It explores all the important aspects of this field in the present day scenario. For all those who are interested in the field of neuroscience, this book can prove to be an essential guide.

Various studies have approached the subject by analyzing it with a single perspective, but the present book provides diverse methodologies and techniques to address this field. This book contains theories and applications needed for understanding the subject from different perspectives. The aim is to keep the readers informed about the progresses in the field; therefore, the contributions were carefully examined to compile novel researches by specialists from across the globe.

Indeed, the job of the editor is the most crucial and challenging in compiling all chapters into a single book. In the end, I would extend my sincere thanks to the chapter authors for their profound work. I am also thankful for the support provided by my family and colleagues during the compilation of this book.

Editor

1

Cell cycle activity of neural precursors in the diseased mammalian brain

Sara Bragado Alonso*[†]*, Max Schulze-Steikow*[†] *and Federico Calegari**

DFG–Research Center and Cluster of Excellence for Regenerative Therapies, Dresden, Germany

Edited by:
Luca Bonfanti, University of Turin, Italy

Reviewed by:
Claudio Giachino, University of Basel, Switzerland
Giovanna Ponti, University of Turin, Italy

***Correspondence:**
Federico Calegari, DFG–Research Center and Cluster of Excellence for Regenerative Therapies, TU-Dresden., Fetscherstrasse 105, 01307 Dresden, Germany
e-mail: federico.calegari@crt-dresden.de
[†]*Joint first authors.*

Basic research during embryonic development has led to the identification of general principles governing cell cycle progression, proliferation and differentiation of mammalian neural stem cells (NSC). These findings were recently translated to the adult brain in an attempt to identify the overall principles governing stemness in the two contexts and allowing us to manipulate the expansion of NSC for regenerative therapies. However, and despite a huge literature on embryonic neural precursors, very little is known about cell cycle parameters of adult neural, or any other somatic, stem cell. In this review, we briefly discuss the long journey of NSC research from embryonic development to adult homeostasis, aging and therapy with a specific focus on their quiescence and cell cycle length in physiological conditions and neurological disorders. Particular attention is given to a new important player in the field, oligodendrocyte progenitors, while discussing the limitation hampering further development in this challenging area.

Keywords: cell cycle, neural stem cells, oligodendrocyte precursor cell (OPC), neurodegenerative diseases, adult neurogenesis

INTRODUCTION

The study of the cell cycle is one of the most prolific areas in developmental neuroscience with hundreds of publications spanning half a century and contributing new methodologies, basic knowledge and a deeper understanding of brain development and evolution (Fujita, 1962; Schultze and Korr, 1981; Takahashi et al., 1995; Dehay and Kennedy, 2007; Salomoni and Calegari, 2010; Borrell and Calegari, in press).

Cell cycle regulation in itself is a huge field and several reviews already discussed its molecular control during brain development and adulthood (Dehay and Kennedy, 2007; Salomoni and Calegari, 2010; Beukelaers et al., 2011b). As one factor fuelling interest in this area, short cell cycles were found to correlate with a higher proliferative potential of neural precursors at the cellular and tissue level and across phylogeny (Borrell and Calegari, in press). This correlation led to functional manipulations showing that the proliferative potential of neural precursors is increased by shortening their cell cycle while, conversely, lengthening it leads to differentiation and neurogenesis (Calegari and Huttner, 2003; Lange et al., 2009; Pilaz et al., 2009; Artegiani et al., 2011; Beukelaers et al., 2011a).

Considering that the first calculation of the cell cycle during development coincided with the first report on adult neurogenesis five decades ago (Altman, 1962; Fujita, 1962) and that immense efforts are currently invested worldwide in stem cell research and regenerative medicine, it comes as a surprise that cell cycle studies during adulthood, contrary to development, are extremely limited with only a handful addressing the diseased brain. Here we summarize our knowledge on cell cycle parameters of adult neural precursors in physiological and pathological conditions with particular attention to a new player in biomedicine, oligodendrocyte progenitors. This is important to identify potential correlations of biological significance and to identify our gaps in knowledge that the field should address in the years to come.

NEUROGENIC PRECURSORS

CELL CYCLE IN PHYSIOLOGICAL CONDITIONS

Mammalian NSC generate neurons and glia throughout life within two restricted areas: the subgranular zone (SGZ) of the dentate gyrus and the subventricular zone (SVZ) of the lateral ventricles (Zhao et al., 2008; Kriegstein and Alvarez-Buylla, 2009). In both niches a pool of NSC, progenitors and neuroblasts coexist in a dynamic system in which the production of neurons is regulated by intrinsic and extrinsic factors (Lois and Alvarez-Buylla, 1994; Cameron and McKay, 2001). Similarly to their embryonic precursors (Merkle et al., 2004; Li et al., 2013), adult NSC maintain a radial morphology (Doetsch et al., 1999; Seri et al., 2001), contact blood vessels (Palmer et al., 2000; Tavazoie et al., 2008) and share common markers (Kriegstein and Alvarez-Buylla, 2009). However, in contrast to embryonic development no unique marker has been identified that exclusively labels one, but not others, precursor types (Ming and Song, 2011). In addition, no positive marker of quiescent cells is available to date. These limitations, together with the fact that a significant proportion of NSC are quiescent, makes it remarkably difficult to assess cell cycle parameters during adulthood.

In the SGZ, dividing NSC (type 1) give rise to intermediate progenitors (type 2) that in turn generate neuroblasts (type 3) producing granule neurons (Seri et al., 2001; Kempermann et al., 2004). The significance of adult hippocampal neurogenesis is not fully understood but evidence points to a role in learning and memory (Kempermann, 2008; Deng et al., 2010). With regard to the lineage of hippocampal NSC, studies have calculated that type 1 cells undergo 3–4 asymmetric divisions before becoming postmitotic astrocytes (Encinas et al., 2011) while others have concluded that at least some type 1 cells can self-renew unlimited times throughout life (Bonaguidi et al., 2011). Despite this controversy, studies attempting to measure the cell cycle in the adult hippocampus found that cycling NSC divide every about 1 day (Lugert et al., 2010; Encinas et al., 2011; Brandt et al., 2012) with S being the most variable phase among progenitors (Brandt et al., 2012). In particular, type 1 cells complete the cell cycle in 23 h with an S-phase of 10 h (Brandt et al., 2012). Subsequently, type 2 cells lengthen to 27 h while type 3 shorten again to 23 h. Although G1, G2, and M were not individually measured, cell cycle differences were found to be almost exclusively due to S-phase (**Table 1**) (Brandt et al., 2012).

The SVZ is the second and most proliferative neurogenic niche of the adult mammalian brain (Kriegstein and Alvarez-Buylla, 2009; Ming and Song, 2011). Here, NSC (B cells) have an apical process intercalating between ependymal cells and contacting the ventricle (Mirzadeh et al., 2008) and a basal process contacting blood vessels (Shen et al., 2008). B cells give rise to amplifying progenitors (C cells) that generate migrating neuroblasts (A cells) dividing along the SVZ and rostral migratory stream toward the olfactory bulb where they ultimately differentiate into neurons (Petreanu and Alvarez-Buylla, 2002; Ming and Song, 2011). At any given time, B cells represent 10% of all cycling cells (Doetsch et al., 2002) with a similar proportion being cycling as opposed to quiescent (Ponti et al., 2013). B cells complete the cell cycle in 18 h and G1 and S in 8 and 5 h, respectively (**Table 1**) (Ponti et al., 2013). Regarding C cells, these represent over 60% of proliferating cells (Doetsch et al., 2002) with nearly 90% of them cycling at any given time (Ponti et al., 2013). C cells are proposed to divide symmetrically 2–3 times before generating A cells and have more heterogeneous cell cycles of 17–22 h, a longer S-phase of 12–15 h and a remarkably short G1 of 2 h (Ponti et al., 2013). Finally, A cells account for 26% of dividing cells in the SVZ (Doetsch et al., 2002), have a cell cycle similar to C cells with perhaps a longer G1 (2–5 h) and shorter S of 10 h (**Table 1**) (Ponti et al., 2013).

Altogether, cell cycle differences within neurogenic niches seem minor with the only consistent change being a lengthening of S-phase from NSC to progenitors and shortening from progenitors to neuroblasts. Not only is the significance of such changes unknown but no parallelism is evident between embryonic and adulthood precursors because in the former S-phase was found to be longer in NSC than in progenitors (Arai et al., 2011) and G1 during adulthood was found to length from C to A cells but not from B to C cells (Ponti et al., 2013).

CELL CYCLE IN PATHOLOGICAL CONDITIONS

Neural progenitors increase their proliferation, meant both as exiting quiescence and shortening the cell cycle, under pathological conditions in both neurogenic niches (Dash et al., 2001; Arvidsson et al., 2002). Most studies focused on the SVZ where neural precursors change their migration and are redirected to the injured area to acquire the phenotype of local cells (Arvidsson et al., 2002), thus, making the SVZ a potential target of therapy. Increased proliferation and altered migration were found in rodent models of multiple sclerosis (Rasmussen et al., 2011; Mecha et al., 2013), Huntington's disease (Tattersfield et al., 2004), Parkinson (Aponso et al., 2008) and stroke (Thored et al., 2006), the latter of which was also shown in humans (Jin et al., 2006; Minger et al., 2007). Among these diseases, the neurogenic response triggered by stroke is the most prominent and best characterized.

Stroke is a cerebrovascular accident resulting in a permanent damage and second leading cause of death worldwide (WHO, 2013). Two days after striatal stroke, SVZ precursors shorten the cell cycle form 19 to 12 h due to a shorter G1 from 13 to 8 h and S from 5 to 2 h (**Table 1**) (Zhang et al., 2006, 2008). Subsequently, cell cycle progressively lengthens reaching normal values 14 days after stroke. Interestingly, the proportion of proliferative, as opposed to differentiative, divisions increases (from 10 to 50%) during the period of short cell cycles and, conversely, decreases (back to 10%) during the long ones (Zhang et al., 2008) although it is important to note that in these studies precursor types were not distinguished and that these values refer to the total SVZ population. Nevertheless, stroke results in an increasing cohort of neuroblasts migrating from the SVZ toward the striatum with a peak at day 14 (Zhang et al., 2004) and lasting for at least 4 months (Arvidsson et al., 2002; Thored et al., 2006; Yamashita et al., 2006). Most of these newborn neurons undergo apoptosis but those that survive functionally integrate (Yamashita et al., 2006; Hou et al., 2008) with evidence indicating that this endogenous neurogenesis can contribute to functional recovery after stroke since, for instance, ablation of neural precursors impairs recovery (Jin et al., 2010; Sun et al., 2013). Yet, it still has to be shown whether an artificial increase in endogenous neurogenesis would favor brain function.

Altogether, cell cycle parameters of precursor cells after stroke recapitulate embryonic development in the sense that short cell cycles are coupled to proliferation and long cell cycles to differentiation. In this context, cell cycle re-entry is likely instrumental to guide the stroke-induced neurogenic response and, in fact, activation of cell cycle regulators is known to occur in both rodents and humans (Love, 2003; Rashidian et al., 2007). Yet, this response in postmitotic neurons is likely to induce apoptosis rather than cell cycle re-entry (Rashidian et al., 2007). This is supported by the fact that injecting a cdk inhibitor in the ischemic area reduces apoptosis and extension of the ischemic core (Osuga et al., 2000) suggesting that cell cycle regulators have different effects in postmitotic neurons or precursors, which should be considered in manipulations aimed to improve recovery. In this context, increasing the endogenous pool of neurogenic precursors by manipulating their cell cycle seems a promising approach to therapy. Moreover, other targets have recently emerged including ependymal cells (Carlen et al., 2009) and glial precursors (Zhang et al., 2011). To our knowledge cell cycle of ependymal cells during neurodegeneration has not been assessed while some groups are now pioneering the study of gliogenesis.

GLIOGENIC PRECURSORS

CELL CYCLE IN PHYSIOLOGICAL CONDITIONS

Astrocytes and oligodendrocytes are the most abundant cell type of the adult brain with the latter gaining more interest for their role and potential use during brain recovery (Richardson et al., 2011; Tsai et al., 2012).

Table 1 | Cell cycle parameters of neurogenic and oligodendrogenic precursors.

precursors	CNS area	cell or tissue type	GF (%)	G1	S	G2+M	cell cycle
neurogenic precursors	hippocampus	type 1	-	-	10 h	-	23 h
		type 2	-	-	14 h	-	27 h
		type 3	-	-	10 h	-	23 h
	SVZ	B cells	9	8 h	5 h	6 h	18 h
		C cells	87	2 h	12-15 h	4 h	17-22 h
		A cells	-	2-5 h	9-11 h	4 h	17-20 h
		total cells	20 / 24	13 h / 8 h	4-5 h / 2 h	2 h / 2 h	19 h / 12 h
oligodendrogenic precursors	brain	white matter	30-99	-	0.8 d	-	10 d
		grey matter	50-98	-	1 d	4 d*	36 d
	spinal cord	white matter	99	-	1.1 d	-	15 d
		grey matter	99	-	0.8 d	-	27 d

*Left to right: precursor types in different areas of the CNS and individual cell types or tissues are indicated with proportion of cycling cells (growth fraction, GF), length of individual phases and total cell cycle in hours (h) or days (d). Split cells indicate values calculated in physiological (left) or pathological (right) conditions. OPC values were acquired at the age of approximately 2 months. *Value calculated from (Simon et al., 2011; Young et al., 2013).*

Oligodendrocyte progenitor cells (OPC) play pivotal roles in CNS development (Richardson et al., 2006) and adulthood where they represent the most abundant and homogeneously distributed cycling cell population of the CNS (Richardson et al., 2011). Oligodendrocytes during development are generated from different regions in consecutive waves but it is unknown whether each population has any specific role in brain function (Kessaris et al., 2006). Adult OPC represent 8 and 2% of the white and gray matter, respectively (Dawson, 2003; Rivers et al., 2008) with resident and migrating OPC in the SVZ and septum giving rise to mature myelinating oligodendrocytes in physiological and pathological conditions (Menn et al., 2006). Maturation of OPC involves changes in morphology and marker expression including Pdgfra, Ng2 for OPC and Olig2 and Sox10 for the whole lineage (Fumagalli et al., 2011). OPC are reactive to neurotransmitters (Bergles et al., 2000; Stevens et al., 2002) and display highly dynamic behavior with regard to migration, filopodia extension, proliferation, differentiation and reaction to injury (Hughes et al., 2013).

Starting at postnatal day 7 and during adulthood, approximately 50–80% of OPC in the whole brain were described as cycling based on BrdU incorporation (Rivers et al., 2008; Psachoulia et al., 2009; Simon et al., 2011). Another report based on EdU however calculated a growth fraction of about 99% (Young et al., 2013) but this thymidine analog has raised concern with regard to toxicity (Ponti et al., 2013). Cell cycle length of OPC differs among brain regions and is significantly longer than that of neurogenic precursors. In the white matter, in particular corpus callosum, OPC cell cycle linearly increases from 2 days at 1 week postnatal to a plateau of 150 days at 8 months (Rivers et al., 2008; Psachoulia et al., 2009; Young et al., 2013) with the spinal cord white matter yielding comparable results (**Table 1**) (Young et al., 2013). In the cortical gray matter cell cycle length was estimated to be about 37 days at 2 months (Simon et al., 2011; Young et al., 2013) with S/G2/M of 5 days (Simon et al., 2011). Cell cycle in the cortex also showed a decrease similar to the corpus callosum with the important difference that a plateau is not reached and cell cycle increases to up to 340 days at 18 months (Psachoulia et al., 2009; Young et al., 2013). This almost linear relationship between age and cell cycle implies a lengthening by about 16 h every day starting at birth (Young et al., 2013), that is, every cell cycle is two thirds longer than the previous one. Finally, cell cycle in the gray matter of the spinal cord is significantly shorter than in the cortex with OPC dividing every 8 or 27 days at 3 weeks or 2 months postnatal, respectively (**Table 1**) (Young et al., 2013). With regard to the proportion of OPC that divide to proliferate as opposed to generate mature oligodendrocytes, different studies led to different estimations while consistently reporting higher values for the white matter both in the brain and spinal cord with both declining during aging (Rivers et al., 2008; Psachoulia et al., 2009; Kang et al., 2010; Simon et al., 2011; Zhu et al., 2011; Young et al., 2013).

In conclusion, OPC exhibit a remarkably longer cell cycle than neurogenic precursors, which to our opinion reflects long periods of quiescence followed by re-entry in a cell cycle that is a fraction of the total inter-mitotic time. Moreover, the cell cycle of OPC differs between gray and white matter, which is possibly explained by region-specific differences as revealed by transplantation experiments (Vigano et al., 2013).

CELL CYCLE IN PATHOLOGICAL CONDITIONS

Accumulating evidence indicates that OPC play key roles during brain injury (Nguyen et al., 2006; Huang et al., 2011; Zhang et al., 2013). Demyelination in multiple sclerosis leads to impaired saltatory signal conduction and loss of axon integrity (Huang et al., 2011). OPC react by migrating into the lesion and differentiate in mature myelinating oligodendrocytes and Schwann cells (Zawadzka et al., 2010). This reaction enhances recovery and is known to decrease with age making it a potential target for regenerative therapies (Nguyen et al., 2006; Zawadzka et al., 2010; Huang et al., 2011; Deshmukh et al., 2013).

Stab wound in the cortex increases proliferation in the whole brain with a five-fold higher response in the ipsilateral compared to contralateral hemisphere 3 days post injury (Simon et al., 2011). In particular, at 1 week 74% of OPC cycle suggesting that cells enter the cell cycle from quiescence and, concomitantly, shorten the G1-phase of their cell cycle (Simon et al., 2011).

Cerebral ischemia has a strong impact on oligodendrocytes since they lack the ability to proliferate and, once damaged, to myelinate axons (McTigue and Tripathi, 2008). After stroke resident and SVZ-derived OPC start to proliferate and migrate to the penumbra where they differentiate into mature oligodendrocytes that myelinate newly sprouted axons thus enhancing neuronal survival and short-term synaptic plasticity (Zhang and Chopp, 2009; Ueno et al., 2012; Zhang et al., 2013) and preclinical studies showed improved healing of stroke after pharmaceutically enhanced oligodendrogenesis (Zhang et al., 2013).

Most studies have focused on neuronal aspects of brain recovery and the role of other cell types awaits further investigation. Only recently studies started to focus on cell cycle parameters of OPC and other cell types such as astrocytes and pericytes playing critical roles in disease including glial scar formation and inflammation (Goritz et al., 2011; Lambertsen et al., 2012).

DISCUSSION

Decades of cell cycle measurements during development have been instrumental to understand and manipulate the contribution of neural precursors in the mammalian brain (Fujita, 1962; Schultze and Korr, 1981; Takahashi et al., 1995; Dehay and Kennedy, 2007; Salomoni and Calegari, 2010; Borrell and Calegari, in press). Studies during adulthood have just begun and parallelisms between the two contexts are hard to identify due to our limited understanding of adult lineages and difficulties in assessing cell cycle and quiescence. Notably, during development progenitors have longer cell cycles than stem cells (Borrell and Calegari, in press). Yet, differences of greater significance were found by comparing cells undergoing proliferative vs. differentiative division within these two populations (Calegari et al., 2005; Arai et al., 2011). Hence, analyses of, say, type 1/B vs. 2/C cells can only reveal part of the truth with identification of proliferative vs. differentiative precursors within each type being perhaps more important. Moreover, independently from physiological correlations between cell cycle and stemness, it is clear that artificial manipulations can still be effective in increasing stem cell expansion since these can override physiological processes as indicated by studies on NSC and OPC (Artegiani et al., 2011; Beukelaers et al., 2011a; Caillava et al., 2011; Nobs et al., 2013).

It is premature to know whether manipulation of neural precursors will ever allow practical and efficient means toward effective therapy, but the history of cell cycle measurements during development suggests that this may pave a promising road. To achieving this goal, technical limitations need first to be overcome including the identification of markers for the relevant cell types, establishing behavioral tests reflecting functional recovery rather than compensatory learning (Hicks et al., 2009) and animal models of disease faithfully recapitulating the human condition. As one example of the latter, models of stroke often involve the striatum whereas human ischemia mainly affects cortical areas while the few that involve the striatum cause mild deficits (Delavaran et al., 2013). Moreover, modeling disease is often done in young mice while most neurodegenerative diseases are relevant during aging, which has major effects on cell cycle and neurogenesis (Artegiani and Calegari, 2012). We envision that improvements in these aspects of biomedical research will have the greatest impact in the field and hope that this review will help readers to identify, hence overcome, some of our current limitations.

ACKNOWLEDGMENTS

The authors were supported by the CRTD, the TU-Dresden, ERA-NET NEURON, BMBF, RENEW IT and the DFG Collaborative Research Center SFB655 (subproject A20). The authors declare no conflict of interest.

REFERENCES

Altman, J. (1962). Are new neurons formed in the brains of adult mammals? *Science* 135, 1127–1128. doi: 10.1126/science.135.3509.1127

Aponso, P. M., Faull, R. L., and Connor, B. (2008). Increased progenitor cell proliferation and astrogenesis in the partial progressive 6-hydroxydopamine model of Parkinson's disease. *Neuroscience* 151, 1142–1153. doi: 10.1016/j.neuroscience.2007.11.036

Arai, Y., Pulvers, J. N., Haffner, C., Schilling, B., Nusslein, I., Calegari, F., et al. (2011). Neural stem and progenitor cells shorten S-phase on commitment to neuron production. *Nat. Commun.* 2, 154. doi: 10.1038/ncomms1155

Artegiani, B., and Calegari, F. (2012). Age-related cognitive decline: can neural stem cells help us? *Aging* 4, 176–186.

Artegiani, B., Lindemann, D., and Calegari, F. (2011). Overexpression of cdk4 and cyclinD1 triggers greater expansion of neural stem cells in the adult mouse brain. *J. Exp. Med.* 208, 937–948. doi: 10.1084/jem.20102167

Arvidsson, A., Collin, T., Kirik, D., Kokaia, Z., and Lindvall, O. (2002). Neuronal replacement from endogenous precursors in the adult brain after stroke. *Nat. Med.* 8, 963–970. doi: 10.1038/nm747

Bergles, D. E., Roberts, J. D., Somogyi, P., and Jahr, C. E. (2000). Glutamatergic synapses on oligodendrocyte precursor cells in the hippocampus. *Nature* 405, 187–191. doi: 10.1038/35012083

Beukelaers, P., Vandenbosch, R., Caron, N., Nguyen, L., Belachew, S., Moonen, G., et al. (2011a). Cdk6-dependent regulation of G(1) length controls adult neurogenesis. *Stem cells* 29, 713–724. doi: 10.1002/stem.616

Beukelaers, P., Vandenbosch, R., Caron, N., Nguyen, L., Moonen, G., and Malgrange, B. (2011b). Cycling or not cycling: cell cycle regulatory molecules and adult neurogenesis. *Cell. Mol. Life Sci.* 69, 1493–1503. doi: 10.1007/s00018-011-0880-6

Bonaguidi, M. A., Wheeler, M. A., Shapiro, J. S., Stadel, R. P., Sun, G. J., Ming, G. L., et al. (2011). *In vivo* clonal analysis reveals self-renewing and multipotent adult neural stem cell characteristics. *Cell* 145, 1142–1155. doi: 10.1016/j.cell.2011.05.024

Borrell, V., and Calegari, F. (in press). Mechanisms of brain evolution: regulation of neural progenitor cell diversity and cell cycle length. *Neurosci Res.*

Brandt, M. D., Hubner, M., and Storch, A. (2012). Brief report: adult hippocampal precursor cells shorten S-phase and total cell cycle length during neuronal differentiation. *Stem cells* 30, 2843–2847. doi: 10.1002/stem.1244

Caillava, C., Vandenbosch, R., Jablonska, B., Deboux, C., Spigoni, G., Gallo, V., et al. (2011). Cdk2 loss accelerates precursor differentiation and remyelination in the adult central nervous system. *J. Cell Biol.* 193, 397–407. doi: 10.1083/jcb.201004146

Calegari, F., Haubensak, W., Haffner, C., and Huttner, W. B. (2005). Selective lengthening of the cell cycle in the neurogenic subpopulation of neural progenitor cells during mouse brain development. *J. Neurosci.* 25, 6533–6538. doi: 10.1523/JNEUROSCI.0778-05.2005

Calegari, F., and Huttner, W. B. (2003). An inhibition of cyclin-dependent kinases that lengthens, but does not arrest, neuroepithelial cell cycle induces premature neurogenesis. *J. Cell Sci.* 116, 4947–4955. doi: 10.1242/jcs.00825

Cameron, H. A., and McKay, R. D. (2001). Adult neurogenesis produces a large pool of new granule cells in the dentate gyrus. *J. Comp. Neurol.* 435, 406–417. doi: 10.1002/cne.1040

Carlen, M., Meletis, K., Goritz, C., Darsalia, V., Evergren, E., Tanigaki, K., et al. (2009). Forebrain ependymal cells are Notch-dependent and generate neuroblasts and astrocytes after stroke. *Nat. Neurosci.* 12, 259–267. doi: 10.1038/nn.2268

Dash, P. K., Mach, S. A., and Moore, A. N. (2001). Enhanced neurogenesis in the rodent hippocampus following traumatic brain injury. *J. Neurosci. Res.* 63, 313–319. doi: 10.1002/1097-4547(20010215)63:4%3C313::AID-JNR1025%3E3.3.CO;2-W

Dawson, M. (2003). NG2-expressing glial progenitor cells: an abundant and widespread population of cycling cells in the adult rat CNS. *Mol. Cell. Neurosci.* 24, 476–488. doi: 10.1016/S1044-7431(03)00210-0

Dehay, C., and Kennedy, H. (2007). Cell-cycle control and cortical development. *Nat. Rev. Neurosci.* 8, 438–450. doi: 10.1038/nrn2097

Delavaran, H., Sjunnesson, H., Arvidsson, A., Lindvall, O., Norrving, B., Van Westen, D., et al. (2013). Proximity of brain infarcts to regions of endogenous neurogenesis and involvement of striatum in ischaemic stroke. *Eur. J. Neurol.* 20, 473–479. doi: 10.1111/j.1468-1331.2012.03877.x

Deng, W., Aimone, J. B., and Gage, F. H. (2010). New neurons and new memories: how does adult hippocampal neurogenesis affect learning and memory? *Nat. Rev. Neurosci.* 11, 339–350. doi: 10.1038/nrn2822

Deshmukh, V. A., Tardif, V., Lyssiotis, C. A., Green, C. C., Kerman, B., Kim, H. J., et al. (2013). A regenerative approach to the treatment of multiple sclerosis. *Nature* 502, 327–332. doi: 10.1038/nature12647

Doetsch, F., Caille, I., Lim, D. A., Garcia-Verdugo, J. M., and Alvarez-Buylla, A. (1999). Subventricular zone astrocytes are neural stem cells in the adult mammalian brain. *Cell* 97, 703–716. doi: 10.1016/S0092-8674(00)80783-7

Doetsch, F., Verdugo, J. M., Caille, I., Alvarez-Buylla, A., Chao, M. V., and Casaccia-Bonnefil, P. (2002). Lack of the cell-cycle inhibitor p27Kip1 results in selective increase of transit-amplifying cells for adult neurogenesis. *J. Neurosci.* 22, 2255–2264.

Encinas, J. M., Michurina, T. V., Peunova, N., Park, J. H., Tordo, J., Peterson, D. A., et al. (2011). Division-coupled astrocytic differentiation and age-related depletion of neural stem cells in the adult hippocampus. *Cell Stem Cell* 8, 566–579. doi: 10.1016/j.stem.2011.03.010

Fujita, S. (1962). Kinetics of cellular proliferation. *Exp. Cell Res.* 28, 52–60. doi: 10.1016/0014-4827(62)90311-7

Fumagalli, M., Daniele, S., Lecca, D., Lee, P. R., Parravicini, C., Fields, R. D., et al. (2011). Phenotypic changes, signaling pathway, and functional correlates of GPR17-expressing neural precursor cells during oligodendrocyte differentiation. *J. Biol. Chem.* 286, 10593–10604. doi: 10.1074/jbc.M110.162867

Goritz, C., Dias, D. O., Tomilin, N., Barbacid, M., Shupliakov, O., and Frisen, J. (2011). A pericyte origin of spinal cord scar tissue. *Science* 333, 238–242. doi: 10.1126/science.1203165

Hicks, A., Schallert, T., and Jolkkonen, J. (2009). Cell-based therapies and functional outcome in experimental stroke. *Cell Stem Cell* 5, 139–140. doi: 10.1016/j.stem.2009.07.009

Hou, S. W., Wang, Y. Q., Xu, M., Shen, D. H., Wang, J. J., Huang, F., et al. (2008). Functional integration of newly generated neurons into striatum after cerebral ischemia in the adult rat brain. *Stroke* 39, 2837–2844. doi: 10.1161/STROKEAHA.107.510982

Huang, J. K., Fancy, S. P., Zhao, C., Rowitch, D. H., Ffrench-Constant, C., and Franklin, R. J. (2011). Myelin regeneration in multiple sclerosis: targeting endogenous stem cells. *Neurotherapeutics* 8, 650–658. doi: 10.1007/s13311-011-0065-x

Hughes, E. G., Kang, S. H., Fukaya, M., and Bergles, D. E. (2013). Oligodendrocyte progenitors balance growth with self-repulsion to achieve homeostasis in the adult brain. *Nat. Neurosci.* 16, 668–676. doi: 10.1038/nn.3390

Jin, K., Wang, X., Xie, L., Mao, X. O., and Greenberg, D. A. (2010). Transgenic ablation of doublecortin-expressing cells suppresses adult neurogenesis and worsens stroke outcome in mice. *Proc. Natl. Acad. Sci. U.S.A.* 107, 7993–7998. doi: 10.1073/pnas.1000154107

Jin, K., Wang, X., Xie, L., Mao, X. O., Zhu, W., Wang, Y., et al. (2006). Evidence for stroke-induced neurogenesis in the human brain. *Proc. Natl. Acad. Sci. U.S.A.* 103, 13198–13202. doi: 10.1073/pnas.0603512103

Kang, S. H., Fukaya, M., Yang, J. K., Rothstein, J. D., and Bergles, D. E. (2010). NG2+ CNS glial progenitors remain committed to the oligodendrocyte lineage in postnatal life and following neurodegeneration. *Neuron* 68, 668–681. doi: 10.1016/j.neuron.2010.09.009

Kempermann, G. (2008). The neurogenic reserve hypothesis: what is adult hippocampal neurogenesis good for? *Trends Neurosci.* 31, 163–169. doi: 10.1016/j.tins.2008.01.002

Kempermann, G., Jessberger, S., Steiner, B., and Kronenberg, G. (2004). Milestones of neuronal development in the adult hippocampus. *Trends Neurosci.* 27, 447–452. doi: 10.1016/j.tins.2004.05.013

Kessaris, N., Fogarty, M., Iannarelli, P., Grist, M., Wegner, M., and Richardson, W. D. (2006). Competing waves of oligodendrocytes in the forebrain and postnatal elimination of an embryonic lineage. *Nat. Neurosci.* 9, 173–179. doi: 10.1038/nn1620

Kriegstein, A., and Alvarez-Buylla, A. (2009). The glial nature of embryonic and adult neural stem cells. *Annu. Rev. Neurosci.* 32, 149–184. doi: 10.1146/annurev.neuro.051508.135600

Lambertsen, K. L., Biber, K., and Finsen, B. (2012). Inflammatory cytokines in experimental and human stroke. *J. Cereb. Blood Flow Metab.* 32, 1677–1698. doi: 10.1038/jcbfm.2012.88

Lange, C., Huttner, W. B., and Calegari, F. (2009). Cdk4/cyclinD1 overexpression in neural stem cells shortens G1, delays neurogenesis, and promotes the generation and expansion of basal progenitors. *Cell Stem Cell* 5, 320–331. doi: 10.1016/j.stem.2009.05.026

Li, G., Fang, L., Fernandez, G., and Pleasure, S. J. (2013). The ventral hippocampus is the embryonic origin for adult neural stem cells in the dentate gyrus. *Neuron* 78, 658–672. doi: 10.1016/j.neuron.2013.03.019

Lois, C., and Alvarez-Buylla, A. (1994). Long-distance neuronal migration in the adult mammalian brain. *Science* 264, 1145–1148. doi: 10.1126/science.8178174

Love, S. (2003). Neuronal expression of cell cycle-related proteins after brain ischaemia in man. *Neurosci. Lett.* 353, 29–32. doi: 10.1016/j.neulet.2003.09.004

Lugert, S., Basak, O., Knuckles, P., Haussler, U., Fabel, K., Gotz, M., et al. (2010). Quiescent and active hippocampal neural stem cells with distinct morphologies respond selectively to physiological and pathological stimuli and aging. *Cell Stem Cell* 6, 445–456. doi: 10.1016/j.stem.2010.03.017

McTigue, D. M., and Tripathi, R. B. (2008). The life, death, and replacement of oligodendrocytes in the adult CNS. *J. Neurochem.* 107, 1–19. doi: 10.1111/j.1471-4159.2008.05570.x

Mecha, M., Feliu, A., Carrillo-Salinas, F. J., Mestre, L., and Guaza, C. (2013). Mobilization of progenitors in the subventricular zone to undergo oligodendrogenesis in the Theiler's virus model of multiple sclerosis: implications for remyelination at lesions sites. *Exp. Neurol.* 250, 348–352. doi: 10.1016/j.expneurol.2013.10.011

Menn, B., Garcia-Verdugo, J. M., Yaschine, C., Gonzalez-Perez, O., Rowitch, D., and Alvarez-Buylla, A. (2006). Origin of oligodendrocytes in the subventricular zone of the adult brain. *J. Neurosci.* 26, 7907–7918. doi: 10.1523/JNEUROSCI.1299-06.2006

Merkle, F. T., Tramontin, A. D., Garcia-Verdugo, J. M., and Alvarez-Buylla, A. (2004). Radial glia give rise to adult neural stem cells in the subventricular zone. *Proc. Natl. Acad. Sci. U.S.A.* 101, 17528–17532. doi: 10.1073/pnas.0407893101

Ming, G. L., and Song, H. (2011). Adult neurogenesis in the mammalian brain: significant answers and significant questions. *Neuron* 70, 687–702. doi: 10.1016/j.neuron.2011.05.001

Minger, S. L., Ekonomou, A., Carta, E. M., Chinoy, A., Perry, R. H., and Ballard, C. G. (2007). Endogenous neurogenesis in the human brain following cerebral infarction. *Regen. Med.* 2, 69–74. doi: 10.2217/17460751.2.1.69

Mirzadeh, Z., Merkle, F. T., Soriano-Navarro, M., Garcia-Verdugo, J. M., and Alvarez-Buylla, A. (2008). Neural stem cells confer unique pinwheel architecture to the ventricular surface in neurogenic regions of the adult brain. *Cell Stem Cell* 3, 265–278. doi: 10.1016/j.stem.2008.07.004

Nguyen, L., Borgs, L., Vandenbosch, R., Mangin, J. M., Beukelaers, P., Moonen, G., et al. (2006). The Yin and Yang of cell cycle progression and differentiation in the oligodendroglial lineage. *Ment. Retard. Dev. Disabil. Res. Rev.* 12, 85–96. doi: 10.1002/mrdd.20103

Nobs, L., Nestel, S., Kulik, A., Nitsch, C., and Atanasoski, S. (2013). Cyclin D1 is required for proliferation of Olig2-expressing progenitor cells in the injured cerebral cortex. *Glia* 61, 1443–1455. doi: 10.1002/glia.22533

Osuga, H., Osuga, S., Wang, F., Fetni, R., Hogan, M. J., Slack, R. S., et al. (2000). Cyclin-dependent kinases as a therapeutic target for stroke. *Proc. Natl. Acad. Sci. U.S.A.* 97, 10254–10259. doi: 10.1073/pnas.170144197

Palmer, T. D., Willhoite, A. R., and Gage, F. H. (2000). Vascular niche for adult hippocampal neurogenesis. *J. Com. Neurol.* 425, 479–494. doi: 10.1002/1096-9861(20001002)425:4%3C479::AID-CNE2%3E3.0.CO;2-3

Petreanu, L., and Alvarez-Buylla, A. (2002). Maturation and death of adult-born olfactory bulb granule neurons: role of olfaction. *J. Neurosci.* 22, 6106–6113.

Pilaz, L. J., Patti, D., Marcy, G., Ollier, E., Pfister, S., Douglas, R. J., et al. (2009). Forced G1-phase reduction alters mode of division, neuron number, and laminar phenotype in the cerebral cortex. *Proc. Natl. Acad. Sci. U.S.A.* 106, 21924–21929. doi: 10.1073/pnas.0909894106

Ponti, G., Obernier, K., Guinto, C., Jose, L., Bonfanti, L., and Alvarez-Buylla, A. (2013). Cell cycle and lineage progression of neural progenitors in the ventricular-subventricular zones of adult mice. *Proc. Natl. Acad. Sci. U.S.A.* 110, E1045–E1054. doi: 10.1073/pnas.1219563110

Psachoulia, K., Jamen, F., Young, K. M., and Richardson, W. D. (2009). Cell cycle dynamics of NG2 cells in the postnatal and ageing brain. *Neuron Glia Biol.* 5, 57–67. doi: 10.1017/S1740925X09990354

Rashidian, J., Iyirhiaro, G. O., and Park, D. S. (2007). Cell cycle machinery and stroke. *Biochim. Biophys. Acta* 1772, 484–493. doi: 10.1016/j.bbadis.2006.11.009

Rasmussen, S., Imitola, J., Ayuso-Sacido, A., Wang, Y., Starossom, S. C., Kivisakk, P., et al. (2011). Reversible neural stem cell niche dysfunction in a model of multiple sclerosis. *Ann. Neurol.* 69, 878–891. doi: 10.1002/ana.22299

Richardson, W. D., Kessaris, N., and Pringle, N. (2006). Oligodendrocyte wars. *Nature Rev. Neurosci* 7, 11–18. doi: 10.1038/nrn1826

Richardson, W. D., Young, K. M., Tripathi, R. B., and McKenzie, I. (2011). NG2-glia as multipotent neural stem cells: fact or fantasy? *Neuron* 70, 661–673. doi: 10.1016/j.neuron.2011.05.013

Rivers, L. E., Young, K. M., Rizzi, M., Jamen, F., Psachoulia, K., Wade, A., et al. (2008). PDGFRA/NG2 glia generate myelinating oligodendrocytes and piriform projection neurons in adult mice. *Nat. Neurosci.* 11, 1392–1401. doi: 10.1038/nn.2220

Salomoni, P., and Calegari, F. (2010). Cell cycle control of mammalian neural stem cells: putting a speed limit on G1. *Trends Cell Biol.* 5, 332–342. doi: 10.1016/j.tcb.2010.01.006

Schultze, B., and Korr, H. (1981). Cell kinetic studies of different cell types in the developing and adult brain of the rat and the mouse: a review. *Cell Tissue Kinet.* 14, 309–325.

Seri, B., Garcia-Verdugo, J. M., McEwen, B. S., and Alvarez-Buylla, A. (2001). Astrocytes give rise to new neurons in the adult mammalian hippocampus. *J. Neurosci.* 21, 7153–7160.

Shen, Q., Wang, Y., Kokovay, E., Lin, G., Chuang, S. M., Goderie, S. K., et al. (2008). Adult SVZ stem cells lie in a vascular niche: a quantitative analysis of niche cell-cell interactions. *Cell Stem Cell* 3, 289–300. doi: 10.1016/j.stem.2008.07.026

Simon, C., Gotz, M., and Dimou, L. (2011). Progenitors in the adult cerebral cortex: cell cycle properties and regulation by physiological stimuli and injury. *Glia* 59, 869–881. doi: 10.1002/glia.21156

Stevens, B., Porta, S., Haak, L. L., Gallo, V., and Fields, R. D. (2002). Adenosine: a neuron-glial transmitter promoting myelination in the CNS in response to action potentials. *Neuron* 36, 855–868. doi: 10.1016/S0896-6273(02)01067-X

Sun, C., Sun, H., Wu, S., Lee, C. C., Akamatsu, Y., Wang, R. K., et al. (2013). Conditional ablation of neuroprogenitor cells in adult mice impedes recovery of poststroke cognitive function and reduces synaptic connectivity in the perforant pathway. *J. Neurosci.* 33, 17314–17325. doi: 10.1523/JNEUROSCI.2129-13.2013

Takahashi, T., Nowakowski, R. S., and Caviness, V. S. Jr. (1995). The cell cycle of the pseudostratified ventricular epithelium of the embryonic murine cerebral wall. *J. Neurosci.* 15, 6046–6057.

Tattersfield, A. S., Croon, R. J., Liu, Y. W., Kells, A. P., Faull, R. L., and Connor, B. (2004). Neurogenesis in the striatum of the quinolinic acid lesion model of Huntington's disease. *Neuroscience* 127, 319–332. doi: 10.1016/j.neuroscience.2004.04.061

Tavazoie, M., van der Veken, L., Silva-Vargas, V., Louissaint, M., Colonna, L., Zaidi, B., et al. (2008). A specialized vascular niche for adult neural stem cells. *Cell Stem Cell* 3, 279–288. doi: 10.1016/j.stem.2008.07.025

Thored, P., Arvidsson, A., Cacci, E., Ahlenius, H., Kallur, T., Darsalia, V., et al. (2006). Persistent production of neurons from adult brain stem cells during recovery after stroke. *Stem Cells* 24, 739–747. doi: 10.1634/stemcells.2005-0281

Tsai, H. H., Li, H., Fuentealba, L. C., Molofsky, A. V., Taveira-Marques, R., Zhuang, H., et al. (2012). Regional astrocyte allocation regulates CNS synaptogenesis and repair. *Science* 337, 358–362. doi: 10.1126/science.1222381

Ueno, Y., Chopp, M., Zhang, L., Buller, B., Liu, Z., Lehman, N. L., et al. (2012). Axonal outgrowth and dendritic plasticity in the cortical peri-infarct area after experimental stroke. *Stroke* 43, 2221–2228. doi: 10.1161/STROKEAHA.111.646224

Vigano, F., Mobius, W., Gotz, M., and Dimou, L. (2013). Transplantation reveals regional differences in oligodendrocyte differentiation in the adult brain. *Nat. Neurosci.* 16, 1370–1372. doi: 10.1038/nn.3503

WHO. (2013). *The Top 10 Causes of Death*. Available on line at: http://www.who.int/mediacentre/factsheets/fs310/en/

Yamashita, T., Ninomiya, M., Hernandez Acosta, P., Garcia-Verdugo, J. M., Sunabori, T., Sakaguchi, M., et al. (2006). Subventricular zone-derived neuroblasts migrate and differentiate into mature neurons in the post-stroke adult striatum. *J. Neurosci.* 26, 6627–6636. doi: 10.1523/JNEUROSCI.0149-06.2006

Young, K. M., Psachoulia, K., Tripathi, R. B., Dunn, S. J., Cossell, L., Attwell, D., et al. (2013). Oligodendrocyte dynamics in the healthy adult CNS: evidence for myelin remodeling. *Neuron* 77, 873–885. doi: 10.1016/j.neuron.2013.01.006

Zawadzka, M., Rivers, L. E., Fancy, S. P., Zhao, C., Tripathi, R., Jamen, F., et al. (2010). CNS-resident glial progenitor/stem cells produce Schwann cells as well as oligodendrocytes during repair of CNS demyelination. *Cell Stem Cell* 6, 578–590. doi: 10.1016/j.stem.2010.04.002

Zhang, R., Chopp, M., and Zhang, Z. G. (2013). Oligodendrogenesis after cerebral ischemia. *Front. Neurosci.* 7:201. doi: 10.3389/fncel.2013.00201

Zhang, R. L., Chopp, M., Roberts, C., Jia, L., Wei, M., Lu, M., et al. (2011). Ascl1 lineage cells contribute to ischemia-induced neurogenesis and oligodendrogenesis. *J. Cereb. Blood Flow Metab.* 31, 614–625. doi: 10.1038/jcbfm.2010.134

Zhang, R. L., Zhang, Z. G., Lu, M., Wang, Y., Yang, J. J., and Chopp, M. (2006). Reduction of the cell cycle length by decreasing G1 phase and cell cycle reentry expand neuronal progenitor cells in the subventricular zone of adult rat after stroke. *J. Cereb. Blood Flow Metab.* 26, 857–863. doi: 10.1038/sj.jcbfm.9600237

Zhang, R. L., Zhang, Z. G., Roberts, C., Letourneau, Y., Lu, M., Zhang, L., et al. (2008). Lengthening the G(1) phase of neural progenitor cells is concurrent with an increase of symmetric neuron generating division after stroke. *J. Cereb. Blood Flow Metab.* 28, 602–611. doi: 10.1038/sj.jcbfm.9600556

Zhang, R., Zhang, Z., Wang, L., Wang, Y., Gousev, A., Zhang, L., et al. (2004). Activated neural stem cells contribute to stroke-induced neurogenesis and neuroblast migration toward the infarct boundary in adult rats. *J. Cereb. Blood Flow Metab.* 24, 441–448. doi: 10.1097/00004647-200404000-00009

Zhang, Z. G., and Chopp, M. (2009). Neurorestorative therapies for stroke: underlying mechanisms and translation to the clinic. *Lancet Neurol.* 8, 491–500. doi: 10.1016/S1474-4422(09)70061-4

Zhao, C., Deng, W., and Gage, F. H. (2008). Mechanisms and functional implications of adult neurogenesis. *Cell* 132, 645–660. doi: 10.1016/j.cell.2008.01.033

Zhu, X., Hill, R. A., Dietrich, D., Komitova, M., Suzuki, R., and Nishiyama, A. (2011). Age-dependent fate and lineage restriction of single NG2 cells. *Development* 138, 745–753. doi: 10.1242/dev.047951

2

Fetal functional imaging portrays heterogeneous development of emerging human brain networks

András Jakab[1]*, Ernst Schwartz[1], Gregor Kasprian[2], Gerlinde M. Gruber[3], Daniela Prayer[2], Veronika Schöpf[2†] and Georg Langs[1,4†]

[1] Computational Imaging Research Lab, Department of Biomedical Imaging and Image-guided Therapy, Medical University of Vienna, Vienna, Austria
[2] Division for Neuroradiology and Musculoskeletal Radiology, Department of Biomedical Imaging and Image-guided Therapy, Medical University of Vienna, Vienna, Austria
[3] Department of Systematic Anatomy, Center for Anatomy and Cell Biology, Medical University of Vienna, Vienna, Austria
[4] Computer Science and Artificial Intelligence Lab, Massachusetts Institute of Technology, Cambridge, MA, USA

Edited by:
Marika Berchicci, University of Rome "Foro Italico," Italy

Reviewed by:
Emmanuel Carrera, Hôpitaux Universitaires de Genève, Switzerland
Lajos R. Kozák, Semmelweis University Budapest, Hungary

***Correspondence:**
András Jakab, Computational Imaging Research Lab, Department of Biomedical Imaging and Image-guided Therapy, Medical University of Vienna, Währinger Gürtel 18-20, Vienna, Austria
e-mail: andras.jakab@meduniwien.ac.at

†Veronika Schöpf and Georg Langs have contributed equally to this work.

The functional connectivity architecture of the adult human brain enables complex cognitive processes, and exhibits a remarkably complex structure shared across individuals. We are only beginning to understand its heterogeneous structure, ranging from a strongly hierarchical organization in sensorimotor areas to widely distributed networks in areas such as the parieto-frontal cortex. Our study relied on the functional magnetic resonance imaging (fMRI) data of 32 fetuses with no detectable morphological abnormalities. After adapting functional magnetic resonance acquisition, motion correction, and nuisance signal reduction procedures of resting-state functional data analysis to fetuses, we extracted neural activity information for major cortical and subcortical structures. Resting fMRI networks were observed for increasing regional functional connectivity from 21st to 38th gestational weeks (GWs) with a network-based statistical inference approach. The overall connectivity network, short range, and interhemispheric connections showed sigmoid expansion curve peaking at the 26–29 GW. In contrast, long-range connections exhibited linear increase with no periods of peaking development. Region-specific increase of functional signal synchrony followed a sequence of occipital (peak: 24.8 GW), temporal (peak: 26 GW), frontal (peak: 26.4 GW), and parietal expansion (peak: 27.5 GW). We successfully adapted functional neuroimaging and image post-processing approaches to correlate macroscopical scale activations in the fetal brain with gestational age. This *in vivo* study reflects the fact that the mid-fetal period hosts events that cause the architecture of the brain circuitry to mature, which presumably manifests in increasing strength of intra- and interhemispheric functional macro connectivity.

Keywords: fetal functional MRI, fetal brain connectivity, prenatal development, connectome, fetal brain development

INTRODUCTION

Human brain development is a finely orchestrated process that relies on the sequential execution of genetic programs, complex cellular interactions, and the formation and resolution of transient organs (Price et al., 2006; Kostovic and Judas, 2010). The protracted telencephalon maturation and the evolutionary expansion of the neocortex are prerequisites for our intellectual capacity (Clancy et al., 2001; Preuss, 2009), and many highly developed cognitive abilities are linked to features that are unique to humans (Bystron et al., 2008; Fjell et al., 2013). Early brain development encompasses the rapid growth of the size of the cerebral cortex and the increase in its cellular variability, associated with the expansion of transient fetal structures, including the subventricular zone and the subplate (Molnár et al., 2006; Rakic, 2009). When compared to the developmental trajectories of great apes, the growth rate of the human brain diverges during mid-gestation, and further expansion of white matter volume is observed in early postnatal life (Rilling, 2014). Specific areas, such as the association areas of the neocortex and areas related to language processing, exhibit exceptionally large subplate zones in humans (Rakic, 2009), and these differences are also mirrored in the cortical expansion during childhood and protracted myelination, which is completed in adulthood (Geschwind, 1964; Hill et al., 2010).

In contrast to our knowledge on brain circuit formation and histogenesis from post mortem studies and functional examinations in early childhood (Johnson, 2001; Price et al., 2006; Huang et al., 2009; Judas et al., 2013), to date, we have only a limited understanding of emerging neural activity during human fetal development. The complex connectional architecture of neural ensembles is a fundamental characteristic of the adult brain, and

---

Abbreviations: BOLD, blood oxygen level dependent contrast; CSF, cerebrospinal fluid; fMRI, functional magnetic resonance imaging; FOV, field of view; FWHM, full width at half maximum; GW, gestational week; ICA, independent component analysis; MRI, magnetic resonance imaging; NBS, network-based statistics; ROI, region of interest; SSE, sum of squares for error; TE, echo time; TR, repetition time.

we are beginning to understand how its variability across individuals is linked to cognitive ability (van den Heuvel et al., 2009), or neuropsychiatric disorders (Greicius, 2008). Some functional networks in the fronto-parietal and ventrolateral frontal cortex seem to be specific to humans (Mantini et al., 2013; Neubert et al., 2014), and the functional variability across the adult cortex correlates with cortical expansion from the primate to human brain (Mueller et al., 2013). To understand normal fetal functional brain development, it is of vital importance to identify critical periods of developmental vulnerability in which harmful environmental agents can manifest as a deterioration of mental capability or cause psychiatric diseases (Rice and Barone, 2000). In these phases of interest, functional assessment of the fetal nervous system would open a novel window on prenatal diagnostics and prognostics (Jakob and Beckmann, 1986; Paul et al., 2007; Schlotz and Phillips, 2009).

Studying fetal behavior with ultrasound has been adopted as a marker for neural development in clinical practice, offering an indirect view of the underlying functional processes (Pugash et al., 2008; Morokuma et al., 2013). MRI in the fetal brain has become increasingly feasible and clinically important due to its higher tissue resolution and better visualization of normal and pathological development of macroscopic anatomy or white matter microstructure and connections (Glenn and Barkovich, 2006; Kasprian et al., 2008; Jokhi and Whitby, 2011). Advanced imaging techniques, such as spectroscopy, serve as indicators of naturally changing metabolite levels during gestation (Kok et al., 2001), and characterize impaired development caused by primary brain malformation, hypoxic-ischemic injury, infection, or a combination of those factors (Mailath-Pokorny et al., 2012). BOLD fMRI has probed macroscopic-scale intrinsic neural activations across the entire life span (Buckner et al., 2013), and has an unsurpassed role in recent population-wide neuroimaging endeavors (Nooner et al., 2012; Uğurbil et al., 2013; Yan et al., 2013). Initial fetal investigation of spontaneous, intrinsic functional activity and functional brain connectivity has established intra-lobar activations (Schöpf et al., 2012) and cross-hemispheric connections in normally developing fetuses (Thomason et al., 2013).

In this paper, we provide a comprehensive view of the developing functional networks in the fetal brain. We capture this process by examining changes in the whole-brain functional connectivity architecture (Achard et al., 2006; Rubinov and Sporns, 2010; Zalesky et al., 2010) during gestation. We measured thalamo-cortical, cortico-cortical, intra-hemispheric, and inter-hemispheric functional connections, and organized them into a whole-brain graph (Fransson, 2005; Bullmore and Sporns, 2009). The graph-based method (Rubinov and Sporns, 2010) detected regional and temporal heterogeneity of functional connectivity development across the cortex before birth, reflecting the possible sequence of maturation in cortical areas.

MATERIALS AND METHODS

ETHICS AND SAFETY OF FETAL MRI ACQUISITIONS

Based on the follow-up studies of infants or children who had been exposed to MR imaging *in utero*, no gross abnormality, disease, or disability likely to be related to MR exposure could be demonstrated (Kok et al., 2004). The study protocol was approved by the local ethics committee, the mothers gave written, informed consent prior to the examination, and research was conducted according to the principles expressed in the Declaration of Helsinki.

STUDY POPULATION

This cross-sectional study included thirty-two singleton fetuses (16 female, 16 male) between GWs 21–37 (mean: 29.2; SD: 4.9) with normal brain development. The distribution of the gestational ages was the following. Second trimester (<26th GW): eight fetuses, early third trimester (26–29th GW): eight fetuses, 29–37th GW: 16 fetuses. Between May 2010 and August 2012, fMRI was performed for 200 fetuses. From of this cohort 141 scans were excluded due to image artifacts, uncontrollable fetal or maternal motion. After retaining the technically successful scans, the next exclusion criterion was the presence of brain abnormalities. Brain abnormalities were confirmed with the use of structural MRI in 27 of the cases. Therefore, 32 scans were retained for further analysis, which had no confirmed brain abnormalities. In the remaining study cohort, the indication for the mothers to undergo fetal MRI included: gastrointestinal pathology (two subjects); maternal clinical conditions (nine subjects); micrognathia or clefts (three subjects); renal and urogenital pathology (six subjects); thoracic pathology (one subject); asymmetry of the lateral ventricles (LVs; six subjects); and pathologies of the diaphragm (five subjects). Our final investigations were restricted to the 32 subjects who were proven negative for these suspected anomalies.

IMAGE ACQUISITION

Functional magnetic resonance imaging was carried out on a 1.5 T clinical scanner (Philips Medical Systems, Best, Netherlands) using a sensitivity encoding (SENSE) cardiac coil with five elements, utilizing single-shot gradient-recalled echo-planar imaging (EPI). The pregnant women were examined in the supine or left decubitus position (feet first), and no contrast agents or sedatives were administered. The MRI scans were acquired between May 2010 and August 2012. All investigations were scheduled between 7 and 9 am. Image matrix size was 144 × 144, with an FOV of 250 mm × 250 mm, a TE/TR of 50/1000 ms, and a flip angle of 90°. The resting-state scan comprised 50 image volumes with slices obtained perpendicular to the fetal brainstem, 10–30 slices were acquired and scan time was 1 min. The fMRI examinations followed the diagnostic (e.g., T2-weighted anatomical) scans, utilizing institutional protocols similar to those of previous reports (Schöpf et al., 2012).

IMAGE PROCESSING

The next paragraphs introduce an optimized work-flow for processing fetal functional images, which required effort in the direction of adapting conventional toolboxes and further extending them by fetal-specific developments. An overview of post-processing steps is given in **Figure 1**.

SPATIAL NORMALIZATION OF FUNCTIONAL MR IMAGES TO GESTATIONAL WEEK-SPECIFIC BRAIN TEMPLATES

A practical way to interrogate the developing fetal neuroanatomy is to pool image datasets of the study cohort according to GW and

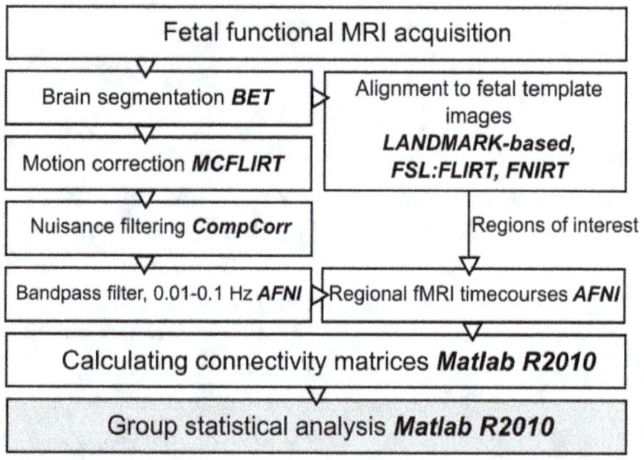

FIGURE 1 | Work diagram of the fMRI processing steps. The names of the respective image processing toolboxes are given in bold. BET, brain extraction tool; FLIRT, FSL linear registration tool; FNIRT, FSL non-linear registration tool; CompCor, component based noise correction method; AFNI, analysis of functional neuroimages.

use templates that depict the mean anatomical configuration of each GW. During the spatial normalization, we used the reference template images provided by Rueckert (2012) which are high-resolution representations of the changing fetal brain from the 23rd to the 37th GW. Template creation procedure described in: (Serag et al., 2012), while the fetal templates were accessed from Rueckert (2012).

Temporally averaged images of the fMRI data guided the registrations to achieve overlap with the T2-weighted templates. Each fMRI image was anatomically aligned to the respective GW-specific template image using the following procedure. We ensured proper orientation and coarse initial alignment by a landmark-based registration procedure using 12 manually annotated corresponding anatomical locations in the source and target images (**Figure 2**). We then relied on a two-step, intensity-based image registration in the FSL software (version 5.0, Linux 64-bit platform; Jenkinson et al., 2012): a linear, affine registration (FLIRT tool) followed by the non-linear matching of images (FNIRT algorithm), thereby coping effectively with the inter-individual anatomical differences. All further image processing steps, such as motion correction, noise reduction, band-pass filtering, and time-course extraction, were performed in the native space of the fMRI images, and the transformations were only used to propagate anatomically defined regions of interest into the subject's space or propagate results through up-sampling to a reference space to aid visualization. Therefore, the possible confounding factor of image interpolation only affected the ROI system, and not the actual fMRI data.

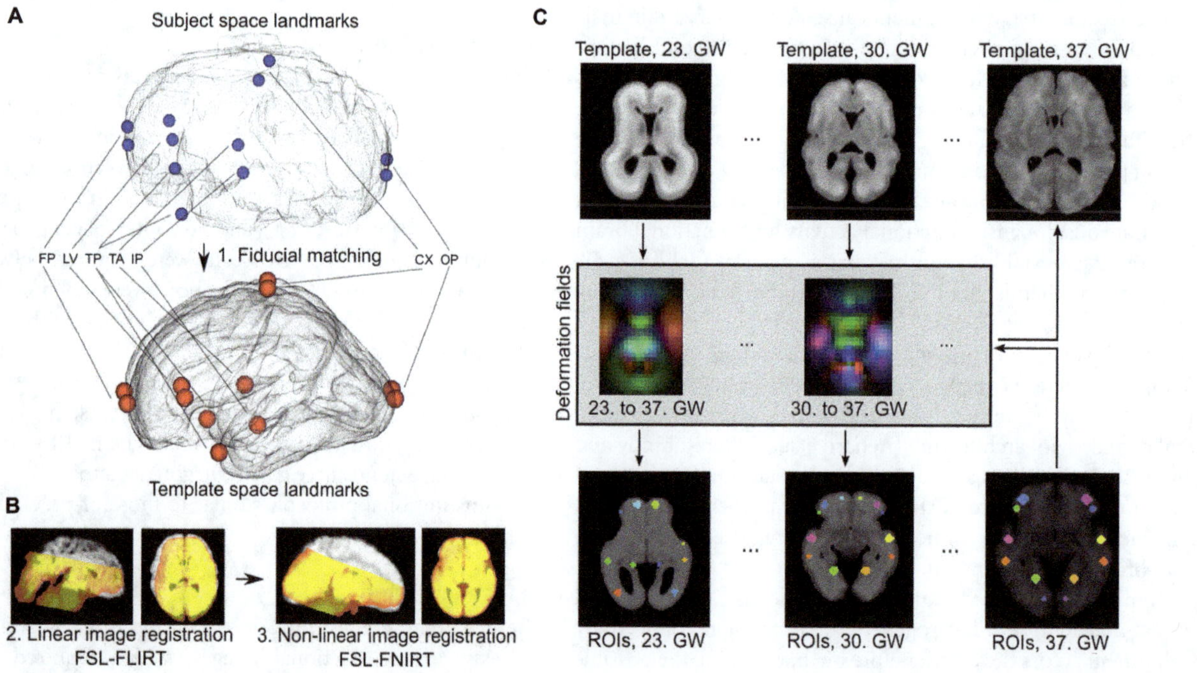

FIGURE 2 | Registration of fetal fMRI data to anatomical standard images and ROI propagation across developmental phases.
(A) Landmark-based initial registration was used to match the averaged BOLD fMRI images of fetuses and GW specific fetal template brains. FP, fontal pole; LV, lateral ventricles, frontal horn; TP, temporal pole; TA, thalamic adhesion (midline); IP, midline point of the interpeduncular cleft in the midbrain; CX, topmost point of the convexities; OP, occipital pole. **(B)** Second step of the fetal to standard image registration, carried out with intensity-based algorithms: linear (FLIRT) and non-linear (FNIRT) registrations in the FSL software.
(C) Establishing GW-specific regions with a longitudinal label propagation approach. First row: for each GW from the 23rd to the 37th, a high-resolution anatomical template was used, between which pair-wise non-linear transformations were calculated (second row). These transformations were used to transform the ROI system into any GW (third and fourth rows).

REGION OF INTEREST DEFINITION, FINDING CORRESPONDENCES ACROSS DEVELOPMENTAL STAGES

A ROI definition is critical when analyzing whole-brain structural or functional connectivity by node-based approaches, as it has a profound influence on network topology (Kelly et al., 2012). Conventionally, it is possible to obtain data-driven parcellations of a given territory or use anatomical priors to define gross landmarks. In the current study, we chose to use the latter. The 37th GW's high-resolution template image was visualized to facilitate the localization of crucial areas that are commonly depicted in adult neuroimaging atlases, such as in the Harvard-Oxford Cortical atlas (Desikan et al., 2006). The labels either matched large surface structures (precentral, postcentral gyrus), or subdivisions of areas with known and assumed diverging connectivity profiles (anterior, lateral, posterior thalamus), or structures that corresponded to functionally defined regions (e.g., the calcarine cortex of the visual system).

As the formation of cortico-cortical and cortico-subcortical circuits is not complete by the mid-fetal period, we placed anatomical regions onto the border of the subplate and the hypothesized future cortical plate position to capture presumably valuable signal from this region as well. In the reference ROI system, the ROI shape was spherical, mainly because little information is available about the volumetric extent of fetal cortical domains in the reference space. In 34.4% of the cases, the field of MR acquisitions did not cover the entire supratentorial area and the fetal cortex, and had limited cranio-caudal brain coverage. Examples for the ROI system, the ROI system matched to individual fetuses and the anatomical reference nomenclature is described in detail in **Figure 3**.

Our assumption was that the ROI system can be propagated into a developmental ensemble of brain reference images. Thus, ROI definition is only performed for the image having the best overall quality (i.e., in the 37th GW reference images, the secondary and tertiary sulci can guide the observer). Pair-wise registrations between the high-resolution templates were created in order to generate a collection of non-linear deformation fields that would feasibly match each GW's space with the 37th GW's template image. The non-linear registration was performed using "FNIRT" algorithm in FSL, with the registration parameters optimized to tackle the small scale of fetal brains. We illustrated this procedure in **Figure 2**. The correspondence between anatomical locations after the deformation in each GW template was checked by an observer with experience in neuroanatomy (András Jakab). The robustness of the ROI propagation method was visually checked by comparing the locations of ROIs with identifiable sulcal structures, such as the lateral, central, or parieto-occipital sulcus.

CORRECTING THE CONFOUNDING EFFECTS OF FETAL HEAD MOTION AND NON-NEURONAL MRI SIGNAL

Significant head rotations and translations can occur during fMRI experiments due to the frequent, spontaneous fetal movements and maternal breathing. Excessive motion in terms of amplitude and duration served as exclusion criteria for fetuses. This decision relied on the subjective observer-driven selection in addition to other imaging artifacts, similar to the approach in previous works (Schöpf et al., 2012). After removing subjects, minor head motion was detectable in almost every case and displacements were estimated and corrected with the MCFLIRT algorithm in FSL (Oakes et al., 2005). This processing step comprised the rigid-body registration of images to the mid-scan frame and removal of those frames that showed excessive motion estimates ("scrubbing" frames with root mean square displacement larger than 2 mm; Power et al., 2012). As displacement induces spurious effects in signal intensity temporal characteristics, we used the motion parameters (translation and rotation) as first-level explanatory variables in signal filtering, as recommended in the literature (Weissenbacher et al., 2009).

Furthermore, the variability of motion patterns can be influenced by gestational age. Hence we included per-subject motion as a covariate in higher-level analysis. This explanatory variable in the general linear model (GLM) putatively diminishes the effect of variable fetal motion among subjects at different developmental stages. We provide an example for typical fetal motion patterns, the effect of motion correction and the relationship to head motion to gestational age in **Figure 4**.

The observed signal during fMRI experiments is known to be coupled with the underlying neural activity due to the BOLD phenomenon (Logothetis and Wandell, 2004). In contrast to the intuitive notion of *structural or axonal connection* in neuroimaging studies, a *functional connection* or co-activation between remote brain areas is assumed when the MR signal fluctuations in the low frequency range are correlated in the temporal domain (Lowe et al., 1998; Greicius et al., 2003). Functional connectivity is thus a purely statistical approach inherently prone to confounding factors, i.e., rhythmic variations in the MR signal not explained by the large-scale activation of neurons. The majority of studies employ a model in which confounding factors are attributed to image noise caused by circulation (Shmueli et al., 2007), respiration (Birn et al., 2008), head motion (Power et al., 2012), or MR equipment-related noise. During nuisance signal reduction, the neural signal is the residual after first-level regression analyses in which we use the time-courses of known non-neural origin and other nuisance variables. Here we adapted the CompCor approach to reduce noise (Behzadi et al., 2007). According to the CompCor noise reduction model, principal MRI signal components from the white matter, CSF, or other "noise" image voxels are used. Time-courses of nuisance signals were derived using anatomical priors, while voxels having the largest SD of signal intensity were segmented as noise voxels. The first five principal components (PCs) of these signals were entered into the confound regression procedure. We illustrate the nuisance confound regression procedure in **Figure 5**. A detailed description of the utilized fetal noise signal model is provided in the Supplementary Material.

PORTRAYING THE DEVELOPING FETAL BRAIN CONNECTOME AS A COMPLEX GRAPH

We built undirected, weighted graphs representing intrinsic functional connectivity, with the set of longitudinally propagated brain regions as nodes. Connectivity value for a network edge was

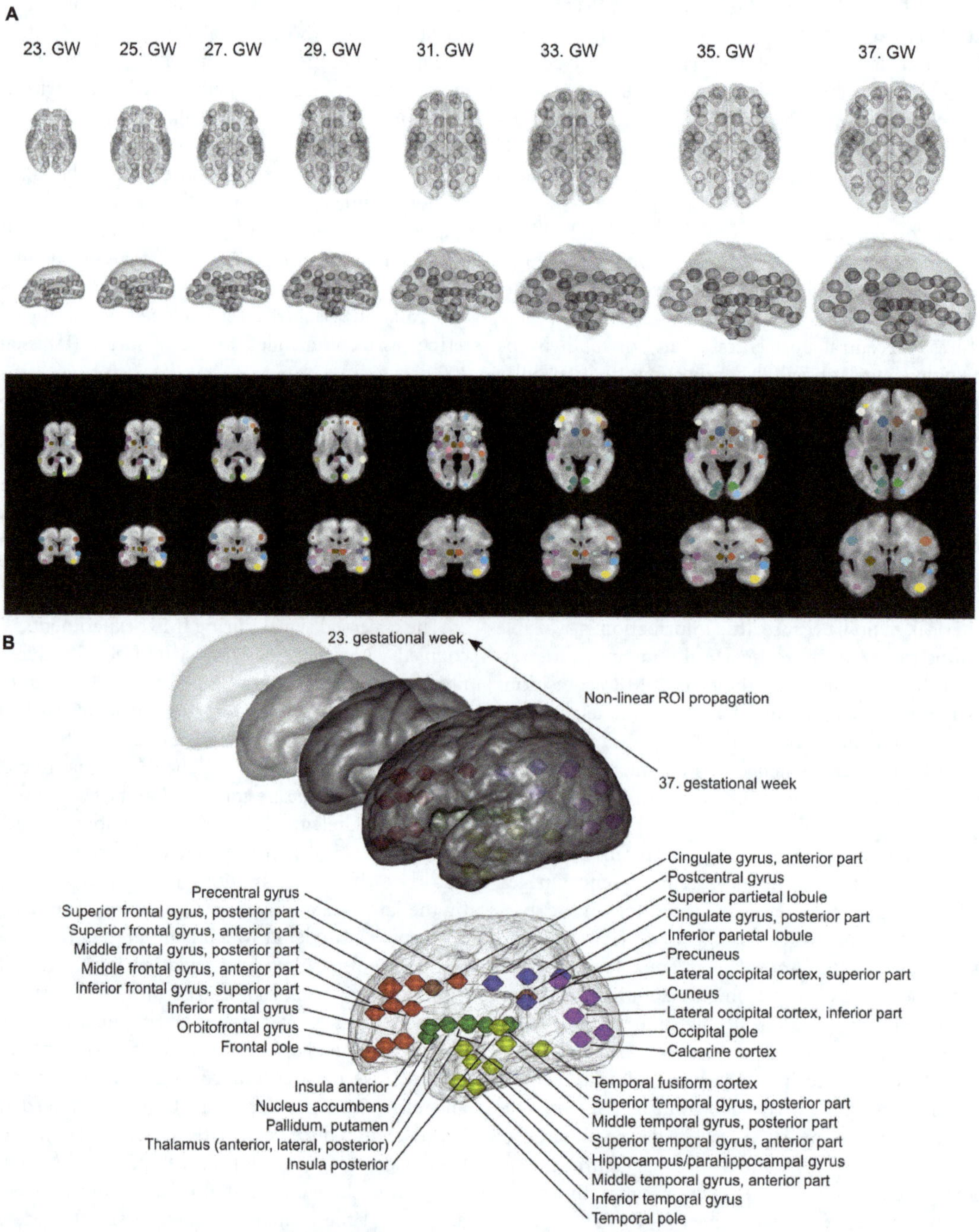

FIGURE 3 | Fetal brain atlas used for fMRI time-course calculation: ROI system and anatomical nomenclature. (A) Illustration of the region propagation procedure. Using high-resolution anatomical templates, we marked 90 anatomically relevant regions on the fetal cortical surface, which was then propagated through the investigated gestational period. Three-dimensional renderings and cross-sectional anatomical images with ROIs are shown. **(B)** Anatomical nomenclature of the ROI system. Correspondence to major lobes or systems is marked with different colors: red = frontal lobe; blue = parietal lobe; purple = occipital lobe; yellow = temporal lobe; green = subcortical; pink = limbic/cingulate gyrus.

defined using the Z-transformed Pearson product-moment correlation coefficient between brain regions. No thresholding or binning of the network was performed. We used the adaptation of graph theoretical measures to weighted nets, as implemented by the Brain Connectivity Toolbox for Matlab (BCT, version: 2012. 12. 04) and described in (Rubinov and Sporns, 2010).

TESTING HYPOTHESES ON COMPLEX NETWORKS: APPLICATION TO FETAL NEURODEVELOPMENT

To test our hypothesis about the developing brain, we modeled the temporal changes of brain connections as the effect of gestational time (gestational days) on the variance of individual connections, $S_{i,j}$. Prior to this model, all connections were evaluated against

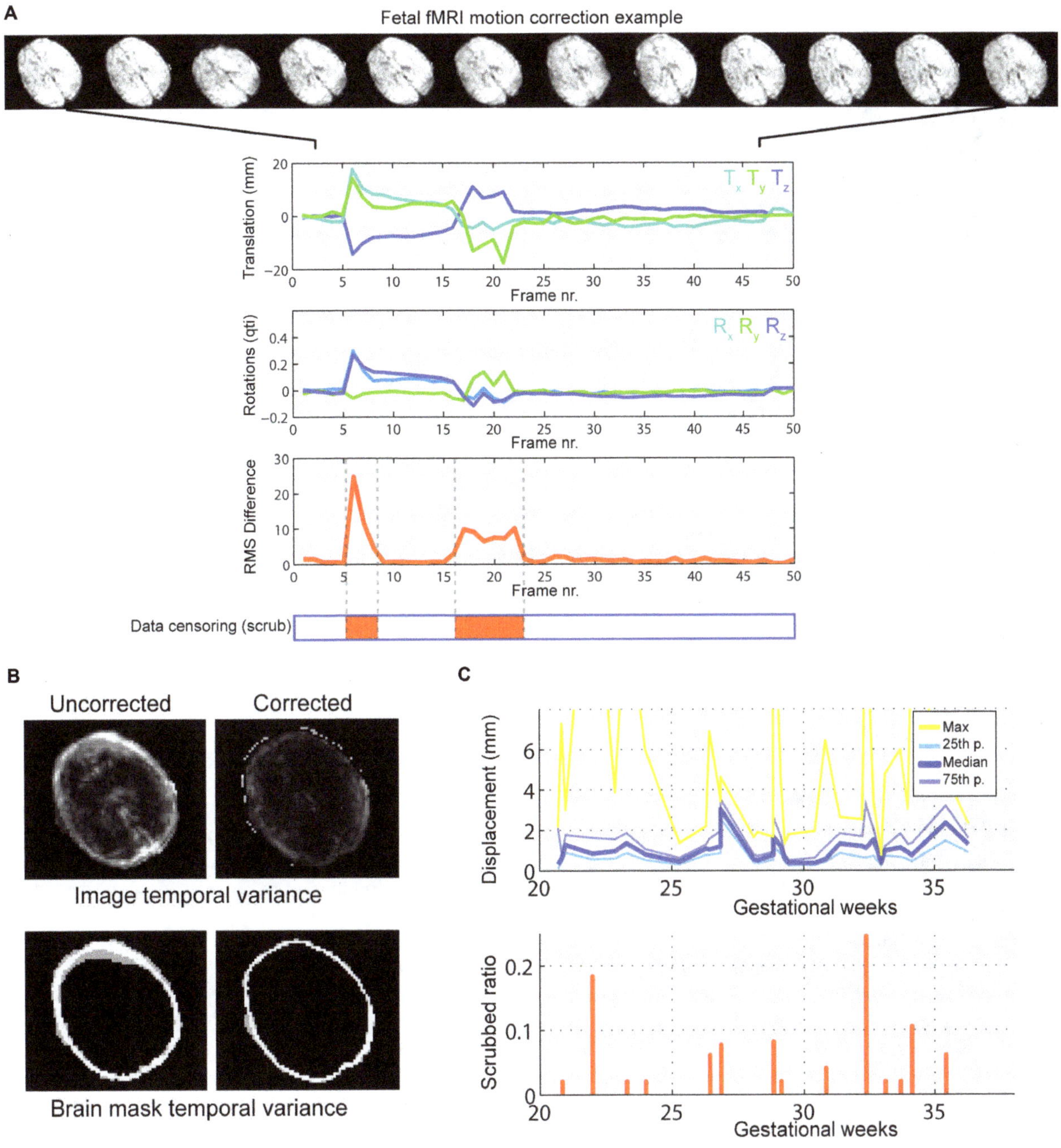

FIGURE 4 | Illustration of typical fetal in-scanner head motion patterns, correlation with gestational age. (A) Fetal head motion during MR scanning is estimated by frame-to-frame linear registrations. We illustrate a fetus with excessive head movements, as indicated by the large peaks in the translation and rotational components. Total displacement was used to censor periods of the scan with large motion (middle panel, red markings). **(B)** The motion correction procedure reduces the temporal variance of peripheral brain voxels, as shown in the cross-sectional panels. Such regions of high, spurious temporal variance give rise to nuisance signals in the functional connectivity patterns. **(C)** Depiction of gestational age-dependent changes of head motion. Top: median, 25th percentile, 75th percentile and maximum displacements of the fetal head vs. GWs. Bottom: the ratio of censored data vs. GWs. In our study cohort, fetal in-scanner head motion does not show correlation with gestational age.

simulated random brain graphs where the intrinsic functional connectivity were assumed to be explained by the spatial closeness of network edges and the consequent sharing of possible nuisance sources. This procedure is detailed in the Supplementary Material.

The application of univariate GLMs to each putative neuronal link (i.e., graph edge) raises the problem of mass multiple comparisons: in general, we cannot simply assume that such links are independent observations. Furthermore, correcting for the family-wise error rate (FWER) with the false discovery rate procedure

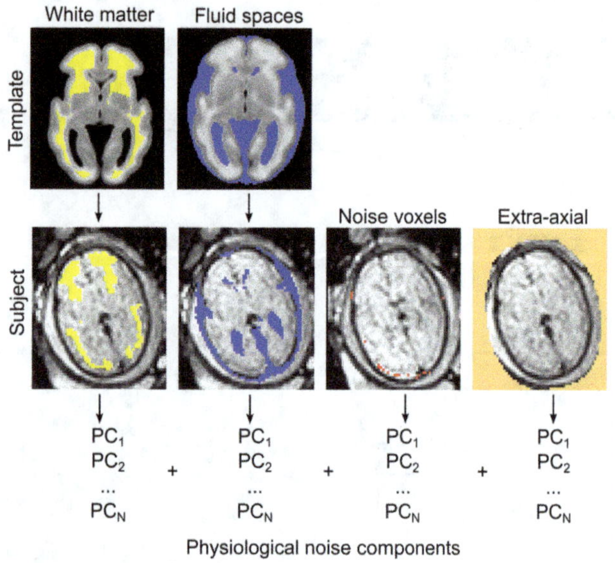

FIGURE 5 | Estimating physiological noise components for the correction of fetal fMRI signal using an adaptation of the CompCor approach. Top row: white matter and CSF components are segmented from the GW-specific anatomical templates. Segmentations are transformed to individual subjects **(bottom row)** while the voxels with highest temporal variation, and other, extra-axial structures, are calculated from the data. These voxels are used to perform the component-based filtering of the nuisance signal, according to the CompCor method described by Behzadi et al. (2007). PCs, principal components.

would inherently result in a loss of statistical power due to the large number of univariate measurements, which, in our case, would mean 2415 individual connections ($n_{i,j} = 70$, therefore the number of total connections is $\frac{70^2-70}{2}$).

The network-based statistics (NBS) method was utilized to tackle the multiple comparisons problem, as described by Zalesky et al. (2010) and implemented in the NBS Toolbox for Matlab R2012. This approach has the advantage of exploiting the internal connectional structure of brain graphs during the correction step for multiple comparisons, and potentially offers a substantial gain in statistical power. For the GLMs in our study, we provide the test statistics (F-test) for each connection in the graph and also for nodes where the test results were averaged over each edge connected with the node.

DETERMINING LOCAL AND GLOBAL GROWTH CHARACTERISTICS

We aimed to determine the trend of overall functional network development (statistical threshold: $F > 5$, NBS-adjusted value) as well as for regional sub-networks. Thus, regional growth characteristics including, but not restricted to the connections in the frontal, parietal, temporal, and occipital lobes, short- and long-range connections, and thalamus connections were evaluated separately. The sub-network of a brain lobe was defined as all the connections that involve regions from that lobe.

Short- and long-range connections were defined by taking the Euclidean distance measures from the ROI-to-ROI distance matrix. For sampling short-range connections, the lowest 25th percentile of the distance matrix was used, while, for long-range connections, we used the highest 75 percentile. This categorization of short- versus long-range connections remained fixed during the gestation, and it was based on the Euclidean distances measured at the 37th week of gestation. We further evaluated the distribution of connectivity lengths across the gestation period.

We fitted two models on the observed network strength values over time: linear (first degree polynomial), and non-linear, sigmoid functions:

$$f(x)_{sub} = \frac{1}{1 + e^{-\frac{x+a}{b}}} c + d$$

where $f(x)_{sub}$ was the predicted value for the mean connectivity strength of the sub-network using the sigma model, x was the predictor variable (gestational age), and a, b, c, and d were the estimated coefficients. Using least squares fitting with robust estimation of outliers in the Curve Fitting Toolbox in Matlab R2012, we determined the goodness of fit for each selected sub-network and the global network. The least absolute residuals (LARs) approach was employed to estimate the statistical outliers during the regression procedure. The two models, i.e., linear and non-linear, were compared by their adjusted R-squared and SSE values. For sigmoid functions, it is possible to determine an inflation point, which is the x value (or the gestational age) that corresponds to the maximum point of its first derivative. Growth characteristics were further evaluated for global brain volumetric changes, head motion, signal intensity, and signal temporal variation.

A bootstrap sampling approach was utilized to test the statistical robustness of curve-fitting for each analyzed brain region. During bootstrapping, 50% of the observations were randomly selected, and the fitting of the linear and sigmoid functions was repeated over 1000 iterations. Two-sample t-tests were performed to compare the goodness of fit between linear and sigmoid fitting.

RESULTS

FETAL FUNCTIONAL MRI: DATA QUALITY AND AGE-RELATED CHANGES

Fetal fMRI is a challenging imaging modality, hindered by potential imaging artifacts. We give examples for fetal fMRI from our study database in **Figure 6**. After removing fMRI time frames with excessive fetal head motion, 46.4 ± 7.8 frames per subject were retained for analysis, while zero to nine frames were removed per case. The ratio of removed (censored) fMRI frames is illustrated in **Figure 4**. Motion correction reduced the image variance in the peripheral brain regions, which is commonly associated by movement artifacts (an example is provided in **Figure 4B.**). Head movement during the examinations (root mean squared displacement of brain voxels by translations and rotations) was not correlated with gestational age [mm, average: 0.643 ± 0.459 (range: 0.158–2.01); linear fit, $R^2 = 0.139$, $p = 0.448$; Illustration: **Figure 4C**].

Next, we describe the potential age-dependent characteristics in our measurement, which may serve as confounding factors. The following quantitative parameters of fetuses changed over the course of gestation. Segmented fetal brain volumes showed significant linear growth [cm^3, average: 266.7 ± 108.5 (range: 77–469.1); linear fit, $R^2 = 0.86$, $p < 0.001$], and this correlation was similar to

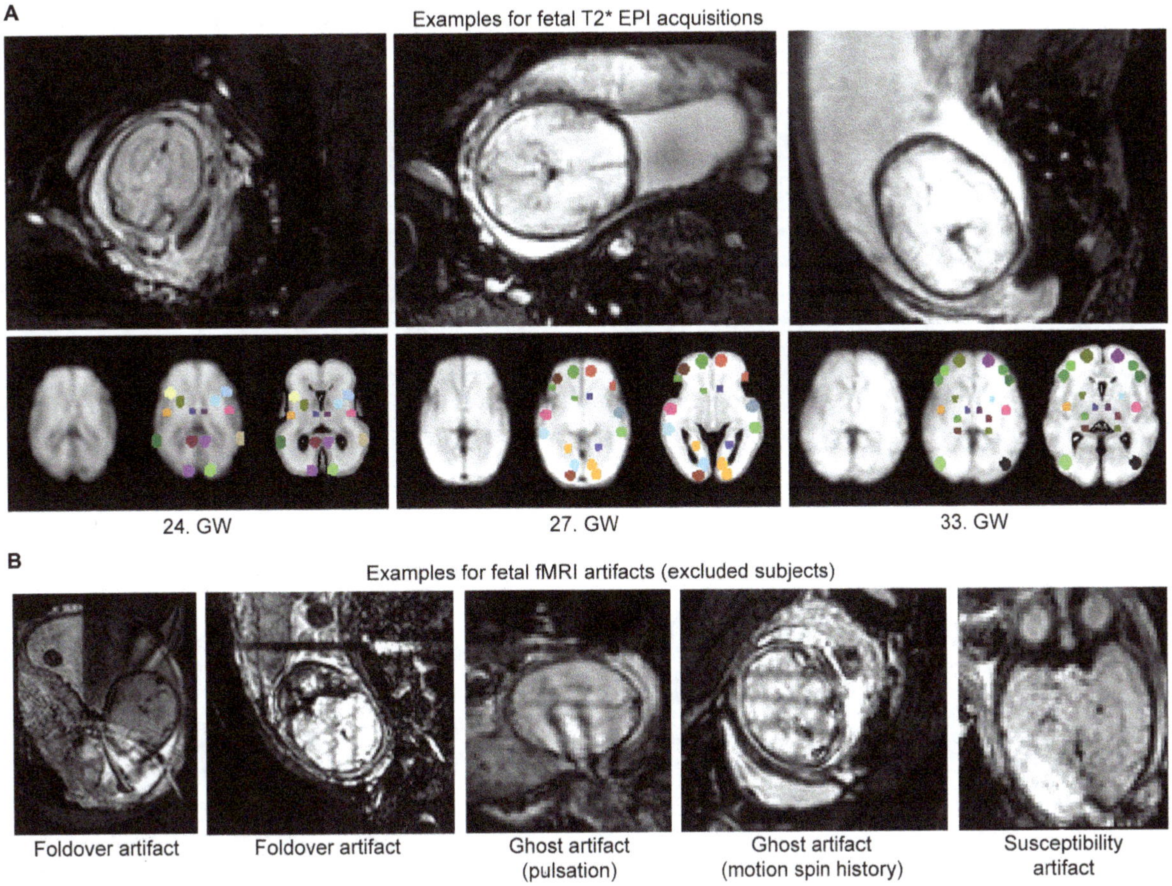

FIGURE 6 | Examples for fetal fMRI and the most common imaging artifacts. **(A)** Fetal fMRI with full FOV. Bottom panels: standardized functional image, ROI system warped to the standardized image and the fetal atlas systems illustrated. We provide 1–1 examples from the GWs 24, 27, and 33. **(B)** Fetal fMRI is a challenging imaging modality with many artifacts to expect. We illustrate this by excluded subjects' cross-sectional images. Examples for fold-over artifact, ghost artifact and susceptibility artifacts are shown.

the increase in the total size of brain ROI over time [cm^3, average: 6.954 ± 2.859 (range: 2.2–11.3); linear fit, $R^2 = 0.856$, $p < 0.001$]. BOLD signal intensities decreased from the 21st to the 37th GW [signal intensity, average: 236.6 ± 66.4 (range: 127.7–387.9); linear fit, $R^2 = -0.207$, $p = 0.256$]. This characteristic change in BOLD signal intensity can be attributed to the slight decrease in water content in fetal brain tissues during gestation and the consequent change of spin relaxivity (Chung et al., 2000). The temporal variation of the filtered and nuisance-corrected BOLD signal decreased over time [signal intensity variation, 6.378 ± 4.532 (1.02–19.06); linear fit, $R^2 = -0.3057$, $p = 0.088$], although this decrease was not significant.

EMERGING INTRINSIC FUNCTIONAL NETWORKS

Network-based statistical inference analysis was performed for 2415 different functional connections (i.e., upper triangle of the brain connectivity matrix; Zalesky et al., 2010). Permutation testing revealed that 850 were different from a random graph, and the intrinsic functional connectivity values of 114 region pairs significantly correlated with gestational age after correcting for multiple comparisons. A linear and a non-linear growth model were tested for the relationship between gestational age and functional connectivity. The variation of each statistical parameter was quantified in terms of the uncertainty calculated during a bootstrapping sampling procedure.

The mean intrinsic functional connectivity of the entire brain network showed a significant increase over gestation (linear model, R^2-adjusted: 0.623 ± 0.0467; SSE: 0.93 ± 0.16; sigmoid model, R^2-adjusted: 0.66 ± 0.063; SSE: 0.875 ± 0.167), and the sigmoid function described the relationship between GW and connectivity more powerfully (difference of SSEs, $p < 0.001$). Until the 25th GW, the mean network connectivity remained close to zero (average connectivity strength range from the 21st–26th GW: −0.163–0.0525). The inflation point of the non-linear strengthening of functional connections was estimated at 26.59 ± 1.19 weeks. The period of connection development in which the connection strengthening rate is larger than 90% of the mean inflation rate was defined as the "expansion period." This interval was calculated from the first derivative of the fitting function. The expansion period of the total functional connectivity network was observed between GWs 25.58–28.69. We illustrate the increase of functional connectivity in **Figure 7B**.

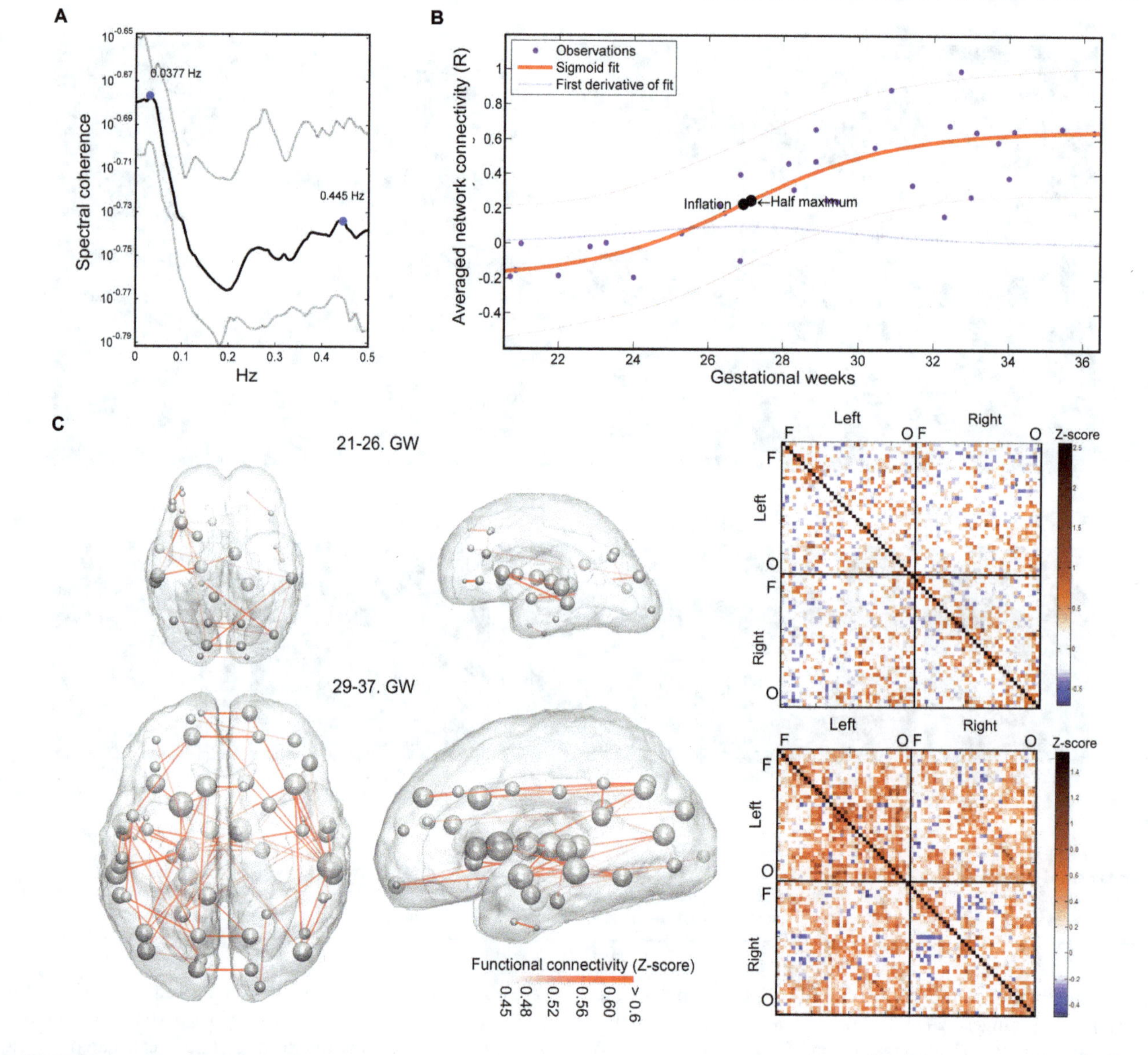

FIGURE 7 | Results of the functional connectivity analysis: spectral coherence of time-courses, developmental trajectory of developing fetal intrinsic functional connectivity. (A) Spectral coherence analysis of fetal fMRI time-courses. The mean coherence plot (black line) was derived for all pairs of fetal functional time-courses at all GWs. Gray line depicts the interquartile range of observation across subjects. The plot is dominated by two peaks, representing low-frequency synchronicity at 0.0377 Hz and possible noise correlation at 0.445 Hz. Bold line: mean coherence, dotted lines: SD. **(B)** Development of the fetal functional brain connectome, gestational age-dependent distribution of functional connections. We illustrate the sigmoid curve-fitting on individual average network connectivity strength measurements. Each point in the graph refers to the mean intrinsic functional connectivity of a fetus, which calculation was restricted to the values that were found to be significantly associated with gestational age. Half-inflation point of the curve is found at the 27th GW and it depicts the gestational age in which the maximum increase of intrinsic functional connectivity is found. **(C)** Developmental expansion of the fetal functional brain connectome, visualization as matrices and 3D graphs. Two stages of the development are depicted: prior to the presumed expansion of functional connectivities (21st–26th GWs) and after this period. This dichotomy was defined using the average intrinsic functional connectivity values **(B)**. The transparence of each edge in the 3D visualization (left images) refers to the population mean of the intrinsic functional connectivity (*Z*-score). The size of nodes in the network depiction is proportional to the sum of connectivity values over all edges that are connected to them. Group-mean network edges were visualized using a threshold of $Z = 0.45$. Graphs were overlaid on anatomical templates from the 23rd and 37th GWs. The mean connectivity networks are also visualized as connectivity matrices, Fs, frontal regions, Os, occipital regions.

Using this concept of expansion, we provide visualizations of the mean fetal functional network structure for pre- and post-expansion periods, and calculated the connectivity values for each of these states of functional connectivity development in **Figure 7C**.

The average intrinsic functional connectivity values in the fetal brain graphs during the expansion period (GW 26–29) were significantly higher than before the 26th GW (pre-expansion: -0.0696 ± 0.0834; expansion: 0.234 ± 0.148; $p = 0.000173$). This difference was also significant for values before and after the expansion state (pre-expansion: −0.0696 ± 0.0834; post-expansion: 0.385 ± 0.159; $p = 0.036$). Our results are summarized in **Table 1**. Between the 21st and 26th GWs, the mean functional network architecture is dominated by occipital and temporal connections, while frontal, parietal, or interhemispheric connections are sparser. After the expansion period (29–37th GW), we observed the increase of functional connectivity strength in the parietal and frontal lobes and long-range correlations between the frontal and temporal lobes.

HETEROGENEOUS AND REGION-SPECIFIC DEVELOPMENTAL CHARACTERISTICS

After separating the entire connectivity network into regions according to brain lobes, we evaluated the developmental trajectories of within-lobe, interhemispheric, and thalamo-cortical connections. Here we use the term "connectivity strength" for the average intrinsic functional connectivity values of a given group of network edges. The estimation of expansion periods revealed a sequential order for how regional functional connectivity becomes increasingly strong. The non-linear sigmoid expansion better described the regional increase of intrinsic network connectivity strength (**Table 2**). The correlation between the gestational time and the connectivity observations was high, with adjusted R-squared values ranging from 0.45 (thalamus connections) to 0.64 (interhemispheric connections).

The inflation time shows a heterogeneous pattern across the fetal cortex. The inflation time of the occipital connections was the earliest (R^2-adjusted: 0.47 ± 0.08, inflation point: 24.83 ± 1.59 GW), while the inflation time for the parietal connections was the latest in the sequence (R^2-adjusted: 0.55 ± 0.07, inflation point: 27.48 ± 0.79 GW). The occipital expansion of functional connectivity was followed by the temporal, frontal, and parietal lobes. Thalamus-cortex interconnections displayed trends of development similar to that of the overall network (expansion of overall network: 26.59 ± 1.19 GW; expansion of thalamic connections: 26.31 ± 1.75 GW).

COMPARING SHORT- AND LONG-RANGE CONNECTIVITY

A further distinction was made according to the region-to-region physical (Euclidean) distances: short- and long-range connections were analyzed separately. Maximum strengthening of all short-range connections occurred at the 27.69 ± 0.94 GW, although we were unable to determine the same for long-range functional coherence where linear strengthening was discovered (SSE of linear model: 0.53 ± 0.1; SSE of non-linear model: 1.47 ± 0.3, $p < 0.0001$). Numeric data of the revealed order of development are summarized in **Table 2**. We provide a visualization of the core regional networks, the developmental curves and the estimated sequence of functional connectivity inflation in **Figure 8**.

After the 26th GW, the proportion of long-range connections becomes significantly higher, as reflected by the larger Euclidean region-to-region distances within the reference network (**Table 1**).

The sigmoid strengthening described the functional connectivity of short-range connections significantly better than the linear, but this observation did not hold for long-range connections. Instead, it appears that long-range connectivities gradually increase from the beginning of the observed gestational period.

SPECTRAL COHERENCE ANALYSIS OF FETAL FUNCTIONAL MRI SIGNALS FROM THE CORTICAL PLATE

Magnitude-squared spectral coherence of BOLD recordings characterized low frequency synchrony of intrinsic signal fluctuations in the fetal brain. Prominent frequency peaks of signal synchronicity were found at 0.0377 ± 0.0599 Hz and 0.427 ± 0.068 Hz, and peak heights were 0.255 ± 0.096 and 0.219 ± 0.047, respectively. This pattern remained consistent at all observed gestational ages. Similar to adult fMRI measurements, it can be assumed that the lower frequency peak corresponds to the neural component, while the higher frequency component is likely to be explained by cardiac effects on the signal (calculated frequency, beats per minute: 144 ± 28, range: 120–216). We illustrated the average spectrum of time-courses and the spectral coherence in **Figure 7A**.

DISCUSSION

CHARACTERISTICS OF THE DEVELOPING FETAL FUNCTIONAL CONNECTOME

In this work, we have employed fMRI to portray the development of the fetal functional brain connectome. The rate of signal synchronicity increase is highest at the transition from the second to the third trimester, with the peak around the 26th GW. MRI

Table 1 | Prenatal development of intrinsic functional connectivity and changes in the region-to-region Euclidean distances.

	Average network connectivity, region-to-region distances (mm)	Average functional connectivity strength of network
Pre-expansion (GW 21–26; $n = 8$)	24.726 ± 1.922 (21.232–27.186)	−0.0696 ± 0.0834 (−0.163–0.0525)
Expansion (GW 26–29; $n = 8$)	27.28 ± 1.608 (25.344–30.526)	0.234 ± 0.148 (−0.0669–0.38)
Post-expansion (GW 29–37; $n = 16$)	26.612 ± 1.459 (23.106–28.626)	0.385 ± 0.159 (0.147–0.6094)
Difference: pre-expansion vs. expansion	Increase: 2.554; $p = 0.0121$	Increase: 0.304; $p = 1.7296e-4$
Difference: post-expansion vs. expansion	Increase: 1.885; $p = 0.0135$	Increase: 0.151; $p = 0.036$

Functional connectivity refers to the Pearson product moment correlation coefficient of the signal time-courses of two brain regions. The average functional connectivity strength is the average correlation coefficient of the network edges that were found to be significantly correlated with gestational age. For optimal comparison, the reported Euclidean distances were fixed for each network edge and these values reflect the distances found at the 37th week of gestation.

Table 2 | Regional characteristics of prenatal intrinsic functional connectivity development: results of the regression analysis.

	Linear model			Sigmoid model				Linear vs. sigmoid
	R^2	Adjusted R^2	SSE	R^2	Adjusted R^2	SSE	Inflation time	
Overall network	0.639 ± 0.045	0.624 ± 0.047	0.93 ± 0.161	0.66 ± 0.064	0.613 ± 0.073	0.878 ± 0.168	26.589 ± 1.196	Sigmoid, $p < 0.0001$
Occipital connections	0.513 ± 0.059	0.492 ± 0.061	1.378 ± 0.219	0.538 ± 0.071	0.473 ± 0.08	1.312 ± 0.251	24.826 ± 1.589	Sigmoid, $p < 0.0001$
Frontal connections	0.563 ± 0.062	0.544 ± 0.065	1.187 ± 0.194	0.649 ± 0.06	0.6 ± 0.069	0.954 ± 0.153	26.434 ± 0.477	Sigmoid, $p < 0.0001$
Temporal connections	0.505 ± 0.054	0.484 ± 0.056	1.601 ± 0.254	0.541 ± 0.063	0.477 ± 0.071	1.468 ± 0.269	25.993 ± 0.929	Sigmoid, $p < 0.0001$
Parietal connections	0.566 ± 0.081	0.547 ± 0.084	1.381 ± 0.31	0.602 ± 0.058	0.547 ± 0.066	1.297 ± 0.22	27.477 ± 0.786	Sigmoid, $p < 0.0001$
Thalamocortical and subcortical connections	0.504 ± 0.0548	0.483 ± 0.057	1.967 ± 0.317	0.519 ± 0.067	0.453 ± 0.077	1.919 ± 0.312	26.31 ± 1.75	Sigmoid, $p < 0.0001$
Short-range connectivity	0.509 ± 0.048	0.488 ± 0.05	1.642 ± 0.251	0.557 ± 0.065	0.495 ± 0.075	1.471 ± 0.251	27.69 ± 0.942	Sigmoid, $p < 0.0001$
Long-range connectivity	0.673 ± 0.052	0.657 ± 0.054	0.532 ± 0.104	0.545 ± 0.07	0.481 ± 0.08	1.471 ± 0.293	25.647 ± 1.445	Linear, $p < 0.0001$
Interhemispheric connections	0.663 ± 0.044	0.649 ± 0.046	0.904 ± 0.144	0.687 ± 0.046	0.643 ± 0.053	0.853 ± 0.132	26.416 ± 1.014	0.084

Two models were tested, we evaluated whether connectivity development was better described with a linear or a non-linear sigmoid growth model. Variance during the bootstrapping analysis is given by the SD. Group comparisons were performed using two-sample, two-sided Student t-tests, assuming equal variances.

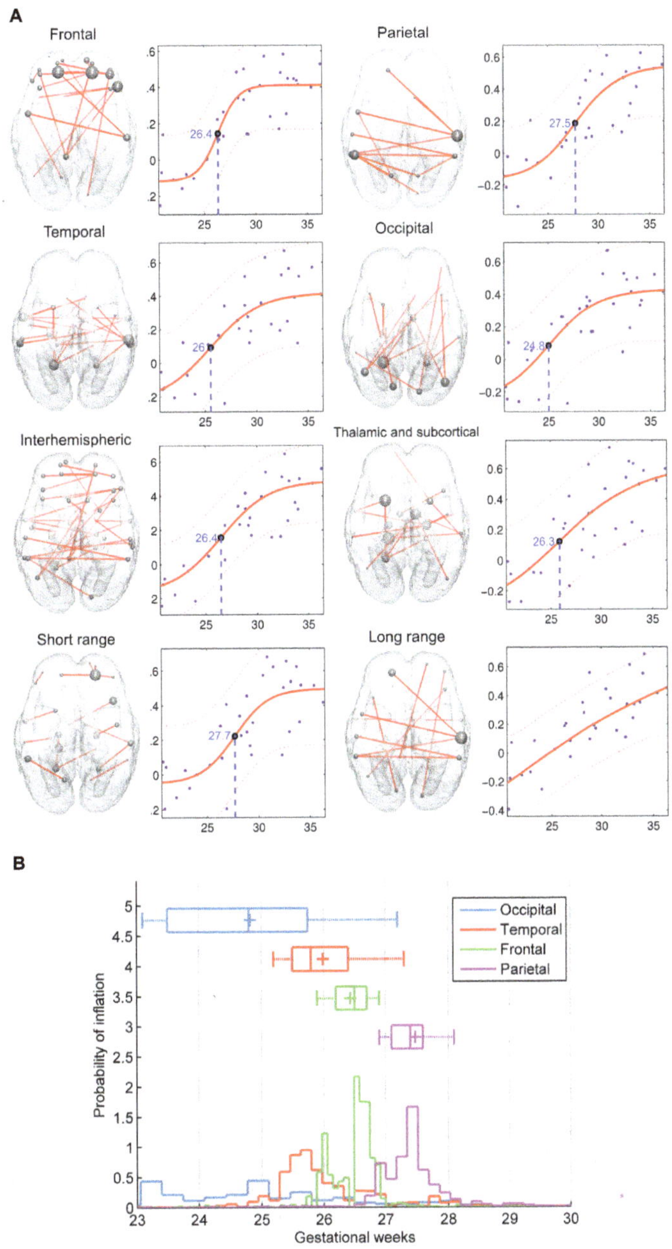

FIGURE 8 | Region-specific development of functional connectivity in the fetal brain. (A) In these visualizations, a regional sub-network was defined to include all connections within a brain lobe, and these were restricted for the edges which connectivity values showed significant correlation with gestational age. Plots depict significant age effects on functional connectivity within each sub-network. Components of sub-networks are depicted as graphs, overlaid onto a 25th-GW brain template model. In this form of visualization, graph edges refer to a functional connection (*Z*-score) between two areas, while the brain areas are represented as nodes. Node size refers to the sum of its connections, weighted by the functional connectivity. **(B)** Regional timing of functional brain connectivity expansion during the late second and third trimester, variability of the observed inflation times during the bootstrapping procedure. According to the hypothesis that functional connectivities exhibit non-linear growth characteristics rather than a linear trend during the mid-fetal period, it is possible to determine the gestational age of inflation by sampling. 50% of the measurement points were sampled randomly during this procedure, and the relative probability estimates of the inflation points of the fitted functions are depicted against the gestational age. The distribution of sampled connections indicates a sequence of occipital, temporal, frontal, and parietal development of intrinsic functional connectivity values.

signal fluctuations were first synchronized in the occipital lobe (e.g., primary visual cortex), followed by the temporal, frontal (including the motor cortex), and parietal lobes. When looking for the optimal characteristics to describe the increase of intrinsic functional connectivity, observations followed a non-linearly increasing trend, the only exception to which were the long-range connections. The proportion of short- and long-range connections was not homogeneous in the evaluated course of gestation: after the expansion period (26th to 29th week), more long-range connections could be observed.

PRENATAL DEVELOPMENT OF FUNCTIONAL BRAIN CONNECTIVITY FOLLOWS POSTERO-ANTERIOR TIMING

The heterogeneous timing of network development across the cortex relates to findings regarding the network variability across adult subjects. Mueller and co-authors found that parietal regions—in particular the association cortex—exhibit high variability compared to primary regions, such as the sensorimotor system (Mueller et al., 2013). The timing suggests that the regions with high inter-individual variability are those regions whose connectivity structure is developed relatively late during gestation. Similarly, these late-developing regions are phylogenetically young cortical areas that exhibit the strongest cortical expansion during late evolution, when comparing the macaque and human cortex (Hill et al., 2010). Buckner and Krienen (2013) discuss the timing of primary cortical areas and subsequent areas, such as the association cortex, relating the complex long-range networks with relatively weak organizational coherence across individuals to the rapid expansion of the corresponding cortical areas during evolution. Although we do not answer the question of whether this is mirrored during early individual brain development, the results suggest that the fetal brain appears to exhibit timing patterns similar to those of cortical evolution.

EMERGENCE OF FETAL NEURAL ACTIVITY: BIOLOGICAL BACKGROUND

The second and third trimester of gestation is critical for the healthy development of cerebral pathways and for the normal functioning of the newborn brain. Here, we interpret findings in the context of major events of telencephalon development within this time frame. Cortical neurons begin to receive their first afferent inputs from the thalamus through a multiple-step process that involves the establishment and resolution of transient connections through the subplate (Price et al., 2006; Kostovic and Judas, 2010). The subplate constitutes a distinct layer of the fetal cortex (Kostovic and Molliver, 1974) and contains a heterogeneous set of early post-migratory neurons, which show the most advanced and mature electrophysiological characteristics compared to other neurons of the fetal brain (Moore et al., 2009). Experimental data indicate an essential role of GABAergic subplate neurons in the generation of early synchronized network activity, and thus, in the establishment of normal neuronal circuits and a regular columnar architecture of the developing cortical plate (Zhang and Poo, 2001; Lopez-Bendito and Molnar, 2003; Kanold, 2009; Luhmann et al., 2009; Judas et al., 2013). Electrical discharges in the human cortex can be demonstrated *in vitro* (Penn and Shatz, 1999; Moore et al., 2009). Moreover, correlates of spontaneous network activity can be identified by early human preterm electrophysiology.

The maturation of thalamocortical afferentation is accompanied by the evolution of a more complex electroencephalography pattern (Vanhatalo and Kaila, 2006), including delta brushes from the 28–30th GWs onward (Khazipov and Luhmann, 2006). Thus, early cortical maturation occurs mainly independent of sensory input, and is driven by spontaneous activity, amplified through subplate neurons (Luhmann et al., 2009). Due to the high water content in the extracellular matrix and the low number of neurons, the subplate displays distinct MRI features, as described *in vitro* and *in vivo* (Maas et al., 2004; Prayer et al., 2006). A spatial and temporal regional morphological variation during development has been described. In the dorsolateral cortical areas, receiving massive cortico-cortical and thalamocortical input, the subplate shows the thickest dimensions, whereas it is diminished in size in the mesocortical regions (Kostovic et al., 2002). There is a developmental peak between 27 and 30 GWs, followed by a stage of dissolution after 30 GWs. Thus, the morphologic dimensions of the fetal subplate mirror the dynamics and grade of the regional connectivity of somatosensory and association cortices. This spatiotemporal anatomic trajectory is in accordance with the results of our functional imaging-based global effects analysis (**Figure 4**). The rapid and significant increase in connectivity between 24 and 31 GWs, with a half-inflation point at 27 GWs correlates with the period of maximum growth of the human fetal subplate and increasing synaptogenesis in the cortical plate. We were able to describe a stage of stabilization of the connectome after 31 GWs, which parallels the process of subplate dissolution and the consolidation of existing networks. The general hierarchy of myelination starts with sensory pathway myelination before the motor and association pathways (Flechsig, 1920). Although myelination mainly occurs postnatally, we were able to demonstrate that functional connections develop first in the occipital and temporal areas at around the 25th GW, whereas the frontal lobe connectivity evolves later. This is consistent with recent neuroimaging and neuropathology data showing an earlier maturation of the optic and acoustic radiations, compared to the frontal lobe pathways traveling through the anterior limb of the internal capsule (Yakovlev and Lecours, 1967; Kinney et al., 1988; Dubois et al., 2008). Trivedi et al. (2009) used diffusion tensor magnetic resonance imaging to demonstrate the region-specific maturation of the fetal brain, concluding that diffusion anisotropy quantifies the microstructural orderedness that reflects the peaking activity of neuronal migration. Coherent with the functional developmental timing in our study, they revealed an initial occipital and temporal increase and peaking of anisotropy.

Moreover, we reported that long-range and interhemispheric connectivity shows a linear increase during development, as opposed to the rapid dynamics of short-range connectivity within certain brain lobes. As long-range association pathways as well as commissural pathways follow a steady and linear developmental trajectory, the dynamics of our functional imaging-based connectome seems to reflect the divergent properties of these processes.

RELATIONSHIP TO PREVIOUS FINDINGS

In utero fMRI came to the forefront only in the last decade to assess stimulation-related activity (Gowland and Fulford, 2004; Jardri et al., 2008) or activation in resting conditions (Schöpf et al., 2012). To date, only a small number of studies have employed this method for the portrayal of functional ontogenesis in normal or pathological circumstances.

A possible way to extend our knowledge in this field is to adapt imaging techniques that are widely used in humans after birth. In this regard, *in vivo* neuroimaging techniques, such as diffusion tensor MR imaging (DTI, Johansen-Berg and Rushworth,

2009; Dennis et al., 2013; Yoshida et al., 2013) or BOLD fMRI have already contributed to significant findings in human developmental neuroscience. The analysis of fetal functional neuroimaging data as an emerging network can be viewed as an extension of previous single-subject or group-based analytical approaches (Schöpf et al., 2012; Thomason et al., 2013).

Observations of fetal behavior *in utero* (Joseph, 2000; Morokuma et al., 2013) outline a fine-tuned arrangement of how functioning neural ensembles emerge that serve basic capacities, like somatomotor functioning, auditory responses, plasticity, or regulatory mechanisms (D'Elia et al., 2001; Partanen et al., 2013a). Evidence for the emergence of fetal auditory processing and simple learning capacities mostly comes from electrophysiological measurements (Holst et al., 2005; Partanen et al., 2013b) or task-related functional imaging (Jardri et al., 2012).

Similarly, fMRI of the immature neonatal brain is restrictive for the characterization of *typical* development: observations are mostly limited to the 26–40th weeks of gestation when the prerequisites for sensory-driven processing are assumed to be already in place (Doria et al., 2010).

Our findings of increasing interhemispheric intrinsic functional connectivity are in line with previously performed studies utilizing prenatal MR imaging, with a notable difference that previous works reported qualitative findings on the emerging activity, or used linear growth models for selected connections (Schöpf et al., 2012; Thomason et al., 2013). The sequence of functional connectivity increase was recently reported to follow a medial–lateral and posterior–anterior trajectory, which is partially supported by our observation of an occipital-temporal-frontal course of network emergence. Using ICA to map the temporo-spatial components of prenatal brain activity, Schöpf et al. (2012) revealed consistent bilateral occipital networks as early as the 22nd GW. Further reproducible components were observed bilaterally in the frontal lobe and unilaterally in the temporal lobe, and, notably, parietal networks were absent. In our developmental model, the pre-expansion period before the 26th week was characterized by bilateral occipital, unilateral temporal connections, and the presence of inter-hemispheric long-range synchrony between non-homotopic areas. The low-frequency MRI signal fluctuations were found to be the most coherent in the 0.01–0.1 Hz range, which matches the commonly assigned filter intervals in adult studies and other prenatal fMRI analyses. In this work, we relied on a more intricate representation of the developing brain activity, compared to previous works on prenatal data: a graph model and network-based inference approach was chosen to capture the overall network properties in a statistically sound framework. In addition, a careful preprocessing pipeline was used to lessen physiological noise and confound the effects of fetal head motion (Power et al., 2012).

The analysis of the developing functional connectome and macroscopic-scale network architecture was previously elucidated using imaging data from immature neonates. According to a report by Doria et al. (2010) preterm neonates seem to exhibit distributed functional connectivity networks at birth. A longitudinal study by Smyser et al. (2010) discovered a variety of network components that resembled their adult counterparts as early as the 26th GW. A consistent component in similar studies is the *default mode network*, whose prenatal existence has been questioned (Lee et al., 2013). This interrogation of developing resting-state functional networks suggests that the period of the most rapid synaptogenesis triggers spontaneous brain activity that is organized into networks, and such networks are similar in spatial extent to those observed in newborns.

By measuring the signal intensity changes coupled with blood oxygenation levels, fMRI indirectly characterizes the time-course of slowly fluctuating neural activation (Logothetis and Wandell, 2004). Physiological measurements suggest that fMRI activations are neuronally driven and more strongly coupled to dendritic activity than action potentials (Lauritzen, 2005). The known mid-gestational shifts of electrical activity in the human cortex correlate with the reported periods of functional connectivity expansion, although a definitive conclusion cannot yet be drawn due to the limitations of *in vivo* imaging technology. Spontaneous brain activity in preterm neonates remains questionable as a model for normal, *in utero* development (Damaraju et al., 2010); a more faithful description about the electrophysiological maturation in healthy subjects would be optimal to explicate our findings on functional activity. So far, such an investigation on normally developing human subjects is not feasible and this problem remains unsolved.

STUDY LIMITATIONS

A number of factors limit the experimental support of our work to describe emerging brain function in human fetuses. Here we report three major categories of possible limitations in fetal fMRI studies: (1) origin of fMRI signals in the developing brain, (2) fetal head motion and age-related confounds, and (3) finding optimal anatomical correspondences during gestation and ROI system creation.

Colonnese and Khazipov (2012) advised a more careful interpretation of pre- and perinatal fMRI studies on the grounds that the coupling of the BOLD signal and neuronal activity is immature or unknown. The relationship between the MRI signal and the underlying neural activity is the topic of extensive debate. However, there is converging evidence that functional connectivity can be explained or predicted by mono- and polysynaptic cortico-cortical interconnections (Honey et al., 2009). Furthermore, spontaneous low-frequency activations in the fetal sensory areas are possibly driven by mechanisms different than that in the adult brain, serving the development of the cortex and not endogenous processing.

Fetal in-scanner head motion is a challenging issue in fMRI, and here in our study this was the primary criteria for excluding otherwise normally developing fetuses. For fMRI experiments with long TR, fetal motion can occur between slices as well, requiring special algorithms for motion correction. In our study, we did not reveal significant dependency of fetal motion patterns with gestational age, although in a larger, unfiltered cohort, this can be expected. Therefore we suggest including total subject-level head displacement as a higher level explanatory variable in group comparisons. As head motion causes not only voxel displacement but signal intensity changes as well, it is important to include motion confound variables in the nuisance regression step.

Here we summarize the following age-related confounds that can hinder the interpretation of our current results. First, fetal brain size significantly grows during gestation, therefore any trend in functional connectivity increase can be a result of merely observing larger ROI. Another consequence of the brain growth is that ROIs are naturally closer to each other in a young brain and this may result in a bias toward stronger short-range connections. In our study, fMRI signal variance did not show significant correlation with gestational age. A further critical step in resting-state fMRI analysis is the nuisance correction, where nuisance means both predictable and random sources of image noise. Here, the steps for MR image analysis were adapted for fetal functional imaging to ensure that maturing macroscopic-scale neural activity contributes to the observed signal intensity fluctuations. Although the current strategy is to obtain noise signals from areas where no neurons reside, the spurious effects of non-neuronal origin cannot be excluded, and, furthermore, monitoring of possible physiological noise sources would be desirable. We experienced a high exclusion rate of clinical cases on the grounds of excessive movement or other artifacts, greatly reducing the data available for analysis.

A possible limiting factor comes from the fact that our study relied on a manually defined ROI system. Localization in the fetal cortex is not directly possible by anatomical atlases, but rather, via the transfer of adult landmarks based on non-linear matching of geometry. This limits the spatial correspondence between subjects. It is possible that the propagation of cortical loci through similarity-based transformations introduces a bias toward later gestational ages when the convoluted surface is more ideal for localization and inter-subject correspondences are better. A possible solution to this problem is the use of functional data-driven parcellation of the cortex, such as demonstrated by Craddock et al. (2012) on the group level. It is possible to use group level ICA to reveal spatially coherent networks within the resting-state fMRI data. Although the transformation of our fetal fMRI data into one reference space for group ICA may suffer from interpolation artifacts due to the large volumetric and anatomical differences.

OUTLOOK AND CONCLUSION

Understanding the formation of functioning neural ensembles in the human brain is particularly important for a model of healthy development, and such a functional, developmental model could be a standard to which pathological conditions can be compared. The assessment of the critical late gestational sculpting of fetal brain activity and macroscopic-scale functional circuitry is feasible with *in utero* neuroimaging. The optimization of imaging sequences and post-processing is crucial and must include strategies to address fetal head motion and non-neuronal sources of fMRI signal. The use of functional connectivity on a ROI basis will allow future investigations on disease development and its correlation to healthy characteristics of connectivity development curves, as shown in this work.

AUTHOR CONTRIBUTIONS

András Jakab has written the manuscript, designed the experiments, performed the analysis and created figures. Ernst Schwartz has performed the analysis and contributed to the manuscript. Gerlinde M. Gruber has acquired data and contributed to the manuscript. Gregor Kasprian has written the manuscript and provided expert consultation. Daniela Prayer has acquired data, written manuscript and provided expert consultation, Veronika Schöpf, Georg Langs has written the manuscript, designed the experiments, provided senior supervision.

ACKNOWLEDGMENTS

This work was supported by the Austrian National Bank Anniversary Fund (FETALMORPHO) to Gregor Kasprian, the EU FP7 projects KHRESMOI to Georg Langs, the Austrian Science Fund (P23205-B09) to Veronika Schöpf. András Jakab is supported by the European Union FP7 Marie Curie IEF Research grant FABRIC – exploring the Formation and Adaptation of the Brain Connectome," grant no. 2012-PIEF-GA-33003.

REFERENCES

Achard, S., Salvador, R., Whitcher, B., Suckling, J., and Bullmore, E. (2006). A resilient, low-frequency, small-world human brain functional network with highly connected association cortical hubs. *J. Neurosci.* 26, 63–72. doi: 10.1523/JNEUROSCI.3874-05.2006

Behzadi, Y., Restom, K., Liau, J., and Liu, T. T. (2007). A component based noise correction method (CompCor) for BOLD and perfusion based fMRI. *Neuroimage* 37, 90–101. doi: 10.1016/j.neuroimage.2007.04.042

Birn, R. M., Murphy, K., and Bandettini, P. A. (2008). The effect of respiration variations on independent component analysis results of resting state functional connectivity. *Hum. Brain Mapp.* 29, 740–750. doi: 10.1002/hbm.20577

Buckner, R. L., and Krienen, F. M. (2013). The evolution of distributed association networks in the human brain. *Trends Cogn. Sci. (Regul. Ed.)* 17, 648–665. doi: 10.1016/j.tics.2013.09.017

Buckner, R. L., Krienen, F. M., and Yeo, B. T. T. (2013). Opportunities and limitations of intrinsic functional connectivity MRI. *Nat. Neurosci.* 16, 832–837. doi: 10.1038/nn.3423

Bullmore, E., and Sporns, O. (2009). Complex brain networks: graph theoretical analysis of structural and functional systems. *Nat. Rev. Neurosci.* 10, 186–198. doi: 10.1038/nrn2575

Bystron, I., Blakemore, C., and Rakic, P. (2008). Development of the human cerebral cortex: boulder committee revisited. *Nat. Rev. Neurosci.* 9, 110–122. doi: 10.1038/nrn2252

Chung, H. W., Chen, C. Y., Zimmerman, R. A., Lee, K. W., Lee, C. C., and Chin, S. C. (2000). T2-Weighted fast MR imaging with true FISP versus HASTE: comparative efficacy in the evaluation of normal fetal brain maturation. *AJR Am. J. Roentgenol.* 175, 1375–1380. doi: 10.2214/ajr.175.5.1751375

Clancy, B., Darlington, R. B., and Finlay, B. L. (2001). Translating developmental time across mammalian species. *Neuroscience* 105, 7–17. doi: 10.1016/S0306-4522(01)00171-3

Colonnese, M., and Khazipov, R. (2012). Spontaneous activity in developing sensory circuits: implications for resting state fMRI. *Neuroimage* 62, 2212–2221. doi: 10.1016/j.neuroimage.2012.02.046

Craddock, R. C., James, G. A., Holtzheimer, P. E. III, Hu, X. P., and Mayberg, H. S. (2012). A whole brain fMRI atlas generated via spatially constrained spectral clustering. *Hum. Brain Mapp.* 33, 1914–1928. doi: 10.1002/hbm.21333

Damaraju, E., Phillips, J. R., Lowe, J. R., Ohls, R., Calhoun, V. D., and Caprihan, A. (2010). Resting-state functional connectivity differences in premature children. *Front. Syst. Neurosci.* 4:23. doi: 10.3389/fnsys.2010.00023

D'Elia, A., Pighetti, M., Moccia, G., and Santangelo, N. (2001). Spontaneous motor activity in normal fetuses. *Early Hum. Dev.* 65, 139–147. doi: 10.1016/S0378-3782(01)00224-9

Dennis, E. L., Jahanshad, N., McMahon, K. L., de Zubicaray, G. I., Martin, N. G., Hickie, I. B., et al. (2013). Development of brain structural connectivity between ages 12 and 30: a 4-tesla diffusion imaging study in 439 adolescents and adults. *Neuroimage* 64, 671–684. doi: 10.1016/j.neuroimage.2012.09.004

Desikan, R. S., Ségonne, F., Fischl, B., Quinn, B. T., Dickerson, B. C., Blacker, D., et al. (2006). An automated labeling system for subdividing the human cerebral cortex on MRI scans into gyral based regions of interest. *Neuroimage* 31, 968–980. doi: 10.1016/j.neuroimage.2006.01.021

Doria, V., Beckmann, C. F., Arichi, T., Merchant, N., Groppo, M., Turkheimer, F. E., et al. (2010). Emergence of resting state networks in the preterm human brain. *Proc. Natl. Acad. Sci. U.S.A.* 107, 20015–20020. doi: 10.1073/pnas.1007921107

Dubois, J., Dehaene-Lambertz, G., Perrin, M., Mangin, J. F., Cointepas, Y., Duchesnay, E., et al. (2008). Asynchrony of the early maturation of white matter bundles in healthy infants: quantitative landmarks revealed noninvasively by diffusion tensor imaging. *Hum. Brain Mapp.* 29, 14–27. doi: 10.1002/hbm.20363

Fjell, A. M., Westlye, L. T., Amlien, I., Tamnes, C. K., Grydeland, H., Engvig, A., et al. (2013). High-expanding cortical regions in human development and evolution are related to higher intellectual abilities. *Cereb. Cortex* doi: 10.1093/cercor/bht201 [Epub ahead of print].

Flechsig, P. E. (1920). *Anatomie des Menschlichen Gehirns und Rückenmarks auf Myelogenetischer Grundlage.* Leipzig: G. Thieme.

Fransson, P. (2005). Spontaneous low-frequency BOLD signal fluctuations: an fMRI investigation of the resting-state default mode of brain function hypothesis. *Hum. Brain Mapp.* 26, 15–29. doi: 10.1002/hbm.20113

Geschwind, N. (1964). "The development of the brain and the evolution of language," in *Monograph Series on Language and Linguistics*, ed. C. I. J. M. Stuart (Washington, DC: Georgetown University Press).

Glenn, O. A., and Barkovich, A. J. (2006). Magnetic resonance imaging of the fetal brain and spine: an increasingly important tool in prenatal diagnosis, part 1. *AJNR Am. J. Neuroradiol.* 27, 1604–1611.

Gowland, P., and Fulford, J. (2004). Initial experiences of performing fetal fMRI. *Exp. Neurol.* 190(Suppl. 1), 22–27. doi: 10.1016/j.expneurol.2004.06.022

Greicius, M. (2008). Resting-state functional connectivity in neuropsychiatric disorders. *Curr. Opin. Neurol.* 21, 424–430. doi: 10.1097/WCO.0b013e328306f2c5

Greicius, M. D., Krasnow, B., Reiss, A. L., and Menon, V. (2003). Functional connectivity in the resting brain: a network analysis of the default mode hypothesis. *Proc. Natl. Acad. Sci. U.S.A.* 100, 253–258. doi: 10.1073/pnas.0135058100

Hill, J., Inder, T., Neil, J., Dierker, D., Harwell, J., and Van Essen, D. (2010). Similar patterns of cortical expansion during human development and evolution. *Proc. Natl. Acad. Sci. U.S.A.* 107, 13135–13140. doi: 10.1073/pnas.1001229107

Holst, M., Eswaran, H., Lowery, C., Murphy, P., Norton, J., and Preissl, H. (2005). Development of auditory evoked fields in human fetuses and newborns: a longitudinal MEG study. *Clin. Neurophysiol.* 116, 1949–1955. doi: 10.1016/j.clinph.2005.04.008

Honey, C. J., Sporns, O., Cammoun, L., Gigandet, X., Thiran, J. P., Meuli, R., et al. (2009). Predicting human resting-state functional connectivity from structural connectivity. *Proc. Natl. Acad. Sci. U.S.A.* 106, 2035–2040. doi: 10.1073/pnas.0811168106

Huang, H., Xue, R., Zhang, J., Ren, T., Richards, L. J., Yarowsky, P., et al. (2009). Anatomical characterization of human fetal brain development with diffusion tensor magnetic resonance imaging. *J. Neurosci.* 29, 4263–4273. doi: 10.1523/JNEUROSCI.2769-08.2009

Jakob, H., and Beckmann, H. (1986). Prenatal developmental disturbances in the limbic allocortex in schizophrenics. *J. Neural Transm.* 65, 303–326. doi: 10.1007/BF01249090

Jardri, R., Houfflin-Debarge, V., Delion, P., Pruvo, J. P., Thomas, P., and Pins, D. (2012). Assessing fetal response to maternal speech using a noninvasive functional brain imaging technique. *Int. J. Dev. Neurosci.* 30, 159–161. doi: 10.1016/j.ijdevneu.2011.11.002

Jardri, R., Pins, D., Houfflin-Debarge, V., Chaffiotte, C., Rocourt, N., Pruvo, J. P., et al. (2008). Fetal cortical activation to sound at 33 weeks of gestation: a functional MRI study. *Neuroimage* 42, 10–18. doi: 10.1016/j.neuroimage.2008.04.247

Jenkinson, M., Beckmann, C. F., Behrens, T. E., Woolrich, M. W., and Smith, S. M. (2012). FSL. *Neuroimage* 62, 782–790. doi: 10.1016/j.neuroimage.2011.09.015

Johansen-Berg, H., and Rushworth, M. F. S. (2009). Using diffusion imaging to study human connectional anatomy. *Annu. Rev. Neurosci.* 32, 75–94. doi: 10.1146/annurev.neuro.051508.135735

Johnson, M. H. (2001). Functional brain development in humans. *Nat. Rev. Neurosci.* 2, 475–483. doi: 10.1038/35081509

Jokhi, R. P., and Whitby, E. H. (2011). Magnetic resonance imaging of the fetus. *Dev. Med. Child Neurol.* 53, 18–28. doi: 10.1111/j.1469-8749.2010.03813.x

Joseph, R. (2000). Fetal brain behavior and cognitive development. *Dev. Rev.* 20, 81–98. doi: 10.1006/drev.1999.0486

Judas, M., Sedmak, G., and Kostovic, I. (2013). The significance of the subplate for evolution and developmental plasticity of the human brain. *Front. Hum. Neurosci.* 7:423. doi: 10.3389/fnhum.2013.00423

Kanold, P. O. (2009). Subplate neurons: crucial regulators of cortical development and plasticity. *Front. Neuroanat.* 3:16. doi: 10.3389/neuro.05.016.2009

Kasprian, G., Brugger, P. C., Weber, M., Krssák, M., Krampl, E., Herold, C., et al. (2008). In utero tractography of fetal white matter development. *Neuroimage* 43, 213–224. doi: 10.1016/j.neuroimage.2008.07.026

Kelly, C., Biswal, B. B., Craddock, R. C., Castellanos, F. X., and Milham, M. P. (2012). Characterizing variation in the functional connectome: promise and pitfalls. *Trends Cogn. Sci. (Regul. Ed.)* 16, 181–188. doi: 10.1016/j.tics.2012.02.001

Khazipov, R., and Luhmann, H. J. (2006). Early patterns of electrical activity in the developing cerebral cortex of humans and rodents. *Trends Neurosci.* 29, 414–418. doi: 10.1016/j.tins.2006.05.007

Kinney, H. C., Brody, B. A., Kloman, A. S., and Gilles, F. H. (1988). Sequence of central nervous system myelination in human infancy. II. Patterns of myelination in autopsied infants. *J. Neuropathol. Exp. Neurol.* 47, 217–234. doi: 10.1097/00005072-198805000-00003

Kok, R. D., de Vries, M. M., Heerschap, A., and van den Berg, P. P. (2004). Absence of harmful effects of magnetic resonance exposure at 1.5 T in utero during the third trimester of pregnancy: a follow-up study. *Magn. Reson. Imaging* 22, 851–854. doi: 10.1016/j.mri.2004.01.047

Kok, R. D., van den Bergh, A. J., Heerschap, A., Nijland, R., and van den Berg, P. P. (2001). Metabolic information from the human fetal brain obtained with proton magnetic resonance spectroscopy. *Am. J. Obstet. Gynecol.* 185, 1011–1015. doi: 10.1067/mob.2001.117677

Kostovic, I., and Judas, M. (2010). The development of the subplate and thalamocortical connections in the human foetal brain. *Acta Paediatr.* 99, 1119–1127. doi: 10.1111/j.1651-2227.2010.01811.x

Kostovic, I., Judas, M., Rados, M., and Hrabac, P. (2002). Laminar organization of the human fetal cerebrum revealed by histochemical markers and magnetic resonance imaging. *Cereb. Cortex* 12, 536–544. doi: 10.1093/cercor/12.5.536

Kostovic, I., and Molliver, M. (1974). New interpretation of laminar development of cerebral-cortex-synaptogenesis in different layers of neopallium in human fetus. *Anat. Rec.* 178:395.

Lauritzen, M. (2005). Reading vascular changes in brain imaging: is dendritic calcium the key? *Nat. Rev. Neurosci.* 6, 77–85. doi: 10.1038/nrn1589

Lee, W., Morgan, B. R., Shroff, M. M., Sled, J. G., and Taylor, M. J. (2013). The development of regional functional connectivity in preterm infants into early childhood. *Neuroradiology* 55(Suppl. 2), 105–111. doi: 10.1007/s00234-013-1232-z

Logothetis, N. K., and Wandell, B. A. (2004). Interpreting the BOLD signal. *Annu. Rev. Physiol.* 66, 735–769. doi: 10.1146/annurev.physiol.66.082602.092845

Lopez-Bendito, G., and Molnar, Z. (2003). Thalamocortical development: how are we going to get there? *Nat. Rev. Neurosci.* 4, 276–289. doi: 10.1038/nrn1075

Lowe, M., Mock, B., and Sorenson, J. (1998). Functional connectivity in single and multislice echoplanar imaging using resting-state fluctuations. *Neuroimage* 7, 119–132. doi: 10.1006/nimg.1997.0315

Luhmann, H. J., Kilb, W., and Hanganu-Opatz, I. L. (2009). Subplate cells: amplifiers of neuronal activity in the developing cerebral cortex. *Front. Neuroanat.* 3:19. doi: 10.3389/neuro.05.019.2009

Maas, L. C., Mukherjee, P., Carballido-Gamio, J., Veeraraghavan, S., Miller, S. P., Partridge, S. C., et al. (2004). Early laminar organization of the human cerebrum demonstrated with diffusion tensor imaging in extremely premature infants. *Neuroimage* 22, 1134–1140. doi: 10.1016/j.neuroimage.2004.02.035

Mailath-Pokorny, M., Kasprian, G., Mitter, C., Schöpf, V., Nemec, U., and Prayer, D. (2012). Magnetic resonance methods in fetal neurology. *Semin. Fetal Neonatal Med.* 17, 278–284. doi: 10.1016/j.siny.2012.06.002

Mantini, D., Corbetta, M., Romani, G. L., Orban, G. A., and Vanduffel, W. (2013). Evolutionarily novel functional networks in the human brain? *J. Neurosci.* 33, 3259–3275. doi: 10.1523/JNEUROSCI.4392-12.2013

Molnár, Z., Métin, C., Stoykova, A., Tarabykin, V., Price, D. J., Francis, F., et al. (2006). Comparative aspects of cerebral cortical development. *Eur. J. Neurosci.* 23, 921–934. doi: 10.1111/j.1460-9568.2006.04611.x

Moore, A. R., Filipovic, R., Mo, Z., Rasband, M. N., Zecevic, N., and Antic, S. D. (2009). Electrical excitability of early neurons in the human cerebral cortex during the second trimester of gestation. *Cereb. Cortex* 19, 1795–1805. doi: 10.1093/cercor/bhn206

Morokuma, S., Fukushima, K., Otera, Y., Yumoto, Y., Tsukimori, K., Ochiai, M., et al. (2013). Ultrasound evaluation of fetal brain dysfunction based on behavioral patterns. *Brain Dev.* 35, 61–67. doi: 10.1016/j.braindev.2012.01.007

Mueller, S., Wang, D., Fox, M. D., Yeo, B. T., Sepulcre, J., Sabuncu, M. R., et al. (2013). Individual variability in functional connectivity architecture of the human brain. *Neuron* 77, 586–595. doi: 10.1016/j.neuron.2012.12.028

Neubert, F., Mars, R., Thomas, A., Sallet, J., and Rushworth, M. S. (2014). Comparison of Human ventral frontal cortex areas for cognitive control and language with areas in monkey frontal cortex. *Neuron* 81, 700–713. doi: 10.1016/j.neuron.2013.11.012

Nooner, K. B., Colcombe, S., Tobe, R., Mennes, M., Benedict, M., Moreno, A., et al. (2012). The NKI-Rockland sample: a model for accelerating the pace of discovery science in psychiatry. *Front. Neurosci.* 6:152. doi: 10.3389/fnins.2012.00152

Oakes, T., Johnstone, T., Ores Walsh, K., Greischar, L., Alexander, A., Fox, A., et al. (2005). Comparison of fMRI motion correction software tools. *Neuroimage* 28, 529–543. doi: 10.1016/j.neuroimage.2005.05.058

Partanen, E., Kujala, T., Naatanen, R., Liitola, A., Sambeth, A., and Huotilainen, M. (2013a). Learning-induced neural plasticity of speech processing before birth. *Proc. Natl. Acad. Sci. U.S.A.* 110, 15145–15150. doi: 10.1073/pnas.1302159110

Partanen, E., Kujala, T., Tervaniemi, M., and Huotilainen, M. (2013b). Prenatal music exposure induces long-term neural effects. *PLoS ONE* 8:e78946. doi: 10.1371/journal.pone.0078946

Paul, L. K., Brown, W. S., Adolphs, R., Tyszka, J. M., Richards, L. J., Mukherjee, P., et al. (2007). Agenesis of the corpus callosum: genetic, developmental and functional aspects of connectivity. *Nat. Rev. Neurosci.* 8, 287–299. doi: 10.1038/nrn2107

Penn, A. A., and Shatz, C. J. (1999). Brain waves and brain wiring: the role of endogenous and sensory-driven neural activity in development. *Pediatr. Res.* 45, 447–458. doi: 10.1203/00006450-199904010-00001

Power, J. D., Barnes, K. A., Snyder, A. Z., Schlaggar, B. L., and Petersen, S. E. (2012). Spurious but systematic correlations in functional connectivity MRI networks arise from subject motion. *Neuroimage* 59, 2142–2154. doi: 10.1016/j.neuroimage.2011.10.018

Prayer, D., Kasprian, G., Krampl, E., Ulm, B., Witzani, L., Prayer, L., et al. (2006). MRI of normal fetal brain development. *Eur. J. Radiol.* 57, 199–216. doi: 10.1016/j.ejrad.2005.11.020

Preuss, T. M. (2009). "The cognitive neuroscience of human uniqueness," in, *The Cognitive Neurosciences*, ed. M. S. Gazzaniga (Cambridge, MA: MIT Press), 49–64.

Price, D. J., Kennedy, H., Dehay, C., Zhou, L., Mercier, M., Jossin, Y., et al. (2006). The development of cortical connections. *Eur. J. Neurosci.* 23, 910–920. doi: 10.1111/j.1460-9568.2006.04620.x

Pugash, D., Brugger, P. C., Bettelheim, D., and Prayer, D. (2008). Prenatal ultrasound and fetal MRI: the comparative value of each modality in prenatal diagnosis. *Eur. J. Radiol.* 68, 214–226. doi: 10.1016/j.ejrad.2008.06.031

Rakic, P. (2009). Evolution of the neocortex: a perspective from developmental biology. *Nat. Rev. Neurosci.* 10, 724–735. doi: 10.1038/nrn2719

Rice, D., and Barone, S. (2000). Critical periods of vulnerability for the developing nervous system: evidence from humans and animal models. *Environ. Health Perspect.* 108(Suppl. 3), 511–533. doi: 10.1289/ehp.00108s3511

Rilling, J. K. (2014). Comparative primate neuroimaging: insights into human brain evolution. *Trends Cogn. Sci. (Regul. Ed.)* 18, 46–55. doi: 10.1016/j.tics.2013.09.013

Rubinov, M., and Sporns, O. (2010). Complex network measures of brain connectivity: uses and interpretations. *Neuroimage* 52, 1059–1069. doi: 10.1016/j.neuroimage.2009.10.003

Rueckert, D. (2012). *A Multi-channel 4D Probabilistic Atlas of the Developing Fetal Brain.* Available at: http://biomedic.doc.ic.ac.uk/brain-development/index.php?n=Main.Fetal (accessed November 1, 2013).

Schlotz, W., and Phillips, D. I. W. (2009). Fetal origins of mental health: evidence and mechanisms. *Brain Behav. Immun.* 23, 905–916. doi: 10.1016/j.bbi.2009.02.001

Schöpf, V., Kasprian, G., Brugger, P. C., and Prayer, D. (2012). Watching the fetal brain at "rest." *Int. J. Dev. Neurosci.* 30, 11–17. doi: 10.1016/j.ijdevneu.2011.10.006

Serag, A., Aljabar, P., Ball, G., Counsell, S. J., Boardman, J. P., Rutherford, M. A., et al. (2012). Construction of a consistent high-definition spatio-temporal atlas of the developing brain using adaptive kernel regression. *Neuroimage* 59, 2255–2265. doi: 10.1016/j.neuroimage.2011.09.062

Shmueli, K., van Gelderen, P., de Zwart, J. A., Horovitz, S. G., Fukunaga, M., Jansma, J. M., et al. (2007). Low-frequency fluctuations in the cardiac rate as a source of variance in the resting-state fMRI BOLD signal. *Neuroimage* 38, 306–320. doi: 10.1016/j.neuroimage.2007.07.037

Smyser, C. D., Inder, T. E., Shimony, J. S., Hill, J. E., Degnan, A. J., Snyder, A. Z., et al. (2010). Longitudinal analysis of neural network development in preterm infants. *Cereb. Cortex* 20, 2852–2862. doi: 10.1093/cercor/bhq035

Thomason, M. E., Dassanayake, M. T., Shen, S., Katkuri, Y., Alexis, M., Anderson, A. L., et al. (2013). Cross-hemispheric functional connectivity in the human fetal brain. *Sci. Transl. Med.* 5:173ra24.

Trivedi, R., Gupta, R. K., Husain, N., Rathore, R. K., Saksena, S., Srivastava, S., et al. (2009). Region-specific maturation of cerebral cortex in human fetal brain: diffusion tensor imaging and histology. *Neuroradiology* 51, 567–576. doi: 10.1007/s00234-009-0533-8

Uğurbil, K., Xu, J., Auerbach, E. J., Moeller, S., Vu, A. T., Duarte-Carvajalino, J. M., et al. (2013). Pushing spatial and temporal resolution for functional and diffusion MRI in the human connectome project. *Neuroimage* 80, 80–104. doi: 10.1016/j.neuroimage.2013.05.012

van den Heuvel, M. P., Stam, C. J., Kahn, R. S., and Hulshoff Pol, H. E. (2009). Efficiency of functional brain networks and intellectual performance. *J. Neurosci.* 29, 7619–7624. doi: 10.1523/JNEUROSCI.1443-09.2009

Vanhatalo, S., and Kaila, K. (2006). Development of neonatal EEG activity: from phenomenology to physiology. *Semin. Fetal Neonatal Med.* 11, 471–478. doi: 10.1016/j.siny.2006.07.008

Weissenbacher, A., Kasess, C., Gerstl, F., Lanzenberger, R., Moser, E., and Windischberger, C. (2009). Correlations and anticorrelations in resting-state functional connectivity MRI: a quantitative comparison of preprocessing strategies. *Neuroimage* 47, 1408–1416. doi: 10.1016/j.neuroimage.2009.05.005

Yakovlev, P. I., and Lecours, A. (1967). "The myelogenetic cycles of regional maturation of the brain," in *Regional Development of the Brain in Early Life*, ed. A. Minkowski (Oxford: Blackwell), 3–70.

Yan, C., Craddock, R. C., Zuo, X., Zang, Y., and Milham, M. P. (2013). Standardizing the intrinsic brain: towards robust measurement of inter-individual variation in 1000 functional connectomes. *Neuroimage* 80, 246–262. doi: 10.1016/j.neuroimage.2013.04.081

Yoshida, S., Oishi, K., Faria, A., and Mori, S. (2013). Diffusion tensor imaging of normal brain development. *Pediatr. Radiol.* 43, 15–27. doi: 10.1007/s00247-012-2496-x

Zalesky, A., Fornito, A., and Bullmore, E. T. (2010). Network-based statistic: identifying differences in brain networks. *Neuroimage* 53, 1197–1207. doi: 10.1016/j.neuroimage.2010.06.041

Zhang, L. I., and Poo, M. M. (2001). Electrical activity and development of neural circuits. *Nat. Neurosci.* 4(Suppl.), 1207–1214. doi: 10.1038/nn753

3

The functional significance of newly born neurons integrated into olfactory bulb circuits

Masayuki Sakamoto[1,2†], Ryoichiro Kageyama[1,3,4*] and Itaru Imayoshi[1,3,5,6*]

[1] Institute for Virus Research, Kyoto University, Kyoto, Japan
[2] Kyoto University Graduate School of Biostudies, Kyoto, Japan
[3] World Premier International Research Initiative–Institute for Integrated Cell-Material Sciences, Kyoto University, Kyoto, Japan
[4] Japan Science and Technology Agency, Core Research for Evolutional Science and Technology, Kyoto, Japan
[5] The Hakubi Center, Kyoto University, Kyoto, Japan
[6] Japan Science and Technology Agency, Precursory Research for Embryonic Science and Technology, Kyoto, Japan

Edited by:
Luca Bonfanti, University of Turin, Italy

Reviewed by:
Francesca Ciccolini, University of Heidelberg, Germany
Liliana Bernardino, University of Beira Interior, Portugal

***Correspondence:**
Ryoichiro Kageyama, Institute for Virus Research, Kyoto University, Shogoin-Kawahara, Sakyo-ku, Kyoto 606-8507, Japan
e-mail: rkageyam@virus.kyoto-u.ac.jp;
Itaru Imayoshi, The Hakubi Center, Institute for Virus Research, Kyoto University, Shogoin-Kawahara, Sakyo-ku, Kyoto 606-8507, Japan
e-mail: iimayosh@virus.kyoto-u.ac.jp

†Present address:
Masayuki Sakamoto, Department of Biological Sciences, Columbia University, New York, USA

The olfactory bulb (OB) is the first central processing center for olfactory information connecting with higher areas in the brain, and this neuronal circuitry mediates a variety of odor-evoked behavioral responses. In the adult mammalian brain, continuous neurogenesis occurs in two restricted regions, the subventricular zone (SVZ) of the lateral ventricle and the hippocampal dentate gyrus. New neurons born in the SVZ migrate through the rostral migratory stream and are integrated into the neuronal circuits of the OB throughout life. The significance of this continuous supply of new neurons in the OB has been implicated in plasticity and memory regulation. Two decades of huge investigation in adult neurogenesis revealed the biological importance of integration of new neurons into the olfactory circuits. In this review, we highlight the recent findings about the physiological functions of newly generated neurons in rodent OB circuits and then discuss the contribution of neurogenesis in the brain function. Finally, we introduce cutting edge technologies to monitor and manipulate the activity of new neurons.

Keywords: neurogenesis, main olfactory bulb, accessory olfactory bulb, granule cell, periglomerular cell, lateral inhibition, behavior, neural stem cell

INTRODUCTION

It was believed that the adult mammalian brain is incapable of producing new neurons. The prominent histologist Cajal proclaimed "Once the development was ended, the founts of growth and regeneration of the axons and dendrites dried up irrevocably. In the adult centers, the nerve paths are something fixed, ended, and immutable. Everything may die, nothing may be regenerated." (Ramon y Cajal, 1928). In 1960's, Altman and his colleague's pioneering study provided the first anatomical evidence of neurogenesis in the postnatal hippocampal region using a [H^3]-thymidine incorporation labeling (Altman and Das, 1965). These [H^3]-thymidine-labeling cells had neuronal morphology (Kaplan and Hinds, 1977). However, these findings were not accepted by Cajal's neuron doctrine that no new neurons are born in the adult brain. In 1980's, adult neurogenesis identified in songbird's brain was found to play a role in song learning (Goldman and Nottebohm, 1983). In 1990's, neural stem/progenitor cells were isolated from adult rodent brain, and adult neurogenesis was discovered in human hippocampus (Reynolds and Weiss, 1992; Eriksson et al., 1998). Since the discovery, adult neurogenesis has now become a well-accepted phenomenon including humans (Sanai et al., 2011; Bergmann et al., 2012; Spalding et al., 2013; Ernst et al., 2014).

In rodents, adult neurogenesis mainly occurs in two brain regions, the subventricular zone (SVZ) of the lateral ventricles and the subgranular zone (SGZ) of the hippocampal dentate gyrus (DG) (Kriegstein and Alvarez-Buylla, 2009; Suh et al., 2009; Aimone et al., 2011; Fuentealba et al., 2012). Adult neural stem/progenitor cells are regulated by many genes and signaling pathways (Kriegstein and Alvarez-Buylla, 2009; Suh et al., 2009). Neurons born in the SGZ migrate into the granule cell layer (GCL) and become granule cells of the DG, while neurons born in the SVZ migrate into the olfactory bulb (OB) through the rostral migratory stream (RMS), the pathway leading to the OB, and become local interneurons, granule cells (GCs) and periglomerular cells (PGCs) (Lledo et al., 2006; Ming and Song, 2011; Lepousez et al., 2013).

The olfactory system, which senses and processes odor information, is one of the oldest and important parts of the brain. Odor information is transferred to local neural circuits in the OB, and then conveyed to various regions of the olfactory cortex via principal neurons (mitral and tufted cells, hereafter referred to these neurons as M/T cells). Unlike most other central nervous system areas, GABAergic inhibitory interneurons greatly outnumber principal neurons, suggesting that odor representations in the OB are shaped by local inhibitory circuits (Yokoi et al., 1995; Isaacson and Strowbridge, 1998; Egger and Urban, 2006). Furthermore, although most neurons comprising the mammalian central nervous system are produced during embryonic development, a large proportion of these interneurons in the OB are generated and continuously renewed throughout life. Why do such continuous neuronal addition and replacement occur in the OB? Two decades of huge investigation revealed the biological importance of integration of new neurons into the olfactory circuits (Lledo et al., 2006; Kelsch et al., 2010; Ming and Song, 2011; Lepousez et al., 2013).

In this review, we highlight recent findings about physiological features of new neurons in rodent OB circuits and then describe the role of new neurons in olfaction-associated behaviors. Finally, we introduce optical techniques to monitor and manipulate the activity of new neurons.

NEURONAL CIRCUIT OF THE OLFACTORY SYSTEM

The OB is the first relay station in the olfactory system that can process odor information (**Figure 1**). Odor information is detected by olfactory sensory neurons (OSNs). OSNs expressing the same odorant receptors project and converge their axons into the same glomeruli (Mori and Sakano, 2011). OSNs form excitatory synapses on primary dendrites of M/T cells. M/T cells project their axons to the olfactory cortex to covey odor information to higher brain areas in the forebrain. Mitral cells project their axons to nearly all areas of the olfactory cortex with a dispersed manner, while tufted cells target densely only to the anterior regions of the olfactory cortex (Ghosh et al., 2011; Miyamichi et al., 2011; Sosulski et al., 2011; Igarashi et al., 2012).

Synaptic connections in the external plexiform layer (EPL) of the OB are dominated by dendrodendritic reciprocal synapses between lateral dendrites of M/T cells and GCs, the latter being most numerous type of inhibitory interneurons in the OB. Unlike the neocortex, GABAergic inhibitory interneurons in the OB grealy outnumber principal neurons by 50–100:1 (Isaacson and Strowbridge, 1998; Egger and Urban, 2006). GCs form dendrodendritic synapses with M/T cells. In a dendrodendritic reciprocal synapse, both sides of the synapse are dendrites. M/T to GC is a glutamatergic excitatory synapse, while GC to M/T is a GABAergic inhibitory synapse (**Figure 1**). This large number of inhibitory synapses onto M/T cells may enable inhibitory circuits to refine odor representations. (Isaacson and Strowbridge, 1998; Egger and Urban, 2006; Lepousez and Lledo, 2013).

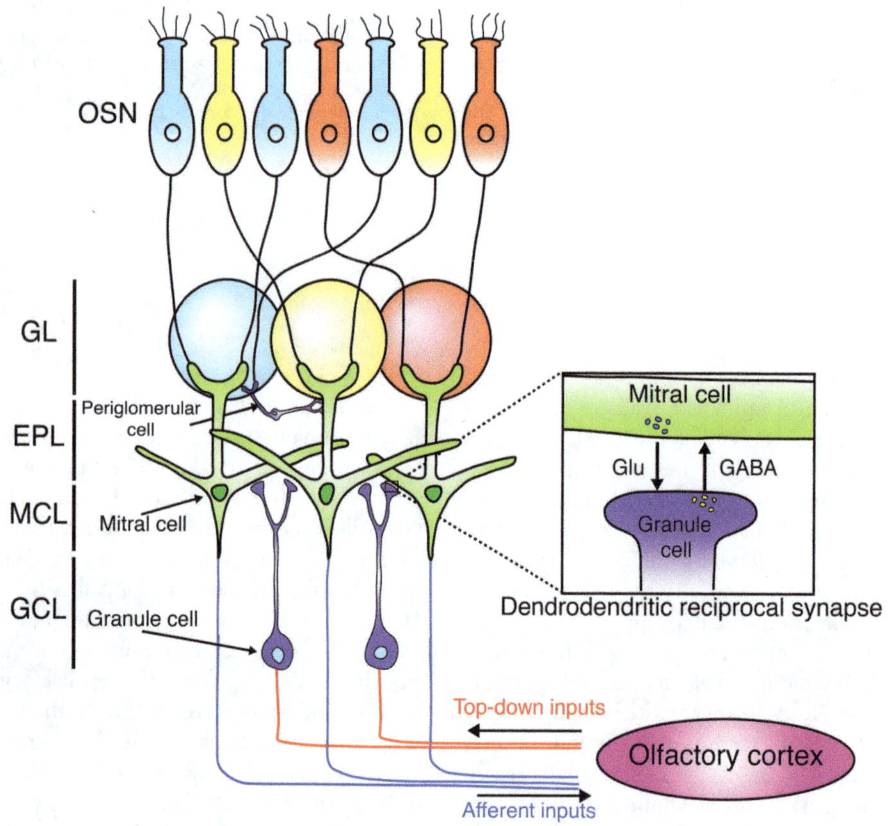

FIGURE 1 | Neural circuit of the olfactory bulb. Schematic diagram of the neuronal circuit of the olfactory bulb. OSNs expressing the same odorant receptors (blue, yellow, red) project and converge their axons into the same glomeruli. OSNs form excitatory synapses with mitral cells. Mitral cells project their axons to the olfactory cortex. Mitral cells form dendrodendritic synapses with granule cells. Granule cells receive centrifugal glutamatergic inputs from the olfactory cortex. OSN, olfactory sensory neuron; GL, glomerular layer; EPL, external plexiform layer; MCL, mitral cell layer; GCL, granule cell layer.

PGCs are another type of major GABAergic interneurons in the OB, and modulate the neural circuit in the glomerulus, consisting of terminals of the olfactory nerve and the dendrites of M/T. PGCs are subdivided into at least three subtypes based on immunoreactivity to calretinin (CalR), calbindin-28K (CalB), and tyrosine hydroxylase (TH) (Kosaka et al., 1998; Pressler and Strowbridge, 2006; Eyre et al., 2008, 2009; Kosaka and Kosaka, 2011). In mice, all three PGC subtypes seem to be GABA-expressing inhibitory neurons, but the definite functional roles of each PGC subtype in odor processing have not been well determined.

In addition to GCs and PGCs, numerous types of GABAergic interneurons have been identified in the OB (Pressler and Strowbridge, 2006; Batista-Brito et al., 2008; Eyre et al., 2008, 2009; Kosaka and Kosaka, 2011; Huang et al., 2013; Kato et al., 2013; Miyamichi et al., 2013), including deep short-axon cells, Blanes cells, and EPL interneurons. Although lineage and turnover analysis of these OB interneuronal populations has just been started (Batista-Brito et al., 2008; Bartolini et al., 2013), dynamic turnover of these interneurons by postnatal/adult neurogenesis may also contribute to the reorganization of OB circuitry.

UNIQUE FEATURES OF NEWLY GENERATED NEURONS

While M/T cells are generated only at an embryonic stage, GCs and PGCs are generated throughout life (Imayoshi et al., 2008; Imamura et al., 2011; Sakamoto et al., 2014). Long-term genetic labeling analysis revealed that the majority of GCs are replaced by newly generated neurons during adult life (Imayoshi et al., 2008). Newly generated GCs are preferentially located in a deep region, while pre-existing GCs are located in a superficial region in the GCL of the OB (Lemasson et al., 2005; Imayoshi et al., 2008; Sakamoto et al., 2014). Interestingly, it has been shown that outer/superficial GCs, whose dendrites preferentially target the superficial lamina of the EPL, establish synapses with tufted cells, whereas deep GCs mainly contact the dendrites of mitral cells in the deep lamina of the EPL (Mori et al., 1983; Orona et al., 1983; Shepherd and Greer, 2004; Imamura et al., 2006). Therefore, one attractive hypotheis is that these two GC subpopulations fundamentally modulate distinct neural circuits. This implies that the activity of tufted cells is under the preferential control of embryonic-born GCs (static, superficial layers), while postnatal-born GCs (turnover, deep layers) provide an inhibitory drive to both mitral and tufted cells.

In rodents, although numerous new neurons reach the OB each day (roughly one percent of the total OB GCs), only half of them are integrated into pre-existing neural circuits. The remains of them are eliminated by apoptosis during their maturation (Lledo et al., 2006). This "survival or death" depends on olfactory sensory experience. Sensory deprivation triggers a decrease in new GC survival, whereas olfactory enrichment and learning boost the survival of these neurons (Petreanu and Alvarez-Buylla, 2002; Rochefort et al., 2002). Interestingly, day 14 to 28 after the generation is a critical period of newly born GCs when their survival is influenced by sensory experience (Yamaguchi and Mori, 2005). This time window overlaps with the period when newly generated neurons make synapses with pre-existing neurons, suggesting that synaptic inputs play a crucial role in the selection of adult born GCs (Kelsch et al., 2008; Yokoyama et al., 2011). Although the number of PGCs is one order smaller than that of GCs, new PGCs are also continuously produced throughout life (Ninkovic et al., 2007; Sakamoto et al., 2014). Like GCs, the survival of newly born PGCs is regulated in an activity-dependent manner. Sensory deprivation triggers a decrease in new PGCs' survival, whereas olfactory enrichment and learning boost the survival of adult generated PGCs (Rochefort et al., 2002; Alonso et al., 2006; Adam and Mizrahi, 2011; Sawada et al., 2011; Livneh and Mizrahi, 2012). A recent work also reported the generation of some glutamatergic short-axon cells at a very low proportion (Brill et al., 2009).

One recent elegant study provided direct evidence of the involvement of adult-born PGCs in olfactory sensory processing (Livneh et al., 2014). By using two-photon-targeted patch recordings, they showed that adult-born PGCs indeed respond to odor input. Interestingly, young adult-born neurons (2–4 weeks of age) have broader odor response profile than that of matured resident PGCs. Furthermore, sensory enrichment during developmental periods of adult-born neurons sharpens their odor response selectivity after maturation. These results indicated that continuous supply of these sensitive adult-born neurons into the olfactory circuit provides it with a mechanism of long-lasting plasticity (Livneh et al., 2014).

The OB receives input not only from OSNs but also from the olfactory cortex (**Figure 1**). This top-down input targets preferentially to the GCL and is important to shape the activity of M/T neurons (Manabe et al., 2011; Boyd et al., 2012; Markopoulos et al., 2012). In addition, recent studies showed that this cortical feedback is necessary for odor discrimination and food-intake (Nunez-Parra et al., 2013; Soria-Gomez et al., 2014). Furthermore, several studies showed the connectivity of newly generated neurons using monosynaptic rabies virus-based tracing system and revealed that newborn neurons in the OB receive glutamatergic inputs from neurons in the olfactory cortex (Arenkiel et al., 2011; Deshpande et al., 2013). Interestingly, new neurons exhibit more synaptic plasticity from centrifugal inputs than mature neurons do (Nissant et al., 2009). Furthermore, top-down inputs on the proximal dendrites of GCs also contribute to the survival/death of new neurons (Yamaguchi et al., 2013). Therefore, these observations imply that top-down glutamatergic input from the olfactory cortex to new GCs has a critical role in generating high plasticity in OB cirucuits.

Adult neurogenesis occurs in human brain as well as in rodents. Radiocarbon dating technologies revealed that adult neurogenesis in the OB is extremely limited though hippocampal neurogenesis occurs at a steady rate (Bergmann et al., 2012; Spalding et al., 2013). Surprisingly, new neurons born SVZ/lateral ventricles migrate and differentiate into striatum interneurons (Ernst et al., 2014). Furthermore, striatum neurogenesis is reduced in patients with Huntington's diseases. These results indicate that adult neurogenesis in humans has a unique pattern, and that these neurons derived from SVZ/lateral ventricles might be involved in brain functions such as cognition and motor coordination.

THE ROLES OF NEWLY GENERATED NEURONS FOR OLFACTION-RELATED BEHAVIORS

While the functional significance of continuous neurogenesis in hippocampus has been extensively studied (Deng et al., 2010; Aimone et al., 2011), the role of newly generated neurons in olfaction-related behaviors remains elusive. As mentioned above, newly born neurons form dendrodendritic synapses with M/T cells and control the activity of M/T cells to shape odor representation. Genetic ablation of newly born neurons in the OB impairs the structure and neural circuits in the OB (Imayoshi et al., 2008; Sakamoto et al., 2011). It was reported that newly generated GCs exhibit long-term synaptic plasticity, and that this ability is gradually lost as these neurons become mature, indicating that newly born GCs play a more important role in plastic change than mature GCs (Nissant et al., 2009). Importantly, electrophysiological recording revealed that ablation of adult born neurons impairs recurrent and lateral dendrodendritic inhibition of M/T cells and reduces the frequency of the induced gamma oscillations in the OB (Breton-Provencher et al., 2009). Furthermore, the survival of newly generated neurons is regulated by sensory experience (Yamaguchi and Mori, 2005; Lledo et al., 2006; Yokoyama et al., 2011). Together, these findings suggest that neurogenesis has a key role in olfaction-related plastic activities in the OB.

To understand the functional role of neurogenesis in the OB, various behavioral analyses have been applied. To address this question, various methodologies for inhibiting neurogenesis have been used: pharmacological, irradiation, and genetic targeting (Gheusi et al., 2000; Kim et al., 2007; Bath et al., 2008; Imayoshi et al., 2008; Breton-Provencher et al., 2009; Lazarini et al., 2009; Sultan et al., 2010; Sakamoto et al., 2011). Conversely, an apoptotic inhibitor was used to suppress cell death of newly born neurons (Mouret et al., 2009; Sultan et al., 2011).

One of the simplest behavioral tests for olfaction is to check spontaneous odor exploration toward a novel odor without any rewards (**Figure 2A**). In this task, the ability of odor discrimination can be assessed by repeated presentations of the same odor (habituation) followed by the presentation of a novel odor (dishabituation). The sniffing time decreases during habituation sessions, but then increases when the odor is recognized as a new one in a dishabituation session. This can be applied to evaluate the odor detection threshold by comparing sniffing times between different concentrations. This test can also assess the short-term olfactory memory by changing time interval between sessions. Blockade of neurogenesis by infusion of an antimitotic drug impairs the ability of odor detection and short-term memory (60 min), suggesting that new neurons are involved in odor detection and processing odor memory (Breton-Provencher et al., 2009). In addition, gene deficient mice, which result in a decrease of new neurons in the OB, could not discriminate between dissimilar odors (Gheusi et al., 2000; Bath et al., 2008). However, not all findings have supported this result. Mice treated with γ-ray irradiation to block neurogenesis showed normal sensitivity (Lazarini et al., 2009), suggesting that spontaneous odor discrimination is not affected in these mice. Similar results were obtained from other studies (Kim et al., 2007; Imayoshi et al., 2008; Sakamoto et al., 2011). The discrepancies between these findings may be due to different ablation methods. Regarding the target specificity, blocking adult neurogenesis by using conventional knock in/out mice is far from specific.

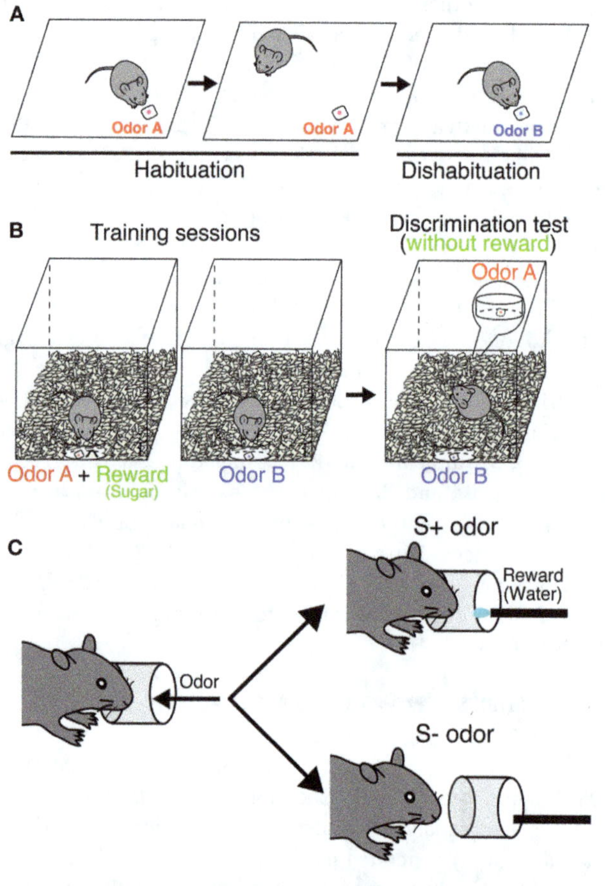

FIGURE 2 | Behavioral paradigm of odor discrimination test. (A) Habituation-dishabituation test. In habituation sessions, odor A (red) is presented repeatedly. A mouse is habituated to this odor, and sniffing time is getting decreased. In a dishabituation session, sniffing time increases when the mouse can recognize a novel odor B (blue). **(B)** Odor-reward association test. During the training, a mouse is associated with one of the odors with reward (sugar). In the test, both odors are placed under the bedding separately without reward. Digging time of each odorant is measured to judge whether the mouse can discriminate between the two odors. In an odor memory retention test, mice are exposed to the same test without further training. **(C)** Go/no-go olfactory conditioning test. A mouse is associated with one of the odors with reward (water). Each trial is counted as correct if the mouse licks continuously upon presentation of a rewarded (S+) odor or does not lick continuously with a non-rewarded (S−) odor.

Odor-reward association learning is another major paradigm that has been used to evaluate the function of neurogenesis in the OB (**Figures 2B,C**). This test can evaluate the capacity to associate an odor with reward (food or water) and the ability of odor discrimination and memory retention. Genetically ablated mice can acquire the odor-associated memory and maintain it for at least 2 months (Imayoshi et al., 2008; Sakamoto et al., 2011). Similar results were obtained from other animal models (Schellinck et al., 2004; Breton-Provencher et al., 2009). These results indicate that continuous neurogenesis is not required for simple discrimination between similar odors or retention of odor-associated memory. Pre-existing granule neurons born in embryonic and neonatal stages may compensate for these functions in the absence of new neurons. However, conflicting results were also reported following odor-reward association learning. Although mice showed normal odor discrimination ability, their long-term odor-associated memory retention was impaired by irradiation- or drug-induced inhibition of neurogenesis (Lazarini et al., 2009; Sultan et al., 2010). This discrepancy likely results from the difference in experimental paradigms. In addition, parameters to evaluate odor memory are totally different depending on behavior tests [digging time (seconds) or correct decision (%)].

These discrepancies may result from the target specificity for blockade of neurogenesis. Strictly speaking, these past methods did not specifically target new neurons in the OB. Neurons in other cortical regions might be affected to some extent. Therefore, there is a need to generate more sophisticated model that can target only newly generated neurons in the OB. One possibility to increase the target specificity is an intersectional strategy with dual site-specific recombinases (Cre and Flp) (Imayoshi et al., 2011; Huang and Zeng, 2013). Most of new neurons in the OB are GABAergic inhibitory neurons, while new neurons in the DG are glutamatergic excitatory neurons. Based on their different transmitter characteristics, new neurons in the OB and DG can be separately targeted. Recently, our group has developed new transgenic mice in which new neurons in the OB and DG can be separately targeted, and found that continuous neurogenesis is important for flexible olfactory associative learning and memory (Sakamoto et al., 2014). Continuous supply of new neurons in the OB is important to rewrite aquired odor memory and modify the value of odor-associated memory.

Adult neurogenesis in the hippocampus is required for pattern separation (Clelland et al., 2009; Sahay et al., 2011a,b; Nakashiba et al., 2012). It seems that odor enrichment improves a recruitment of newly born neurons and the olfactory discrimination ability. Blockade of neurogenesis with AraC impaired the improvement of odor discrimination, suggesting that neurogenesis is required for perceptual learning (Moreno et al., 2009). This result implies that neurogenesis in the OB also contributes to pattern separation. It would be interesting to examine the relationship between OB neurogenesis and pattern separation (Sahay et al., 2011b).

OB NEUROGENESIS IN INNATE BEHAVIORS

Adult neurogenesis is physiologically linked to reproductive behaviors, suggesting that continuous neurogenesis plays a pivotal role in pheromone-associated behaviors (Shingo et al., 2003; Mak et al., 2007; Mak and Weiss, 2010; Nunez-Parra et al., 2011). Pregnancy and lactation increase the number of both new GCs and PGCs (Shingo et al., 2003). Around gestation day 7, the proliferation reaches a peak in the SVZ/lateral ventricles. After the delivery, the number of new neurons integrated into OB circuits increases, and their dendritic spines exhibit stable features (Shingo et al., 2003; Kopel et al., 2012). These phenomena during early pregnancy and parenting might be important for fine-tuning of olfactory response to mating partners and pups. This induction of neurogenesis is mediated by prolactin (Shingo et al., 2003; Larsen and Grattan, 2010). Reducing the prolactin levels decreases neurogenesis in the SVZ/lateral ventricles and impairs maternal behaviors (Larsen and Grattan, 2010). Neurogenesis in females is also induced by pheromones of dominant males (but not other males) and is important for sexual behaviors (Mak et al., 2007; Oboti et al., 2009, 2011). Relevant increase of new neurons also occurs in male mice when they interact with their postnatal offspring (Mak and Weiss, 2010). This increase of neurogenesis mediated by prolactin appears to depend on the odor of their offspring and is involved in offspring recognition (Mak and Weiss, 2010).

These results indicate that OB neurogenesis is really related to sexual and maternal behaviors, suggesting that neurogenesis plays an important role in such pheromone-associated innately-programmed behaviors. Genetic inhibition of adult neurogenesis revealed that new neurons are essential for mating and maternal behaviors (Sakamoto et al., 2011). Blocking neurogenesis by injecting antimitotic drugs also impairs mating behaviors (Oboti et al., 2011). Pregnancy block (Bruce effect) is a well-known phenomenon; females terminate their pregnancy when they are exposed to the scent of unfamiliar males (Bruce, 1959). Although the detailed mechanism of this pregnancy block remains to be determined, it was shown that the pregnancy failure rate is highly increased by the blockade of continuous neurogenesis (Sakamoto et al., 2011). These results indicate that continuous neurogenesis is essential for pheromone-associated innately-programmed behaviors and activities. However, conflicting results were also reported. Disruption of neurogenesis in the OB by γ-ray irradiation left sexual and maternal behaviors unaffected (Feierstein et al., 2010). The discrepancy between these studies might derive from different models and target specificity as described above. One possibility is that newly born neurons in the DG might be involved in such behaviors. Moreover, because current available methods ablate new neurons in both the main and accessory olfactory bulb, it is difficult to conclude which is important for these pheromone-associated behaviors. More restricted ablating method will be required to address these questions.

Although the majority of newly born neurons are incorporated into the main olfactory bulb (MOB), a small number of new neurons migrate into the accessory olfactory bulb (AOB) (Oboti et al., 2009, 2011; Sakamoto et al., 2011). Genetic ablation of newly born neurons revealed that continuous neurogenesis is required for the maintenance of neuronal circuits in the AOB, as observed in the MOB (Sakamoto et al., 2011). However, unlike the MOB, adult neurogenesis does not lead to substantial replacement of GCs in the AOB. This result highlighted a unique integration mode of new neurons in the AOB, suggesting that intrinsic cellular and molecular properties of GCs may be different between the AOB and MOB. Further studies are necessary to elucidate cellular and molecular mechanisms underlying distinct features of GCs in the AOB.

OPTICAL IMAGING AND MANIPULATION OF NEW NEURONS

Odor information processing is influenced by the activity of OB interneurons, including pre-existing neurons and newly born neurons. As mentioned above, neurogenesis contributes to various olfaction-related behaviors. However, how new neurons contribute to such behaviors is still unclear. New technologies are required to monitor and manipulate the activity of new neurons during such behaviors. Neuronal imaging technologies can help to tackle this issue. During the past decade, two-photon microscope has become a key tool for monitoring the structure, function, and plasticity of neurons *in vivo*. Calcium imaging is widely used to image the activity of many neurons simultaneously (Grienberger and Konnerth, 2012). In addition, two-photon calcium imaging can monitor the activity of OB GCs in the head-fixed awake state (Kato et al., 2012). However, calcium imaging operates too slowly to track the rapid firing of neurons and is also unable to measure the inhibitory signals. An alternative technique, voltage imaging, has a potential to overcome these problems and may ultimately enable to monitor spatiotemporal activity patterns with millisecond order (Peterka et al., 2011). Various kinds of genetically encoded voltage indicators have been developed (Knopfel, 2012). Recently, Akemann and his colleagues succeeded in voltage imaging at a single cell resolution with two-photon microscope *in vivo* (Akemann et al., 2013). It would be interesting to apply these technologies to examine physiological functions of newly born neurons in the OB. Because most OB newborn neurons are inhibitory interneurons, voltage imaging of M/T cells may help to clarify the contribution of GCs in olfactory circuitry more precisely than calcium imaging.

Optogenetics is also a powerful tool in the field of OB neurogenesis. Over the last decade, a wide variety of different kinds of opsins have been developed and become available, and now optogenetic approach is a standard methodology for investigating the functional properties of neurons at the circuit and behavioral level (Fenno et al., 2011). Recently, it was reported that the activation of newly born neurons by channelrhodopsin can accelerate difficult odor discrimination learning and improved odor-associated memory (Alonso et al., 2012). This strategy may also be useful to examine how newly born neurons contribute to pheromone-associated behaviors. Furthermore, optogenetic tools can control centrifugal input from the olfactory cortex to the OB (Boyd et al., 2012; Markopoulos et al., 2012). It will be interesting to examine how the top-down input affects the survival of new neurons and the effect of odor-associated learning (Yamaguchi et al., 2013). It would be also useful to express optogenetic probes in neurons under activity-dependent control. This approach can allow the reactivation or inactivation of only the subset of neurons that had been activated during a training phase and identify minimal ensemble that are required for behaviors. Light-reactivation of hippocampal neurons that are activated during the training can recall the fear memory of training task (Liu et al., 2012). Because new neurons express immediate-early genes in response to odor stimulation, this approach might be able to identify and manipulate newly born neurons that have been activated by odor stimulation (Magavi et al., 2005).

Although neurogenesis continues throughout life, newly generated neurons dramatically decrease in number with age, and this decline may be involved in memory deficit (Seki and Arai, 1995; Cameron and McKay, 1999; Encinas et al., 2011). In addition, aged mice are impaired at fine olfactory discrimination (Enwere et al., 2004). Furthermore, neurodegenerative diseases are relevant to OB function and adult neurogenesis. For instance, olfactory dysfunction is well known as an early symptom in Parkinson's disease although there is no specific change in the olfactory epithelium (Braak et al., 2003; Haehner et al., 2009). In Parkinson's disease model (α-synuclein overexpressing mice), the ability of odor discrimination is impaired and the survival of adult born neurons is reduced (Neuner et al., 2014). The next key challenge is to increase neurogenesis in aged/neurodegenerative brain and restore brain functions. Light-sensitive promoter system has a strong potential to achieve it (Wang et al., 2012; Imayoshi et al., 2013; Imayoshi and Kageyama, 2014). This system can control gene expression by blue-light illumination with reversibility. By applying this method *in vivo*, it might be possible to promote adult neurogenesis even in aged brains and lead to restore brain functions.

CONCLUSION

Olfaction is indispensable in mammalian life. GCs are the most common GABAergic inhibitory neurons in the OB and modulate the activity of M/T cells to shape odor representations. The OB neural circuits are reorganized by incorporation and elimination of newly generated granule neurons throughout life. Furthermore, blockade of neurogenesis results in various olfaction-related behavior defects. Therefore, continuous neurogenesis is important to acquire plasticity in the olfactory system and thereby adapt neural circuits to environmental changes. However, there are still a lot of problems about adult neurogenesis to be solved. For example, molecular mechanisms integrating new neurons into the OB neural circuits is still unclear. In addition, there are some discrepancies about behavioral analyses. More sophisticated animal model and standardized behavior paradigms should be established. Further studies will contribute to solution of these problems and lead to the development of therapies and drugs for treatment of neurodegenerative diseases.

ACKNOWLEDGMENTS

Some works reviewed here were conducted in collaboration with M. Yamaguchi and K. Mori at the University of Tokyo. This work was supported by research grants from the Ministry of Education, Culture, Sports, Science, and the Technology of Japan and Japan Science and Technology Agency (JST) as well as Research Fellowships of the Japan Society for the Promotion of Science for Young Scientists (Masayuki Sakamoto), Young Investigator Grants of the Human Frontier Science Program (Itaru Imayoshi), and the JST PRESTO program (Itaru Imayoshi).

REFERENCES

Adam, Y., and Mizrahi, A. (2011). Long-term imaging reveals dynamic changes in the neuronal composition of the glomerular layer. *J. Neurosci.* 31, 7967–7973. doi: 10.1523/JNEUROSCI.0782-11.2011

Aimone, J. B., Deng, W., and Gage, F. H. (2011). Resolving new memories: a critical look at the dentate gyrus, adult neurogenesis, and pattern separation. *Neuron* 70, 589–596. doi: 10.1016/j.neuron.2011.05.010

Akemann, W., Sasaki, M., Mutoh, H., Imamura, T., Honkura, N., and Knopfel, T. (2013). Two-photon voltage imaging using a genetically encoded voltage indicator. *Sci. Rep.* 3:2231. doi: 10.1038/srep02231

Alonso, M., Lepousez, G., Sebastien, W., Bardy, C., Gabellec, M. M., Torquet, N., et al. (2012). Activation of adult-born neurons facilitates learning and memory. *Nat. Neurosci.* 15, 897–904. doi: 10.1038/nn.3108

Alonso, M., Viollet, C., Gabellec, M. M., Meas-Yedid, V., Olivo-Marin, J. C., and Lledo, P. M. (2006). Olfactory discrimination learning increases the survival of adult-born neurons in the olfactory bulb. *J. Neurosci.* 26, 10508–10513. doi: 10.1523/JNEUROSCI.2633-06.2006

Altman, J., and Das, G. D. (1965). Autoradiographic and histological evidence of postnatal hippocampal neurogenesis in rats. *J. Comp. Neurol.* 124, 319–335. doi: 10.1002/cne.901240303

Arenkiel, B. R., Hasegawa, H., Yi, J. J., Larsen, R. S., Wallace, M. L., Philpot, B. D., et al. (2011). Activity-induced remodeling of olfactory bulb microcircuits revealed by monosynaptic tracing. *PLoS ONE* 6:e29423. doi: 10.1371/journal.pone.0029423

Bartolini, G., Ciceri, G., and Marin, O. (2013). Integration of GABAergic interneurons into cortical cell assemblies: lessons from embryos and adults. *Neuron* 79, 849–864. doi: 10.1016/j.neuron.2013.08.014

Bath, K. G., Mandairon, N., Jing, D., Rajagopal, R., Kapoor, R., Chen, Z. Y., et al. (2008). Variant brain-derived neurotrophic factor (Val66Met) alters adult olfactory bulb neurogenesis and spontaneous olfactory discrimination. *J. Neurosci.* 28, 2383–2393. doi: 10.1523/JNEUROSCI.4387-07.2008

Batista-Brito, R., Close, J., Machold, R., and Fishell, G. (2008). The distinct temporal origins of olfactory bulb interneuron subtypes. *J. Neurosci.* 28, 3966–3975. doi: 10.1523/JNEUROSCI.5625-07.2008

Bergmann, O., Liebl, J., Bernard, S., Alkass, K., Yeung, M. S., Steier, P., et al. (2012). The age of olfactory bulb neurons in humans. *Neuron* 74, 634–639. doi: 10.1016/j.neuron.2012.03.030

Boyd, A. M., Sturgill, J. F., Poo, C., and Isaacson, J. S. (2012). Cortical feedback control of olfactory bulb circuits. *Neuron* 76, 1161–1174. doi: 10.1016/j.neuron.2012.10.020

Braak, H., Del Tredici, K., Rub, U., De Vos, R. A. I., Steur, E. N. H. J., and Braak, E. (2003). Staging of brain pathology related to sporadic Parkinson's disease. *Neurobiol. Aging* 24, 197–211. doi: 10.1016/S0197-4580(02)00065-9

Breton-Provencher, V., Lemasson, M., Peralta, M. R. 3rd., and Saghatelyan, A. (2009). Interneurons produced in adulthood are required for the normal functioning of the olfactory bulb network and for the execution of selected olfactory behaviors. *J. Neurosci.* 29, 15245–15257. doi: 10.1523/JNEUROSCI.3606-09.2009

Brill, M. S., Ninkovic, J., Winpenny, E., Hodge, R. D., Ozen, I., Yang, R., et al. (2009). Adult generation of glutamatergic olfactory bulb interneurons. *Nat. Neurosci.* 12, 1524–1533. doi: 10.1038/nn.2416

Bruce, H. M. (1959). An exteroceptive block to pregnancy in the mouse. *Nature* 184, 105. doi: 10.1038/184105a0

Cameron, H. A., and McKay, R. D. (1999). Restoring production of hippocampal neurons in old age. *Nat. Neurosci.* 2, 894–897. doi: 10.1038/13197

Clelland, C. D., Choi, M., Romberg, C., Clemenson, G. D. Jr., Fragniere, A., Tyers, P., et al. (2009). A functional role for adult hippocampal neurogenesis in spatial pattern separation. *Science* 325, 210–213. doi: 10.1126/science.1173215

Deng, W., Aimone, J. B., and Gage, F. H. (2010). New neurons and new memories: how does adult hippocampal neurogenesis affect learning and memory? *Nat. Rev. Neurosci.* 11, 339–350. doi: 10.1038/nrn2822

Deshpande, A., Bergami, M., Ghanem, A., Conzelmann, K. K., Lepier, A., Gotz, M., et al. (2013). Retrograde monosynaptic tracing reveals the temporal evolution of inputs onto new neurons in the adult dentate gyrus and olfactory bulb. *Proc. Natl. Acad. Sci. U.S.A.* 110, 1152–1161. doi: 10.1073/pnas.1218991110

Egger, V., and Urban, N. N. (2006). Dynamic connectivity in the mitral cell-granule cell microcircuit. *Semin. Cell Dev. Biol.* 17, 424–432. doi: 10.1016/j.semcdb.2006.04.006

Encinas, J. M., Michurina, T. V., Peunova, N., Park, J. H., Tordo, J., Peterson, D. A., et al. (2011). Division-coupled astrocytic differentiation and age-related depletion of neural stem cells in the adult hippocampus. *Cell Stem Cell* 8, 566–579. doi: 10.1016/j.stem.2011.03.010

Enwere, E., Shingo, T., Gregg, C., Fujikawa, H., Ohta, S., and Weiss, S. (2004). Aging results in reduced epidermal growth factor receptor signaling, diminished olfactory neurogenesis, and deficits in fine olfactory discrimination. *J. Neurosci.* 24, 8354–8365. doi: 10.1523/JNEUROSCI.2751-04.2004

Eriksson, P. S., Perfilieva, E., Bjork-Eriksson, T., Alborn, A. M., Nordborg, C., Peterson, D. A., et al. (1998). Neurogenesis in the adult human hippocampus. *Nat. Med.* 4, 1313–1317. doi: 10.1038/3305

Ernst, A., Alkass, K., Bernard, S., Salehpour, M., Perl, S., Tisdale, J., et al. (2014). Neurogenesis in the striatum of the adult human brain. *Cell* 156, 1072–1083. doi: 10.1016/j.cell.2014.01.044

Eyre, M. D., Antal, M., and Nusser, Z. (2008). Distinct deep short-axon cell subtypes of the main olfactory bulb provide novel intrabulbar and extrabulbar GABAergic connections. *J. Neurosci.* 28, 8217–8229. doi: 10.1523/JNEUROSCI.2490-08.2008

Eyre, M. D., Kerti, K., and Nusser, Z. (2009). Molecular diversity of deep short-axon cells of the rat main olfactory bulb. *Eur. J. Neurosci.* 29, 1397–1407. doi: 10.1111/j.1460-9568.2009.06703.x

Feierstein, C. E., Lazarini, F., Wagner, S., Gabellec, M. M., De Chaumont, F., Olivo-Marin, J. C., et al. (2010). Disruption of adult neurogenesis in the olfactory bulb affects social interaction but not maternal behavior. *Front. Behav. Neurosci.* 4:176. doi: 10.3389/fnbeh.2010.00176

Fenno, L., Yizhar, O., and Deisseroth, K. (2011). The development and application of optogenetics. *Annu. Rev. Neurosci.* 34, 389–412. doi: 10.1146/annurev-neuro-061010-113817

Fuentealba, L. C., Obernier, K., and Alvarez-Buylla, A. (2012). Adult neural stem cells bridge their niche. *Cell Stem Cell* 10, 698–708. doi: 10.1016/j.stem.2012.05.012

Gheusi, G., Cremer, H., McLean, H., Chazal, G., Vincent, J. D., and Lledo, P. M. (2000). Importance of newly generated neurons in the adult olfactory bulb for odor discrimination. *Proc. Natl. Acad. Sci. U.S.A.* 97, 1823–1828. doi: 10.1073/pnas.97.4.1823

Ghosh, S., Larson, S. D., Hefzi, H., Marnoy, Z., Cutforth, T., Dokka, K., et al. (2011). Sensory maps in the olfactory cortex defined by long-range viral tracing of single neurons. *Nature* 472, 217–220. doi: 10.1038/nature09945

Goldman, S. A., and Nottebohm, F. (1983). Neuronal production, migration, and differentiation in a vocal control nucleus of the adult female canary brain. *Proc. Natl. Acad. Sci. U.S.A.* 80, 2390–2394. doi: 10.1073/pnas.80.8.2390

Grienberger, C., and Konnerth, A. (2012). Imaging calcium in neurons. *Neuron* 73, 862–885. doi: 10.1016/j.neuron.2012.02.011

Haehner, A., Hummel, T., and Reichmann, H. (2009). Olfactory dysfunction as a diagnostic marker for Parkinson's disease. *Expert Rev. Neurother.* 9, 1773–1779. doi: 10.1586/ern.09.115

Huang, L., Garcia, I., Jen, H. I., and Arenkiel, B. R. (2013). Reciprocal connectivity between mitral cells and external plexiform layer interneurons in the mouse olfactory bulb. *Front. Neural Circuits* 7:32. doi: 10.3389/fncir.2013.00032

Huang, Z. J., and Zeng, H. (2013). Genetic approaches to neural circuits in the mouse. *Annu. Rev. Neurosci.* 36, 183–215. doi: 10.1146/annurev-neuro-062012-170307

Igarashi, K. M., Ieki, N., An, M., Yamaguchi, Y., Nagayama, S., Kobayakawa, K., et al. (2012). Parallel mitral and tufted cell pathways route distinct odor information to different targets in the olfactory cortex. *J. Neurosci.* 32, 7970–7985. doi: 10.1523/JNEUROSCI.0154-12.2012

Imamura, F., Ayoub, A. E., Rakic, P., and Greer, C. A. (2011). Timing of neurogenesis is a determinant of olfactory circuitry. *Nat. Neurosci.* 14, 331–337. doi: 10.1038/nn.2754

Imamura, F., Nagao, H., Naritsuka, H., Murata, Y., Taniguchi, H., and Mori, K. (2006). A leucine-rich repeat membrane protein, 5T4, is expressed by a subtype of granule cells with dendritic arbors in specific strata of the mouse olfactory bulb. *J. Comp. Neurol.* 495, 754–768. doi: 10.1002/cne.20896

Imayoshi, I., Isomura, A., Harima, Y., Kawaguchi, K., Kori, H., Miyachi, H., et al. (2013). Oscillatory control of factors determining multipotency and fate in mouse neural progenitors. *Science* 342, 1203–1208. doi: 10.1126/science.1242366

Imayoshi, I., and Kageyama, R. (2014). bHLH factors in self-renewal, multipotency, and fate choice of neural progenitor cells. *Neuron* 82, 9–23. doi: 10.1016/j.neuron.2014.03.018

Imayoshi, I., Sakamoto, M., and Kageyama, R. (2011). Genetic methods to identify and manipulate newly born neurons in the adult brain. *Front. Neurosci.* 5:64. doi: 10.3389/fnins.2011.00064

Imayoshi, I., Sakamoto, M., Ohtsuka, T., Takao, K., Miyakawa, T., Yamaguchi, M., et al. (2008). Roles of continuous neurogenesis in the structural and functional integrity of the adult forebrain. *Nat. Neurosci.* 11, 1153–1161. doi: 10.1038/nn.2185

Isaacson, J. S., and Strowbridge, B. W. (1998). Olfactory reciprocal synapses: dendritic signaling in the CNS. *Neuron* 20, 749–761. doi: 10.1016/S0896-6273(00)81013-2

Kaplan, M. S., and Hinds, J. W. (1977). Neurogenesis in the adult rat: electron microscopic analysis of light radioautographs. *Science* 197, 1092–1094. doi: 10.1126/science.887941

Kato, H. K., Chu, M. W., Isaacson, J. S., and Komiyama, T. (2012). Dynamic sensory representations in the olfactory bulb: modulation by wakefulness and experience. *Neuron* 76, 962–975. doi: 10.1016/j.neuron.2012.09.037

Kato, H. K., Gillet, S. N., Peters, A. J., Isaacson, J. S., and Komiyama, T. (2013). Parvalbumin-expressing interneurons linearly control olfactory bulb output. *Neuron* 80, 1218–1231. doi: 10.1016/j.neuron.2013.08.036

Kelsch, W., Lin, C. W., and Lois, C. (2008). Sequential development of synapses in dendritic domains during adult neurogenesis. *Proc. Natl. Acad. Sci. U.S.A.* 105, 16803–16808. doi: 10.1073/pnas.0807970105

Kelsch, W., Sim, S., and Lois, C. (2010). Watching synaptogenesis in the adult brain. *Annu. Rev. Neurosci.* 33, 131–149. doi: 10.1146/annurev-neuro-060909-153252

Kim, W. R., Kim, Y., Eun, B., Park, O. H., Kim, H., Kim, K., et al. (2007). Impaired migration in the rostral migratory stream but spared olfactory function after the elimination of programmed cell death in Bax knock-out mice. *J. Neurosci.* 27, 14392–14403. doi: 10.1523/JNEUROSCI.3903-07.2007

Knopfel, T. (2012). Genetically encoded optical indicators for the analysis of neuronal circuits. *Nat. Rev. Neurosci.* 13, 687–700. doi: 10.1038/nrn3293

Kopel, H., Schechtman, E., Groysman, M., and Mizrahi, A. (2012). Enhanced synaptic integration of adult-born neurons in the olfactory bulb of lactating mothers. *J. Neurosci.* 32, 7519–7527. doi: 10.1523/JNEUROSCI.6354-11.2012

Kosaka, K., Toida, K., Aika, Y., and Kosaka, T. (1998). How simple is the organization of the olfactory glomerulus?: the heterogeneity of so-called periglomerular cells. *Neurosci. Res.* 30, 101–110. doi: 10.1016/S0168-0102(98)00002-9

Kosaka, T., and Kosaka, K. (2011). "Interneurons" in the olfactory bulb revisited. *Neurosci. Res.* 69, 93–99. doi: 10.1016/j.neures.2010.10.002

Kriegstein, A., and Alvarez-Buylla, A. (2009). The glial nature of embryonic and adult neural stem cells. *Annu. Rev. Neurosci.* 32, 149–184. doi: 10.1146/annurev.neuro.051508.135600

Larsen, C. M., and Grattan, D. R. (2010). Prolactin-induced mitogenesis in the subventricular zone of the maternal brain during early pregnancy is essential for normal postpartum behavioral responses in the mother. *Endocrinology* 151, 3805–3814. doi: 10.1210/en.2009-1385

Lazarini, F., Mouthon, M. A., Gheusi, G., De Chaumont, F., Olivo-Marin, J. C., Lamarque, S., et al. (2009). Cellular and behavioral effects of cranial irradiation of the subventricular zone in adult mice. *PLoS ONE* 4:e7017. doi: 10.1371/journal.pone.0007017

Lemasson, M., Saghatelyan, A., Olivo-Marin, J. C., and Lledo, P. M. (2005). Neonatal and adult neurogenesis provide two distinct populations of newborn neurons to the mouse olfactory bulb. *J. Neurosci.* 25, 6816–6825. doi: 10.1523/JNEUROSCI.1114-05.2005

Lepousez, G., and Lledo, P. M. (2013). Odor discrimination requires proper olfactory fast oscillations in awake mice. *Neuron* 80, 1010–1024. doi: 10.1016/j.neuron.2013.07.025

Lepousez, G., Valley, M. T., and Lledo, P. M. (2013). The impact of adult neurogenesis on olfactory bulb circuits and computations. *Annu. Rev. Physiol.* 75, 339–363. doi: 10.1146/annurev-physiol-030212-183731

Liu, X., Ramirez, S., Pang, P. T., Puryear, C. B., Govindarajan, A., Deisseroth, K., et al. (2012). Optogenetic stimulation of a hippocampal engram activates fear memory recall. *Nature* 484, 381–385. doi: 10.1038/nature11028

Livneh, Y., Adam, Y., and Mizrahi, A. (2014). Odor processing by adult-born neurons. *Neuron* 81, 1097–1110. doi: 10.1016/j.neuron.2014.01.007

Livneh, Y., and Mizrahi, A. (2012). Experience-dependent plasticity of mature adult-born neurons. *Nat. Neurosci.* 15, 26–28. doi: 10.1038/nn.2980

Lledo, P. M., Alonso, M., and Grubb, M. S. (2006). Adult neurogenesis and functional plasticity in neuronal circuits. *Nat. Rev. Neurosci.* 7, 179–193. doi: 10.1038/nrn1867

Magavi, S. S., Mitchell, B. D., Szentirmai, O., Carter, B. S., and Macklis, J. D. (2005). Adult-born and preexisting olfactory granule neurons undergo distinct experience-dependent modifications of their olfactory responses *in vivo*. *J. Neurosci.* 25, 10729–10739. doi: 10.1523/JNEUROSCI.2250-05.2005

Mak, G. K., Enwere, E. K., Gregg, C., Pakarainen, T., Poutanen, M., Huhtaniemi, I., et al. (2007). Male pheromone-stimulated neurogenesis in the adult female brain: possible role in mating behavior. *Nat. Neurosci.* 10, 1003–1011. doi: 10.1038/nn1928

Mak, G. K., and Weiss, S. (2010). Paternal recognition of adult offspring mediated by newly generated CNS neurons. *Nat. Neurosci.* 13, 753–758. doi: 10.1038/nn.2550

Manabe, H., Kusumoto-Yoshida, I., Ota, M., and Mori, K. (2011). Olfactory cortex generates synchronized top-down inputs to the olfactory bulb during slow-wave sleep. *J. Neurosci.* 31, 8123–8133. doi: 10.1523/JNEUROSCI.6578-10.2011

Markopoulos, F., Rokni, D., Gire, D. H., and Murthy, V. N. (2012). Functional properties of cortical feedback projections to the olfactory bulb. *Neuron* 76, 1175–1188. doi: 10.1016/j.neuron.2012.10.028

Ming, G. L., and Song, H. (2011). Adult neurogenesis in the mammalian brain: significant answers and significant questions. *Neuron* 70, 687–702. doi: 10.1016/j.neuron.2011.05.001

Miyamichi, K., Amat, F., Moussavi, F., Wang, C., Wickersham, I., Wall, N. R., et al. (2011). Cortical representations of olfactory input by trans-synaptic tracing. *Nature* 472, 191–196. doi: 10.1038/nature09714

Miyamichi, K., Shlomai-Fuchs, Y., Shu, M., Weissbourd, B. C., Luo, L., and Mizrahi, A. (2013). Dissecting local circuits: parvalbumin interneurons underlie broad feedback control of olfactory bulb output. *Neuron* 80, 1232–1245. doi: 10.1016/j.neuron.2013.08.027

Moreno, M. M., Linster, C., Escanilla, O., Sacquet, J., Didier, A., and Mandairon, N. (2009). Olfactory perceptual learning requires adult neurogenesis. *Proc. Natl. Acad. Sci. U.S.A.* 106, 17980–17985. doi: 10.1073/pnas.0907063106

Mori, K., Kishi, K., and Ojima, H. (1983). Distribution of dendrites of mitral, displaced mitral, tufted, and granule cells in the rabbit olfactory bulb. *J. Comp. Neurol.* 219, 339–355. doi: 10.1002/cne.902190308

Mori, K., and Sakano, H. (2011). How is the olfactory map formed and interpreted in the mammalian brain? *Annu. Rev. Neurosci.* 34, 467–499. doi: 10.1146/annurev-neuro-112210-112917

Mouret, A., Lepousez, G., Gras, J., Gabellec, M. M., and Lledo, P. M. (2009). Turnover of newborn olfactory bulb neurons optimizes olfaction. *J. Neurosci.* 29, 12302–12314. doi: 10.1523/JNEUROSCI.3383-09.2009

Nakashiba, T., Cushman, J. D., Pelkey, K. A., Renaudineau, S., Buhl, D. L., McHugh, T. J., et al. (2012). Young dentate granule cells mediate pattern separation, whereas old granule cells facilitate pattern completion. *Cell* 149, 188–201. doi: 10.1016/j.cell.2012.01.046

Neuner, J., Filser, S., Michalakis, S., Biel, M., and Herms, J. (2014). A30P alpha-Synuclein interferes with the stable integration of adult-born neurons into the olfactory network. *Sci. Rep.* 4:3931. doi: 10.1038/srep03931

Ninkovic, J., Mori, T., and Gotz, M. (2007). Distinct modes of neuron addition in adult mouse neurogenesis. *J. Neurosci.* 27, 10906–10911. doi: 10.1523/JNEUROSCI.2572-07.2007

Nissant, A., Bardy, C., Katagiri, H., Murray, K., and Lledo, P. M. (2009). Adult neurogenesis promotes synaptic plasticity in the olfactory bulb. *Nat. Neurosci.* 12, 728–730. doi: 10.1038/nn.2298

Nunez-Parra, A., Maurer, R. K., Krahe, K., Smith, R. S., and Araneda, R. C. (2013). Disruption of centrifugal inhibition to olfactory bulb granule cells impairs olfactory discrimination. *Proc. Natl. Acad. Sci. U.S.A.* 110, 14777–14782. doi: 10.1073/pnas.1310686110

Nunez-Parra, A., Pugh, V., and Araneda, R. C. (2011). Regulation of adult neurogenesis by behavior and age in the accessory olfactory bulb. *Mol. Cell. Neurosci.* 47, 274–285. doi: 10.1016/j.mcn.2011.05.003

Oboti, L., Savalli, G., Giachino, C., De Marchis, S., Panzica, G. C., Fasolo, A., et al. (2009). Integration and sensory experience-dependent survival of newly-generated neurons in the accessory olfactory bulb of female mice. *Eur. J. Neurosci.* 29, 679–692. doi: 10.1111/j.1460-9568.2009.06614.x

Oboti, L., Schellino, R., Giachino, C., Chamero, P., Pyrski, M., Leinders-Zufall, T., et al. (2011). Newborn interneurons in the accessory olfactory bulb promote mate recognition in female mice. *Front. Neurosci.* 5:113. doi: 10.3389/fnins.2011.00113

Orona, E., Scott, J. W., and Rainer, E. C. (1983). Different granule cell populations innervate superficial and deep regions of the external plexiform layer in rat olfactory bulb. *J. Comp. Neurol.* 217, 227–237. doi: 10.1002/cne.902170209

Peterka, D. S., Takahashi, H., and Yuste, R. (2011). Imaging voltage in neurons. *Neuron* 69, 9–21. doi: 10.1016/j.neuron.2010.12.010

Petreanu, L., and Alvarez-Buylla, A. (2002). Maturation and death of adult-born olfactory bulb granule neurons: role of olfaction. *J. Neurosci.* 22, 6106–6113.

Pressler, R. T., and Strowbridge, B. W. (2006). Blanes cells mediate persistent feed-forward inhibition onto granule cells in the olfactory bulb. *Neuron* 49, 889–904. doi: 10.1016/j.neuron.2006.02.019

Ramon y Cajal, S. (1928). *Degeneration and Regeneration of the Nervous System.* London: Oxford University Press.

Reynolds, B. A., and Weiss, S. (1992). Generation of neurons and astrocytes from isolated cells of the adult mammalian central nervous system. *Science* 255, 1707–1710. doi: 10.1126/science.1553558

Rochefort, C., Gheusi, G., Vincent, J. D., and Lledo, P. M. (2002). Enriched odor exposure increases the number of newborn neurons in the adult olfactory bulb and improves odor memory. *J. Neurosci.* 22, 2679–2689.

Sahay, A., Scobie, K. N., Hill, A. S., O'Carroll, C. M., Kheirbek, M. A., Burghardt, N. S., et al. (2011a). Increasing adult hippocampal neurogenesis is sufficient to improve pattern separation. *Nature* 472, 466–470. doi: 10.1038/nature09817

Sahay, A., Wilson, D. A., and Hen, R. (2011b). Pattern separation: a common function for new neurons in hippocampus and olfactory bulb. *Neuron* 70, 582–588. doi: 10.1016/j.neuron.2011.05.012

Sakamoto, M., Ieki, N., Miyoshi, G., Mochimaru, D., Miyachi, H., Imura, T., et al. (2014). Continuous postnatal neurogenesis contributes to formation of the olfactory bulb neural circuits and flexible olfactory associative learning. *J. Neurosci.* 34, 5788–5799. doi: 10.1523/JNEUROSCI.0674-14.2014

Sakamoto, M., Imayoshi, I., Ohtsuka, T., Yamaguchi, M., Mori, K., and Kageyama, R. (2011). Continuous neurogenesis in the adult forebrain is required for innate olfactory responses. *Proc. Natl. Acad. Sci. U.S.A.* 108, 8479–8484. doi: 10.1073/pnas.1018782108

Sanai, N., Nguyen, T., Ihrie, R. A., Mirzadeh, Z., Tsai, H. H., Wong, M., et al. (2011). Corridors of migrating neurons in the human brain and their decline during infancy. *Nature* 478, 382–386. doi: 10.1038/nature10487

Sawada, M., Kaneko, N., Inada, H., Wake, H., Kato, Y., Yanagawa, Y., et al. (2011). Sensory input regulates spatial and subtype-specific patterns of neuronal turnover in the adult olfactory bulb. *J. Neurosci.* 31, 11587–11596. doi: 10.1523/JNEUROSCI.0614-11.2011

Schellinck, H. M., Arnold, A., and Rafuse, V. F. (2004). Neural cell adhesion molecule (NCAM) null mice do not show a deficit in odour discrimination learning. *Behav. Brain Res.* 152, 327–334. doi: 10.1016/j.bbr.2003.10.011

Seki, T., and Arai, Y. (1995). Age-related production of new granule cells in the adult dentate gyrus. *Neuroreport* 6, 2479–2482. doi: 10.1097/00001756-199512150-00010

Shepherd, G., and Greer, C. (2004). *Olfactory Bulb in the Synaptic Organization of the Brain*. New York, NY: Oxford University Press. doi: 10.1093/acprof:oso/9780195159561.001.1

Shingo, T., Gregg, C., Enwere, E., Fujikawa, H., Hassam, R., Geary, C., et al. (2003). Pregnancy-stimulated neurogenesis in the adult female forebrain mediated by prolactin. *Science* 299, 117–120. doi: 10.1126/science.1076647

Soria-Gomez, E., Bellocchio, L., Reguero, L., Lepousez, G., Martin, C., Bendahmane, M., et al. (2014). The endocannabinoid system controls food intake via olfactory processes. *Nat. Neurosci.* 17, 407–415. doi: 10.1038/nn.3647

Sosulski, D. L., Bloom, M. L., Cutforth, T., Axel, R., and Datta, S. R. (2011). Distinct representations of olfactory information in different cortical centres. *Nature* 472, 213–216. doi: 10.1038/nature09868

Spalding, K. L., Bergmann, O., Alkass, K., Bernard, S., Salehpour, M., Huttner, H. B., et al. (2013). Dynamics of hippocampal neurogenesis in adult humans. *Cell* 153, 1219–1227. doi: 10.1016/j.cell.2013.05.002

Suh, H., Deng, W., and Gage, F. H. (2009). Signaling in adult neurogenesis. *Annu. Rev. Cell Dev. Biol.* 25, 253–275. doi: 10.1146/annurev.cellbio.042308.113256

Sultan, S., Mandairon, N., Kermen, F., Garcia, S., Sacquet, J., and Didier, A. (2010). Learning-dependent neurogenesis in the olfactory bulb determines long-term olfactory memory. *FASEB J.* 24, 2355–2363. doi: 10.1096/fj.09-151456

Sultan, S., Rey, N., Sacquet, J., Mandairon, N., and Didier, A. (2011). Newborn neurons in the olfactory bulb selected for long-term survival through olfactory learning are prematurely suppressed when the olfactory memory is erased. *J. Neurosci.* 31, 14893–14898. doi: 10.1523/JNEUROSCI.3677-11.2011

Wang, X., Chen, X., and Yang, Y. (2012). Spatiotemporal control of gene expression by a light-switchable transgene system. *Nat. Methods* 9, 266–269. doi: 10.1038/nmeth.1892

Yamaguchi, M., Manabe, H., Murata, K., and Mori, K. (2013). Reorganization of neuronal circuits of the central olfactory system during postprandial sleep. *Front. Neural Circuits* 7:132. doi: 10.3389/fncir.2013.00132

Yamaguchi, M., and Mori, K. (2005). Critical period for sensory experience-dependent survival of newly generated granule cells in the adult mouse olfactory bulb. *Proc. Natl. Acad. Sci. U.S.A.* 102, 9697–9702. doi: 10.1073/pnas.0406082102

Yokoi, M., Mori, K., and Nakanishi, S. (1995). Refinement of odor molecule tuning by dendrodendritic synaptic inhibition in the olfactory bulb. *Proc. Natl. Acad. Sci. U.S.A.* 92, 3371–3375. doi: 10.1073/pnas.92.8.3371

Yokoyama, T. K., Mochimaru, D., Murata, K., Manabe, H., Kobayakawa, K., Kobayakawa, R., et al. (2011). Elimination of adult-born neurons in the olfactory bulb is promoted during the postprandial period. *Neuron* 71, 883–897. doi: 10.1016/j.neuron.2011.05.046

4

Glial cells, but not neurons, exhibit a controllable response to a localized inflammatory microenvironment *in vitro*

Salah Sommakia[1,2], Jenna L. Rickus[1,2,3] and Kevin J. Otto[1,4,5] *

[1] Weldon School of Biomedical Engineering, Purdue University, West Lafayette, IN, USA
[2] Physiological Sensing Facility at the Bindley Bioscience Center and Birck Nanotechnology Center, Purdue University, West Lafayette, IN, USA
[3] Department of Agricultural and Biological Engineering, Purdue University, West Lafayette, IN, USA
[4] Department of Biological Sciences, Purdue University, West Lafayette, IN, USA
[5] J. Crayton Pruitt Family Department of Biomedical Engineering, University of Florida, Gainesville, FL, USA

Edited by:
Ulrich G. Hofmann, Albert-Ludwigs-University Freiburg, Germany

Reviewed by:
Hugues Berry, INRIA, France
Ian D. Dryg, University of Washington, USA

***Correspondence:**
Kevin J. Otto, J. Crayton Pruitt Family Department of Biomedical Engineering, University of Florida, 1064 Center Drive, NEB 363, Gainesville, FL 32611, USA
e-mail: kevin.otto@bme.ufl.edu

The ability to design long-lasting intracortical implants hinges on understanding the factors leading to the loss of neuronal density and the formation of the glial scar. In this study, we modify a common *in vitro* mixed cortical culture model using lipopolysaccharide (LPS) to examine the responses of microglia, astrocytes, and neurons to microwire segments. We also use dip-coated polyethylene glycol (PEG), which we have previously shown can modulate impedance changes to neural microelectrodes, to control the cellular responses. We find that microglia, as expected, exhibit an elevated response to LPS-coated microwire for distances of up to 150 μm, and that this elevated response can be mitigated by co-depositing PEG with LPS. Astrocytes exhibit a more complex, distance-dependent response, whereas neurons do not appear to be affected by the type or magnitude of glial response within this *in vitro* model. The discrepancy between our *in vitro* responses and typically observed *in vivo* responses suggest the importance of using a systems approach to understand the responses of the various brain cell types in a chronic *in vivo* setting, as well as the necessity of studying the roles of cell types not native to the brain. Our results further indicate that the loss of neuronal density observed *in vivo* is not a necessary consequence of elevated glial activation.

Keywords: intracortical microelectrodes, foreign body response, primary cortical cultures

INTRODUCTION

Implantable intracortical microelectrodes hold great potential as neural prostheses for the treatment of a wide range of traumatic and degenerative injuries to the central nervous system, but suffer from unreliability in chronic settings. This decline in chronic device performance correlates with a reactive response of brain tissue (Vetter et al., 2004). Designing therapeutic approaches to counter this decline in device performance is complicated by the lack of detailed mechanistic understanding of the progression of the reactive tissue. Dural and vascular damage appear to be major factors contributing to the reactive tissue response (Karumbaiah et al., 2013; Saxena et al., 2013). Using novel device capture techniques (Woolley et al., 2011, 2013a,b), this reactive tissue response has been shown to be non-uniform and depth dependent, with stronger scarring closer to the surface of the brain (Woolley et al., 2013c). Transdural implants elicit a much greater response than implants dwelling completely within the brain (Markwardt et al., 2013). These findings collectively suggest that the introduction of non-native cellular and molecular components into the brain amplifies inflammatory pathway activation, and that this activation is strongest at the site of injury to respective structures. Recently, potential therapeutic targets such as reactive oxygen species and toll-like receptor 4 (TL4) have been identified (Potter et al., 2013; Ravikumar et al., 2014), but the complexity underlying *in vivo* conditions can obscure investigations of biological mechanisms.

These obstacles can be somewhat overcome by studying simpler models, such as *in vitro* cell cultures. The most widely used model, first described by Polikov et al. (2006, 2009), presents microscale foreign bodies to primary mixed neural cultures., and has been applied to test biocompatibility of various materials as neural interfaces (Achyuta et al., 2010; Tien et al., 2013). This model requires the modification of the culture media to achieve a globally elevated activation state. We posit that a more localized inflammatory microenvironment may better represent the non-uniform reactive tissue response, and propose a modification to the model whereby the foreign objects are dip-coated in lipopolysaccharide (LPS) to simulate a localized inflammatory microenvironment. LPS is a known upregulator of microglial activation through TL4 binding (Lehnardt et al., 2003; Tzeng et al., 2005), and as such is an attractive option for modifying the Polikov model to test cellular responses to localized targeting of TL4 receptors. In contrast to the previous model, the creation of a localized inflammatory microenvironment also enables the analysis of neuronal responses.

Previous research in the neurotrauma field has also found that, due its surfactant properties, soluble polyethylene glycol (PEG) can induce membrane sealing of damaged cells and reduce edema

(Borgens et al., 2002). This effect significantly improves recovery from both spinal cord and traumatic brain injuries by inducing cellular and behavioral recovery (Koob et al., 2005, 2008; Koob and Borgens, 2006). Additionally, we have recently showed that a dip-coated PEG film can modulate impedance changes caused by non-cellular components both *in vitro* and *in vivo* (Sommakia et al., 2014). In this regard, a non-grafted dip-coated PEG film is a technically and economically attractive option to achieve both antifouling and membrane sealing. Our hypothesis is that a dip-coated layer of high molecular weight PEG will exhibit sufficient short term stability to modulate cellular responses to microelectrodes *in vitro*. Given the importance of the early stages of the injury response in shaping the later chronic stages, this approach might prove highly beneficial *in vivo*.

In this work we test our PEG hypothesis using the local inflammation-modified Polikov model. We show that, as expected, coating segments of microwire with LPS results in an increase in microglial activation at distances up to 150 μm, and, importantly, co-depositing LPS with a PEG solution prevents observed increases in microglial activation. We also observe a slight increase in astrocyte activation in response to LPS-coated microwire, but not at the same magnitude or spatial distribution as microglia. Interestingly, neuronal responses in this *in vitro* paradigm do not appear to be influenced by corresponding glial responses.

MATERIALS AND METHODS

CELL CULTURE AND MICROWIRE PLACEMENT

The experimental procedures complied with the Guide for the Care and Use of Laboratory Animals and were approved by The Purdue Animal Care and Use Committee (PACUC). Forebrains from E17 embryonic rat pups were received suspended in 5 ml of Solution 1 (NaCl 7.24 g/L; KCl 0.4 g/L; NaH2PO4 0.14 g/L; Glucose 2.61 g/L; HEPES 5.96 g/L; MgSO4 0.295 g/L; Bovine Serum Albumin 3 g/L) in a 50 ml centrifuge tube. Under sterile conditions, the tissue was gently triturated with an added 18 μl of trypsin solution (Sigma-Aldrich, St. Louis, MO) (7.5 mg/ml in 0.9% saline) and incubated for 20 min in a 37°C water bath. Following the incubation step, 100 μl of trypsin inhibitor/DNAase solution (Sigma-Aldrich, St. Louis, MO) (2.5 mg/ml trypsin inhibitor, 400 μg/ml DNAase in 0.9% saline) was added and tissue was again gently triturated. The tissue was then centrifuged at 1,000 rpm for 5 min at room temperature and supernatant was poured off. Cells were re-suspended in 16 ml of Hibernate-E (Brainbits, Springfield, IL) and triturated once again. Cells were filtered through a 70 μm cell strainer (Fisher Scientific) and centrifuged at 1,400 rpm for 5 min at room temperature. Supernatant was poured off and cells were re-suspended in a culture medium consisting of Dulbecco's modified Eagle's Medium (DMEM) with 10% Fetal Bovine Serum (FBS) and 10% horse serum (HS). The cells were then seeded in 96 well plates at a density of 500,000 cells/cm^2, and cultured for 7 days at 37°C and 5% CO_2, with the cell media being replaced every 48 h. At day 7 *in vitro*, lengths of 50 μm-diameter tungsten microwire (California Fine Wire Co., Grover Beach, CA) were autoclaved then cut into small segments of 5–7 mm in length using carbide scissors. The microwire segments were treated by dip coating with one of four treatments: LPS (50 ng/ml) only, PEG (20% aqueous solution, 4000 MW) only, a 1:1 mixture of LPS and PEG, or uncoated. A relatively low LPS concentration was chosen based on reported literature values (Das et al., 1995; Wang et al., 2005) in order to achieve localized activation of microglia, but prevent a generalized activation that might result from a higher concentration of LPS diffusing rapidly throughout the well. PEG concentration is based on our previous work demonstrating a proof of concept for using PEG to modulate impedance changes to neural microelectrodes (Sommakia et al., 2014). In each well, one segment of microwire was dropped into the medium and allowed to sink to the bottom of the well. The plates were then placed in the incubator for an additional 7 days.

CELL FIXING AND LABELING

At day 14 *in vitro*, the cultures were fixed with 4% paraformaldehyde for 10 min, rinsed 3× with HEPES Buffered Hank's saline (HBHS) (in g/L; 7.5 g NaCl, 0.3 g KCl, 0.06 g KH2PO4, 0.13 g Na2HPO4, 2 g Glucose, 2.4 g HEPES, 0.05 g MgCl2:6H2O, 0.05 g MgSO4:7H2O, 0.165 g CaCl2, 90 mg NaN3, at pH 7.4), then permeabilized with 0.2% Triton-X (Sigma-Aldrich, St. Louis, MO). The cultures were then blocked with 10% normal goat serum (Jackson Immunoresearch, West Grove, PA) for 1 h, after which primary antibodies to beta-3-tubulin (β-3-tub) (Covance, Princeton, NJ), which labels neurons; Glial Fibrillary Acidic Protein (GFAP) (Millipore, Billerica, MA), which labels astrocytes; and Ionized Calcium binding adaptor molecule 1 (Iba1) (Wako, Osaka, Japan), which labels microglia, were added, and the cultures incubated in a 4°C refrigerator overnight. The wells were then aspirated, rinsed in HBHS 3×, and the following secondary antibodies were added: Alexa Fluor 488 Goat anti-mouse, Alexa Fluor 555 Goat anti-chicken, and Alexa Fluor 635 Goat anti-rabbit (Invitrogen, Carlsbad, CA). After a 2 h incubation at room temperature, the secondary antibodies were rinsed 3× with HBHS, and a final volume of 100 μl of HBHS was left in the wells for imaging. Special care was taken to ensure the microwire segments remained attached to the bottom of the wells.

IMAGE ACQUISITION AND ANALYSIS

Fluorescent images (512 × 512 pixels) were obtained on a confocal microscope fitted with a long working distance 10× air objective using Fluoview software (Olympus, Center Valley, PA). The different channels were imaged sequentially, and noise reduction was achieved by applying a Kalman filter built into the acquisition software to 3 scans for each channel. Each plate was imaged using the same set of imaging parameters (laser power, aperture, acquisition time) to ensure uniformity. Source images were imported into ImageJ (ImageJ, U. S. National Institutes of Health, Bethesda, MD), visually inspected and rotated to place the microwire in a vertical orientation. When possible, two adjacent rectangular selections, 480 pixels high by 240 pixels wide (equivalent to 994 μm by 496 μm), were made with the long edge running on the center of the wire. If that was not possible due to excessive proximity to wall of the well, only a single rectangular selection was made facing the interior of the well. Each of these selections was considered a single sample for analysis purposes. From these selections, intensity profiles of average brightness of each vertical line were generated, as shown in **Figure 1C**. Microwire segments were also imaged in three empty wells, and an average intensity profile was obtained and subtracted from the intensity profile generated from cell-containing wells. One response index (RI) per cell type was obtained for each region by summing the area underneath the intensity profile line between the distance points corresponding to the region boundaries and dividing by 10000. Statistical analysis was performed using the SAS 9.3 statistical package (SAS Institute Inc., Cary, NC). A general linear model (GLM) procedure was used perform to a one way ANOVA with block, to remove the effects of variations between the plates by treating the plates as a statistical block. *Post hoc* Tukey tests were used to determine statistical significance between the treatment groups at a significance level of $\alpha = 0.05$. The error bars plotted

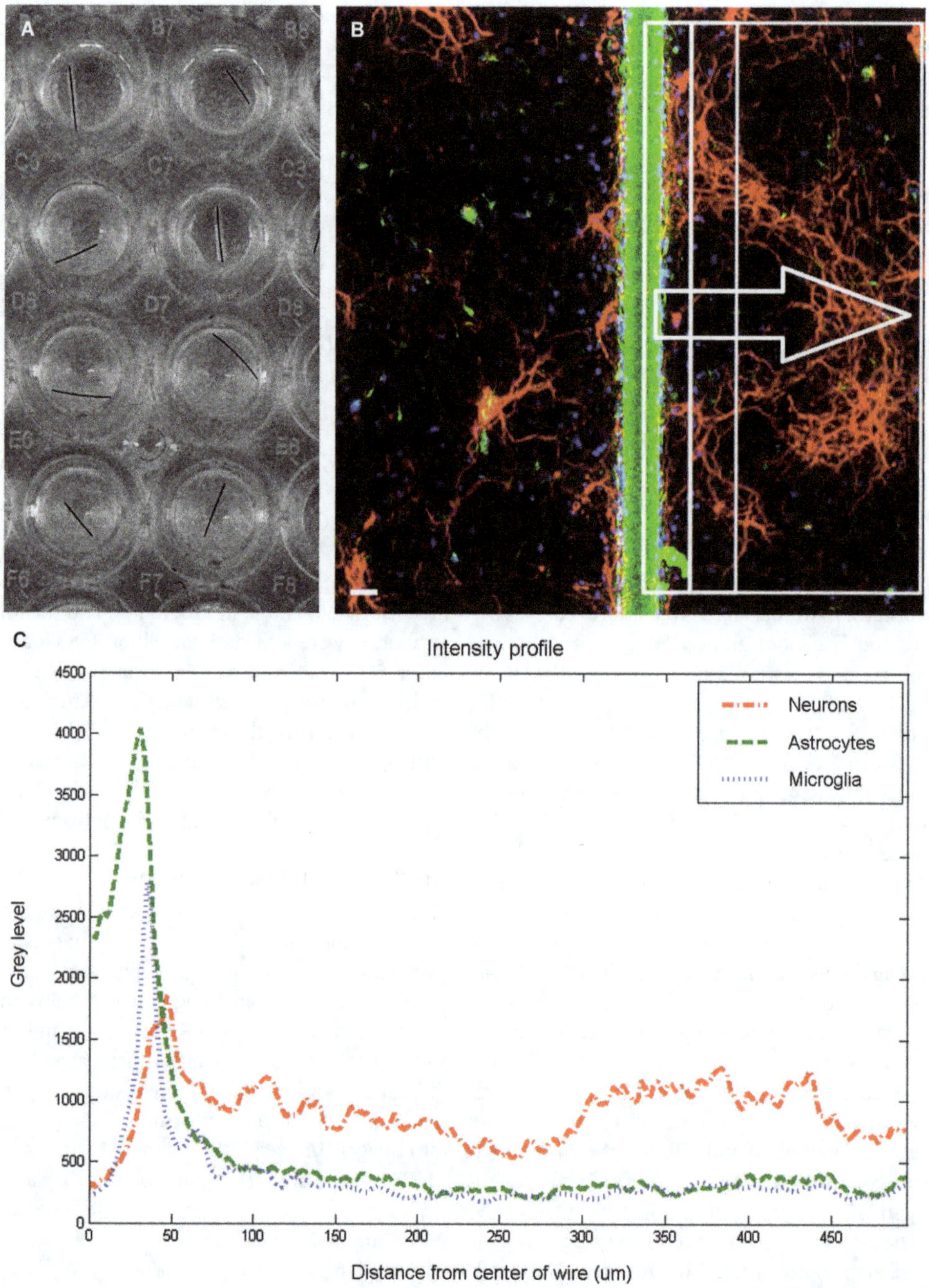

FIGURE 1 | Image quantification. Wells in 96 well plate **(A)** were imaged to produce a fluorescent image **(B)** and extract intensity profiles for each channel. The fluorescent image is pseudocolored to show neurons in red, astrocytes in green, and microglia in blue. Scale bar is 50 μm. For each examined region (examples shown within rectangles), three intensity profiles **(C)** are generated, and response indices calculated by summing the area under the graph corresponding to the chosen distances and dividing by 10000.

represent the standard error of the means. *P*-values less than 0.05 are denoted in the figures by a single asterisk, while *p*-values less than 0.001 are denoted by double asterisks. Plots were generated using MATLAB (The MathWorks Inc., Natick, MA).

RESULTS

Figure 1 shows an overview of the methodology employed to analyze the cellular responses to microwire segments. Microwire segments placed in the wells (**Figure 1A**) were imaged, resulting in sets of images such as the one shown in **Figure 1B**. Intensity profiles (**Figure 1C**) of areas of various widths were analyzed to obtain the results described below.

MICROGLIA

Figure 2 shows the different levels of aggregate microglial response in interface areas of different sizes. In the interface area containing only the microwire (i.e., 25 μm), the only significant difference in the microglial RI was between the PEG coated microwire and LPS coated microwire (RI = 1.37 vs. 2.2, $p = 0.007$). For the interface area containing the wire and extending over an adjacent 25 μm, significant pairwise differences were observed between the LPS coated wire (RI = 5.84) and the other wires (uncoated RI = 4.92, $p = 0.041$; PEG RI = 4.26, $p < 0.0001$; LPS + PEG RI = 4.82, $p = 0.022$). For a wider interface area containing the microwire and extending over the adjacent 50 μm, these pairwise differences get stronger between the LPS coated wire (RI = 8.27) and the other wires (uncoated RI = 6.58, $p = 0.0007$; PEG RI = 5.8, $p < 0.0001$; LPS + PEG RI = 6.4, $p = 0.0002$). Notably, the relative pattern of the microglia response indices for the different conditions is the same for all three regions. Only the overall magnitude of the responses increase as the anti-Iba1 fluorescence is summed over larger areas. This indicates that all three size regions up to the wire plus 50 microns are representative of interface. In all three cases LPS induced microglia activation rises to a level statistical significance. As more distance is included in the interface measurement, the ability of the PEG to relieve microglia activation by LPS rises to statistical significance.

Figure 3 shows the microglial responses at more distant regions. For the closest distant bin extending from 50 to 150 μm from edge of wire, the RI for LPS coated wire (RI = 5.62) was significantly higher than all the other treatments (uncoated RI = 4.21, $p = 0.0001$; PEG RI = 3.71, $p < 0.0001$; LPS + PEG RI = 3.91, $p < 0.0001$). For the next three distant 100 μm wide bins, the only significant difference observed was between LPS coated wire and PEG coated wire in all 3 bins. These calculated RI are as follows: for the bin extending from 150 to 250 μm from edge of wire: LPS RI = 4.5 vs. PEG 3.12, $p = 0.0001$; for the bin extending 250–350 μm from edge of wire: RI = 5.12 vs. 3.8, $p = 0.0003$; for the bin extending 350–450 μm from edge of wire): RI = 4.98 vs. 3.9, $p = 0.01$. Again the pattern of relative RI's is consistent at all distances in the distant regions and matches that of the interface region. In this case the size of each measurement area is the same across cases and is always 100 microns. Again LPS induces an increased RI in all regions reaching statistical significance when comparing LPS to the PEG coated wire and in the most near distant region (50–150 microns) when comparing LPS to an uncoated wire. The wire likely induces some basal level of microglial attachment or activation, which is reduced by PEG alone, therefore the effect of LPS is most pronounced when we compare the PEG wire. These results are consistent with a diffusion based model whereby the effect of LPS will decrease with increasing distance from the wire.

ASTROCYTES

Figure 4 shows the astrocyte RI at interface areas. For the interface area containing only the microwire, the astrocyte RI for LPS

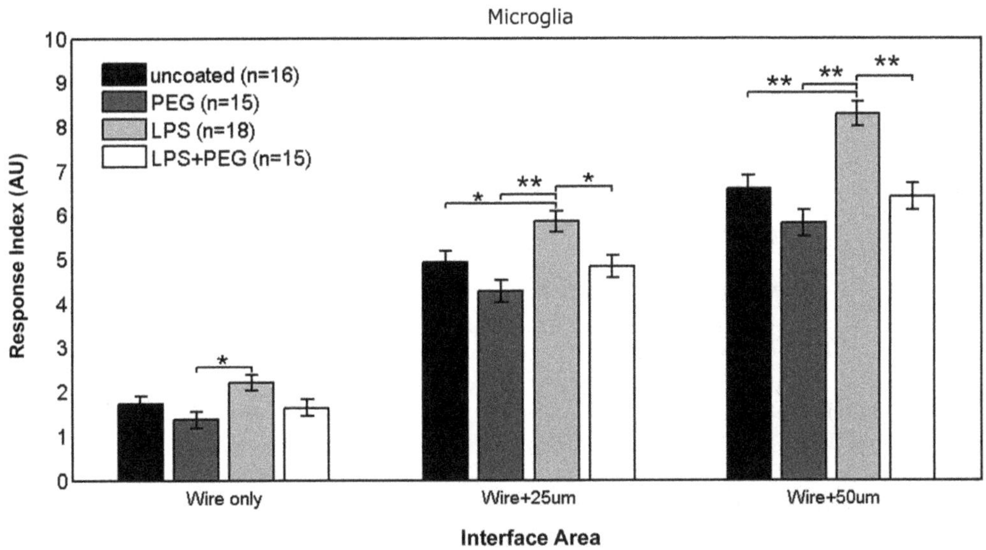

FIGURE 2 | LPS-coated microwire elicits higher microglial response in interface areas, and co-deposition of PEG with LPS reduces microglial response to control levels.

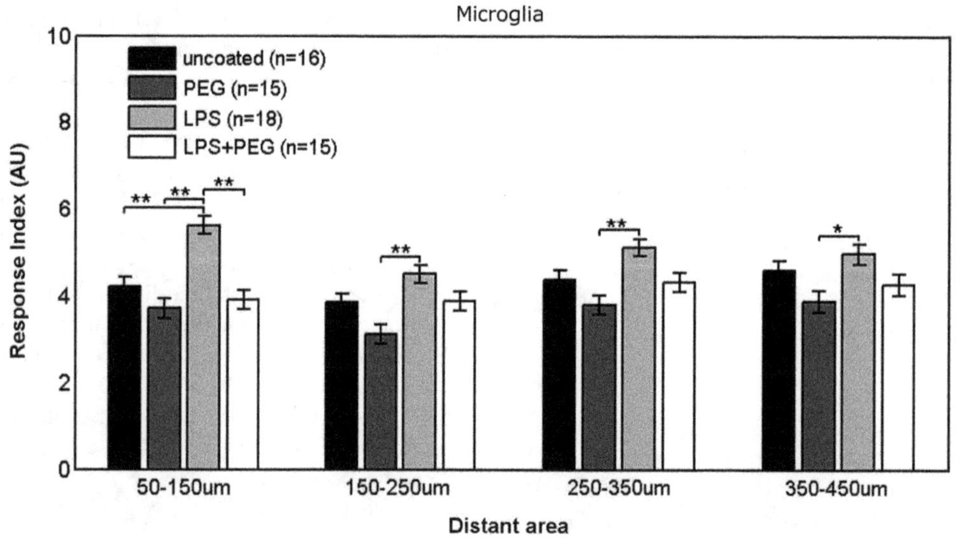

FIGURE 3 | Microglial response to LPS-coated microwire compared to all other treatments is elevated at distances up to 150 μm, after which a tiered response is observed.

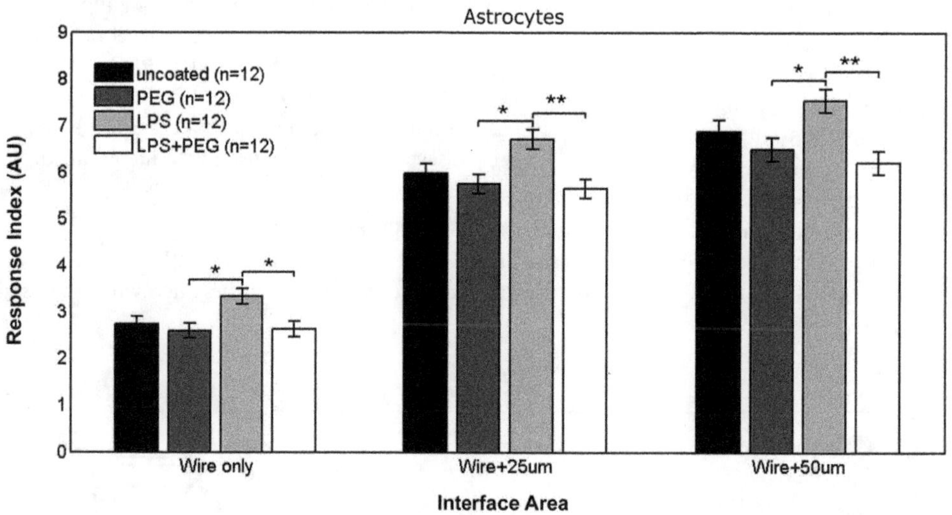

FIGURE 4 | Astrocytes in interface areas of varying width exhibit a tiered response to microwires coated with PEG, with or without LPS.

coated wire (RI = 3.33) was significantly higher than PEG coated and LPS + PEG coated wire (PEG RI = 2.59, $p = 0.015$; LPS + PEG RI = 2.63, $p = 0.02$). For the interface area containing the wire and extending an adjacent 25 μm, the same pairwise difference were observed, but with a stronger difference between the LPS coated wire (RI = 6.7) and the LPS + PEG coated wire (PEG RI = 5.75, $p = 0.012$; LPS + PEG RI = 5.64, $p = 0.0045$). For the interface area containing the microwire and extending an adjacent 50 μm, the same observation of the LPS astrocyte RI being higher than both PEG and LPS + PEG was noticed (LPS RI = 7.54, PEG RI = 6.49, $p = 0.02$; LPS + PEG RI = 6.19, $p = 0.002$). Overall the astrocytes show a similar pattern in the interface as the microglia, but to a lesser extent. Importantly, for all three interface sizes (at the wire, within 25 μm of the wire, and within 50 μm of the wire), the PEG coating is able to significantly reduce the LPS-induced astrocyte response.

Figure 5 shows the astrocyte RI at distant areas. No significant differences were observed between the different treatments for the closest distant bin extending from 50 to 150 μm from edge of microwire. For the middle two distant bins, a slightly significant difference was observed between LPS coated wire and LPS + PEG coated wire [bin 2 (150–250 μm from edge of wire): LPS RI = 2.31, LPS + PEG RI = 1.37, $p = 0.012$; bin 3 (250–350 μm from edge of wire): LPS RI = 2.73, LPS + PEG RI = 1.73, $p = 0.03$].

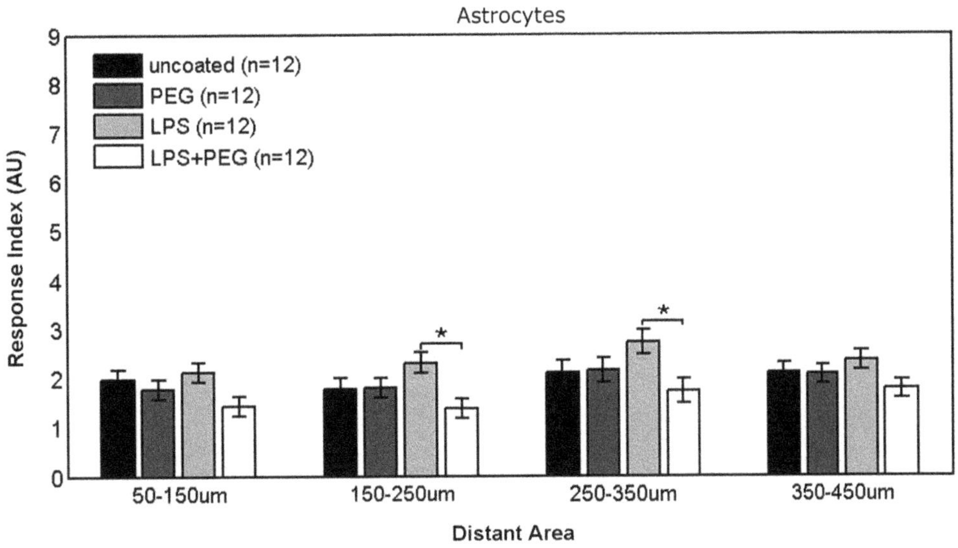

FIGURE 5 | Differences in astrocyte responses in distant areas appear between LPS and LPS + PEG coated microwires at the middle of the distance range analyzed.

NEURONS

Figures 6, 7 show the neuron RI in interface and distant regions respectively. No significant differences in the neuron response were found between any of the treatment conditions in either interface or distant region. In contrast to microglia and astrocytes, where the RI was higher in distant areas in comparison to the widest interface area examined, the neuron RI in distant areas was roughly equal to that in the widest interface area examined.

DISCUSSION

VALIDITY OF MODEL SYSTEM

To test the effects of a dip coated PEG film on the cellular responses to implanted electrodes, we modified a robust and frequently replicated *in vitro* mixed cortical culture model pioneered by Polikov et al. (2006, 2009, 2010; Achyuta et al., 2010; Tien et al., 2013). The anatomical and physiological complexity *in vivo* obscures mechanistic investigations into the reactive tissue response to implanted microelectrodes. Using an *in vitro* model allows us to simplify the biological system under study, and isolate particular components of interest. The challenge with *in vitro* models is to simulate physiological conditions in the absence of particular anatomical structures. In this particular model of primary cortical cell cultures, the cells exist in isolation from supporting vasculature, structural extra-cellular matrix components, and meninges. These aforementioned structures are heavily damaged during microelectrode insertion, which has been shown to strongly affect the chronic response of the brain to implanted microelectrodes (Karumbaiah et al., 2013; Markwardt et al., 2013; Saxena et al., 2013). The original model (Polikov et al., 2006) did not elicit a consistent glial scar, and it was necessary to alter the composition of the culture media to place all glial cells in the culture in an elevated reactive state, thereby ensuring a consistent glial scar (Polikov et al., 2009). By coating LPS directly onto microwire, we are able to create a localized inflammatory microenvironment that more closely mimics the reality of an indwelling cortical implant, rather than placing the glial cells in the culture in a globally activated state. This localized inflammatory microenvironment enables us to examine distance related effects on the cultured cells. For the LPS + PEG condition, concerns about cross contamination and the potential to disrupt the dip-coated PEG film led to the decision to co-deposit PEG and LPS via dip-coating from a single pot. While polymeric films containing PEG have the potential for prolonged drug release, they are typically crosslinked to form hydrogels (Peppas, 1997; Lin and Anseth, 2009) or composites (Ramakrishna et al., 2001). Dip-coated films of a pure hydrophilic polymer, such as PEG, are rarely used for prolonged drug release due to their burst release characteristics and potential for dissolution over timescales shorter than is therapeutically beneficial (Acharya and Park, 2006). PEG, in various conformations, has been shown to accelerate the release of small hydrophobic molecules similar to LPS (Ooya et al., 2003; Kang et al., 2007). For these aforementioned reasons, we were confident that our codeposition of PEG and LPS would not hinder the exposure of the cells to LPS.

To examine microglial response, we chose to quantify Iba1 fluorescence across relatively wide bins. The choice of Iba1 was due to its high specificity to the microglia/macrophage cell type. The function and level of Iba1 expression is directly related to the classic morphological changes associated with microglial activation (Ito et al., 1998). Iba1 crosslinks actin and is involved in the formation of membrane ruffles and rapid motility (Sasaki et al., 2001). Additionally, Iba1 levels correlate directly with morphological feature changes associated with microglial activation (Kozlowski and Weimer, 2012). While current morphological analysis methods have been found lacking (Beynon and Walker,

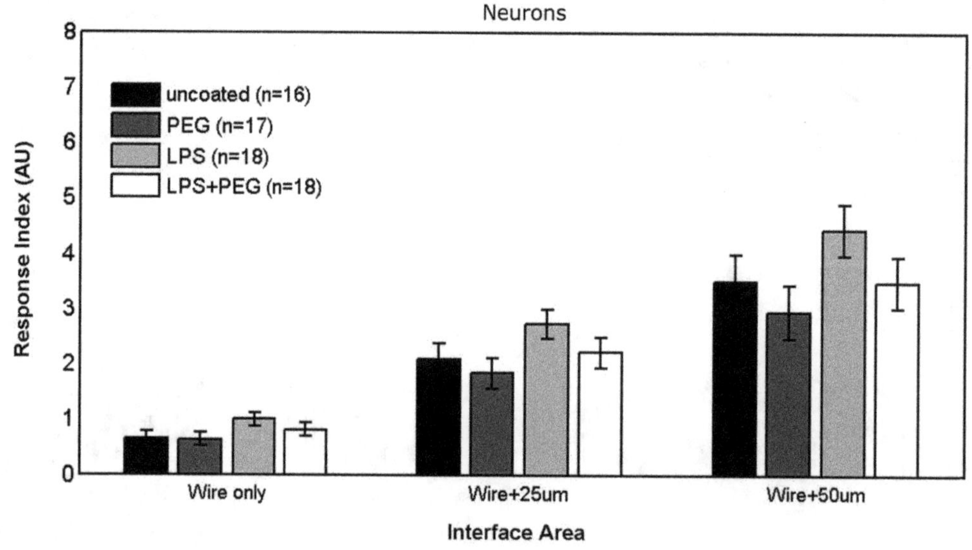

FIGURE 6 | No differences are observed in neuronal responses in interface areas of various widths.

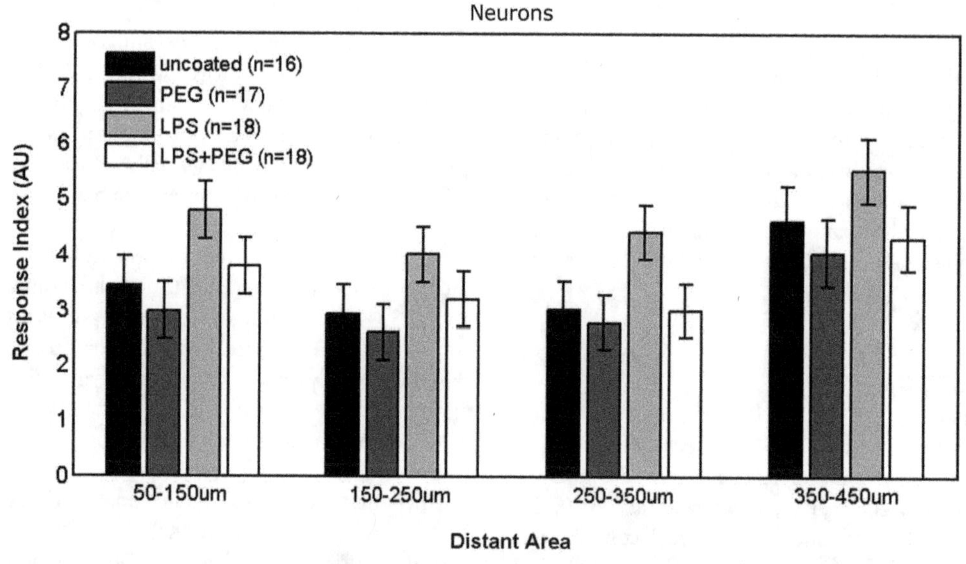

FIGURE 7 | No differences are observed in neuronal responses in distant areas.

2012), the method of quantification we employ is not without its shortcomings. Given our bin sizing, an increase in fluorescence in a bin could be attributed to either an increase in microglial cell numbers, or a higher level of Iba1 expression, or both. However, proliferation, migration, and morphological changes are all important components of microglial activation. Quantification of Iba1 fluorescence in a given area can therefore capture an aggregate of these aspects of microglial activation, but cannot distinguish between the individual components. We chose our method of quantification of Iba1fluorescence using bin sizes of up to 100 μm as an indicator of microglial response because we were most interested in quantifying gross activation across an extended distance from the foreign body. This resulted in a tradeoff against smaller bin sizes and higher magnification examination of individual microglia. Similar image analysis approaches quantifying fluorescence levels have been used *in vitro* (Polikov et al., 2009, 2010; Achyuta et al., 2010; Tien et al., 2013) and *in vivo* (Azemi et al., 2011; Potter et al., 2013, 2014) to analyze responses to microelectrodes and microscale foreign bodies., while presenting similar shortcomings in terms of elucidating separate aspects of microglial activation. Additional markers of microglial activation, such as secreted cytokines, are also a major factor of interest when studying microglial responses. Commercially available biochemical assays are not sensitive enough to detect secreted cytokines in this particular *in vitro* injury model. Future studies should examine improved experimental and analysis methodologies to combine gross microglial responses with morphological changes and biochemical expression patterns.

ANALYSIS OF CELLULAR RESPONSES

Microglia

The microglial response in a narrow interface region comprising only the area under the microwire exhibits a three tiered response where a significant difference exists between the LPS only and the PEG only treatments, but not between the other conditions. This tiered response might be attributed to the difference between increased activation caused by the LPS and reduced cellular adhesion caused by PEG. The three data sets from the interfacial region included in **Figure 2** (wire only, wire + 25 μm, wire +50 μm) examine the RI of the microglia near the wire by summing the fluorescence over progressively increasing areas. We note that all three sets have the same relative trend when we compare each condition (bare wire, PEG only, LPS, LPS + PEG), only the magnitudes increase as the sets progress because the summation area increases. We observe a microglial monolayer forming at the surface of the wire, explaining the lack of a significant difference between the different treatments. The difference becomes significant only at the wire +50 μm because the magnitudes of the fluorescence become large enough to detect the differences given the variance of the assay. Even though this effect is not statistically significant when we analyze the wire only and wire +25 μm, the trend is consistent. The same is true for LPS vs. a bare wire, although this effect becomes significant at both wire +25 μm and wire +50 μm. We therefore think that the effect of LPS to locally activate microglia and mitigate that activation by a PEG coating is happening throughout the entire interfacial area. This increase in microglial response might be explained by elevated activation of microglia through amplification of inflammatory pathways precipitated by TL4 binding, leading to an increase in microglial response at distance. The observed elevation of Iba1 fluorescence persists in the next 100 μm wide distant region, again indicating an extended inflammatory response, potentially mediated by secreted cytokines produced by activated microglia but dissipates in further distant regions, reverting to a tiered response, where the only significant pairwise difference is between LPS and PEG. This tiered response can again be attributed to distinct pathway amplification between the two treatments; the difference appearing only between the increased upregulation of microglial activation due to LPS and the reduced microglial activation due to PEG.

Astrocytes

In interface regions of varying width, the astrocyte response also exhibits a three tiered response, where an elevated astrocyte response is observed with LPS, and a reduction occurs with both PEG conditions (with LPS and without). In the distant regions, the first and fourth 100 μm wide distant bin do not exhibit any differences between the different treatments, but we observe a difference between LPS and LPS + PEG in the middle two 100 μm wide bins, but surprisingly no difference between LPS and PEG in these distant areas. A potential explanation is that the astrocytes are exhibiting a dose dependent response to LPS. Under this explanation, the increased activation in the interface area for the LPS only treatment results in both astrocyte migration from distant regions and increased overall proliferation; delivering the LPS with PEG results in astrocyte migration without an accompanying equivalent increase in proliferation, resulting in a depletion of distant astrocytes; while PEG only results in even less astrocyte activation in interface areas, which in turn does not signal migration of distant astrocytes. Because we did not directly test for whether the LPS was acting through direct binding to receptors on astrocyte surfaces, we are merely discussing correlative effects. It is unclear whether the astrocyte response is due to direct action by LPS, or if it they are reacting to cytokines and chemokines secreted by microglia. While astrocytes are not typically thought to express TL4 receptors, there is some evidence to the contrary (Bowman et al., 2003). Additionally, while GFAP-positive astrocytes are observed in primary cultures, a considerable portion of them differentiate *in vitro* from astrocyte precursors (Abney et al., 1981). It is possible that due to these culture conditions that astrocyte response is altered from normally developing astrocytes *in vivo*.

Neurons

No significant differences were detected in neuron response to any of the treatments, in either interface or distant regions. While not statistically significant, a coupling between neuron and astrocyte response can be noticed, where slightly higher (but not significantly different) neuron growth was observed for the LPS treatment. Neuronal growth has been consistently shown to occur on a supporting substrate of astrocytes (Noble et al., 1984; Tomaselli et al., 1988). In contrast to the microglia and astrocytes, where the response in the widest interface bin was considerably higher than the first adjacent distant bin, the neuron RI in the first distant bin was comparable to the neuron RI in the wide interface bin, and we did not observe a decline in neuron density over distance. One explanation mirrors the concern expressed earlier about the maturity of the astrocytes, where immature astrocytes in culture provided a better substrate for neuron outgrowth compared to mature astrocytes (Smith et al., 1990). An alternative explanation is that elevated glial activation is not in and of itself neurotoxic or neurodegenerative within a foreign body reactive tissue response paradigm. If the latter explanation is correct, then the loss of neural density *in vivo* following implantation of a microelectrode might be better explained by displacement of neurons following insertion trauma and edema which fail to reoccupy depleted zones because of the glial scar formation, or that *in vivo* neurotoxicity occurs due to direct contact between neurons and extrabrain components.

CONCLUSIONS

We have shown that microglial response in a primary mixed cortical culture can be manipulated by dip-coated treatments. Microglial response can be increased by coating the surface of the foreign body with LPS, and this increase can be prevented by co-depositing LPS and PEG. We hypothesize that the film of high molecular weight PEG, while allowing for LPS release, presents a hydrated physical barrier that disrupts cytokine, chemokine and adsorbed protein gradients that typically guide pathological responses. Astrocyte response also increased for LPS coated foreign bodies, but it is unclear whether this response is directly mediated by LPS or whether it is caused by other microglia-secreted factors. Neuron response was not negatively correlated with microglial response, suggesting mechanisms other than glial activation causing *in vivo* neuronal density loss. Our results highlight the importance of considering the *in vivo* chronic foreign body response as a complex phenomenon with multiple, interconnected yet parallel processes. Attempts to target an individual brain cell type to reduce the overall chronic response are unlikely to be successful. The differences between our findings and typical *in vivo* responses indicate the importance of components other than native brain cells in the progression of the reactive tissue response. Our findings additionally point to a viable alternative hypothesis regarding neuronal density depletion following microelectrode implantation in the brain.

ACKNOWLEDGMENTS

Funding for this research was provided by the Purdue Research Foundation, the Indiana Spinal Cord and Brain Injury Research Grant Program (Fund # 00015115), and the Defense Advanced Research Projects Agency (DARPA) Microsystems Technology Office (MTO), under the auspices of Dr. Jack W. Judy (jack.judy@darpa.mil) and Dr. Doug Weber (douglas.weber@darpa.mil) as part of the Reliable Neural Technology Program, through the Space and Naval Warfare Systems Command (SPAWAR) Systems Center (SSC) Pacific grant No. N66001-11-1-4013. Thanks to members of the Neuroprostheses Research Laboratory for feedback on the manuscript.

REFERENCES

Abney, E. R., Bartlett, P. P., and Raff, M. C. (1981). Astrocytes, ependymal cells and oligodendrocytes develop on schedule in dissociated cell cultures of embryonic rat brain. *Dev. Biol.* 83, 301–310. doi: 10.1016/0012-1606(81)90476-0

Acharya, G., and Park, K. (2006). Mechanisms of controlled drug release from drug-eluting stents. *Adv. Drug Deliv. Rev.* 58, 387–401. doi: 10.1016/j.addr.2006.01.016

Achyuta, A. K. H., Polikov, V. S., White, A. J., Lewis, H. G. P., and Murthy, S. K. (2010). Biocompatibility assessment of insulating silicone polymer coatings using an in vitro glial scar assay. *Macromol. Biosci.* 10, 872–880. doi: 10.1002/mabi.200900451

Azemi, E., Lagenaur, C. F., and Cui, X. T. (2011). The surface immobilization of the neural adhesion molecule L1 on neural probes and its effect on neuronal density and gliosis at the probe/tissue interface. *Biomaterials* 32, 681–692. doi: 10.1016/j.biomaterials.2010.09.033

Beynon, S. B., and Walker, F. R. (2012). Microglial activation in the injured and healthy brain: what are we really talking about? Practical and theoretical issues associated with the measurement of changes in microglial morphology. *Neuroscience* 225, 162–171. doi: 10.1016/j.neuroscience.2012.07.029

Borgens, R. B., Shi, R., and Bohnert, D. (2002). Behavioral recovery from spinal cord injury following delayed application of polyethylene glycol. *J. Exp. Biol.* 205, 1–12.

Bowman, C. C., Rasley, A., Tranguch, S. L., and Marriott, I. (2003). Cultured astrocytes express toll-like receptors for bacterial products. *Glia* 43, 281–291. doi: 10.1002/glia.10256

Das, K. P., McMillian, M. K., Bing, G., and Hong, J.-S. (1995). Modulatory effects of [Met^5]-enkephalin on interleukin-1β secretion from microglia in mixed brain cell cultures. *J. Neuroimmunol.* 62, 9–17. doi: 10.1016/0165-5728(95)00083-e

Ito, D., Imai, Y., Ohsawa, K., Nakajima, K., Fukuuchi, Y., and Kohsaka, S. (1998). Microglia-specific localisation of a novel calcium binding protein, Iba1. *Brain Res. Mol. Brain Res.* 57, 1–9. doi: 10.1016/s0169-328x(98)00040-0

Kang, E., Robinson, J., Park, K., and Cheng, J.-X. (2007). Paclitaxel distribution in poly (ethylene glycol)/poly (lactide-co-glycolic acid) blends and its release visualized by coherent anti-Stokes Raman scattering microscopy. *J. Control. Release* 122, 261–268. doi: 10.1016/j.jconrel.2007.05.007

Karumbaiah, L., Saxena, T., Carlson, D., Patil, K., Patkar, R., Gaupp, E. A., et al. (2013). Relationship between intracortical electrode design and chronic recording function. *Biomaterials* 34, 8061–8074. doi: 10.1016/j.biomaterials.2013.07.016

Koob, A. O., and Borgens, R. B. (2006). Polyethylene glycol treatment after traumatic brain injury reduces beta-amyloid precursor protein accumulation in degenerating axons. *J. Neurosci. Res.* 83, 1558–1563. doi: 10.1002/jnr.20837

Koob, A. O., Colby, J. M., and Borgens, R. B. (2008). Behavioral recovery from traumatic brain injury after membrane reconstruction using polyethylene glycol. *J. Biol. Eng.* 2:9. doi: 10.1186/1754-1611-2-9

Koob, A. O., Duerstock, B. S., Babbs, C. F., Sun, Y., and Borgens, R. B. (2005). Intravenous polyethylene glycol inhibits the loss of cerebral cells after brain injury. *J. Neurotrauma* 22, 1092–1111. doi: 10.1089/neu.2005.22.1092

Kozlowski, C., and Weimer, R. M. (2012). An automated method to quantify microglia morphology and application to monitor activation state longitudinally in vivo. *PLoS One* 7:e31814. doi: 10.1371/journal.pone.0031814

Lehnardt, S., Massillon, L., Follett, P., Jensen, F. E., Ratan, R., Rosenberg, P. A., et al. (2003). Activation of innate immunity in the CNS triggers neurodegeneration through a toll-like receptor 4-dependent pathway. *Proc. Natl. Acad. Sci. U S A* 100, 8514–8519. doi: 10.1073/pnas.1432609100

Lin, C.-C., and Anseth, K. S. (2009). PEG hydrogels for the controlled release of biomolecules in regenerative medicine. *Pharm. Res.* 26, 631–643. doi: 10.1007/s11095-008-9801-2

Markwardt, N. T., Stokol, J., and Rennaker, R. L. 2nd (2013). Sub-meninges implantation reduces immune response to neural implants. *J. Neurosci. Methods* 214, 119–125. doi: 10.1016/j.jneumeth.2013.01.020

Noble, M., Fok-Seang, J., and Cohen, J. (1984). Glia are a unique substrate for the in vitro growth of central nervous system neurons. *J. Neurosci.* 4, 1892–1903.

Ooya, T., Lee, J., and Park, K. (2003). Effects of ethylene glycol-based graft, star-shaped and dendritic polymers on solubilization and controlled release of paclitaxel. *J. Control. Release* 93, 121–127. doi: 10.1016/j.jconrel.2003.07.001

Peppas, N. A. (1997). Hydrogels and drug delivery. *Curr. Opin. Colloid Interface Sci.* 2, 531–537. doi: 10.1016/S1359-0294(97)80103-3

Polikov, V. S., Block, M. L., Fellous, J.-M. M., Hong, J.-S. S., and Reichert, W. M. (2006). In vitro model of glial scarring around neuroelectrodes chronically implanted in the CNS. *Biomaterials* 27, 5368–5376. doi: 10.1016/j.biomaterials.2006.06.018

Polikov, V. S., Hong, J.-S., and Reichert, W. M. (2010). Soluble factor effects on glial cell reactivity at the surface of gel-coated microwires. *J. Neurosci. Methods* 190, 180–187. doi: 10.1016/j.jneumeth.2010.05.002

Polikov, V. S., Su, E. C., Ball, M. A., Hong, J.-S., and Reichert, W. M. (2009). Control protocol for robust in vitro glial scar formation around microwires: essential roles of bFGF and serum in gliosis. *J. Neurosci. Methods* 181, 170–177. doi: 10.1016/j.jneumeth.2009.05.002

Potter, K. A., Buck, A. C., Self, W. K., Callanan, M. E., Sunil, S., and Capadona, J. R. (2013). The effect of resveratrol on neurodegeneration and blood brain barrier stability surrounding intracortical microelectrodes. *Biomaterials* 34, 7001–7015. doi: 10.1016/j.biomaterials.2013.05.035

Potter, K. A., Jorfi, M., Householder, K. T., Johan Foster, E., Weder, C., and Capadona, J. R. (2014). Curcumin-releasing mechanically-adaptive intracortical implants improve the proximal neuronal density and blood-brain barrier stability. *Acta Biomater.* 10, 2209–2222. doi: 10.1016/j.actbio.2014.01.018

Ramakrishna, S., Mayer, J., Wintermantel, E., and Leong, K. W. (2001). Biomedical applications of polymer-composite materials: a review. *Compos. Sci. Technol.* 61, 1189–1224. doi: 10.1016/s0266-3538(00)00241-4

Ravikumar, M., Hageman, D. J., Tomaszewski, W. H., Chandra, G. M., Skousen, J. L., Capadona, J. R., et al. (2014). The effect of residual endotoxin contamination on the neuroinflammatory response to sterilized intracortical microelectrodes. *J. Mater. Chem. B Mater. Biol. Med.* 2, 2517–2529. doi: 10.1039/c3tb21453b

Sasaki, Y., Ohsawa, K., Kanazawa, H., Kohsaka, S., and Imai, Y. (2001). Ibal is an actin-cross-linking protein in macrophages/microglia. *Biochem. Biophys. Res. Commun.* 286, 292–297. doi: 10.1006/bbrc.2001.5388

Saxena, T., Karumbaiah, L., Gaupp, E. A., Patkar, R., Patil, K., Betancur, M., et al. (2013). The impact of chronic blood—brain barrier breach on intracortical electrode function. *Biomaterials* 34, 4703–4713. doi: 10.1016/j.biomaterials.2013.03.007

Smith, G. M., Rutishauser, U., Silver, J., and Miller, R. H. (1990). Maturation of astrocytes in vitro alters the extent and molecular basis of neurite outgrowth. *Dev. Biol.* 138, 377–390. doi: 10.1016/0012-1606(90)90204-v

Sommakia, S., Gaire, J., Rickus, J. L., and Otto, K. J. (2014). Resistive and reactive changes to the impedance of intracortical microelectrodes can be mitigated with polyethylene glycol under acute in vitro and in vivo settings. *Front. Neuroeng.* 7:33. doi: 10.3389/fneng.2014.00033

Tien, L. W., Wu, F., Tang-Schomer, M. D., Yoon, E., Omenetto, F. G., and Kaplan, D. L. (2013). Silk as a multifunctional biomaterial substrate for reduced Glial scarring around brain-penetrating electrodes. *Adv. Funct. Mater.* 23, 3185–3193. doi: 10.1002/adfm.201203716

Tomaselli, K. J., Neugebauer, K. M., Bixby, J. L., Lilien, J., and Reichard, L. F. (1988). N-cadherin and integrins: two receptor systems that mediate neuronal process outgrowth on astrocyte surfaces. *Neuron* 1, 33–43. doi: 10.1016/0896-6273(88)90207-3

Tzeng, S. F., Huang, H. Y., Lee, T. I., and Jwo, J. K. (2005). Inhibition of lipopolysaccharide-induced microglial activation by preexposure to neurotrophin-3. *J. Neurosci. Res.* 81, 666–676. doi: 10.1002/jnr.20586

Vetter, R. J., Williams, J. C., Hetke, J. F., Nunamaker, E. A., and Kipke, D. R. (2004). Chronic neural recording using silicon-substrate microelectrode arrays implanted in cerebral cortex. *IEEE Trans. Biomed. Eng.* 51, 896–904. doi: 10.1109/tbme.2004.826680

Wang, A. L., Yu, A. C. H., Lau, L. T., Lee, C., Wu, L. M., Zhu, X., et al. (2005). Minocycline inhibits LPS-induced retinal microglia activation. *Neurochem. Int.* 47, 152–158. doi: 10.1016/j.neuint.2005.04.018

Woolley, A. J., Desai, H. A., Gaire, J., Ready, A. L., and Otto, K. J. (2013a). A systemic triple label strategy for fluorescent microscopy of inflammation in CNS and Non-CNS tissue. *Microsc. Microanal.* 19, 196–197. doi: 10.1017/S1431927611001607

Woolley, A. J., Desai, H. A., Gaire, J., Ready, A. L., and Otto, K. J. (2013b). Intact histological characterization of brain-implanted microdevices and surrounding tissue. *J. Vis. Exp.* 72, 50126. doi: 10.3791/50126

Woolley, A. J., Desai, H. A., and Otto, K. J. (2013c). Chronic intracortical microelectrode arrays induce non-uniform, depth-related tissue responses. *J. Neural Eng.* 10:026007. doi: 10.1088/1741-2560/10/2/026007

Woolley, A. J., Desai, H. A., Steckbeck, M. A., Patel, N. K., and Otto, K. J. (2011). In situ characterization of the brain-microdevice interface using device-capture histology. *J. Neurosci. Methods* 201, 67–77. doi: 10.1016/j.jneumeth.2011.07.012

5

NG2 cells (polydendrocytes) in brain physiology and repair

Akiko Nishiyama *, Ryusuke Suzuki and Xiaoqin Zhu

Department of Physiology and Neurobiology, University of Connecticut, Storrs, CT, USA

Edited by:
Luca Bonfanti, University of Turin, Italy

Reviewed by:
Brahim Nait Oumesmar, Inserm, France
Kaylene M. Young, University of Tasmania, Australia

***Correspondence:**
Akiko Nishiyama, Department of Physiology and Neurobiology, University of Connecticut, 75 North Eagleville Road, Storrs, CT 06269-3156, USA
e-mail: akiko.nishiyama@uconn.edu

NG2 cells, also referred to as oligodendrocyte precursor cells (OPCs) or polydendrocytes, represent a major resident glial cell population that is distinct from mature astrocytes, oligodendrocytes, microglia, and neural stem cells and exist throughout the gray and white matter of the developing and mature central nervous system (CNS). While their most established fate is the oligodendrocyte, they retain lineage plasticity in an age- and region-specific manner. During development, they contribute to 36% of protoplasmic astrocytes in the ventral forebrain. Despite intense investigation on the neuronal fate of NG2 cells, there is no definitive evidence that they contribute substantially to the neuronal population. NG2 cells have attributes that suggest that they have functions other than to generate oligodendrocytes, but their exact role in the neural network remains unknown. Under pathological states, NG2 cells not only contribute to myelin repair, but they become activated in response to a wide variety of insults and could play a primary role in pathogenesis.

Keywords: NG2, polydendrocyte, oligodendrocyte, myelin, demyelination, cell fate, subventricular zone

INTRODUCTION

NG2 cells represent a resident glial progenitor cell population that exists throughout the gray and white matter of the developing and mature mammalian central nervous system (CNS) and are distinct from astrocytes, mature oligodendrocytes, microglia, and neural stem cells (reviewed in Nishiyama et al., 2009; Hill and Nishiyama, 2014). Their widespread existence in the CNS began to be recognized in the 1990s by immunohistochemical labeling for NG2 and the alpha receptor for platelet-derived growth factor (Pdgfra). Currently, NG2 cells are considered as the fourth major glial cell type in the CNS, comprising 2–8% of all the cells in the adult CNS (Dawson et al., 2003; Peters, 2004). These cells are often equated with oligodendrocyte precursor cells (OPCs) because of their ability to generate myelinating and non-myelinating oligodendrocytes. However, not all NG2 cells differentiate into oligodendrocytes, and oligodendrocytes are not their only fate, as discussed below. Different names have been used to refer to these cells. The term OPCs is used when discussing their role in oligodendrocyte production, while the terms "NG2 cells" and "NG2 glia" are used when discussing their property that is not directly related to their OPC role, even though NG2, which is also expressed on vascular pericytes, is not an absolute marker for these cells. To avoid using different names to refer to the same cells in different biological contexts, the word "polydendrocytes" has been suggested as a unified name for these cells, in keeping with the names of other types of glia that are loosely associated with their morphology. This perspective article will discuss recent findings and unsolved questions related to the astrocyte and neuronal fate of NG2 cells and their role in brain pathophysiology, primarily in the rodent CNS.

THE FATE OF NG2 CELLS

NG2 cells expand their population by extensive self-renewal. After their peak proliferation during the perinatal period, they retain their proliferative ability throughout life (**Figure 1**).

OLIGODENDROCYTE FATE

The general consensus from a series of Cre-loxP-mediated genetic fate mapping studies is that under normal physiological conditions, NG2 cells in the adult CNS generate oligodendrocytes as they continue to self renew (**Figure 1**) (Dimou et al., 2008; Rivers et al., 2008; Kang et al., 2010; Zhu et al., 2011; Young et al., 2013). It is unlikely, however, that every NG2 cell will differentiate into an oligodendrocyte at some point during the life of the animal, as their uniform distribution does not parallel the distribution of oligodendrocytes (Dawson et al., 2000; Tomassy et al., 2014). It remains to be explored whether all NG2 cells are equivalent in their ability to generate oligodendrocytes or whether there is a subpopulation that is fated to permanently remain as NG2 cells.

ASTROCYTE FATE AND LINEAGE PLASTICITY OF NG2 CELLS

During development, the fate of NG2 cells is not restricted to oligodendrocytes. NG2 cells contribute to 40% of the protoplasmic astrocytes in the gray matter of the ventral forebrain (Zhu et al., 2008, 2011; Huang et al., 2014). The magnitude and the temporal and spatial distribution of protoplasmic astrocytes observed in these studies are quite distinct from the other observations where a small number (1~5%) of sporadically distributed reporter+ astrocytes were seen from Olig2-creER and Pdgfra-CreER fate mapping in adult (Dimou et al., 2008; Tripathi et al., 2010). Two independently generated tamoxifen-inducible NG2-creER transgenic mouse lines (BAC transgenic

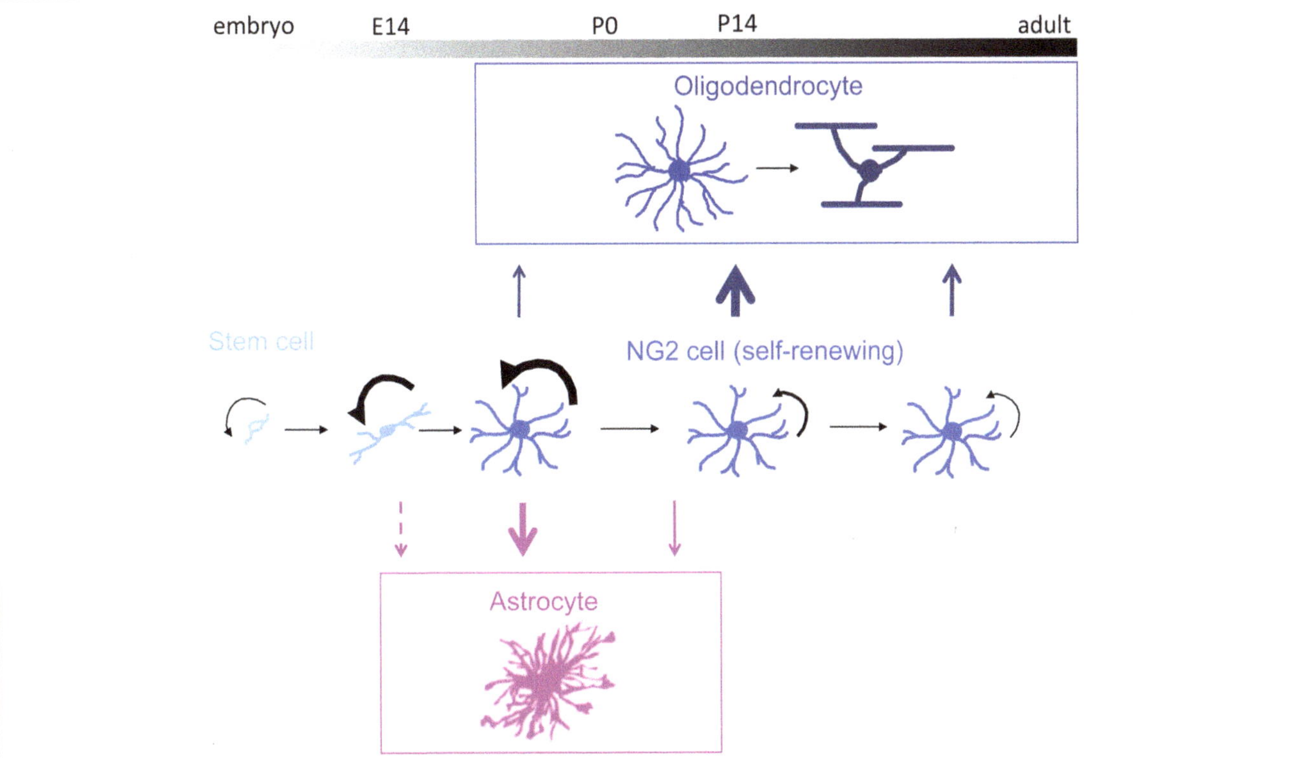

FIGURE 1 | A schematic showing the fate of NG2 cells throughout development. The middle diagram depicts self-renewing NG2 cells, with a chronological scale across the top. Black arrows indicate the rate of proliferation, which is greatest perinatally. Blue upward arrows indicate oligodendrocyte differentiation, peaking during the third postnatal week. Purple downward arrows indicate astrocyte differentiation, which occurs predominantly before birth and gradually ceases shortly after birth. The thickness of the arrows denotes the extent of differentiation. Modified from Nishiyama (2007).

and knock-in) indicate that astrocyte generation from NG2 cells is most robust prenatally and tapers off during the first postnatal week (**Figure 1**) (Zhu et al., 2011; Huang et al., 2014), consistent with the chronology of astrocyte development. This suggests that the astrocyte fate of NG2 cells is a physiological developmental function and not due to radial glial expression of NG2 as suggested in Richardson et al. (2011). None of the other fate mapping studies had attempted to induce Cre prenatally. The reason why NG2 cells lose their astrogliogenic ability shortly after birth could be due to a density-dependent mechanism that regulates astrocyte production (Nakatsuji and Miller, 2001; Zhu et al., 2012).

Are NG2 cells that do not generate astrocytes during early development permanently committed to generating oligodendrocytes? The following observation suggests that under normal conditions, they are restricted to the oligodendrocyte lineage, but that they retain the ability to become astrocytes under certain conditions. When the oligodendrocyte transcription factor Olig2 that is required for NG2 cell specification (Rowitch, 2004; Richardson et al., 2006), was deleted in all NG2 cells, there was a complete fate switch from oligodendrocytes to astrocytes in the neocortex but not in the ventral forebrain, resulting in severe hypomyelination (Zhu et al., 2012). When Olig2 was deleted in early postnatal NG2 cells, only 50% of the Olig2-deleted neocortical NG2 cells switched their fate to astrocytes (Zhu et al., 2012). In the adult, deletion of Olig2 did not convert them into astrocytes, even in response to a stab wound (Komitova et al., 2011), nor was there increased astrocyte generation from NG2 cells in Olig2-creER heterozygous mice (Dimou et al., 2008), although the former study had used an inefficient Cre reporter. Thus, lineage restriction of NG2 cells appears to occur gradually during the first few postnatal weeks. Even after oligodendrocyte specification has occurred during embryogenesis, NG2 cells in certain regions retain some degree of context-dependent lineage plasticity, which is gradually lost in later postnatal life.

NEURONAL FATE OF NG2 CELLS

The neuronal fate of NG2 cells has been one of the most highly debated topics, and Cre-loxP-mediated genetic fate mapping studies have produced inconsistent findings. For example, two studies using Pdgfra-CreER or PLP (proteolipid protein)-CreER transgenic mouse lines observed reporter+ neurons in the piriform cortex (Rivers et al., 2008; Guo et al., 2010), while a subsequent study using an independent line of Pdgfra-CreER mice did not find any evidence for a neuronal fate (Kang et al., 2010). Earlier studies using NG2- and Olig2-Cre driver mice showed no evidence for neurogenesis (Dimou et al., 2008; Zhu et al., 2008; Komitova et al., 2009; Zhu et al., 2011), while a recent study using the same NG2-creER mice showed a few reporter+ neurons in the hypothalamus (Robins et al., 2013). What is the significance of detecting reporter+ neurons in these fate mapping studies? Is the extent of neurogenesis from NG2 cells sufficiently large to bring about a physiological effect in the neural network? The findings must be interpreted in proper context without overemphasizing observations where sporadic reporter+ neurons are found.

The following example illustrates one of the caveats of the Cre-loxP technology that spurious transient activation of Cre in an unrelated cell could lead to reporter expression in that cell in the absence of lineage progression. In NG2-cre:zeg mice generated by crossing constitutively active NG2-cre mice (Zhu et al., 2008) to the zeg reporter mice (Novak et al., 2000), a significant number of reporter+ neurons appeared in the neocortex after P45 but not at P14 (**Figures 2A,B**). To determine whether reporter+ neurons arose as a result of lineage progression from NG2 cells or due to direct Cre expression in neurons, the zeg reporter plasmid was in utero electroporated directly into neuronal precursors of NG2-cre single transgenic mice at E13.5, and the appearance of reporter+ neurons was examined (**Figure 2C**). The plasmid would be retained in neurons that are undergoing their last cell division and lost from glial cells as they undergo multiple divisions (Bai et al., 2003). The expression of the reporter in neurons would suggest direct Cre activation in neurons. A DsRed plasmid was co-electroporated to mark the transfected cells. When the electroporated mice were sacrificed at P70, all the DsRed+ neurons also expressed EGFP (**Figures 2D–F**), and no NG2 cells expressed EGFP or DsRed. This suggests that there was transient Cre (and possibly NG2) expression in neurons, and that the duration of Cre expression was sufficient for Cre-mediated recombination to allow EGFP expression from the zeg plasmid but not sufficiently long-lasting to be detected by Cre immunohistochemistry or in situ hybridization. It is possible that certain physiological conditions cause a spike in NG2 transcription, which is too transient to be detected in NG2-DsRed transgenic mice (Zhu et al., 2008). Furthermore, no transitional forms between NG2 cells and neurons could be observed, unlike the case for NG2 cells transitioning into astrocytes (Zhu et al., 2012) or oligodendrocytes (**Figure 2G**).

In the new NG2 cell fate mapping study using the NG2creER knockin mice crossed to ROSA-tdTomato reporter, Huang et al. (2014) observed reporter+ neurons with electrophysiological and morphological properties of neurons in the non-neuronogenic regions of the forebrain. By contrast, very few reporter+ neurons were found when the same mice were crossed to the less efficient RSOA-YFP reporter. Since these neurons appeared without evidence of proliferation, it is unlikely that they arose from NG2 cells, as previously reported (Clarke et al., 2012), but rather by some form of Cre-dependent DNA recombination that had occurred in neuronal cells. The Huang study also highlights the different outcomes of studies using Cre reporter lines with different efficiencies. Development of a novel, Cre-independent method is needed to resolve the question of the neuronal fate of NG2 cells.

RELATIONSHIP OF NG2 CELLS TO NEURAL STEM CELLS

The adult SVZ consists of a heterogeneous population including GFAP+ neural stem cells (type B cells), transit-amplifying cells (type C cells), and neuroblasts that migrate to the olfactory bulb via the rostral migratory stream (type A cells) (Gonzalez-Perez and Alvarez-Buylla, 2011). Many early studies were focused on testing the then attractive hypothesis that NG2 cells corresponded to multipotential neural stem cells in the SVZ (Nunes et al., 2003; Aguirre and Gallo, 2004), based on the observation that they could be induced to differentiate into astrocytes and neurons under certain culture conditions (Roy et al., 1999; Kondo and Raff, 2000). However, further examination of NG2 cells and the SVZ revealed that NG2 cells comprise a minority of cells, located mostly at the periphery of the SVZ, and are distinct from the Dlx2-expressing type C cells or neuroblasts that express Doublecortin (Komitova et al., 2009; Platel et al., 2009; Richardson et al., 2011). These studies also showed that NG2 cells are distinct from GFAP+ neural stem cells (type B cells) (Rivers et al., 2008; Komitova et al., 2009; Chojnacki et al., 2011), in contrast to an earlier study that showed expression of Pdgfra on type B cells (Jackson et al., 2006). Neural stem cells do generate NG2 cells, but this fate of neural stem cells seems to be a minor fate compared with their neurogenic fate and is highly region-specific. Interestingly, a recent real-time imaging study of the fate of single cells unequivocally demonstrated that neural stem cell clones that generate NG2 cells do not generate neurons and are primarily found in the dorsal SVZ, while those that generate neurons are more enriched in the lateral SVZ and do not generate NG2 cells (Ortega et al., 2013). Thus, there appears to be an early segregation of neuronal and oligodendrocyte lineages in the SVZ. Under normal conditions, only SVZ type C cells, but not NG2 cells, proliferate in response to epidermal growth factor (EGF) (Doetsch et al., 2002; Hill et al., 2013). However, under pathological conditions such as EGF overexpression or demyelination, EGF can redirect SVZ type C cells to become NG2 cells (Aguirre et al., 2007; Ivkovic et al., 2008; Jablonska et al., 2010; Galvez-Contreras et al., 2013). These observations can be explained if EGF receptor becomes upregulated on a small population of cells that are in transit from SVZ type C cells to becoming NG2 cells.

THE ROLE OF NG2 CELLS IN THE NORMAL CNS

Why has the mammalian brain evolved to maintain such a uniformly distributed glial cell type? Recent studies have revealed that new oligodendrocytes and myelin continue to be produced in the mature CNS (Zhu et al., 2011; Young et al., 2013) and a significant amount of activity-dependent myelin plasticity occurs in the adult (Zatorre et al., 2012; Hill and Nishiyama, 2014). NG2 cells also generate non-myelinating perineuronal oligodendrocytes whose somata lie apposed to neuronal somata (Penfield, 1924). Although the role of the perineuronal oligodendrocytes is not clear, they can produce myelin in response to demyelination (Ludwin, 1979) and could be providing neurotrophic and metabolic support for neurons (Taniike et al., 2002; Fünfschilling et al., 2012; Lee et al., 2012).

NG2 cells are evenly distributed to cover the entire mature CNS parenchyma (Dawson et al., 2000). *In vivo* imaging in 2–3-month-old neocortex revealed non-overlapping territories occupied by adjacent NG2 cells, and their processes appeared to be contact-inhibited (Hughes et al., 2013). Another study using fixed hippocampi from 3–4-week-old rats showed that NG2 cells

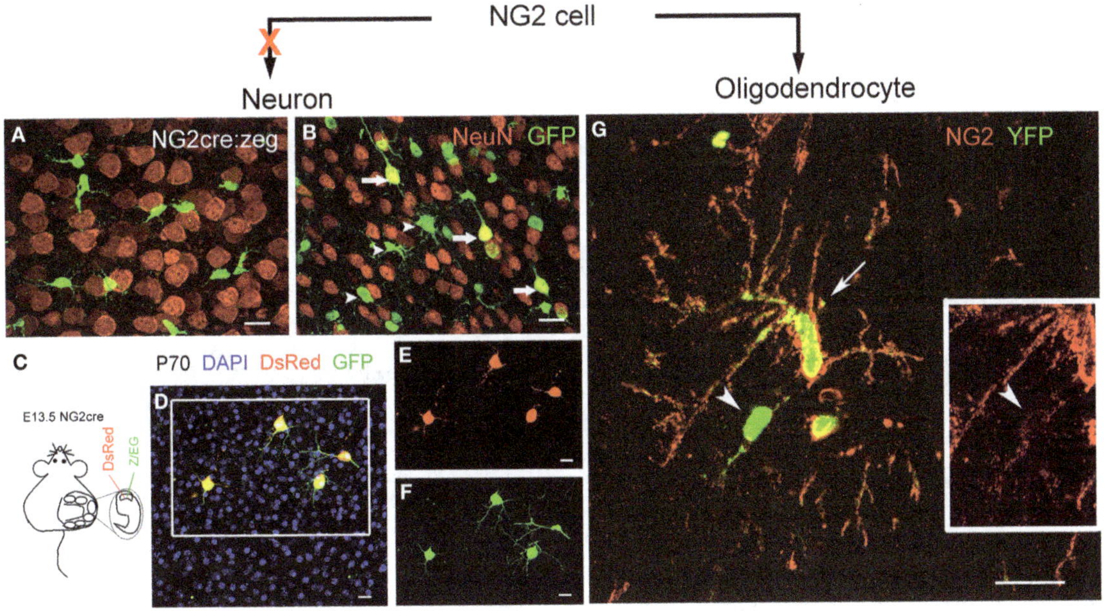

FIGURE 2 | Lineage-dependent and independent reporter expression in Cre-loxP fate mapping. (A,B) Double labeling for GFP and the neuronal marker NeuN in the neocortex of NG2cre:zeg mice at P14 **(A)** and P70 **(B)**. NeuN+ GFP+ cells with mature neuronal morphology (arrows) are seen as well as NeuN- GFP+ NG2 cells (arrowheads) in P70 but not in P14 cortex. **(C–F)** Transfection of zeg reporter plasmid into neuronal precursor cells in NG2cre single transgenic mice. **(C)** Scheme showing co-transfection of DsRed and zeg plasmid DNA into the lateral ventricles of E13.5 NG2cre single transgenic mice by in utero electroporation and positioning the electrodes to target the dorsal pallium. **(D–F)** GFP expression in electroporated neurons at P70. All the GFP+ cells were neurons that had been electroporated (DsRed+), and no GFP+ glial cells were detected. This experiment demonstrates that Cre is activated directly in neocortical neurons of NG2cre mice at some point between P14 and P70, leading to GFP expression in neurons. Unlike the case for oligodendrocytes shown in G, there were no GFP+ cells that appeared to be in transition from NG2 cells to neurons. **(G)** Corpus callosum from P70 NG2creER:YFP mice 14 days after Cre induction with 4-hydroxytamoxifen. A cell that appears to be transitioning from an NG2 cell (NG2+ YFP+) into an NG2- oligodendrocyte (NG2- YFP+) with weak NG2 immunoreactivity in the processes (arrowheads) is seen next to a typical NG2 cell that robustly expresses NG2 (arrow). Inset shows single labeling of the cell marked by arrowhead for NG2.

were tiled but shared approximately 5% of the volume with adjacent NG2 cells (Xu et al., 2013). It is not clear whether the extent of overlap between processes of neighboring NG2 cells changes as the brain matures. Regardless, the uniform distribution of NG2 cells would suggest a yet uncovered homeostatic role in the CNS.

NG2 cells interact uniquely with neurons in that they depolarize in response to receiving direct synaptic input from neuronal axons (Bergles et al., 2000). However, the extent of depolarizations is not sufficient to elicit repetitive action potentials, and thus NG2 cells are still considered as non-excitable glial cells. While the physiological consequences and significance of neuron-NG2 cell synapses remain unknown, and the nature of neuron-NG2 cell communication changes with age and differentiation (Maldonado and Angulo, 2014), it is likely that local increases in intracellular calcium play an important role in mediating downstream cellular effects (Bergles et al., 2000; Ge et al., 2006; Hamilton et al., 2010; Haberlandt et al., 2011).

THE ROLE OF NG2 CELLS IN PATHOLOGY

REPAIR OF DEMYELINATING LESIONS

It is well established that NG2 cells proliferate and differentiate into myelinating oligodendrocytes and repair demyelinated lesions (Di Bello et al., 1999; Watanabe et al., 2002; Tripathi et al., 2010). It still remains to be shown whether replenishment of the NG2 cell population can be a cause for remyelination failure under certain conditions. While repeated acutely demyelinated lesions undergo successful remyelination (Penderis et al., 2003), other studies suggest that NG2 cells can become depleted after acute demyelination (Keirstead et al., 1998) and their repopulation may not occur fast enough to meet the demands of chronic ongoing demyelination (Mason et al., 2004). Recruitment of new NG2 cells could occur by proliferation of local NG2 cells and/or migration and differentiation of cells from the SVZ (Nait-Oumesmar et al., 1999; Picard-Riera et al., 2002; Etxeberria et al., 2010; Tepavcevic et al., 2011). However, evidence is not yet strong that these SVZ-derived cells are capable of fully differentiating into remyelinating cells to the extent that local NG2 cells are.

ACTIVATION OF NG2 CELLS IN OTHER TYPES OF LESIONS

NG2 cells undergo increased proliferation and dramatic morphological changes in response to a wide variety of acute CNS insults besides demyelination, including spinal cord injury (McTigue et al., 2001; Jones et al., 2002), ischemia (Zhang et al., 2013), excitotoxic injury (Bu et al., 2001; Wennström et al., 2004), and viral infection (Levine et al., 1998). The time course of their "activation" and their "reactive morphology" or the extent of proliferation varies depending on the nature of the insult, but the functional significance for these diverse morphological and proliferative changes is not known. For example, it is not known whether the shorter, thicker processes reflect increased uptake of extracellular fluid/ions or increased phagocytic activity. Nor is it known whether the increased number of thin, elongated process after viral infection reflect a search for something or deregulated cytoskeleton. *In vivo* imaging has revealed that NG2 cell processes are highly dynamic (Hughes et al., 2013; Hill et al., under revision), but it is not known what they are seeking besides axons to myelinate.

In most cases of acute injury, NG2 cell responses occur early, within 24 h (Watanabe et al., 2002; Horky et al., 2006; Simon et al., 2011), which is similar to or slightly lags behind the time course of microglial response and a few days before reactive astrogliosis becomes apparent. Some forms of insult such as excitotoxic injury seem to elicit a greater microglial response than NG2 cell response. NG2 cells exhibit a close spatial relation to astrocyte processes and microglial somata (Nishiyama et al., 2002; Hamilton et al., 2010; Xu et al., 2013), and the latter becomes more pronounced in response to injury (Nishiyama et al., 1997; Bu et al., 2001; Wu et al., 2010). Future studies can be directed to studying how the three types of reactive glia signal to each other to achieve a concerted response specifically tailored to each type of injury.

NG2 CELLS IN PATHOGENESIS

The inherent ability of NG2 cells to remain in cell cycle through life also makes them susceptible to neoplastic transformation. Although the cell of origin of glioblastoma multiforme continues to be debated, cell fate mapping of neural stem cells or NG2 cells with deletions in p53 and NF1 genes revealed that neoplastic changes begin to occur in NG2 cells and not in neural stem cells (Liu et al., 2011). Intriguingly, early proliferative foci arise in perineuronal locations in gray matter rather than in white matter tracts where glioma cells are known to expand and disseminate, suggesting a proliferative paracrine signal imparted by neurons.

Several recent studies have shown that metabolic defects in oligodendrocytes can precede neurodegeneration in amyotrophic lateral sclerosis (ALS) (Lee et al., 2012; Kang et al., 2013; Philips et al., 2013), strongly suggesting a pathogenic role for oligodendrocytes. In addition, a direct pathogenic role for NG2 cells has been shown at the neurovascular interface. In a cerebral hypoperfusion model, metalloproteinase-9 (MMP-9) is secreted from NG2 cells in the vicinity of vascular endothelial cells, leading to degradation of the endothelial tight junction protein ZO-1 and breakdown of the blood-brain barrier (Seo et al., 2013). These findings highlight the importance of the oligovascular niche in normal and pathological conditions that could be an important topic of future investigations (Maki et al., 2013; Miyamoto et al., 2014).

REFERENCES

Aguirre, A., Dupree, J. L., Mangin, J. M., and Gallo, V. (2007). A functional role for EGFR signaling in myelination and remyelination. *Nat. Neurosci.* 10, 990–1002. doi: 10.1038/nn1938

Aguirre, A., and Gallo, V. (2004). Postnatal neurogenesis and gliogenesis in the olfactory bulb from NG2-expressing progenitors of the subventricular zone. *J. Neurosci.* 24, 10530–10541. doi: 10.1523/JNEUROSCI.3572-04.2004

Bai, J., Ramos, R. L., Ackman, J. B., Thomas, A. M., Lee, R. V., and LoTurco, J. J. (2003). RNAi reveals doublecortin is required for radial migration in rat neocortex. *Nat. Neurosci.* 6, 1277–1283. doi: 10.1038/nn1153

Bergles, D. E., Roberts, J. D., Somogyi, P., and Jahr, C. E. (2000). Glutamatergic synapses on oligodendrocyte precursor cells in the hippocampus. *Nature* 405, 187–191. doi: 10.1038/35012083

Bu, J., Akhtar, N., and Nishiyama, A. (2001). Transient expression of the NG2 proteoglycan by a subpopulation of activated macrophages in an excitotoxic hippocampal lesion. *Glia* 34, 296–310. doi: 10.1002/glia.1063

Chojnacki, A., Mak, G., and Weiss, S. (2011). PDGFRalpha expression distinguishes GFAP-expressing neural stem cells from PDGF-responsive neural precursors in the adult periventricular area. *J. Neurosci.* 31, 9503–9512. doi: 10.1523/JNEUROSCI.1531-11.2011

Clarke, L. E., Young, K. M., Hamilton, N. B., Li, H., Richardson, W. D., and Attwell, D. (2012). Properties and fate of oligodendrocyte progenitor cells in the corpus callosum, motor cortex, and piriform cortex of the mouse. *J. Neurosci.* 32, 8173–8185. doi: 10.1523/JNEUROSCI.0928-12.2012

Dawson, M. R., Levine, J. M., and Reynolds, R. (2000). NG2-expressing cells in the central nervous system: are they oligodendroglial progenitors? *J. Neurosci. Res.* 61, 471–479. doi: 10.1002/1097-4547(20000901)61:53.3.CO;2-E

Dawson, M. R., Polito, A., Levine, J. M., and Reynolds, R. (2003). NG2-expressing glial progenitor cells: an abundant and widespread population of cycling cells in the adult rat CNS. *Mol. Cell Neurosci.* 24, 476–488. doi: 10.1016/S1044-7431(03)00210-0

Di Bello, C. I., Dawson, M. R., Levine, J. M., and Reynolds, R. (1999). Generation of oligodendroglial progenitors in acute inflammatory demyelinating lesions of the rat brain stem is associated with demyelination rather than inflammation. *J. Neurocytol.* 28, 365–381. doi: 10.1023/A:1007069815302

Dimou, L., Simon, C., Kirchhoff, F., Takebayashi, H., and Gotz, M. (2008). Progeny of Olig2-expressing progenitors in the gray and white matter of the adult mouse cerebral cortex. *J. Neurosci.* 28, 10434–10442. doi: 10.1523/JNEUROSCI.2831-08.2008

Doetsch, F., Petreanu, L., Caille, I., Garcia-Verdugo, J. M., and Alvarez-Buylla, A. (2002). EGF converts transit-amplifying neurogenic precursors in the adult brain into multipotent stem cells. *Neuron* 36, 1021–1034. doi: 10.1016/S0896-6273(02)01133-9

Etxeberria, A., Mangin, J. M., Aguirre, A., and Gallo, V. (2010). Adult-born SVZ progenitors receive transient synapses during remyelination in corpus callosum. *Nat. Neurosci.* 13, 287–289. doi: 10.1038/nn.2500

Fünfschilling, U., Supplie, L. M., Mahad, D., Boretius, S., Saab, A. S., Edgar, J., et al. (2012). Glycolytic oligodendrocytes maintain myelin and long-term axonal integrity. *Nature* 485, 517–521. doi: 10.1038/nature11007

Galvez-Contreras, A. Y., Quinones-Hinojosa, A., and Gonzalez-Perez, O. (2013). The role of EGFR and ErbB family related proteins in the oligodendrocyte specification in germinal niches of the adult mammalian brain. *Front. Cell. Neurosci.* 7:258. doi: 10.3389/fncel.2013.00258

Ge, W. P., Yang, X. J., Zhang, Z., Wang, H. K., Shen, W., Deng, Q. D., et al. (2006). Long-term potentiation of neuron-glia synapses mediated by Ca2+-permeable AMPA receptors. *Science* 312, 1533–1537. doi: 10.1126/science.1124669

Gonzalez-Perez, O., and Alvarez-Buylla, A. (2011). Oligodendrogenesis in the subventricular zone and the role of epidermal growth factor. *Brain Res. Rev.* 67, 147–156. doi: 10.1016/j.brainresrev.2011.01.001

Guo, F., Maeda, Y., Ma, J., Xu, J., Horiuchi, M., Miers, L., et al. (2010). Pyramidal neurons are generated from oligodendroglial progenitor cells in adult piriform cortex. *J. Neurosci.* 30, 12036–12049. doi: 10.1523/JNEUROSCI.1360-10.2010

Haberlandt, C., Derouiche, A., Wyczynski, A., Haseleu, J., Pohle, J., Karram, K., et al. (2011). Gray matter NG2 cells display multiple Ca2+-signaling pathways and highly motile processes. *PLoS ONE* 6:e17575. doi: 10.1371/journal.pone.0017575

Hamilton, N., Vayro, S., Wigley, R., and Butt, A. M. (2010). Axons and astrocytes release ATP and glutamate to evoke calcium signals in NG2-glia. *Glia* 58, 66–79. doi: 10.1002/glia.20902

Hill, R. A., and Nishiyama, A. (2014). NG2 cells (polydendrocytes): listeners to the neural network. *Glia* 62, 1195–1210. doi: 10.1002/glia.22664

Hill, R. A., Patel, K. D., Medved, J., Reiss, A. M., and Nishiyama, A. (2013). NG2 cells in white matter but not gray matter proliferate in response to PDGF. *J. Neurosci.* 33, 14558–14566. doi: 10.1523/JNEUROSCI.2001-12.2013

Horky, L. L., Galimi, F., Gage, F. H., and Horner, P. J. (2006). Fate of endogenous stem/progenitor cells following spinal cord injury. *J. Comp. Neurol.* 498, 525–538. doi: 10.1002/cne.21065

Huang, W., Zhao, N., Bai, X., Karram, K., Trotter, J., Goebbels, S., et al. (2014). Novel NG2-CreERT2 knock-in mice demonstrate heterogeneous differentiation potential of NG2 glia during development. *Glia* 62, 896–913. doi: 10.1002/glia.22648

Hughes, E. G., Kang, S. H., Fukaya, M., and Bergles, D. E. (2013). Oligodendrocyte progenitors balance growth with self-repulsion to achieve homeostasis in the adult brain. *Nat. Neurosci.* 16, 668–676. doi: 10.1038/nn.3390

Ivkovic, S., Canoll, P., and Goldman, J. E. (2008). Constitutive EGFR signaling in oligodendrocyte progenitors leads to diffuse hyperplasia in postnatal white matter. *J. Neurosci.* 28, 914–922. doi: 10.1523/JNEUROSCI.4327-07.2008

Jablonska, B., Aguirre, A., Raymond, M., Szabo, G., Kitabatake, Y., Sailor, K. A., et al. (2010). Chordin-induced lineage plasticity of adult SVZ neuroblasts after demyelination. *Nat. Neurosci.* 13, 541–550. doi: 10.1038/nn.2536

Jackson, E. L., Garcia-Verdugo, J. M., Gil-Perotin, S., Roy, M., Quinones-Hinojosa, A., VandenBerg, S., et al. (2006). PDGFR alpha-positive B cells are neural stem cells in the adult SVZ that form glioma-like growths in response to increased PDGF signaling. *Neuron* 51, 187–199. doi: 10.1016/j.neuron.2006.06.012

Jones, L. L., Yamaguchi, Y., Stallcup, W. B., and Tuszynski, M. H. (2002). NG2 is a major chondroitin sulfate proteoglycan produced after spinal cord injury and is expressed by macrophages and oligodendrocyte progenitors. *J. Neurosci.* 22, 2792–2803.

Kang, S. H., Fukaya, M., Yang, J. K., Rothstein, J. D., and Bergles, D. E. (2010). NG2+ CNS glial progenitors remain committed to the oligodendrocyte lineage in postnatal life and following neurodegeneration. *Neuron* 68, 668–681. doi: 10.1016/j.neuron.2010.09.009

Kang, S. H., Li, Y., Fukaya, M., Lorenzini, I., Cleveland, D. W., Ostrow, L. W., et al. (2013). Degeneration and impaired regeneration of gray matter oligodendrocytes in amyotrophic lateral sclerosis. *Nat. Neurosci.* 16, 571–579. doi: 10.1038/nn.3357

Keirstead, H. S., Levine, J. M., and Blakemore, W. F. (1998). Response of the oligodendrocyte progenitor cell population (defined by NG2 labelling) to demyelination of the adult spinal cord. *Glia* 22, 161–170.

Komitova, M., Serwanski, D. R., Lu, Q. R., and Nishiyama, A. (2011). NG2 cells are not a major source of reactive astrocytes after neocortical stab wound injury. *Glia* 59, 800–809. doi: 10.1002/glia.21152

Komitova, M., Zhu, X., Serwanski, D. R., and Nishiyama, A. (2009). NG2 cells are distinct from neurogenic cells in the postnatal mouse subventricular zone. *J. Comp. Neurol.* 512, 702–716. doi: 10.1002/cne.21917

Kondo, T., and Raff, M. (2000). Oligodendrocyte precursor cells reprogrammed to become multipotential CNS stem cells. *Science* 289, 1754–1757. doi: 10.1126/science.289.5485.1754

Lee, Y., Morrison, B. M., Li, Y., Lengacher, S., Farah, M. H., Hoffman, P. N., et al. (2012). Oligodendroglia metabolically support axons and contribute to neurodegeneration. *Nature* 487, 443–448. doi: 10.1038/nature11314

Levine, J. M., Enquist, L. W., and Card, J. P. (1998). Reactions of oligodendrocyte precursor cells to alpha herpesvirus infection of the central nervous system. *Glia* 23, 316–328.

Liu, C., Sage, J. C., Miller, M. R., Verhaak, R. G., Hippenmeyer, S., Vogel, H., et al. (2011). Mosaic analysis with double markers reveals tumor cell of origin in glioma. *Cell* 146, 209–221. doi: 10.1016/j.cell.2011.06.014

Ludwin, S. K. (1979). The perineuronal satellite oligodendrocyte. *Acta Neuropathol.* 47, 49–53. doi: 10.1007/BF00698272

Maki, T., Liang, A. C., Miyamato, N., Lo, E. H., and Arai, K. (2013). Mechanisms of oligodendrocyte regeneration from ventricular-subventricular zone-derived progenitor cells in white matter diseases. *Front. Cell. Neurosci.* 7:275. doi: 10.3389/fncel.2013.00275

Maldonado, P. P., and Angulo, M. C. (2014). Multiple modes of communication between neurons and oligodendrocyte precursor cells. *Neuroscientist.* doi: 10.1177/1073858414530784. [Epub ahead of print].

Mason, J. L., Toews, A., Hostettler, J. D., Morell, P., Suzuki, K., Goldman, J. E., et al. (2004). Oligodendrocytes and progenitors become progressively depleted within chronically demyelinated lesions. *Am. J. Pathol.* 164, 1673–1682. doi: 10.1016/S0002-9440(10)63726-1

McTigue, D. M., Wei, P., and Stokes, B. T. (2001). Proliferation of NG2-positive cells and altered oligodendrocyte numbers in the contused rat spinal cord. *J. Neurosci.* 21, 3392–3400.

Miyamoto, N., Pham, L. D., Seo, J. H., Kim, K. W., Lo, E. H., and Arai, K. (2014). Crosstalk between cerebral endothelium and oligodendrocyte. *Cell. Mol. Life Sci.* 71, 1055–1066. doi: 10.1007/s00018-013-1488-9

Nait-Oumesmar, B., Decker, L., Lachapelle, F., Avellana-Adalid, V., Bachelin, C., and Van Evercooren, A. B. (1999). Progenitor cells of the adult mouse subventricular zone proliferate, migrate and differentiate into oligodendrocytes after demyelination. *Eur. J. Neurosci.* 11, 4357–4366. doi: 10.1046/j.1460-9568.1999.00873.x

Nakatsuji, Y., and Miller, R. H. (2001). Density dependent modulation of cell cycle protein expression in astrocytes. *J. Neurosci. Res.* 66, 487–496. doi: 10.1002/jnr.1240

Nishiyama, A. (2007). Polydendrocytes: NG2 cells with many roles in development and repair of the CNS. *Neuroscientist* 13, 62–76. doi: 10.1177/1073858406295586

Nishiyama, A., Komitova, M., Suzuki, R., and Zhu, X. (2009). Polydendrocytes (NG2 cells): multifunctional cells with lineage plasticity. *Nat. Rev. Neurosci.* 10, 9–22. doi: 10.1038/nrn2495

Nishiyama, A., Watanabe, M., Yang, Z., and Bu, J. (2002). Identity, distribution, and development of polydendrocytes: NG2-expressing glial cells. *J. Neurocytol.* 31, 437–455. doi: 10.1023/A:1025783412651

Nishiyama, A., Yu, M., Drazba, J. A., and Tuohy, V. K. (1997). Normal and reactive NG2+ glial cells are distinct from resting and activated microglia. *J. Neurosci. Res.* 48, 299–312.

Novak, A., Guo, C., Yang, W., Nagy, A., and Lobe, C. G. (2000). Z/EG, a double reporter mouse line that expresses enhanced green fluorescent protein upon Cre-mediated excision. *Genesis* 28, 147–155. doi: 10.1002/1526-968X(200011/12)28:3/4<147::AID-GENE90>3.0.CO;2-G

Nunes, M. C., Roy, N. S., Keyoung, H. M., Goodman, R. R., McKhann, G. 2nd., Jiang, L., et al. (2003). Identification and isolation of multipotential neural progenitor cells from the subcortical white matter of the adult human brain. *Nat. Med.* 9, 439–447. doi: 10.1038/nm837

Ortega, F., Gascon, S., Masserdotti, G., Deshpande, A., Simon, C., Fischer, J., et al. (2013). Oligodendrogliogenic and neurogenic adult subependymal zone neural stem cells constitute distinct lineages and exhibit differential responsiveness to Wnt signalling. *Nat. Cell Biol.* 15, 602–613. doi: 10.1038/ncb2736

Penderis, J., Shields, S. A., and Franklin, R. J. (2003). Impaired remyelination and depletion of oligodendrocyte progenitors does not occur following repeated episodes of focal demyelination in the rat central nervous system. *Brain* 126, 1382–1391. doi: 10.1093/brain/awg126

Penfield, W. (1924). Oligodendroglia and its relation to classic neuroglia. *Brain* 47, 430–452. doi: 10.1093/brain/47.4.430

Peters, A. (2004). A fourth type of neuroglial cell in the adult central nervous system. *J. Neurocytol.* 33, 345–357. doi: 10.1023/B:NEUR.0000044195.64009.27

Philips, T., Bento-Abreu, A., Nonneman, A., Haeck, W., Staats, K., Geelen, V., et al. (2013). Oligodendrocyte dysfunction in the pathogenesis of amyotrophic lateral sclerosis. *Brain* 136, 471–482. doi: 10.1093/brain/aws339

Picard-Riera, N., Decker, L., Delarasse, C., Goude, K., Nait-Oumesmar, B., Liblau, R., et al. (2002). Experimental autoimmune encephalomyelitis mobilizes neural progenitors from the subventricular zone to undergo oligodendrogenesis in adult mice. *Proc. Natl. Acad. Sci. U.S.A.* 99, 13211–13216. doi: 10.1073/pnas.192314199

Platel, J. C., Gordon, V., Heintz, T., and Bordey, A. (2009). GFAP-GFP neural progenitors are antigenically homogeneous and anchored in their enclosed mosaic niche. *Glia* 57, 66–78. doi: 10.1002/glia.20735

Richardson, W. D., Kessaris, N., and Pringle, N. (2006). Oligodendrocyte wars. *Nat. Rev. Neurosci.* 7, 11–18. doi: 10.1038/nrn1826

Richardson, W. D., Young, K. M., Tripathi, R. B., and McKenzie, I. (2011). NG2-glia as multipotent neural stem cells: fact or fantasy? *Neuron* 70, 661–673. doi: 10.1016/j.neuron.2011.05.013

Rivers, L. E., Young, K. M., Rizzi, M., Jamen, F., Psachoulia, K., Wade, A., et al. (2008). PDGFRA/NG2 glia generate myelinating oligodendrocytes and piriform projection neurons in adult mice. *Nat. Neurosci.* 11, 1392–1401. doi: 10.1038/nn.2220

Robins, S. C., Trudel, E., Rotondi, O., Liu, X., Djogo, T., Kryzskaya, D., et al. (2013). Evidence for NG2-glia derived, adult-born functional neurons in the hypothalamus. *PLoS ONE* 8:e78236. doi: 10.1371/journal.pone.0078236

Rowitch, D. H. (2004). Glial specification in the vertebrate neural tube. *Nat. Rev. Neurosci.* 5, 409–419. doi: 10.1038/nrn1389

Roy, N. S., Wang, S., Harrison-Restelli, C., Benraiss, A., Fraser, R. A. R., Gravel, M., et al. (1999). Identification, isolation, and promoter-defined separation of mitotic oligodendrocyte progenitor cells from the adult human subcortical white matter. *J. Neurosci.* 19, 9986–9995.

Seo, J. H., Miyamoto, N., Hayakawa, K., Pham, L. D., Maki, T., Ayata, C., et al. (2013). Oligodendrocyte precursors induce early blood-brain barrier opening after white matter injury. *J. Clin. Invest.* 123, 782–786. doi: 10.1172/JCI65863

Simon, C., Götz, M., and Dimou, L. (2011). Progenitors in the adult cerebral cortex: cell cycle properties and regulation by physiological stimuli and injury. *Glia* 59, 869–881. doi: 10.1002/glia.21156

Taniike, M., Mohri, I., Eguchi, N., Beuckmann, C. T., Suzuki, K., and Urade, Y. (2002). Perineuronal oligodendrocytes protect against neuronal apoptosis through the production of lipocalin-type prostaglandin D synthase in a genetic demyelinating model. *J. Neurosci.* 22, 4885–4896.

Tepavcevic, V., Lazarini, F., Alfaro-Cervello, C., Kerninon, C., Yoshikawa, K., Garcia-Verdugo, J. M., et al. (2011). Inflammation-induced subventricular zone dysfunction leads to olfactory deficits in a targeted mouse model of multiple sclerosis. *J. Clin. Invest.* 121, 4722–4734. doi: 10.1172/JCI59145

Tomassy, G. S., Berger, D. R., Chen, H. H., Kasthuri, N., Hayworth, K. J., Vercelli, A., et al. (2014). Distinct profiles of myelin distribution along single axons of pyramidal neurons in the neocortex. *Science* 344, 319–324. doi: 10.1126/science.1249766

Tripathi, R. B., Rivers, L. E., Young, K. M., Jamen, F., and Richardson, W. D. (2010). NG2 glia generate new oligodendrocytes but few astrocytes in a murine experimental autoimmune encephalomyelitis model of demyelinating disease. *J. Neurosci.* 30, 16383–16390. doi: 10.1523/JNEUROSCI.3411-10.2010

Watanabe, M., Toyama, Y., and Nishiyama, A. (2002). Differentiation of proliferated NG2-positive glial progenitor cells in a remyelinating lesion. *J. Neurosci. Res.* 69, 826–836. doi: 10.1002/jnr.10338

Wennström, M., Hellsten, J., and Tingström, A. (2004). Electroconvulsive seizures induce proliferation of NG2-expressing glial cells in adult rat amygdala. *Biol. Psychiatry* 55, 464–471. doi: 10.1016/j.biopsych.2003.11.011

Wu, J., Yoo, S., Wilcock, D., Lytle, J. M., Leung, P. Y., Colton, C. A., et al. (2010). Interaction of NG2(+) glial progenitors and microglia/macrophages from the injured spinal cord. *Glia* 58, 410–422. doi: 10.1002/glia.20932

Xu, G., Wang, W., and Zhou, M. (2013). Spatial organization of NG2 glial cells and astrocytes in rat hippocampal CA1 region. *Hippocampus* 24, 383–395. doi: 10.1002/hipo.22232

Young, K. M., Psachoulia, K., Tripathi, R. B., Dunn, S. J., Cossell, L., Attwell, D., et al. (2013). Oligodendrocyte dynamics in the healthy adult CNS: evidence for myelin remodeling. *Neuron* 77, 873–885. doi: 10.1016/j.neuron.2013.01.006

Zatorre, R. J., Fields, R. D., and Johansen-Berg, H. (2012). Plasticity in gray and white: neuroimaging changes in brain structure during learning. *Nat. Neurosci.* 15, 528–536. doi: 10.1038/nn.3045

Zhang, R., Chopp, M., and Zhang, Z. G. (2013). Oligodendrogenesis after cerebral ischemia. *Front. Cell. Neurosci.* 7:201. doi: 10.3389/fncel.2013.00201

Zhu, X., Bergles, D. E., and Nishiyama, A. (2008). NG2 cells generate both oligodendrocytes and gray matter astrocytes. *Development* 135, 145–157. doi: 10.1242/dev.004895

Zhu, X., Hill, R. A., Dietrich, D., Komitova, M., Suzuki, R., and Nishiyama, A. (2011). Age-dependent fate and lineage restriction of single NG2 cells. *Development* 138, 745–753. doi: 10.1242/dev.047951

Zhu, X., Zuo, H., Maher, B. J., Serwanski, D. R., LoTurco, J. J., Lu, Q. R., et al. (2012). Olig2-dependent developmental fate switch of NG2 cells. *Development* 139, 2299–2307. doi: 10.1242/dev.078873

6

Bio-inspired hybrid microelectrodes: a hybrid solution to improve long-term performance of chronic intracortical implants

Sara De Faveri[1,2] *, Emma Maggiolini[1], Ermanno Miele[3], Francesco De Angelis[3], Fabrizia Cesca[2], Fabio Benfenati[2,4†] and Luciano Fadiga[1,5†]

[1] *Department of Robotics, Brain and Cognitive Science, Istituto Italiano di Tecnologia, Genova, Italy*
[2] *Department of Neuroscience and Brain Technologies, Istituto Italiano di Tecnologia, Genova, Italy*
[3] *Department of Nanostructures, Istituto Italiano di Tecnologia, Genova, Italy*
[4] *Department of Experimental Medicine, University of Genova, Genova, Italy*
[5] *Section of Human Physiology, University of Ferrara, Ferrara, Italy*

Edited by:
Ulrich G. Hofmann, Albert-Ludwigs-University Freiburg, Germany

Reviewed by:
Christian K. E. Moll, University Clinic Hamburg-Eppendorf, Germany
Jürgen Krüger, University of Freibourg, Germany

***Correspondence:**
Sara De Faveri, Department of Robotics, Brain and Cognitive Science, Istituto Italiano di Tecnologia, via Morego 30, Genova 16163, Italy
e-mail: sara.defaveri@iit.it

[†] Fabio Benfenati and Luciano Fadiga have contributed equally to this work.

The use of implants that allow chronic electrical stimulation and recording in the brain of human patients is currently limited by a series of events that cause the deterioration over time of both the electrode surface and the surrounding tissue. The main reason of failure is the tissue inflammatory reaction that eventually causes neuronal loss and glial encapsulation, resulting in a progressive increase of the electrode-electrolyte impedance. Here, we describe a new method to create bio-inspired electrodes to mimic the mechanical properties and biological composition of the host tissue. This combination has a great potential to increase the implant lifetime by reducing tissue reaction and improving electrical coupling. Our method implies coating the electrode with reprogrammed neural or glial cells encapsulated within a hydrogel layer. We chose fibrin as a hydrogel and primary hippocampal neurons or astrocytes from rat brain as cellular layer. We demonstrate that fibrin coating is highly biocompatible, forms uniform coatings of controllable thickness, does not alter the electrochemical properties of the microelectrode and allows good quality recordings. Moreover, it reduces the amount of host reactive astrocytes – over time – compared to a bare wire and is fully reabsorbed by the surrounding tissue within 7 days after implantation, avoiding the common problem of hydrogels swelling. Both astrocytes and neurons could be successfully grown onto the electrode surface within the fibrin hydrogel without altering the electrochemical properties of the microelectrode. This bio-hybrid device has therefore a good potential to improve the electrical integration at the neuron-electrode interface and support the long-term success of neural prostheses.

Keywords: gliosis, intracortical microelectrodes, fibrin, bio-inspired, *in-vivo*, chronic implants

INTRODUCTION

Patients with various neurological disorders could benefit from the stereotaxic implant of chronic intracerebral microelectrodes to record endogenous activity and/or to electrically stimulate specific brain areas (Donoghue et al., 2007; Larson, 2008; Truccolo et al., 2008; Velliste et al., 2008; Benabid et al., 2009; Normann et al., 2009; Hemm and Wårdell, 2010). To be functional and safe, the implant should keep a stable electric interface with the tissue, enabling an efficient recording and/or activation of neurons over time. However, the long-term functionality of implanted electrodes has been very critical, because of the progressive deterioration of both the electrode surface and the surrounding neural tissue.

Electrode insertion is a traumatic event that induces acute injury to the brain tissue (Polikov et al., 2005; Grill et al., 2009; Marin and Fernández, 2010). The tissue is cut, stretched or compressed by the penetration of the electrode and neurons and glial cells within and around the electrode path are killed or severely injured during insertion. Since the first day of implantation, microglial cells -that are extremely sensitive to even small pathological changes- start to be activated to scavenge damaged neurons and cell debris. Moreover, activated microglia also releases pro-inflammatory cytokines that propagate the inflammatory reaction. The deepening of the electrode into the brain pushes aside the tissue and increases the local pressure of the surrounding tissue. Blood vessels and capillaries are disrupted and the blood–brain barrier is compromised (Bjornsson et al., 2006), leading to plasma extravasation and local edema, that further increase the intracranial pressure (Unterberg et al., 2004).

This initial acute tissue reaction triggers, and is followed by, a more adverse long-term response mainly operated by activated astrocytes that is dependent on the extension of the injury and ends up in the generation of a glial scar, neuronal loss and impairment of the regrowth of neuronal processes (Fawcett and Asher, 1999; Polikov et al., 2005; Grill et al., 2009; Marin and Fernández, 2010). The glial encapsulation surrounding the electrode becomes denser and organized over time pushing away neurons from the tip of the probe (the so-called "kill zone"). This leads to a progressive increase of the electrode-electrolyte impedance and to a deterioration of the recordings. All these events reduce the long-term performance of the electrodes, making the long-term application of this type of technology to human subjects almost unfeasible.

The physical properties of the electrodes such as surface composition, size, shape and stiffness, the mechanical connection between the probe and the recording system, the functionalization of the electrode and the implantation method all have some impact on the intensity of the tissue reaction (Edell et al., 1992). Different approaches have been proposed to solve or reduce the inflammatory reaction. One is the reduction of the electrode size. Minimizing the device footprint is important to reduce the insertion trauma. A smaller device induces a much smaller increase in the local pressure and minimizes tissue displacement (Kozai et al., 2012). However, miniaturization of the electrode worsens its electrochemical characteristics in terms of contact impedance and signal-to-noise ratio (SNR). To circumvent this effect, various groups have used conductive polymers such as poly(3,4-ethylenedioxythiophene, PEDOT) or nanostructured materials (e.g., carbon nanotubes) to reduce the impedance of the recording site (Richardson-Burns et al., 2007; Kim et al., 2010b; Ansaldo et al., 2011; Baranauskas et al., 2011).

Other solutions employing untethered or flexible probes (Rousche et al., 2001; Takeuchi et al., 2005; Kim et al., 2010a; Castagnola et al., 2013; Zhang et al., 2013) have been adopted to decrease the formation of the glial scar. Indeed, when an electrode is tethered to the skull or the device has a different compliance with respect to the adjacent brain tissue, the brain, subject to normal movement induced by respiration and circulation, moves around the probe causing chronic trauma as well as instability of the recording (Kim et al., 2004b; Biran et al., 2007; Thelin et al., 2011).

Approaches aimed at reducing the mechanical mismatch at the interface between the stiff intracortical electrode and the soft brain tissue have been proposed. Intracortical wires were covered with soft materials (Kim et al., 2010b) or with polymeric nano-composite materials that switch from a stiff to a compliant state when inside the cerebral tissue (Harris et al., 2011). The soft coating, matching the host tissue softness, was shown to play an important role in limiting the severity of the inflammatory reaction over time in terms of the amount of reactive astrocytes, neuronal death, and density of active microglial cells around the probe (Harris et al., 2011). The use of hydrogel scaffolds has also been introduced to contrast the consequences due to the inflammatory and immune responses by astrocytes and oligodendrocytes involved in the assembly of the glial scar. Both biologically derived hydrogels (e.g., alginate, Frampton et al., 2011; hyaluronic acid, Hou et al., 2005) and synthetic hydrogels (e.g., polyethylene glycol Bjugstad et al., 2010) have provided promising results in terms of repair and regeneration after surgical implants (Nisbet et al., 2008; Green et al., 2010). Bioactive materials such as L1, growth factors, dextran or laminin, have also been used to functionalize the probe improving its tolerability (He et al., 2006; Klaver and Caplan, 2007; Azemi et al., 2011). Furthermore, cell-coated interfaces were proposed to increase the biocompatibility of the device and minimize the reaction of the host tissue (Purcell et al., 2009; Richter et al., 2011).

Although all the above-mentioned approaches may lead to potentially interesting results, the preservation of the performance of intracortical devices still remains an unresolved issue. To contribute to this challenge, we developed a strategy to improve the biocompatibility of the implant by coating microelectrodes with soft hydrogel and live cells to mimic both the mechanical properties and the biological composition of the host tissue. We used fibrin as hydrogel and either glial cells or neurons to immunologically hide the foreign object to the host tissue. By using such approach we obtained: (i) a strong adhesion of hydrogel and cells to the microelectrode without altering its electrochemical properties; (ii) a small and transient tissue reaction to the implant; and (iii) high quality of electrophysiological recordings.

MATERIALS AND METHODS

IMPLANTABLE WIRES

Quartz-coated metal microelectrodes

Single core quartz-insulated metal microelectrodes (Thomas Recording, Giessen, Germany) were prepared in-house by mechanically grinding 95% platinum, 5% tungsten microwires of 20 μm diameter coated with 30 μm of quartz (see **Figure 1A**). The measured impedance of these electrodes, measured in saline at 1 kHz, was typically between 500 and 700 kΩ (Ansaldo et al., 2011).

This probe was used as a seeding substrate and to evaluate the grip of the hydrogel to the electrode surface during intra-cortical insertion.

Black-lead sticks

Black-lead sticks were 350 μm in diameter and 3 mm long (see **Figure 1B**). The tip was mechanically ground. This probe was used to evaluate the time of hydrogel in-vivo reabsorption and the extent of tissue reaction to the implant without removing it from the brain, thanks to the possibility to cut the stick inserted in the brain with the microtome.

FIBRIN HYDROGEL COATING

Human fibrin (TISSEEL, Baxter, Deerfield, IL, USA) from pooled human plasma was used. It was composed by two sterile components, namely the sealer protein solution (aprotinin and fibrinogen) and thrombin solution (thrombin, $CaCl_2$ and factor XIII). To form a cross-linked fibrin gel, fibrinogen was dipped in the thrombin solution to generate fibrin monomers that were subsequently cross-linked by factor XIII (soluble transglutaminase). Wires were coated by alternate dippings in the two components of the fibrin sealant. The resulting electrode coating was uniform and its thickness was controllable by the number of dippings (Kim et al., 2010b). The radial thickness of the coating was evaluated by measuring the hemi-diameter of the covered probe in five points and subtracting the probe diameter. Thin films of fibrin were prepared by dropping 50 μl of the first component of the fibrin sealant and 50 μl of the second component over sterile glass slides. The drops broadened and they were left drying in air for 15 min in a laminar hood.

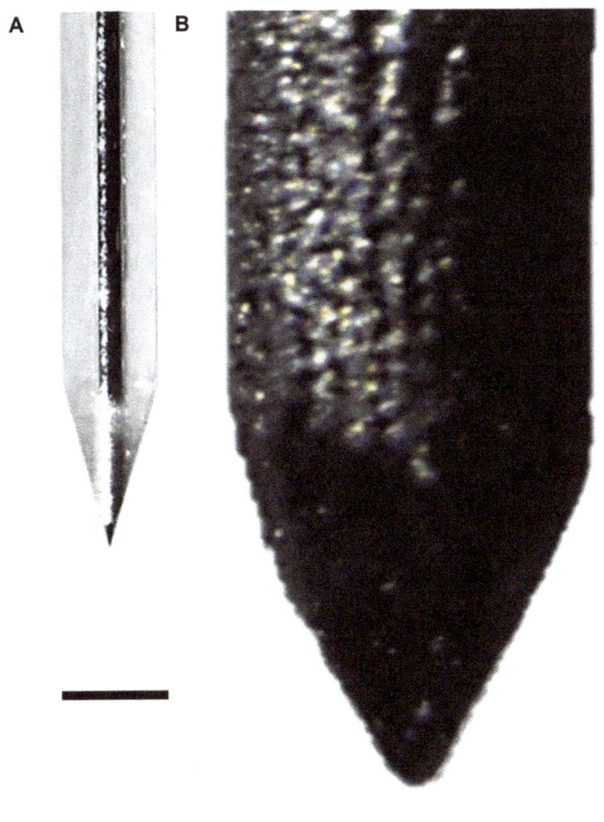

FIGURE 1 | Implantable wires used in this study. (A) Single-core quartz insulated metal microelectrode (Thomas Recording, Giessen, Germany). **(B)** Black-lead wire. Scale bar 100 μm.

EVALUATION OF THE ELECTROCHEMICAL PROPERTIES OF THE FIBRIN-COATED DEVICE

The electrochemical properties of the microelectrode were studied via electrochemical impedance spectroscopy (EIS) in a physiological aqueous solution (NaCl 0.9%). For the measurements, a sine wave (10 mV root mean square amplitude) was superimposed on the open circuit potential while varying the frequency from 1 Hz to 100 kHz. The electrochemical characterization was carried out using a potentiostat/galvanostat/ZRA (Reference 600, Gamry Instruments, Philadelphia, PA, USA) connected to a standard electrochemical cell used in a three-electrode configuration with a platinum counter-electrode (35 mm^2 area) and an Ag/AgCl reference electrode.

MODIFICATION OF THE MICROELECTRODE QUARTZ SURFACE

The roughness of the microelectrode quartz surface was manipulated by using an argon ion plasma etching. Sputter-coated and annealed nanometric gold islands acted as masks for quartz surface milling. The ions hit all the surface, etching both quartz and gold but where quartz was not covered, the generated holes were deeper than where it was covered by gold. The process stopped when all the gold coating was removed. Thanks to this etching, the peak-to-peak average distance was about 500 nm (Goyal et al., 2006).

EXPERIMENTAL ANIMALS

Adult Sprague-Dawley rats (from Charles River, Calco, Italy) and Long-Evans rats (born in house) were used. All experiments were carried out in accordance with the guidelines established by the European Communities Council (Directive 2010/63/EU of September 22nd, 2010), and were approved by the Italian Ministry of Health.

Neurons

Neurons were isolated from E18 rat embryos. Briefly, embryos were removed, placed in cold Hank's balanced salts solution (HBSS) and hippocampi were dissected under sterile conditions. Subsequently, the tissue was enzymatically digested with 0.125% Trypsin for 20 min at 37°C and disaggregated with a pipette. The cells were incubated with 1% Glutamax, penicillin-streptomycin, 2% B-27 supplemented Neurobasal medium in a humidified 5% CO_2 atmosphere at 37°C. Half of the medium was changed every week. All culture media and reagents were from Invitrogen (Milano, Italy).

Glial cells

Glial cells were isolated from the cerebral cortex of P0 rat pups. Cortices were dissected in cold HBSS, broken into small fragments by pipetting and enzymatically digested with 0.25% Trypsin – 1 mg/ml DNase for 15 min at 37°C. After centrifugation at 1200 rpm for 5 min at 8°C, the digestion medium was removed and the pellet was suspended in 10% horse serum, penicillin-streptomycin and 33 mM glucose-supplemented minimum essential medium. Cells were plated in culture flasks and half of the medium was changed every week.

SEEDING OF CELLS OVER THE MICROELECTRODES

Microelectrodes were fixed in a silicon cap by the end opposite to the tip and coated with 0.1% poly-D-lysine, which created a positively charged layer enhancing cell adhesion. Microelectrodes were dipped inside a vial containing the cells suspended in the medium (300000 cells/500 μl). Half of the medium was harvested from a high concentration cell culture, the so-called conditioned medium. The vials were kept in slow and continuous rotation in an incubator (2.31 rpm; relative centrifugal force 0.013 × *g*).

EVALUATION OF THE BIOCOMPATIBILITY OF THE FIBRIN FILM

Approximately 5000 astrocytes or neurons in 100 μl of medium were plated over a thin layer of fibrin. After the cells attached to the surface, the coverslip was covered by culture medium and the cell viability was analyzed at 1, 5, 7, and 11 days. Viability was evaluated by rating the surviving cells over the total number of cells. Samples were incubated for 3 min at room temperature in Ringer-Locke solution containing propidium iodide (PI; Sigma-Aldrich, Milano, Italy; 15 μg/ml), fluorescein diacetate (FDA; Sigma–Aldrich, Milano, Italy; 5 mg/ml) and Hoechst-33342 (Sigma-Aldrich, Milano, Italy; 3.3 μg/ml). After incubation, samples were washed once in Ringer-Locke solution and immediately imaged. At least 15 different fields of view were acquired for each sample. For each field, the ratio of PI-positive cells over the total number of nuclei, identified by Hoechst-33342, was calculated (Limongi et al., 2013).

ANIMAL SURGERY

Male Long Evans rats were anesthetized with a cocktail of Zoletil (Virbac, Carros cedex, France; 30 mg/kg) and Xylazine (Bayer, Leverkusen, Germany; 5 mg/kg) administered intraperitoneally. Their heads were then shaved and swabbed with ethanol. The anesthetized animal was placed in a stereotaxic apparatus (Myneurolab, St Louis, MO, USA). Lacrigel (Farmigea, Pisa, Italy) was distributed over the eyes to avoid dryness. An approximately 2 cm incision was made along the midline of the cranium. The underlying muscle and connective tissue were retracted to expose the skull. A craniotomy (5 mm × 3mm) was made in the parietal bone to expose the somatosensory cortex. Sterile saline was applied during pauses while drilling to help dissipate any local heating and to clean the surfaces. The exposed dura mater was wetted with saline, and carefully incised using surgical micro-scissors. Pia mater was incised too. Implantable wires were lowered perpendicularly through the cortical surface using a hydraulic microdrive (David Kopf Instruments, Tujunga, CA, USA) to 2800 μm from the surface of the brain (layer V). To minimize the variability associated with the surgery, all implants – both quartz-coated metal microelectrodes for acute experiments and black-lead sticks for chronic experiments – were performed by the same subject. During the surgery, the depth of anesthesia was monitored by testing for the absence of hindlimb withdrawal reflex and was maintained by additional doses of anesthetic (i.p. or i.m.), while the rat body temperature was kept at 36–38°C by positioning the animal onto a thermostatic heating pad.

ACUTE NEURAL RECORDING

Acute recordings in layer V of rat cortex were performed to characterize *in vivo* the electrical performance of the fibrin-coated microelectrodes. Recordings were acquired for 20 min using a custom-made, low-power recording system (Bonfanti et al., 2008; Borghi et al., 2008) composed of a compact headstage (amplification gain = 62 dB) and a control unit for data acquisition. Raw traces were band-pass filtered between 3 Hz (first-order Butterworth) and 8 kHz (fourth-order Butterworth). The amplified signals were multiplexed, digitally converted (10-bit, 40 k sample/s) and sent via USB to a PC for subsequent analysis. LabView-based (National Instruments, Austin, TX, USA) acquisition software was used for real-time data visualization and storage. All experimental sessions were conducted inside a Faraday cage to reduce the electromagnetic noise interference.

EVALUATION OF THE SIGNAL-TO-NOISE RATIO

To evaluate the SNR, each acquired trace was high-pass digitally filtered above 300 Hz. The signal was wavelet decomposed and thresholded to 3.5 standard deviations (SD) above and below the mean of the sample distribution to discriminate signal from noise. Waveforms were clustered using Run-Valley seeking sort method (Offline-Sorter; Plexon Inc., Dallas, TX, USA). Signal amplitude was defined as the peak-to-peak amplitude of the mean waveform for each cluster. Noise was defined as two times the calculated rms noise voltage. The SNR was calculated as follows:

$$SNR = \frac{S}{2Vrms_n} \quad (1)$$

where S is the signal amplitude and $Vrms_n$ is the voltage root mean square of the noise. SNR values were sorted into categories (Ludwig et al., 2006, 2009; Abidian et al., 2009; Kim et al., 2010b). Clusters with a SNR greater than 4 were categorized as high-quality units, while clusters with a SNR between 3 and 4 were categorized as moderate units.

IMMUNOHISTOCHEMICAL AND IMMUNOCYTOCHEMICAL TECHNIQUES

Animals were anesthetized and transcardially perfused with cold fixative (2% paraformaldehyde, 1.25% glutaraldehyde, 2% sucrose in phosphate-buffered saline, PBS) 3, 7, and 30 days after the insertion. The brain was removed with the probe in place, fixed for an additional 24 h in the same fixative and then cryoprotected in 30% sucrose solution. Brain horizontal slices were cut (thickness, 50 μm) up to approximately 3 mm of cortical depth. Tissue sections were hydrated in PBS, blocked and permeabilized with 4% goat serum, 2% bovine serum albumin (BSA) and 0.5% Triton X-100 in PBS for 1 h with gentle rocking. Sections were then incubated overnight with primary antibodies against human fibrinogen (1:200; Dako, Milano, Italy) to visualize the presence of fibrin and glial fibrillary acidic protein (GFAP; 1:500; Sigma-Aldrich, Milano, Italy) to visualize reactive glia. The next day, sections were rinsed in PBS and incubated in secondary antibody (1:500; Invitrogen, Milano, Italy) for 3 h. All sections were mounted with ProLong^{TM} Gold Antifade reagent with DAPI (Invitrogen, Milano, Italy) to stain nuclei.

Cultured cells were fixed in cold fixative (2% paraformaldehyde, PFA, 1.25% glutaraldehyde, 2% sucrose in PBS) for 20 min. Cell-coated substrates were rinsed in cold PBS, blocked and permeabilized with 10% goat serum, 2% BSA and 0.5% Triton X-100 in PBS for 1 h with gentle rocking agitation. Samples were later incubated for 90 min with the following primary antibodies in blocking solution: anti-GFAP (1:500; Sigma-Aldrich, Milano, Italy), anti-NeuN (1:500; Millipore, Milano, Italy) and anti-βIII tubulin (1:500; Sigma-Aldrich, Milano, Italy). The seeded microelectrodes were rinsed in PBS and then incubated for 3 h with Alexa-Fluor 633 goat anti-rabbit and Alexa Fluor 488 goat anti-mouse (1:500; Invitrogen, Milano, Italy). All samples were mounted with ProLong^{TM} Gold Antifade reagent with DAPI (Invitrogen, Milano, Italy).

QUANTITATIVE IMMUNOFLUORESCENCE ANALYSES

Images were acquired using an Olympus BX51 fluorescence microscope (Melville, NY, USA) equipped with X-Cite 120 fluorescence illumination system (EXFO, Canada, USA) and with a color digital camera (MBF Bioscience, Williston, VT, USA). Images for the specific antibody were taken by keeping the same exposure time and gain. Fluorescence intensity profiles were obtained by using the custom written MATLAB program MINUTE (Microelectrode INterface Universal Tool for Evaluation; Potter et al., 2012). The mean intensity of fluorescence at discrete distances was compared by one-way repeated measures ANOVA followed by the Bonferroni's *post hoc* test when more than two groups were involved. Significance for all tests was determined at $P < 0.05$.

RESULTS

ELECTROCHEMICAL PROPERTIES AND QUALITY OF THE RECORDINGS OF FIBRIN-COATED MICROELECTRODES

We analyzed the effect of the fibrin layer on the electrical properties of the coated electrode. Coating thickness was progressively increased by dipping the electrode in both fibrinogen and thrombin from 2 to 7 times. **Figure 2A** shows that increasing the fibrin sheath did not significantly affect the electrochemical properties of the microelectrode at 1 kHz, that is the fundamental frequency of neuronal action potentials (Williams et al., 2007) both in terms of impedance modulus (**Figure 2A**) and impedance phase (**Figure 2B**). The lack of alteration of the electrical properties of the electrodes is likely due to the swelling of the hydrogel and to the associated absorption of water and ions from the saline solution that maintain an optimal conductivity (Kim et al., 2004a).

However, once the electrode is implanted in-vivo, the swelling of the fibrin hydrogel coating increases the distance between the tissue and the electrode. Under our conditions, the fibrin coating displayed a smaller swelling than other types of hydrogels, such as alginate (Kong et al., 2004; Kim et al., 2010b) and was controllable in thickness.

To obtain the desired thickness of coating, the following constraints had to be considered: (i) the hydrogel thickness should be less than 100 μm to avoid oxygen deprivation of cells seeded over the probe (Kim et al., 2004a); (ii) the thicker the hydrogel layer, the smaller the gap between the Young modulus of the device and that of the host tissue at the interface; (iii) the thicker the coating, the greater the damage of the host tissue; and, finally, (iv) the swollen hydrogel layer should be thinner than 140 μm to allow activity recordings with high SNR

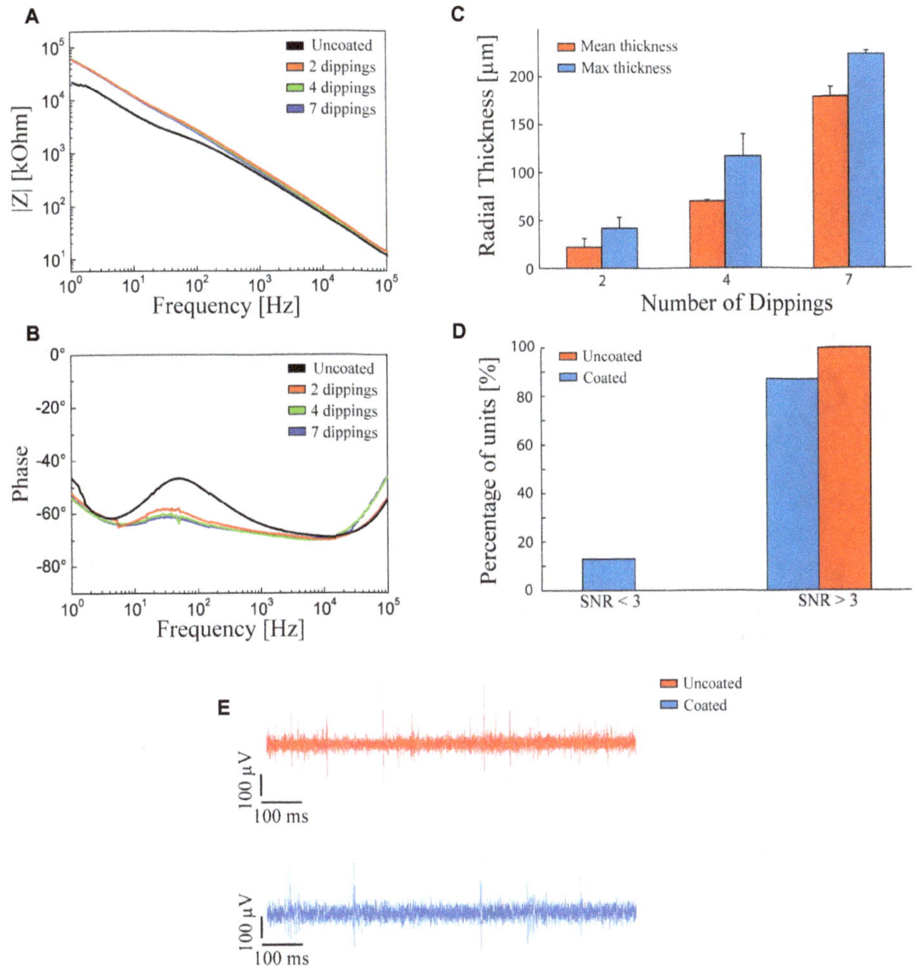

FIGURE 2 | Fibrin coated microelectrodes. (A,B) Electrochemical impedance spectroscopy. Impedance modulus **(A)** and phase **(B)** with respect to the frequency between 1 Hz and 100 kHz. The black line refers to the bare microelectrode. The red, green, and blue lines represent the behavior of fibrin-coated microelectrodes dipped two, four, and seven times into the two sealant components, respectively. **(C)** Thickness of the swollen fibrin coating deposited by two, four, and seven dippings into the two sealant components. Red and blue bars represent the mean and maximum (±SD) radial thickness of the coating, respectively. The procedure with four dippings allowed getting close to the optimal radial thickness of 100 μm, a critical value for the survival of underlying cells and the quality of neural recordings. **(D)** Signal-to-noise ratio in the recordings. Percentage of units with SNR < 3 (poor units), SNR > 3 (moderate or quality units) recorded with uncoated (red bars) and fibrin-coated (blue bars) microelectrodes. **(E)** Examples of recording traces with uncoated (red) and fibrin-coated (blue) microelectrodes. **(D,E)** The measurements were taken immediately after surgery.

(Henze et al., 2000). According to this evaluation, we decided to adopt a thickness of about 100 μm after swelling. **Figure 2C** shows the relationships between the number of dippings of the electrode in the two components of the fibrin sealant and the average and maximum thickness of the coating. Four dippings were found to be optimal to obtain the desired hydrogel thickness.

Recording capabilities of the coated versus non-coated electrodes were evaluated by calculating the SNR of neural waveforms recorded from rat cerebral cortex (see Methods). 85% of the waveforms recorded with fibrin-coated electrodes showed a SNR > 3. This performance is comparable (no statistically significant difference) to that of non-coated microelectrodes (**Figures 2D,E**).

BIOCOMPATIBILITY OF THE FIBRIN LAYER

A viability assay was used to assess the biocompatibility of the fibrin hydrogel deposited as a thin film for primary neurons and glial cells seeded onto the sample. Both astrocytes (**Figure 3A**) and primary neurons (**Figure 3B**) grew well onto the fibrin layer. The assay (**Figures 3C,D**) demonstrated that the viability of both types of cells over time in culture was comparable although, one day after seeding, the mortality of neurons was slightly higher than that of glial cells (86% of surviving glial cells versus 72% of surviving neurons; **Figure 3E**). Viability progressively increased up to 7 days in culture (98% of glial cells versus 95% of neurons; **Figure 3E**) and remained high up to 11 days in culture (95% of glial cells versus 94% of neurons; **Figure 3E**). The extent of viability was in

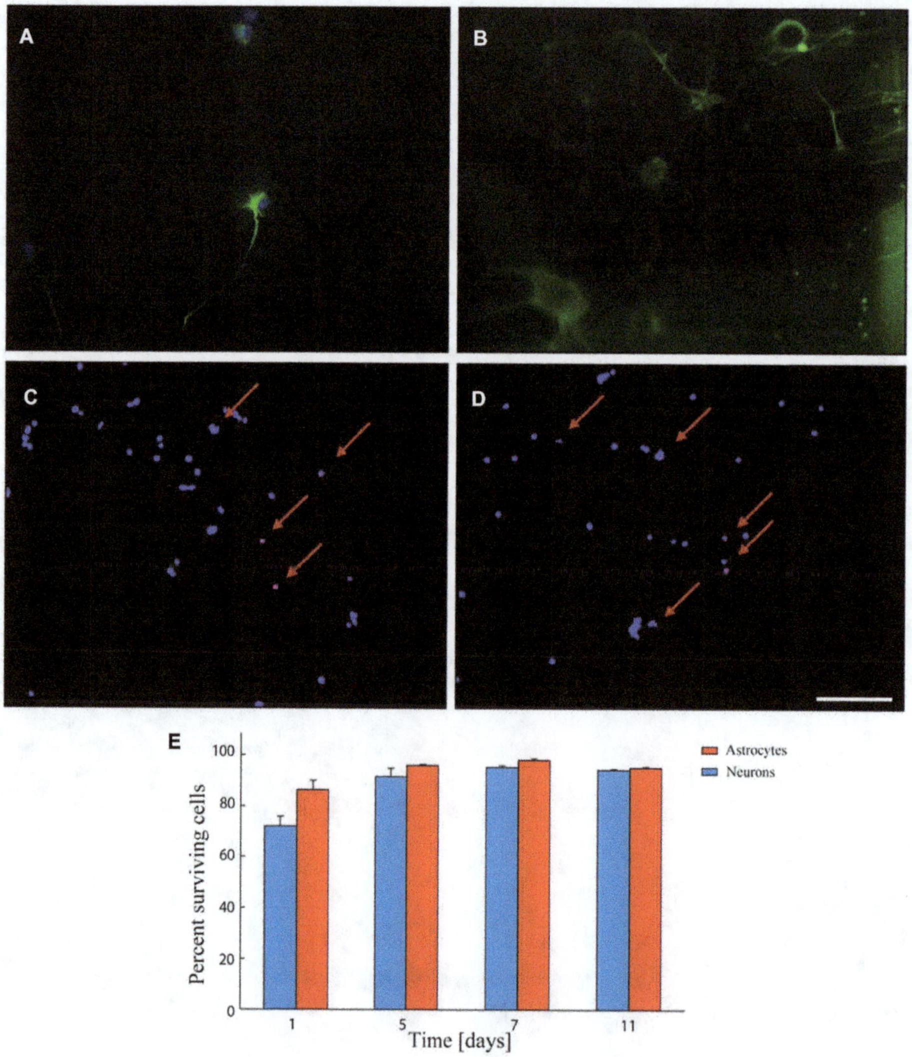

FIGURE 3 | Biocompatibility of the fibrin layer. (A,B) Representative immunofluorescence image of glial cells in fibrin layer **(A)** stained for GFAP (green) and DAPI (blue) and of primary neurons in fibrin layer stained for βIII-tubulin (green; **B**). **(C,D)** Representative images of glial cells **(C)** and primary neurons **(D)** grown in fibrin layer stained with Hoechst (blue-stained nuclei) and propidium iodide (red-stained nuclei). Red arrows indicate the PI-positive nuclei. Scale bar: 50 μm in **A**; 100 μm in **B–D**. **(E)** Quantitative analysis of the viability of primary neurons (blue bars) and astrocytes (red bars) cultured in the presence of fibrin at 1, 5, 7, and 11 days *in vitro*. The percentages of surviving cells (means ± SD) were calculated based on the ratio of total (Hoechst-positive) nuclei minus PI-positive nuclei divided by the total nuclei. Viability values increase and approach the 100% 7 days after seeding.

the same range of that obtained under standard conditions in the absence of the fibrin layer (Ghezzi et al., 2011).

MODIFICATION OF THE MICROELECTRODE SURFACE

The results of the preliminary experiments indicate that the fibrin coating seems to be ideal both in terms of modulation of the coat thickness and biocompatibility for primary cells. However, smoothness of the electrode quartz surface somehow prevented a tight anchorage of the hydrogel to the electrode surface. Thus, during implantation of the electrode into the brain tissue, the fibrin coating (**Figures 4A,B**) could not resist to the shear stress during insertion through the dura mater and detached from the electrode surface in 90% of the cases (**Figures 4C,D**). Also, after the removal of the dura mater, the hydrogel stayed attached to the microelectrode surface only in 40% of the penetrations. As these initial results were poorly reproducible and not sufficiently satisfactory, we etched the quartz surface of the microelectrode to increase its roughness and thereby the grip of the hydrogel to the surface (**Figures 5A,B**). After this treatment, microscopic inspections demonstrated that the fibrin layer was still firmly adherent to the quartz surface in the 100% of cases when the coated microelectrode was inserted and extracted from the somato-sensory cortex deprived of dura mater (**Figures 5C,D**).

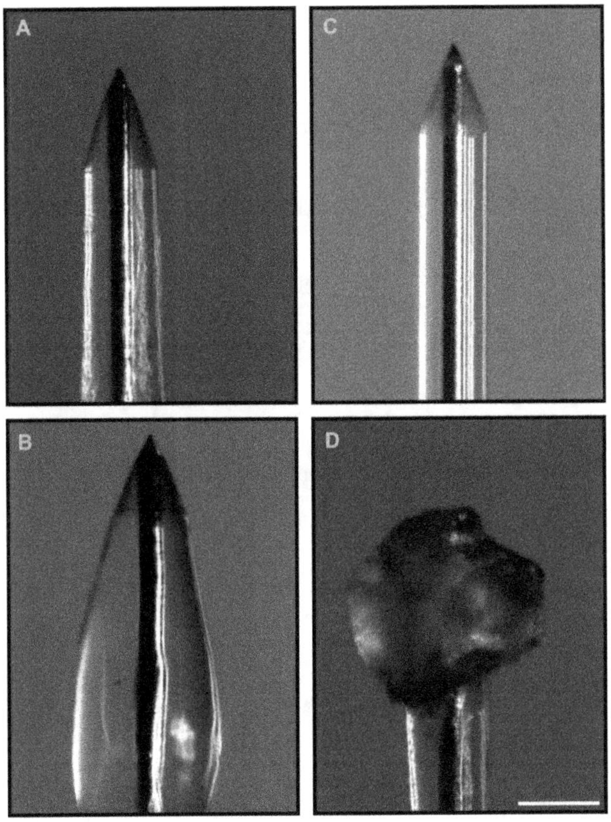

FIGURE 4 | Adhesion of the hydrogel to the microelectrode during the surgical procedure. Optical images of the coated microelectrodes before **(A,B)** and after **(C,D)** the insertion in the brain. Fibrin coating did not resist the shear stress during insertion through the dura mater and detached from the electrode surface in 90% of cases (60% of cases after removal of the dura mater). **(C,D)** Representative images of the adhesion of the hydrogel to the microelectrode before the treatment that increases the microelectrode roughness: during insertion the coating was entirely peeled **(C)** or partially piled up on the tip **(D)**. Scale bar 100 μm.

IN-VIVO REABSORPTION OF THE HYDROGEL AND TISSUE REACTION TO THE COATED ELECTRODE

To evaluate the time of reabsorption of the hydrogel in-vivo and the related tissue reaction, it was necessary to extract the implanted electrode before sectioning. However, during extraction of the implant from the perfused brain, part of the tissue could remain attached to the implant and be distorted or removed together with the probe, thus altering the evaluation of the electrode coating and of the surrounding tissue. To circumvent these problems, we implanted graphite sticks (black-lead rods) that, although thicker than quartz/tungsten microelectrodes, can be easily cut in the microtome, thus allowing to avoid their extraction from the brain before histochemical examination.

Fibrin reabsorption was determined by immunofluorescence after 3, 7, and 30 days from implant (**Figure 6A**). Quantitative analysis of fibrin immunoreactivity as a function of time and distance from the electrode edge (**Figure 6B**) revealed that the intensity of fluorescence steadily decreased in the days immediately after the insertion and that the coating was almost completely reabsorbed, in agreement with previous reports (de Vries et al., 2002). The intensity of the fibrin marker was significantly lower already 7 days after the insertion compared to the values obtained after 3 days, at any distance from the microelectrode edge, up to 90 μm ($P < 0.05$ after 7 days from the insertion; one-way repeated measures ANOVA followed by the Bonferroni's *post hoc* test), while no differences in the extent of fibrin reabsorption were present between 7 and 30 days up to 90 μm from the brain-microelectrode interface.

As astrocytes play a dominant role in the tissue reaction and in the formation of the glial scar, we investigated the glial reaction by monitoring the expression of GFAP around the implantation site. The implant of a bare electrode elicited a strong astrocytic reaction as determined 7 days after the insertion, that became denser and thinner over time, leading to a full encapsulation of the electrode (**Figure 7A**). In contrast, the implant of a fibrin-coated electrode elicited a weaker astrocyte reaction at 7 days, which further decreased to very low levels after 30 days (**Figure 7A**). Quantification of the immunostaining after 7 (**Figure 7B**) and 30 (**Figure 7C**) days as a function of the distance from the electrode-tissue interface revealed that GFAP expression was markedly more pronounced in response to the implant of a bare electrode than that of a fibrin-coated one at both 7 and 30 days post-implant at any distance from the brain-microelectrode interface ($P < 0.05$ after 7 or 30 days of implant; one-way repeated measures ANOVA). In the case of a bare electrode, the peak of GFAP immunoreactivity, localized at 50 μm from the wire-host tissue interface at 7 days became more intense and moved closer to the electrode edge at 30 days (distance: 30 μm). In contrast, in the case of fibrin-coated microelectrodes, the astrocyte reaction in the acute phase (7 days) was milder and evenly distributed around the implant, extending up to 250 μm, while it strongly decreased with time being barely detectable only for 90 μm from the electrode at 30 days.

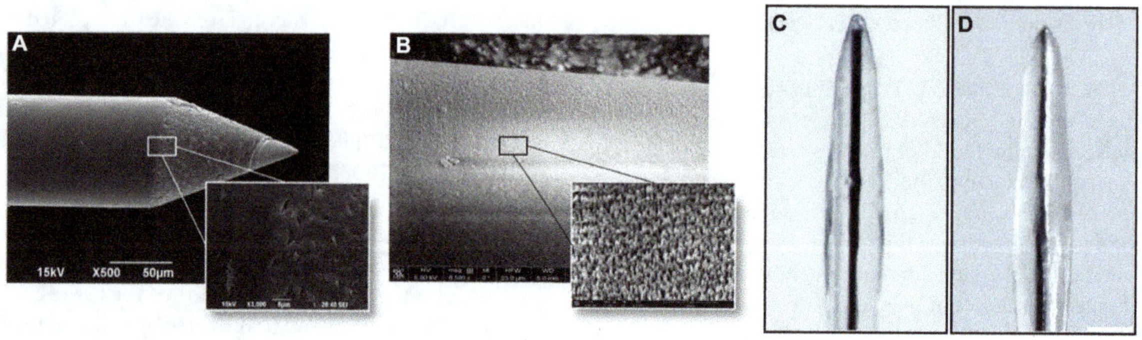

FIGURE 5 | Increase in roughness of the microelectrode surface. **(A)** Scanning electron micrographs of the microelectrodes before the etching treatment. **(B)** Scanning electron micrographs of the microelectrodes after the treatment. Scale bar 50 µm. The obtained peak-to-peak average distance was about 500 nm. **(C,D)** Microelectrodes with increased surface roughness are imaged before **(C)** and after **(D)** the insertion in the cerebral cortex. Coated nanostructured microelectrodes could be effectively inserted in the cerebral cortex deprived of dura mater without any noticeable damage or shift of the coating in the 100% of cases. Scale bar 100 µm.

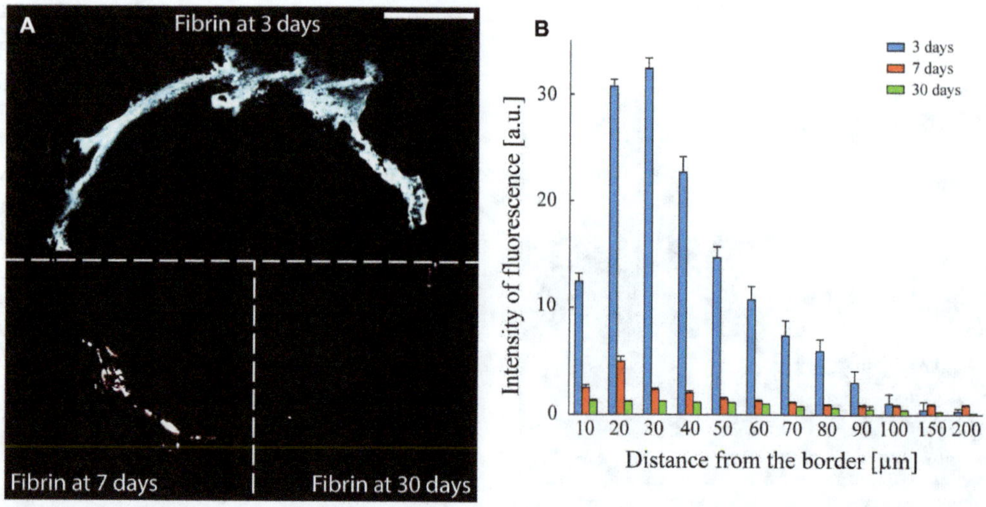

FIGURE 6 | Fibrin reabsorption after implantation. **(A)** Representative images to illustrate the presence of the fibrin over time. The three sectors of the panel represent the three analyzed implant times: 3, 7, and 30 days. Scale bar 100 µm. **(B)** Quantitative evaluation of fibrin immunoreactivity (a.u., arbitrary units; means ± SEM) as a function of distance from the tissue-implant interface after 3 (blue bars), 7 (red bars), and 30 (green bars) days from surgery. An almost complete dissolution of the fibrin hydrogel is already observed after 7 days *in vivo*. One-way repeated measures ANOVA followed by the Bonferroni *post hoc* test; $P < 0.05$ the intensity of fibrin immunoreactivity at 7 or 30 days *versus* 3 days in the distance range 10–90 µm from the implant-tissue interface ($n = 41$, 52, and 58 slices for 3, 7, and 30 days, respectively, from three implants/time point).

COATING MICROELECTRODES WITH CELLS AND FIBRIN HYDROGEL

We next attempted to seed and grow live cells on the electrode surface with the aim of making the artificial device well tolerated by the host tissue after the reabsorption of the fibrin layer. Both primary neurons and glial cells were seeded. The cells seeded with the method illustrated in this paper grew vigorously and formed a uniform compact monolayer on the curved surface of the electrode (**Figure 8A**). Specific staining of primary neurons with either NeuN or βIII-tubulin (**Figure 8B**) and of astrocytes with GFAP (**Figures 8C,D**) revealed that, using conditioned medium, both types of primary cells can grow on the device.

Cells adhered to the microelectrodes were partially stripped during device insertion into the brain (**Figures 9A–D**). Richter et al. (2011) quantified the effects due to the pulling force acting onto a cell layer and demonstrated the abrasion of the adhered cells and a protective role played by fibrin coating. We therefore decided to protect the cell layer by embedding the cells into a fibrin layer which could also increase the mechanical compliance of the inserted microelectrode (**Figures 10A–C**).

Although previous experiments demonstrated that hydrogel coating does not affect the electrochemical properties of the microelectrodes, we repeated these measures with the hybrid cell/hydrogel-coated electrodes, as the cell layer covering the device could alter the current passage. We demonstrated that the combined coating did not significantly affect either the impedance modulus or phase at 1 kHz with respect to uncoated or fibrin-coated electrodes (**Figures 11A,B**).

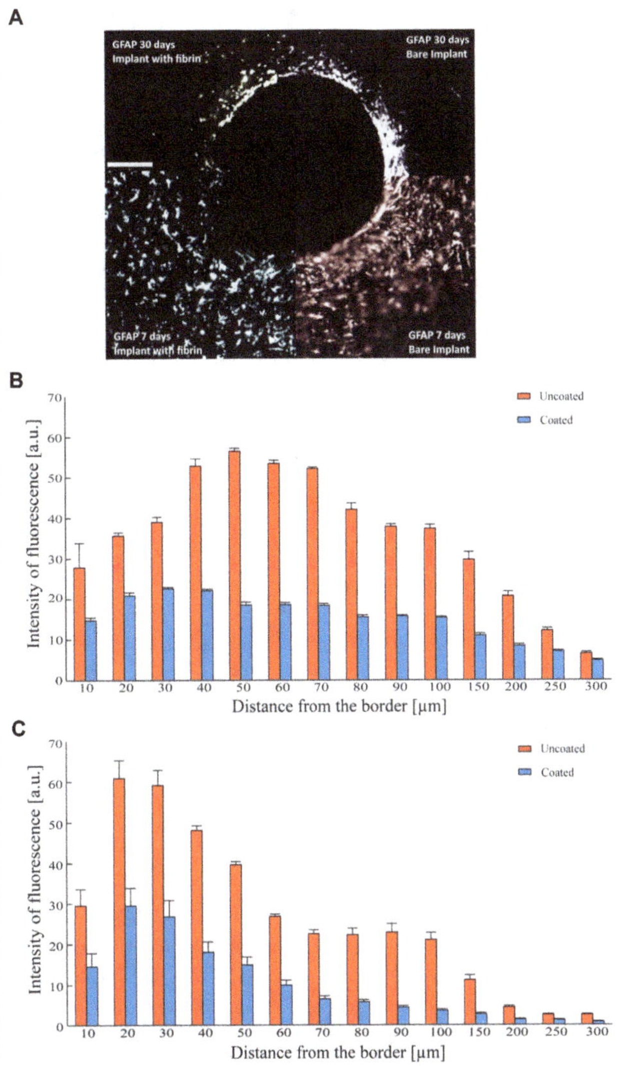

FIGURE 7 | Astrocyte reaction to the implant. (A) Representative images of GFAP immunoreactivity detected 7 (lower quadrants) and 30 days (upper quadrants) after the implant of uncoated (right quadrants) and fibrin-coated (left quadrants) black-lead wires. Scale bar 100 μm. **(B,C)** Analysis of GFAP-positive reactive astrocytes as a function of the distance from the tissue-implant interface. Mean (±SEM) intensity of GFAP immunoreactivity (a.u.) at 7 **(B)** and 30 **(C)** days from the implant. Red and blue bars refer to uncoated and fibrin-coated microelectrodes, respectively. One-way repeated measures ANOVA; $P < 0.05$ coated *versus* uncoated electrodes at all distances for both 7 and 30 days post-implant ($n = 54$ and 58 slices for 7 and 30 days, respectively from 3 implants/time point).

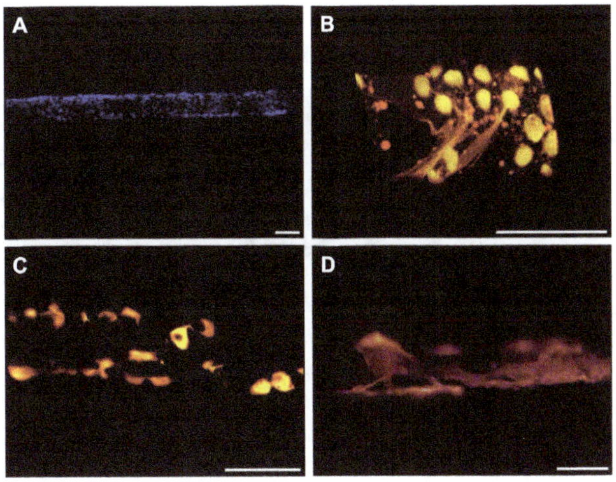

FIGURE 8 | Cell-coated microelectrodes. (A) Representative fluorescent image illustrating the layer of cells adhered to the microelectrode. DAPI staining (blue) reveals cell nuclei. **(B)** Three-dimensional reconstruction of a representative microelectrode coated with neurons. Cells were stained for NeuN (green) and βIII-tubulin (red). **(C,D)** Representative fluorescent images of astrocytes grown on the microelectrode. Cells were stained for GFAP (red) and DAPI (blue). Scale bars 100 μm.

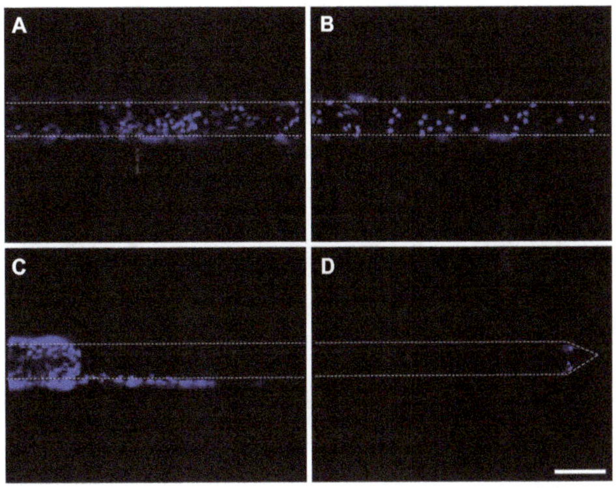

FIGURE 9 | Insertion of cell-coated microelectrodes. (A,B) Representative fluorescent images illustrating the layer of glial cells adhered to a microelectrode. DAPI staining (blue) reveals cell nuclei. The cell-coated microelectrode was inserted 2 mm in depth and the images were acquired from the non-inserted segment of the probe. **(C,D)** Representative fluorescent images of the same microelectrode, illustrating the effects of the insertion of the probe on the adhered glial cells (images acquired along the wire from the inserted segment of the wire). DAPI staining (blue) reveals cell nuclei. Scale bar 100 μm. Dot lines point out the microelectrode shape.

DISCUSSION

The aim of this study was to realize a bio-inspired hybrid device. We developed a strategy to improve the biocompatibility of microelectrodes mimicking the properties of the host tissue in order to increase the biocompatibility over time. To this aim, we modified the device surface to decrease the tissue reaction against the implant and thus increase the working life of the intra-cortical implant. The two main goals we achieved were: (i) to minimize the mechanical difference between the rigid microelectrode shaft and the soft and expanding-retracting brain tissue and (ii) to coat the electrode with a live and tissue-friendly autologous cell layer to improve the tissue tolerance to the foreign body. These aims were obtained by coating the microelectrode with a soft layer of fibrin hydrogel and by coupling it with a layer of living cells (either astrocytes or neurons). While both coatings did not alter the electrochemical properties of the electrode, the combination

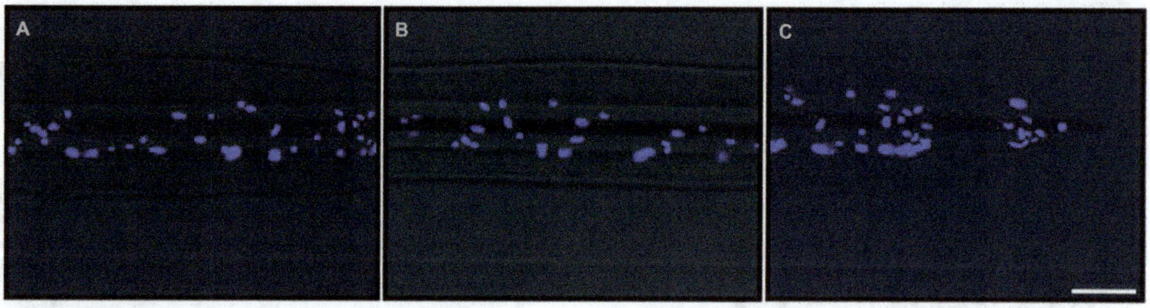

FIGURE 10 | Double-coating of microelectrodes with astrocytes and fibrin hydrogel. Representative images of the final prototype of the bio-inspired hybrid microelectrode: 3 mm far from the tip **(A)**, 1.5 mm far from the tip **(B)** and the tip **(C)**. Fluorescence images (DAPI staining of neuronal nuclei) were merged with the optical image of the microelectrode. The images revealed the microelectrode structure, the fibrin hydrogel sheath surrounding it and the layer of glial cells embedded within the hydrogel. Scale bar 100 μm.

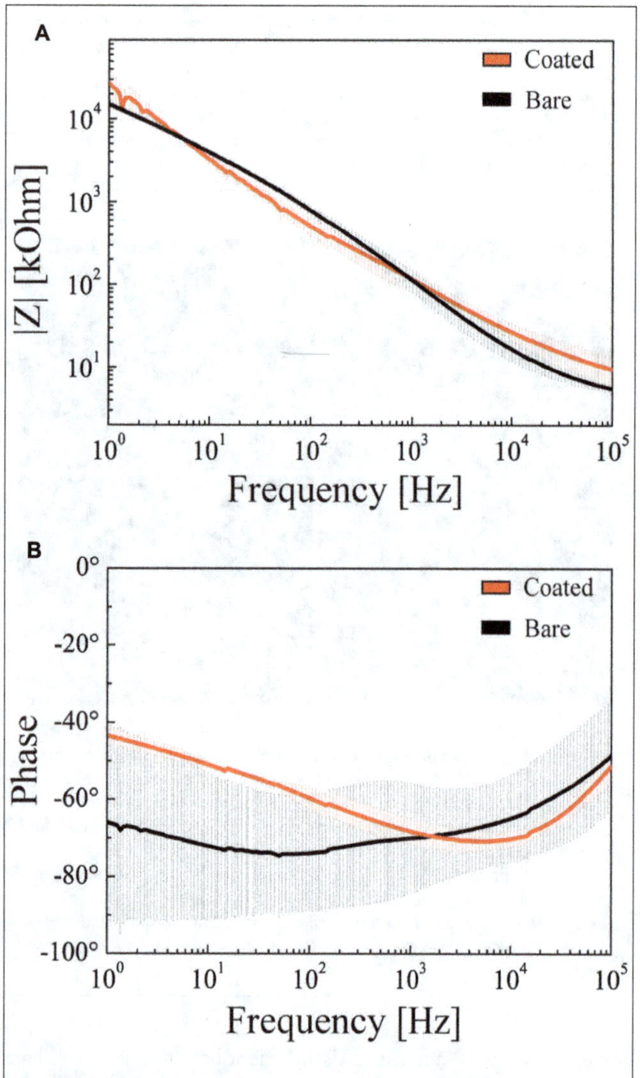

FIGURE 11 | Electrochemical properties of double-coated microelectrodes. Impedance modulus **(A)** and phase **(B)** as a function of the frequency in the 1 Hz–100 kHz range (mean ± SD). Black and red lines refer to the bare microelectrode and to the microelectrode coated with glial cells and hydrogel, respectively.

of the two seems particularly advantageous. In fact, the hydrogel minimizes the continuous trauma due to the different compliance of the electrode and the brain tissue and, at the same time, protects the cell layer from the stress due to the device insertion inside the brain. This can prevent the typical foreign body-dependent inflammation that ends up with a glial scar encapsulating and electrically insulating the device.

The thickness of the soft coating turned out to be a key point. In fact, while the compliance increases with the thickness of the hydrogel, the coating should not be too thick to allow for oxygen supply to the cells seeded on the probe and reliable extracellular recordings of spike activity over the background noise. Another important point is that hydrogels swell when immersed in a saline solution such as the extracellular fluid, and swelling *per se* can compress the surrounding tissue and increase the distance between the brain and the recording site. To comply with these requirements, we exploited fibrin as a hydrogel for the following reasons: (i) coating thickness can be precisely controlled by the number of dippings during the deposition procedure; (ii) it does not affect the electrochemical properties of the microelectrode; (iii) it allows a good quality of recordings (85% of the fibrin-coated electrodes recorded high-quality brain signals with SNR > 3); and (iv) its swelling is moderate with respect to other types of hydrogel (i.e., alginate swelling is such that the recording from target neurons is prevented; Kim et al., 2010b).

Biocompatibility of the fibrin hydrogel was also an important issue. We demonstrated that fibrin coating markedly reduces the extent of astrocyte reaction at both 7 and 30 days after the implant, compared to the bare wire. The astrocyte activation following the implantation of coated wires is more diffuse and less intense, yielding to a significant lesser extent of glial scar and device encapsulation.

Another advantage of the fibrin hydrogel besides its biocompatibility is the progressive, almost complete enzymatic degradation by the host tissue over time. While the hydrogel thickness is an important issue to prevent acute reactions, the progressive degradation does not pose limitations for chronic recordings. While the soft fibrin layer is reabsorbed, cells seeded onto the electrode surface might have integrated with the host tissue both by exchange of extracellular messengers (such as growth factors or neurotransmitters) and by growth of processes and establishment of new connections. Thus, after the disappearance of the fibrin hydrogel, the electrode could already be interfaced and well tolerated by the host tissue.

Another important point was to verify the integrity of the coating upon insertion of the device into the tissue. The shear stress of insertion not only had critical consequences on the unprotected cell coating of the electrode, but was also effective, in a large percentage of cases, in stripping the fibrin hydrogel from the smooth surface of the electrode. We set-up a treatment to increase the roughness of the quartz electrode surface, achieving a better grip for both the cell layer and the fibrin sheath.

Our study has demonstrated the possibility to produce tissue-friendly microelectrodes well-tolerated and functional over time. This is fundamental to realize electrodes for chronic recordings. Additionally, the use of materials that can be withdrawn directly from the individual patient before the implant is a fundamental approach to reduce the immunoreaction to the minimum. Our solution, using fibrin and cells fulfills both these requirements. The fibrin precursor, fibrinogen, can be easily extracted from the patient's blood. Neurons and glial cells can be reprogrammed from patient's fibroblasts either from iPS cell clones or, more safely, by direct reprogramming. The latter procedure has been successfully obtained for dopaminergic neurons (Broccoli et al., 2011; Caiazzo et al., 2011).

CONCLUSIONS

The properties of the tissue-electrode interface, including electrical and mechanical integration, are crucial in determining long-term reliability and functionality of neural implants. The major problems of chronic neural prostheses are the immune and inflammatory tissue responses that occur after device implantation. This causes a significant increase of the electric impedance because of the growth of a dense fibrous sheath. Additionally, target neurons are pushed away by the scar so that the electrode becomes isolated from the surrounding tissue.

In this work, we developed a new method to control the biological response to electrode implantation and promote a more efficient integration of implanted microelectrodes. We developed a bio-inspired hybrid probe obtained with the seeding of a compact sheath of cells encapsulated in a thin re-absorbable fibrin layer and demonstrated that such a device is biocompatible, does not alter the electrochemical properties of the electrode, allows recordings of good quality and markedly reduces the tissue inflammatory reaction. This device has therefore a good potential to improve the electrical integration at the neuron-electrode interface and support the long-term success of neural prostheses.

ACKNOWLEDGMENTS

The study was supported by research grants from the Italian Ministry of University and Research (PRIN to Fabio Benfenati and Luciano Fadiga) and from the EU grants FP7-NMP-2013-EU-China "NEUROSCAFFOLDS"(Grant Agreement No: NMP3-SL-2013-604263; to Fabio Benfenati).

REFERENCES

Abidian, M. R., Ludwig, K. A., Marzullo, T. C., Martin, D. C., and Kipke, D. R. (2009). Interfacing conducting polymer nanotubes with the central nervous system: chronic neural recording using poly(3,4-ethylenedioxythiophene) nanotubes. *Adv. Mater.* 21, 3764–3770. doi: 10.1002/adma.200900887

Ansaldo, A., Castagnola, E., Maggiolini, E., Fadiga, L., and Ricci, D. (2011). Superior electrochemical performance of carbon nanotubes directly grown on sharp microelectrodes. *ACS Nano* 5, 2206–2214. doi: 10.1021/nn103445d

Azemi, E., Lagenaur, C. F., and Cui, X. T. (2011). The surface immobilization of the neural adhesion molecule L1 on neural probes and its effect on neuronal density and gliosis at the probe/tissue interface. *Biomaterials* 32, 681–692. doi: 10.1016/j.biomaterials.2010.09.033

Baranauskas, G., Maggiolini, E., Castagnola, E., Ansaldo, A., Mazzoni, A., Angotzi, G. N., et al. (2011). Carbon nanotube composite coating of neural microelectrodes preferentially improves the multiunit signal-to-noise ratio. *J. Neural Eng.* 8:066013. doi: 10.1088/1741-2560/8/6/066013

Benabid, A. L., Chabardes, S., Mitrofanis, J., and Pollak, P. (2009). Deep brain stimulation of the subthalamic nucleus for the treatment of Parkinson's disease. *Lancet Neurol.* 8, 67–81. doi: 10.1016/S1474-4422(08)70291-6

Biran, R., Martin, D. C., and Tresco, P. A. (2007). The brain tissue response to implanted silicon microelectrode arrays is increased when the device is tethered to the skull. *J. Biomed. Mater. Res. A* 82, 169–178. doi: 10.1002/jbm.a

Bjornsson, C. S., Oh, S. J., Al-Kofahi, Y. A., Lim, Y. J., Smith, K. L., Turner, J. N., et al. (2006). Effects of insertion conditions on tissue strain and vascular damage during neuroprosthetic device insertion. *J. Neural Eng.* 3:196–207. doi: 10.1088/1741-2560/3/3/002

Bjugstad, K. B., Lampe, K., Kern, D. S., and Mahoney, M. (2010). Biocompatibility of poly(ethylene glycol)-based hydrogels in the brain: an analysis of the glial response across space and time. *J. Biomed. Mat. Res. A* 95, 79–91. doi: 10.1002/jbm.a.32809

Bonfanti, A., Borghi, T., Gusmeroli, R., Zambra, G., Spinelli, A. S., Oliynyk, A., et al. (2008). "A Low-power integrated circuit for analog spike detection and sorting in neural prosthesis systems," in *Proceedings of the Biomedical Circuits and Systems Conference, 2008* (Baltimore: IEEE), 257–260. doi: 10.1109/BIOCAS.2008.4696923

Borghi, T., Bonfanti, A., Gusmeroli, R., Zambra, G., and Spinelli, A. S. (2008). A power-efficient analog integrated circuit for amplification and detection of neural signals. *Conf. Proc. IEEE Eng. Med. Biol. Soc.* 2008, 4911–4915. doi: 10.1109/IEMBS.2008.4650315

Broccoli, V., Caiazzo, M., and Dell'Anno, M. T. (2011). Setting a highway for converting skin into neurons. *J. Mol. Cell Biol.* 3, 322–323. doi: 10.1093/jmcb/mjr029

Caiazzo, M., Dell'Anno, M. T., Dvoretskova, E., Lazarevic, D., Taverna, S., Leo, D., et al. (2011). Direct generation of functional dopaminergic neurons from mouse and human fibroblasts. *Nature* 476, 224–227. doi: 10.1038/nature10284

Castagnola, E., Maiolo, L., Maggiolini, E., Minotti, A., Marrani, M., Maita, F., et al. (2013). "Ultra-flexible and brain-conformable micro-electrocorticography device with low impedance PEDOT-carbon nanotube coated microelectrodes," in *Proceedings of the Sixth Annual International IEEE EMBS Conference on Neural Engineering*, San Diego, CA, 6–8.

de Vries, J., Menovsky, T., van Gulik, S., and Wesseling, P. (2002). Histological effects of fibrin glue on nervous tissue: a safety study in rats. *Surg. Neurol.* 57, 415–422. doi: 10.1016/S0090-3019(02)00736-X

Donoghue, J. P., Nurmikko, A., Black, M., and Hochberg, L. R. (2007). Assistive technology and robotic control using motor cortex ensemble-based neural interface systems in humans with tetraplegia. *J. Physiol.* 579(Pt 3), 603–611. doi: 10.1113/jphysiol.2006.127209

Edell, D. J., Toi, V. V., McNeil, V. M., and Clark, L. D. (1992). Factors influencing the biocompatibility of insertable silicon microshafts in cerebral cortex. *IEEE Trans. Biomed. Eng.* 39, 635–643. doi: 10.1109/10.141202

Fawcett, J. W., and Asher, R. A. (1999). The glial scar and central nervous system repair. *Brain Res. Bull.* 49, 377–391. doi: 10.1016/S0361-9230(99)00072-6

Frampton, J. P., Hynd, M. R., Shuler, M. L., and Shain, W. (2011). Fabrication and optimization of alginate hydrogel constructs for use in 3D neural cell culture. *Biomed. Mater.* 6:015002. doi: 10.1088/1748-6041/6/1/015002

Ghezzi, D., Antognazza, M. R., Dal Maschio, M., Lanzarini, E., Benfenati, F., and Lanzani, G. (2011). A hybrid bioorganic interface for neuronal photoactivation. *Nat. Commun.* 2, 166. doi: 10.1038/ncomms1164

Goyal, A., Hood, V., and Tadigadapa, S. (2006). "High speed anisotropic etching of quartz using SF6/C4F8/Ar/O2 based chemistry in inductively coupled plasma reactive ion etching system," in *Proceedings of SPIE, the International Society for Optical Engineering*, eds D. M. Tanner and R. Ramesham (San Jose, CA: Society of Photo-Optical Instrumentation Engineers), 61110. doi: 10.1117/12.657730

Green, R. A., Baek, S., Poole-Warren, L. A., and Martens, P. J. (2010). Conducting polymer-hydrogels for medical electrode applications. *Sci. Technol. Adv. Mater.* 11, 014107. doi: 10.1088/1468-6996/11/1/014107

Grill, W. M., Norman, S. E., and Bellamkonda, R. V. (2009). Implanted neural interfaces: biochallenges and engineered solutions. *Annu. Rev. Biomed. Eng.* 11, 1–24. doi: 10.1146/annurev-bioeng-061008-124927

Harris, J. P., Capadona, J. R., Miller, R. H., Healy, B. C., Shanmuganathan, K., Rowan, S. J., et al. (2011). Mechanically adaptive intracortical implants improve the proximity of neuronal cell bodies. *J. Neural Eng.* 8:066011. doi: 10.1088/1741-2560/8/6/066011

He, W., McConnell, G. C., and Bellamkonda, R. V. (2006). Nanoscale laminin coating modulates cortical scarring response around implanted silicon microelectrode arrays. *J. Neural Eng.* 3, 316–326. doi: 10.1088/1741-2560/3/4/009

Hemm, S., and Wårdell, K. (2010). Stereotactic implantation of deep brain stimulation electrodes: a review of technical systems, methods and emerging tools. *Med. Biol. Eng. Comput.* 48, 611–624. doi: 10.1007/s11517-010-0633-y

Henze, D. A., Borhegyi, Z., Csicsvari, J., Mamiya, A., Harris, K. D., and Buzsáki, G. (2000). Intracellular features predicted by extracellular recordings in the hippocampus *in vivo*. *J. Neurophysiol.* 84, 390–400.

Hou, S., Xu, Q., Tian, W., Cui, F., Cai, Q., Ma, J., et al. (2005). The repair of brain lesion by implantation of hyaluronic acid hydrogels modified with laminin. *J. Neurosci. Methods* 148, 60–70. doi: 10.1016/j.jneumeth.2005.04.016

Kim, D. H., Abidian, M., and Martin, D. C. (2004a). Conducting polymers grown in hydrogel scaffolds coated on neural prosthetic devices. *J. Biomed. Mater. Res. A* 71, 577–585. doi: 10.1002/jbm.a.30124

Kim, Y. T., Hitchcock, R. W., Bridge, M. J., and Tresco, P. A. (2004b). Chronic response of adult rat brain tissue to implants anchored to the skull. *Biomaterials* 25, 2229–2237. doi: 10.1016/j.biomaterials.2003.09.010

Kim, D. H., Viventi, J., Amsden, J. J., Xiao, J., Vigeland, L., Kim, Y. S., et al. (2010a). Dissolvable films of silk fibroin for ultrathin conformal bio-integrated electronics. *Nat. Mater.* 9, 511–517. doi: 10.1038/nmat2745

Kim, D. H., Wiler, J. A., Anderson, D. J., Kipke, D. R., and Martin, D. C. (2010b). Conducting polymers on hydrogel-coated neural electrode provide sensitive neural recordings in auditory cortex. *Acta Biomater.* 6, 57–62. doi: 10.1016/j.actbio.2009.07.034

Klaver, C. L., and Caplan, M. R. (2007). Bioactive surface for neural electrodes: decreasing astrocyte proliferation via transforming growth factor-beta1. *J. Biomed. Mat. Res. A* 81, 1011–1016. doi: 10.1002/jbm.a.31153

Kong, H. J., Kaigler, D., Kim, K., and Mooney, D. J. (2004). Controlling rigidity and degradation of alginate hydrogels via molecular weight distribution. *Biomacromolecules* 5, 1720–1727. doi: 10.1021/bm049879r

Kozai, T. D. Y., Langhals, N. B., Patel, P. R., Deng, X., Zhang, H., Smith, K. L., et al. (2012). Ultrasmall implantable composite microelectrodes with bioactive surfaces for chronic neural interfaces. *Nat. Mater.* 11, 1065–1073. doi: 10.1038/nmat3468

Larson, P. S. (2008). Deep brain stimulation for psychiatric disorders. *Neurotherapeutics* 5, 50–58. doi: 10.1016/j.nurt.2007.11.006

Limongi, T., Cesca, F., Gentile, F., Marotta, R., Ruffilli, R., Barberis, A., et al. (2013). Nanostructured superhydrophobic substrates trigger the development of 3D neuronal networks. *Small* 9:402–412. doi: 10.1002/smll.201201377

Ludwig, K. A., Miriani, R. M., Langhals, N. B., Joseph, M. D., Anderson, D. J., and Kipke, D. R. (2009). Using a common average reference to improve cortical neuron recordings from microelectrode arrays. *J. Neurophysiol.* 101, 1679–1689. doi: 10.1152/jn.90989.2008

Ludwig, K. A., Uram, J. D., Yang, J., Martin, D. C., and Kipke, D. R. (2006). Chronic neural recordings using silicon microelectrode arrays electrochemically deposited with a poly(3,4-ethylenedioxythiophene) (PEDOT) film. *J. Neural Eng.* 3:59–70. doi: 10.1088/1741-2560/3/1/007

Marin, C., and Fernández, E. (2010). Biocompatibility of intracortical microelectrodes: current status and future prospects. *Front. Neuroeng.* 3:1–6. doi: 10.3389/fneng.2010.00008

Nisbet, D. R., Crompton, K. E., Horne, M. K., Finkelstein, D. I., and Forsythe, J. S. (2008). Neural tissue engineering of the CNS using hydrogels. *J. Biomed. Mater. Res. B Appl. Biomater.* 87, 251–263. doi: 10.1002/jbm.b.31000

Normann, R. A., Greger, B., Greger, B. A., House, P., Romero, S. F., Pelayo, F., et al. (2009). Toward the development of a cortically based visual neuroprosthesis. *J. Neural Eng.* 6:035001. doi: 10.1088/1741-2560/6/3/035001

Polikov, V. S., Tresco, P. A., and Reichert, W. M. (2005). Response of brain tissue to chronically implanted neural electrodes. *J. Neurosci. Methods* 148, 1–18. doi: 10.1016/j.jneumeth.2005.08.015

Potter, K. A., Simon, J. S., Velagapudi, B., and Capadona, J. R. (2012). Reduction of autofluorescence at the microelectrode-cortical tissue interface improves antibody detection. *J. Neurosci. Methods* 203, 96–105. doi: 10.1016/j.jneumeth.2011.09.024

Purcell, E. K., Seymour, J. P., Yandamuri, S., and Kipke, D. R. (2009). *In vivo* evaluation of a neural stem cell-seeded prosthesis. *J. Neural Eng.* 6:026005. doi: 10.1088/1741-2560/6/2/026005

Richardson-Burns, S. M., Hendricks, J. L., and Martin, D. C. (2007). Electrochemical polymerization of conducting polymers in living neural tissue. *J. Neural Eng.* 4:L6–L13. doi: 10.1088/1741-2560/4/2/L02

Richter, A., Kruse, C., Moser, A., Hofmann, U. G., and Danner, S. (2011). Cellular modulation of polymeric device surfaces: promise of adult stem cells for neuro-prosthetics. *Front. Neurosci.* 5:1–10. doi: 10.3389/fnins.2011.00114

Rousche, P. J., Pellinen, D. S., Pivin, D. P., Williams, J. C., Vetter, R. J., and Kipke, D. R. (2001). Flexible polyimide-based intracortical electrode arrays with bioactive capability. *IEEE Trans. Biomed. Eng.* 48, 361–371. doi: 10.1109/10.914800

Takeuchi, S., Ziegler, D., Yoshida, Y., Mabuchi, K., and Suzuki, T. (2005). Parylene flexible neural probes integrated with microfluidic channels. *Lab Chip* 5, 519–523. doi: 10.1039/b417497f

Thelin, J., Jörntell, H., Psouni, E., Garwicz, M., Schouenborg, J., Danielsen, N., et al. (2011). Implant size and fixation mode strongly influence tissue reactions in the CNS. *PLoS ONE* 6:e16267. doi: 10.1371/journal.pone.0016267

Truccolo, W., Friehs, G. M., Donoghue, J. P., and Hochberg, L. R. (2008). Primary motor cortex tuning to intended movement kinematics in humans with tetraplegia. *J. Neurosci.* 28, 1163–1178. doi: 10.1523/JNEUROSCI.4415-07.2008

Unterberg, A. W., Stover, J., Kress, B., and Kiening, K. L. (2004). Edema and brain trauma. *Neuroscience* 129, 1021–1029. doi: 10.1016/j.neuroscience.2004.06.046

Velliste, M., Perel, S., Spalding, M. C., Whitford, A. S., and Schwartz, A. B. (2008). Cortical control of a prosthetic arm for self-feeding. *Nature* 453, 1098–1101. doi: 10.1038/nature06996

Williams, J. C., Hippensteel, J. A., Dilgen, J., Shain, W., and Kipke, D. R. (2007). Complex impedance spectroscopy for monitoring tissue responses to inserted neural implants. *J. Neural Eng.* 4:410–423. doi: 10.1088/1741-2560/4/4/007

Zhang, H., Patel, P. R., Xie, Z., Swanson, S. D., Wang, X., and Kotov, N. A. (2013). Tissue-compliant neural implants from microfabricated carbon nanotube multilayer composite. *ACS Nano* 7, 7619–7629. doi: 10.1021/nn402074y

New insights into the role of histamine in subventricular zone-olfactory bulb neurogenesis

Maria F. Eiriz[1], Jorge Valero[1], João O. Malva[2] and Liliana Bernardino[3]*

[1] Center for Neuroscience and Cell Biology of Coimbra, University of Coimbra (CNC-UC), Coimbra, Portugal
[2] Faculty of Medicine, Institute of Biomedical Imaging and Life Sciences (IBILI), University of Coimbra, Coimbra, Portugal
[3] Faculty of Health Sciences, Health Sciences Research Center, University of Beira Interior, Covilhã, Portugal

Edited by:
Luca Bonfanti, University of Turin, Italy

Reviewed by:
Joanne C. Conover, University of Connecticut, USA
Carlos Vicario-Abejón, Instituto Cajal, Consejo Superior de Investigaciones Científicas (CSIC), Spain

***Correspondence:**
Liliana Bernardino, Health Sciences Research Center, University of Beira Interior, Av. Infante D. Henrique, 6200-506 Covilhã, Portugal
e-mail: libernardino@gmail.com

The subventricular zone (SVZ) contains neural stem cells (NSCs) that generate new neurons throughout life. Many brain diseases stimulate NSCs proliferation, neuronal differentiation and homing of these newborns cells into damaged regions. However, complete cell replacement has never been fully achieved. Hence, the identification of proneurogenic factors crucial for stem cell-based therapies will have an impact in brain repair. Histamine, a neurotransmitter and immune mediator, has been recently described to modulate proliferation and commitment of NSCs. Histamine levels are increased in the brain parenchyma and at the cerebrospinal fluid (CSF) upon inflammation and brain injury, thus being able to modulate neurogenesis. Herein, we add new data showing that *in vivo* administration of histamine in the lateral ventricles has a potent proneurogenic effect, increasing the production of new neuroblasts in the SVZ that ultimately reach the olfactory bulb (OB). This report emphasizes the multidimensional effects of histamine in the modulation of NSCs dynamics and sheds light into the promising therapeutic role of histamine for brain regenerative medicine.

Keywords: subventricular zone, olfactory bulb, neural stem cells, histamine, neurogenesis

INTRODUCTION

Brain diseases represent a very demanding worldwide health challenge. Nevertheless, no effective cure exists for the majority of these disorders. The discovery of NSCs in restricted regions of the adult brain redefined it as a plastic organ. Thus, the search for new drug candidates that may enhance stem cells properties and a full knowledge of NSCs biology are crucial to fulfil the actual healthcare and scientific demands.

NSCs reside in two niches of the adult brain: the SVZ lining the lateral ventricles and the subgranular zone (SGZ) in the dentate gyrus (DG) of the hippocampus. Newly born neurons generated in the SGZ migrate short distances toward the granular cell layer, whereas SVZ-derived neuroblasts migrate long distances through the rostral migratory stream (RMS) toward the OB (Eiriz et al., 2011). Interestingly, upon brain injury, some neuroblasts can leave the SVZ/RMS axis to migrate toward damaged areas and differentiate into the specific neuronal/glial phenotype of the injured region. Therefore, a great effort has been taken on the design of stem cells-based strategies to promote brain repair (Ruan et al., 2014). For that purpose it is crucial to identify new factors that can enhance NSCs capabilities to produce new neurons. Herein, we comment on recent data supporting the role of histamine as a robust proneurogenic factor *in vivo* and we also discuss the profits vs. challenges for its usage in stem cell-based brain repair therapies.

GENERAL ROLE OF HISTAMINE IN THE CENTRAL NERVOUS SYSTEM

Histamine is an amine that has been classically associated with peripheral inflammatory reactions (Dale and Laidlaw, 1910). However, new evidences also highlight its function as a neuromodulator and neuroinflammatory agent. Four receptors mediate the effects driven by histamine: two postsynaptic (H1R, H2R), one presynaptic (H3R), and a forth receptor mainly present in the immune system (H4R). All receptors belong to the family of rhodopsin-like class A receptors coupled to guanine nucleotide-binding proteins (Brown et al., 2001). Neurons, microglia and mast cells are the three cellular reservoirs of histamine in the adult brain (Brown et al., 2001; Katoh et al., 2001). Histaminergic neurons, present in the tuberomammillary nucleus, project numerous ramifications throughout the entire adult brain, allowing histamine to be involved in a broad range of physiological functions, such as sleep-wake control, emotions, learning and memory (Panula and Nuutinen, 2013). Histamine is found at nanomolar levels in the healthy brain (Soya et al., 2008; Croyal et al., 2011; Bourgogne et al., 2012). However, several brain pathological conditions may be associated with an increased degranulation of mast cells in the *choroid plexus*, leading to a massive release of histamine in the CSF and the consequent increase of the blood brain barrier (BBB) permeability. Histaminergic neuronal activity (analyzed by positron emission tomography) was also found to be increased in the lesioned brain parenchyma (Vizuete et al., 2000; Motoki et al., 2005; Yanai and Tashiro, 2007; Kallweit et al., 2013). Importantly, histamine has been described to be involved in several brain pathologies such as seizures (Bhowmik et al., 2012), stroke (Fan et al., 2011), multiple sclerosis (Ballerini et al., 2013; Krementsov et al., 2013), Parkinson and Alzheimer's disease (Shan et al., 2013). Remarkably, histamine may have a dual role and exert either neuroprotective or neurotoxic effects depending on the animal disease model, the receptor/signaling pathway activated and the diversity of histamine and histamine agonists/antagonists administration protocols. A clinically relevant therapeutic platform should take in account all of these distinct criteria, to be successful. Regarding neurogenesis, and although a recent review (Panula et al., 2014) highlights the role of histamine as a stem cell modulator during brain development, very few research studies on the role of histamine as a proneurogenic factor within the postnatal and adult brain were reported.

HISTAMINE EFFECTS ON NEURAL STEM CELL CULTURES

It is currently clear that histamine is involved in several brain functions but just recently its role as a modulator of stem cell biology has been revealed. We and others have shown that histamine transiently increases intracellular free calcium levels ($[Ca^{2+}]_i$) in SVZ stem/progenitor cells, embryonic stem cells and carcinoma cells (Tran et al., 2004; Agasse et al., 2008), suggesting the presence of functional histamine receptors in undifferentiated stem/progenitor cells. Particularly, we found that SVZ cells express the three types of histamine receptors, H1R, H2R, and H3R, being H1R the one responsible for the selective increase of $[Ca^{2+}]_i$ in immature cells (Agasse et al., 2008).

Recently, it was shown that histamine has a strong proneurogenic effect in neonatal SVZ (Bernardino et al., 2012) and in embryonic cortical cell cultures (Molina-Hernández and Velasco, 2008; Rodríguez-Martínez et al., 2012; Molina-Hernández et al., 2013) *via* H1R activation. Histamine may trigger increased transcription of FGFR1 and increased cell proliferation culminating in the differentiation of FOXP2 neuronal cells both *in vitro* and *in vivo* (Rodríguez-Martínez et al., 2012; Molina-Hernández et al., 2013) (**Figure S1A**). We also showed that histamine induces an increase of the expression of Mash1, Dlx2 and Ngn1 proneurogenic genes and ultimately favors the GABAergic neuronal phenotype. Thus, histamine may be used as an efficient inductor of neuronal differentiation *in vitro* prior NSCs transplantation. In fact, SVZ cells pretreated with poly(lactic-*co*-glycolic) acid (PLGA) microparticles that release histamine succeeded to survive, integrate and differentiate into newly born doublecortin (DCX)-neurons when transplanted into organotypic hippocampal slice cultures and into the DG or striatum of adult mice (Bernardino et al., 2012). Altogether, these data showed that histamine may be a key player in the priming of NSCs toward the neuronal phenotype.

ROLE OF HISTAMINE IN THE ADULT SVZ NEUROGENIC NICHE *IN VIVO*

Despite the absence of *in vivo* studies disclosing the role of histamine in the regulation of the SVZ neurogenic niche, *in vitro* studies have already shown that SVZ NSCs express functional H1R receptors that may be involved in neuronal commitment (Agasse et al., 2008; Bernardino et al., 2012). The relevance of investigating the effects of histamine on SVZ neurogenesis *in vivo* relies on the fact that both inflammation or brain injury may elicit *choroid plexus* mast cells degranulation, increasing the levels of histamine in the CSF and brain parenchyma leading to increased BBB permeability (Anichtchik et al., 2000; Yoshitake et al., 2003; Soya et al., 2008; Kanbayashi et al., 2009; Kallweit et al., 2013). The presence of histamine in the CSF that baths the SVZ neurogenic niche may affect SVZ GFAP-positive stem cells (type B cells) and its progeny *in vivo* by the direct contact of their cilia with the lumen of the lateral ventricles or by the interaction of stem/progenitor cells with the monolayer of ependymal cells (paracrine effect). Interestingly, it was observed that histamine is part of the adult mouse *choroid plexus* transcriptome signature (Marques et al., 2011). Taking into account these considerations, herein we disclose the role of chronic histamine administration in the adult SVZ neurogenic niche *in vivo*. For that, sustained intraventricular infusion of histamine was performed by using mini osmotic pumps that delivered histamine at the CSF for 21 days. All experiments were performed in accordance with the European Community guidelines for the care and use of laboratory animals (86/609/EEC; 2010/63/EU). Weight matched wild-type C57BL/6 8-10 week old male mice were infused at the right lateral ventricle (Anterior-posterior: −0.5 mm, Medial-lateral: 0.7 mm, Dorso-ventral: 3.0 mm) with osmotic mini pumps (Alzet 1004, Charles River, flow rate: 0.10 μl/h) containing histamine (0.8 mg/Kg, Sigma-Aldrich) dissolved in artificial cerebrospinal fluid (aCSF: 150 mM NaCl, 3 mM KCl, 1.3 mM $CaCl_2$, 0.8 mM $MgCl_2$, 0.8 mM Na_2HPO_4, and 0.2 mM NaH_2PO_4) or aCSF alone, as vehicle for 21 days. To ensure stable releasing rates, pumps were incubated before implantation in sterile 0.9% saline at 37°C for 48 h. During the first 3 days after surgery, 50 mg/Kg BrdU was administered intraperitoneally twice a day (**Figure 1A**). After brain fixation in 4% PFA and cryopreservation in 30% sucrose, 40 μm coronal slices were then cut and stained against Ki67, BrdU, DCX, and NeuN (1:1000 Rabbit polyclonal anti-Ki67—Abcam; 1:1000 Rat monoclonal anti-BrdU—Serotec; 1:1000 Rabbit polyclonal anti-DCX—BD Pharmingen; 1:4000 Mouse monoclonal anti-NeuN—Millipore). Sections were then rinsed and incubated with the appropriate AlexaFluor-conjugated secondary antibodies, stained for Hoechst-33342 and mounted. Confocal digital images were obtained on a LSM 510 Meta; Carl Zeiss microscope. The Software used was Axiovision, release 4.6 (Carl Zeiss) and Image J. Cell counting was performed in confocal images from five slices at 240 μm intervals, both at the SVZ and OB. Only counts performed in the contralateral hemispheres (left) are shown in order to exclude any possible bias induced by inflammatory reactions and/or lesion due to the cannulation at the ipsilateral hemisphere (right).

We found that the intracerebroventricular (i.c.v.) infusion of histamine in the lateral ventricles for 21 days induced a trend increase in the number of BrdU retaining cells (BrdU+DCX−) at the SVZ (Control: 25.8 ± 2.7; Histamine: 34.4 ± 4.7; statistically not-significant). This increase is statistically significant if we consider the BrdU+DCX+ double positive cells (Control: 4.6 ± 0.4; Histamine: 10.1 ± 1.9; $p < 0.05$; **Figure S1B** and **Figures 1B,C**). Accordingly, the number of DCX+ cells increased from 67.6 ± 3.9 in control to 129.1 ± 7.9 in histamine treated mice ($p < 0.001$, **Figure 1C**). No significant differences were found in counts of

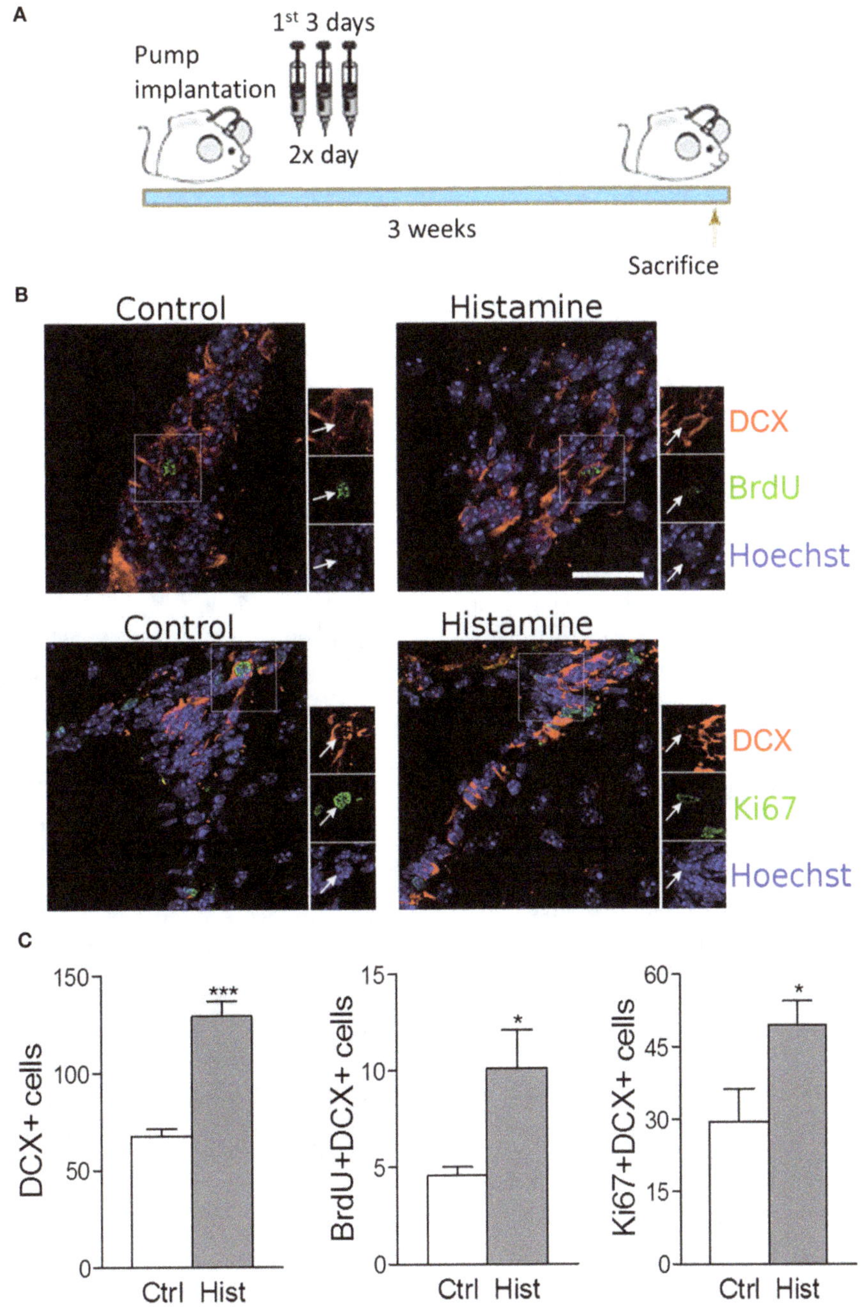

FIGURE 1 | Intracerebroventricular infusion of histamine triggers neuronal commitment in the SVZ. (A) Design of the 3 weeks experiment, consisting in 3-day BrdU treatment (twice daily with 12 h interval) starting at the day after surgery. Animals were sacrificed 3 weeks after surgery. **(B)** Representative fluorescent confocal digital images of BrdU (green; upper panel), Ki67 (green; lower panel) and DCX (red) positive cells observed in the SVZ of control and histamine treated animals *in vivo*, 21 days after pump installation. Scale bar = 20 μm. Arrows highlight double BrdU+DCX+ (upper panel) or Ki67+DCX+ (lower panel) positive cells. Hoechst staining (blue) labels cell nuclei. **(C)** From left to right: bargraphs represent the total DCX+ positive cells, total BrdU+DCX+ double positive cells and total Ki67+DCX+ double positive cells in both control and histamine *in vivo* treated animals, 21 days after pump installation. Ctrl: Control; Hist: Histamine. Data are expressed as mean ± SEM ($n = 5$–7 mice; $^{*}p < 0.05$; $^{***}p < 0.001$). Statistical analysis was performed using Student's unpaired *t*-test.

BrdU+DCX− and BrdU+DCX+ cells between both ipsilateral and contralateral hemispheres (regarding the same experimental condition) and, most importantly, both hemispheres showed the same relative differences between control and histamine treated animals (data not shown), excluding a putative influence of inflammation and/or tissue damage in the ipsilateral hemisphere. These data confirms previous *in vitro* data identifying histamine as a relevant inductor of neuronal commitment.

Curiously, some BrdU+DCX+ cells were retained at the SVZ 21 days upon histamine i.c.v. administration. We may hypothesize that this BrdU+DCX+ cell population at SVZ is derived from BrdU retaining cells, such as quiescent NSCs (B cells) that produce intermediate highly proliferating progenitor cells (C cells). Thus, further studies are also needed to disclose whether this increase of neuroblasts (A cells, BrdU+DCX+ cells) production induced by histamine is due to the activation of B cells which contact with CSF through their apical cilia, or by an increase in the proliferation of C or/and A cells.

Since histamine induced an increase in the number of BrdU+DCX+ cells at the SVZ, we then performed the Ki67 labeling to disclose if histamine had an effect in neuroblast proliferation. Ki67 is a cell marker associated with G1, G2, S and M phases of cell cycle. At the SVZ, Ki67 labelling showed a trend to increase upon histamine treatment (Control: 86.2 ± 24.6; Histamine: 133.0 ± 19.5; statistically not-significant) that was significant when looking to Ki67+DCX+ cells only (Control: 29.4 ± 6.8; Histamine: 49.3 ± 5.0; $p < 0.05$; **Figure S1B,** and **Figures 1B,C**). Interestingly, histamine increased the number of BrdU+DCX+ and Ki67+DCX+ cells but did not significantly affected the population of BrdU+DCX− or Ki67+DCX− cells. Altogether, these data indicate that histamine does not induce an overall increase of cell proliferation in the SVZ, but instead may trigger neuronal commitment (as previously showed by us—Bernardino et al., 2012) and/or induce neuroblast proliferation as previously reported (Rodríguez-Martínez et al., 2012; Molina-Hernández et al., 2013).

We also found that SVZ NSCs labelled with BrdU have differentiated into migrating neuroblasts that reached the OB in control and more densely in histamine treated animals (**Figure S1B,** and **Figure 2**). An increased number of BrdU+DCX+ cells was found in both the granular cell layer (GCL) and glomerular layers (GL) of the OB (Control GCL: 60.0 ± 3.5; Histamine GCL: 117.7 ± 7.4, $p < 0.001$; Control GL: 2.2 ± 0.2; Histamine GL: 5.5 ± 1.0, $p < 0.05$; **Figures 2A,C**). A significant increase of the DCX+ cells was also found in the GCL upon histamine infusion (Control GCL: 583.3 ± 11.5; Histamine GCL: 798.4 ± 33.0, $p < 0.001$; Control GL: 86.0 ± 7.1; Histamine GL: 117.3 ± 12.1; **Figure 2B**). In accordance with the SVZ data, the total number of BrdU+DCX− cells was not significantly different between control and histamine-treated animals in either OB layers (Control GCL: 286.0 ± 29.0; Histamine GCL: 362.6 ± 34.0; Control GL 22.5 ± 5.4; Histamine GL: 33.4 ± 5.3; statistically not-significant). Moreover, Ki67 labeling was almost inexistent at the OB (data not shown). These data may suggest that histamine is not interfering with the overall OB cell proliferation, but, instead, it increases the number of neuroblasts that reach the OB and, therefore, the final population of newly-generated OB neurons (**Figure S1B**). Additionally, some BrdU+ cells found at GL and GCL of control and histamine-treated animals generated NeuN-mature neurons (**Figure 2D**).

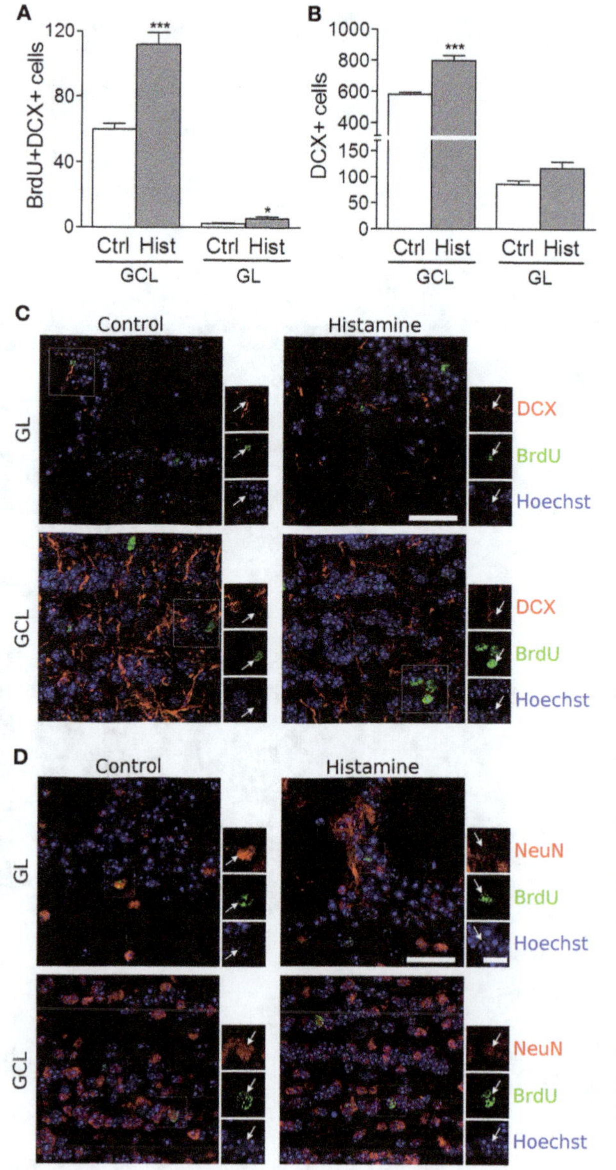

FIGURE 2 | Olfactory bulb integration of newly differentiated neuroblasts upon histamine long-term treatment. Bargraphs represent the total BrdU+DCX+ cells **(A)** and total DCX+ positive cells **(B)** counted in the granular cell layer (GCL) and in the glomerular layer (GL). Ctrl, Control; Hist, Histamine. Data are expressed as mean ± SEM (n = 5–7 mice; $^*p < 0.05$; $^{***}p < 0.001$). Statistical analysis was performed using Student's unpaired t-test. Representative fluorescent confocal digital images of BrdU (green) and DCX (red; **C**) or NeuN (red; **D**) positive cells observed in the granule cell layer (GCL) and glomerular layer (GL) of control and histamine treated animals *in vivo*, 21 days after pump installation. White arrows point to double positive BrdU+DCX+ **(C)** or BrdU+NeuN+ **(D)** cells. Hoechst staining (blue) labels cell nuclei. Scale bars = 30 μm.

In fact, histamine is responsible for the priming of NSCs at the SVZ toward the neuronal phenotype, which ultimately will reach the OB. The SVZ-derived progenitor cells are committed to the GCL and GL of the OB, where they differentiate mainly into GABAergic (Bédard and Parent, 2004; De Marchis et al., 2004) but also glutamatergic (Brill et al., 2009) and dopaminergic interneurons (Saino-Saito et al., 2004). Although we do not know the neuronal phenotypes generated by DCX+ neuroblasts found in the OB, we do know that, as expected, the majority of them differentiate into SVZ-derived cells located at the GCL instead of the GL, a structure that mostly contains GABAergic interneurons. Accordingly, we found that histamine induces GABAergic neuronal differentiation in murine SVZ stem cell cultures (Bernardino et al., 2012). Furthermore, the morphology and disposition of DCX+ cells in the GCL and GL of the OB suggest that they are indeed young granule and periglomerular cells (Merkle et al., 2007).

Taken together, our data reveals that histamine is a crucial modulator of neuronal differentiation at the SVZ-OB neurogenic axis. However, we may anticipate some obstacles in using histamine to boost intrinsic regenerative properties of endogenous NSCs. Histamine was also shown to modulate the growth and specification of several cancer types, including gliomas. Increased activity of histidine decarboxylase (HDC), the enzyme involved in histamine synthesis, was found at the surrounding extracellular space of several cancer types, which is suggestive that it may be a crucial factor involved in tumorigenesis. Experiments performed in malignant cell lines and experimental tumors *in vivo* suggest that histamine modulates diverse biological responses related to tumor growth, such as proliferation, survival, and modulation of inflammation and angiogenesis (Eiriz et al., 2014). We could postulate that histamine have the ability to deregulate NSCs dynamics favouring proliferation and boosting the appearance of cancer stem cells especially nearby the neurogenic niches. However, some contradictory reports showed that histamine does not modulate cancer cell proliferation and instead induce their differentiation. Previously, we have shown that histamine does not support proliferation of SVZ stem/progenitor cells *in vitro* (Bernardino et al., 2012). Herein, we showed that the i.c.v. administration of histamine does not induce a significant increase in the total number of BrdU+DCX- or Ki67+DCX- cells at the SVZ, suggesting that, at least after 21 days, histamine does not induce a cancer-like profile of SVZ NSCs cells *in vivo*.

Another limiting factor responsible for the intrinsic difficulties of endogenous brain repair therapies relies on exacerbated inflammatory reactions occurring upon brain lesion that may create a hostile environment for the survival of neural stem/progenitors and neuroblasts. Microglia cells are the main cellular players involved in the innate immune response against brain injury or infection. Microglia phenotypes vary among neurogenic and non-neurogenic regions (Goings et al., 2006) and it may modulate SVZ neurogenesis (Shigemoto-Mogami et al., 2014). In this sense, we recently showed that histamine *per se* stimulates microglia motility and interleukin-1 beta release *via* H4R activation (Ferreira et al., 2012). But, on the other side, in an inflammatory context, histamine inhibited LPS-stimulated microglia activation *via* the same receptor. This dual role of histamine mediating microglial inflammatory responses highlights the need for further studies on the immunomodulatory effects of histamine within neurogenic niches. Increased levels of histamine found upon injury or inflammation can influence the overall cellular micro-environment, including mast cells, ependyma, neurons and microglia, favouring (or not) the survival, proliferation, and differentiation of new cells. This may depend on histamine levels and its distinct actions on different cellular populations present at SVZ-OB neurogenic niches vs. lesioned brain regions.

Recently, Kallweit et al. (2013) have shown that histamine is increased in the CSF of multiple sclerosis patients. In this line, and although we do not show a clear lack of effect of histamine in other neural cell types, such as oligodendrocytes or astrocytes, we have previously shown that histamine did not change NG2 or GFAP expression within the SVZ *in vitro* (Bernardino et al., 2012). Still, more detailed analysis of the effects induced by histamine at the neurogenic niche *in vivo* needs to be accomplished for further therapeutically relevant conclusions.

Upon brain injury, normal cellular dynamics is disturbed and NSCs are de-routed from their quiescent undifferentiated state to an active proliferative state so that new NSCs differentiate into neuroblasts that migrate to the damaged area (Kaneko and Sawamoto, 2009; Grade et al., 2013). Brain repair therapies involving the administration of proneurogenic factors (e.g., histamine) to boost endogenous mobilization of these neuronal precursors is less aggressive than the transplantation of NSCs, but requires a full control of the external booster in order to achieve a fine-tune of the endogenous resources. Alternatively, the transplantation of exogenous stem cells, or stem cell-based progenies at various stages of maturation (e.g., neuroblasts), to replace lost neurons, also raise several limitations, including the possible death of transplanted cells, low number of cells typically available for therapy, inadequate cell differentiation, erroneous cell integration into the host circuitry, immune rejection and variability in the functional outcome of the transplanted cells. Therefore, it is imperative to take in consideration these limitations (endogenous sources vs. exogenous transplantation) to find new effective platforms aiming the repair of damaged brain regions.

Neurogenesis occurring at the SVZ is well documented in rodents, and has also been demonstrated in primates and humans. However, both the cellular organization and the physiologic mechanisms involved on NSCs biology are distinct among these species. The SVZ NSCs found in the human brain younger than 18 months of age actively produce neurons which fate is the OB and the prefrontal cortex (Sanai et al., 2011). However, despite several controversies, a recent report showed that during adulthood human SVZ-derived NSCs lose the ability to migrate toward the OB and, instead, are found in the striatum (Ernst et al., 2014). Importantly, SVZ stem cells extracted from the adult human brain retain the capacities to produce neurons *in vitro*, suggesting that neurogenesis in the SVZ may be boosted under proper stimulation. In fact, several reports showed an increase of striatal neurogenesis in postmortem brains of Huntington disease and stroke patients (Curtis et al., 2003; Macas et al., 2006; Martí-Fàbregas et al., 2010). With our experimental protocol we showed that histamine increased the generation of newly-born neurons at the SVZ that ultimately migrate toward the OB. Thus, differences between human and mouse SVZ niches should be taken in consideration before extrapolating the proneurogenic effect of histamine found in mouse SVZ-OB axis to the potential application in human brain repair strategies. Further studies should disclose whether histamine may also boost neurogenesis under a pathologic condition, such as ischemia, eventually inducing the migration of SVZ-neuroblasts toward the lesioned striatum. Thus, in spite of the potential bottlenecks in triggering an efficient endogenous brain repair, we may asset that histamine efficiently prime NSCs toward the neuronal phenotype, a phenomenon that may support its application in future brain regenerative medicine therapies.

AUTHOR CONTRIBUTIONS

Maria F. Eiriz: Conception and design; Collection and assembly of data; Data analysis and interpretation; Manuscript writing. Jorge Valero: Conception and design; Collection and assembly of data; Data analysis and interpretation, Manuscript writing. João O. Malva: Conception and design; Provision of study material; Data analysis and interpretation; Administrative support; Critical reading of manuscript. Liliana Bernardino: Conception and design; Provision of study material; Data analysis and interpretation; Financial support; Administrative support; Manuscript writing; Final approval of manuscript.

ACKNOWLEDGMENTS

The work was funded by Fundação para a Ciência e Tecnologia (FCT)—Portugal projects PTDC/SAU-NEU/104415/2008, Fundação Calouste Gulbenkian (project n° 96542) and by L'Oréal-UNESCO Portugal for Women in Science. Maria F. Eiriz was supported by fellowship SFRH/BD/42848/2008, Liliana Bernardino was supported by fellowship SFRH/BPD/34841/2007, all from FCT. Maria Francisca Eiriz acknowledge the MIT-Portugal Program, focus in Bio-engineering Systems. The authors acknowledge Cristina Soares from the animal facility of the CNC-UC for her help with the animal care. We also acknowledge Tiago Santos for the graphical design of the Figures.

SUPPLEMENTARY MATERIAL

Figure S1 | Integrative scheme of the effects driven by histamine in stem/progenitor cells both *in vitro* and *in vivo*. (A) Histamine has been reported to modulate both neuronal differentiation and cell proliferation in diverse types of stem/progenitor cells cultures. Red cells: neurons; Yellow cells: progenitor cells; Blue cell: stem cell. **(B)** Our *in vivo* results showed that histamine increases the number of neuroblasts at the SVZ that reach the OB.

REFERENCES

Agasse, F., Bernardino, L., Silva, B., Ferreira, R., Grade, S., and Malva, J. O. (2008). Response to histamine allows the functional identification of neuronal progenitors, neurons, astrocytes, and immature cells in subventricular zone cell cultures. *Rejuven. Res.* 11, 187–200. doi: 10.1089/rej.2007.0600

Anichtchik, O. V., Rinne, J. O., Kalimo, H., and Panula, P. (2000). An altered histaminergic innervation of the substantia nigra in Parkinson's disease. *Exp. Neurol.* 163, 20–30. doi: 10.1006/exnr.2000.7362

Ballerini, C., Aldinucci, A., Luccarini, I., Galante, A., Manuelli, C., Blandina, P., et al. (2013). Antagonism of histamine H4 receptors exacerbates clinical and pathological signs of experimental autoimmune encephalomyelitis. *Br. J. Pharmacol.* 170, 67–77. doi: 10.1111/bph.12263

Bédard, A., and Parent, A. (2004). Evidence of newly generated neurons in the human olfactory bulb. *Brain Res. Dev. Brain Res.* 151, 159–168. doi: 10.1016/j.devbrainres.2004.03.021

Bernardino, L., Eiriz, M. F., Santos, T., Xapelli, S., Grade, S., Rosa, A. I., et al. (2012) Histamine stimulates neurogenesis in the rodent subventricular zone. *Stem Cells* 30, 773–784. doi: 10.1002/stem.1042

Bhowmik, M., Khanam, R., and Vohora, D. (2012). Histamine H3 receptor antagonists in relation to epilepsy and neurodegeneration: a systemic consideration of recent progress and perspectives. *Br. J. Pharmacol.* 167, 1398–1414. doi: 10.1111/j.1476-5381.2012.02093.x

Bourgogne, E., Mathy, F. X., Boucaut, D., Boekens, H., and Laprevote, O. (2012). Simultaneous quantitation of histamine and its major metabolite 1-methylhistamine in brain dialysates by using precolumn derivatization prior to HILIC-MS/MS analysis. *Anal. Bioanal. Chem.* 402, 449–459. doi: 10.1007/s00216-011-5224-8

Brill, M. S., Ninkovic, J., Winpenny, E., Hodge, R. D., Ozen, I., Yang, R., et al. (2009). Adult generation of glutamatergic olfactory bulb interneurons. *Nat. Neurosci.* 12, 1524–1533. doi: 10.1038/nn.2416

Brown, R. E., Stevens, D. R., and Haas, H. L. (2001) The physiology of brain histamine. *Prog. Neurobiol.* 63, 637–672. doi: 10.1016/S0301-0082(00)00039-3

Croyal, M., Dauvilliers, Y., Labeeuw, O., Capet, M., Schwartz, J. C., and Robert, P. (2011). Histamine and tele-methylhistamine quantification in cerebrospinal fluid from narcoleptic subjects by liquid chromatography tandem mass spectrometry with precolumn derivatization. *Anal. Biochem.* 409, 28–36. doi: 10.1016/j.ab.2010.09.045

Curtis, M. A., Connor, B., and Faull, R. L. (2003). Neurogenesis in the diseased adult human brain–new therapeutic strategies for neurodegenerative diseases. *Cell Cycle* 2, 428–430. doi: 10.4161/cc.2.5.526

Dale, H. H., and Laidlaw, P. P. (1910). The physiological action of beta-iminazolylethylamine. *J. Physiol.* 41, 318–344.

De Marchis, S., Temoney, S., Erdelyi, F., Bovetti, S., Bovolin, P., Szabo, G., et al. (2004). GABAergic phenotypic differentiation of a subpopulation of subventricular derived migrating progenitors. *Eur. J. Neurosci.* 20, 1307–1317. doi: 10.1111/j.1460-9568.2004.03584.x

Eiriz, M. F., Grade, S., Rosa, A., Xapelli, S., Bernardino, L., Agasse, F., et al. (2011). Functional evaluation of neural stem cell differentiation by single cell calcium imaging. *Curr. Stem Cell Res. Ther.* 6, 288–296. doi: 10.2174/157488811796575387

Eiriz, M. F., Malva, J. O., Agasse, F., and Bernardino, L. (2014). "Histamine in the neural and cancer stem cell niches," in *Therapeutic Applications in Disease and Injury- Series: Stem Cells and Cancer Stem Cells*, Vol. 12, ed M. A. Hayat (Springer), 3–17.

Ernst, A., Alkass, K., Bernard, S., Salehpour, M., Perl, S., Tisdale, J., et al. (2014). Neurogenesis in the striatum of the adult human brain. *Cell* 156, 1072–1083. doi: 10.1016/j.cell.2014.01.044

Fan, Y. Y., Hu, W. W., Dai, H. B., Zhang, J. X., Zhang, L. Y., He, P., et al. (2011). Activation of the central histaminergic system is involved in hypoxia-induced stroke tolerance in adult mice. *J. Cereb. Blood Flow. Metab.* 31, 305–314. doi: 10.1038/jcbfm.2010.94

Ferreira, R., Santos, T., Gonçalves, J., Baltazar, G., Ferreira, L., Agasse, F., et al. (2012). Histamine modulates microglia function. *J. Neuroinflamm.* 9:90. doi: 10.1186/1742-2094-9-90

Goings, G. E., Kozlowski, D. A., and Szele, F. G. (2006). Differential activation of microglia in neurogenic versus non-neurogenic regions of the forebrain. *Glia* 54, 329–342. doi: 10.1002/glia.20381

Grade, S., Weng, Y. C., Snapyan, M., Kriz, J., Malva, J. O., and Saghatelyan, A. (2013). Brain-derived neurotrophic factor promotes vasculature-associated migration of neuronal precursors toward the ischemic striatum. *PLoS ONE* 8:e55039. doi: 10.1371/journal.pone.0055039

Kallweit, U., Aritake, K., Bassetti, C. L., Blumenthal, S., Hayaishi, O., Linnebank, M., et al. (2013). Elevated CSF histamine levels in multiple sclerosis patients. *Fluids Barriers CNS* 10:19. doi: 10.1186/2045-8118-10-19

Kanbayashi, T., Kodama, T., Kondo, H., Satoh, S., Inoue, Y., Chiba, S., et al. (2009). CSF histamine contents in narcolepsy, idiopathic hypersomnia and obstructive sleep apnea syndrome. *Sleep* 32, 181–187.

Kaneko, N., and Sawamoto, K. (2009). Adult neurogenesis and its alteration under pathological conditions. *Neurosci. Res.* 63, 155–164. doi: 10.1016/j.neures.2008.12.001

Katoh, Y., Niimi, M., Yamamoto, Y., Kawamura, T., Morimoto-Ishizuka, T., Sawada, M., et al. (2001). Histamine production by cultured microglial cells of the mouse. *Neurosci. Lett.* 305, 181–184. doi: 10.1016/S0304-3940(01)01835-3

Krementsov, D. N., Wall, E. H., Martin, R. A., Subramanian, M., Noubade, R., Del Rio, R., et al. (2013). Histamine H(3) receptor integrates peripheral inflammatory signals in the neurogenic control of immune responses and autoimmune disease susceptibility. *PLoS ONE* 8:e62743. doi: 10.1371/journal.pone.0062743

Macas, J., Nern, C., Plate, K. H., and Momma, S. (2006). Increased generation of neuronal progenitors after ischemic injury in the aged adult human forebrain. *J. Neurosci.* 26, 13114–13119. doi: 10.1523/JNEUROSCI.4667-06.2006

Marques, F., Sousa, J. C., Coppola, G., Gao, F., Puga, R., Brentani, H., et al. (2011) Transcriptome signature of the adult mouse choroid plexus. *Fluids Barriers CNS* 8:10. doi: 10.1186/2045-8118-8-10

Martí-Fàbregas, J., Romaguera-Ros, M., Gómez-Pinedo, U., Martínez-Ramírez, S., Jiménez-Xarrié, E., Marín, R., et al. (2010) Proliferation in the human ipsilateral subventricular zone after ischemic stroke. *Neurology* 74, 357–365. doi: 10.1212/WNL.0b013e3181cbccec

Merkle, F. T., Mirzadeh, Z., and Alvarez-Buylla, A. (2007). Mosaic organization of neural stem cells in the adult brain. *Science* 317, 381–384. doi: 10.1126/science.1144914

Molina-Hernández, A., Rodríguez-Martínez, G., Escobedo-Ávila, I., and Velasco, I. (2013). Histamine up-regulates fibroblast growth factor receptor 1 and increases FOXP2 neurons in cultured neural precursors by histamine type 1 receptor activation: conceivable role of histamine in neurogenesis during cortical development *in vivo*. *Neural Dev.* 8:4. doi: 10.1186/1749-8104-8-4

Molina-Hernández, A., and Velasco, I. (2008). Histamine induces neural stem cell proliferation and neuronal differentiation by activation of distinct histamine receptors. *J. Neurochem* 106, 706–717. doi: 10.1111/j.1471-4159.2008.05424.x

Motoki, A., Adachi, N., Semba, K., Liu, K., and Arai, T. (2005). Reduction in brain infarction by augmentation of central histaminergic activity in rats. *Brain Res.* 1066, 172–178. doi: 10.1016/j.brainres.2005.10.059

Panula, P., and Nuutinen, S. (2013) The histaminergic network in the brain: basic organization and role in disease. *Nat. Rev. Neurosci.* 14. 472–487. doi: 10.1038/nrn3526

Panula, P., Sundvik, M., and Karlstedt, K. (2014). Developmental roles of brain histamine. *Trends Neurosci.* 37, 159–168. doi: 10.1016/j.tins.2014.01.001

Rodríguez-Martínez, G., Velasco, I., García-López, G., Solís, K. H., Flores-Herrera, H., Díaz, N. F., et al. (2012). Histamine is required during neural stem cell proliferation to increase neuron differentiation. *Neuroscience* 216, 10–17. doi: 10.1016/j.neuroscience.2012.04.049

Ruan, L., Lau, B. W., Wang, J., Huang, L., Zhuge, Q., Wang, B., et al. (2014). Neurogenesis in neurological and psychiatric diseases and brain injury: from bench to bedside. *Prog. Neurobiol.* 115C, 116–137. doi: 10.1016/j.pneurobio.2013.12.006

Saino-Saito, S., Sasaki, H., Volpe, B. T., Kobayashi, K., Berlin, R., and Baker, H. (2004). Differentiation of the dopaminergic phenotype in the olfactory system of neonatal and adult mice. *J. Comp. Neurol.* 479, 389–398. doi: 10.1002/cne.20320

Sanai, N., Nguyen, T., Ihrie, R. A., Mirzadeh, Z., Tsai, H. H., Wong, M., et al. (2011). Corridors of migrating neurons in the human brain and their decline during infancy. *Nature* 478, 382–386. doi: 10.1038/nature10487

Shan, L., Swaab, D. F., and Bao, A. M. (2013). Neuronal histaminergic system in aging and age-related neurodegenerative disorders. *Exp. Gerontol.* 48, 603–607. doi: 10.1016/j.exger.2012.08.002

Shigemoto-Mogami, Y., Hoshikawa, K., Goldman, J. E., Sekino, Y., and Sato, K. (2014). Microglia enhance neurogenesis and oligodendrogenesis in the early postnatal subventricular zone. *J. Neurosci.* 34, 2231–2243. doi: 10.1523/JNEUROSCI.1619-13.2014

Soya, A., Song, Y. H., Kodama, T., Honda, Y., Fujiki, N., and Nishino, S. (2008). CSF histamine levels in rats reflect the central histamine neurotransmission. *Neurosci. Lett.* 430, 224–229. doi: 10.1016/j.neulet.2007.11.002

Tran, P. B., Ren, D., Veldhouse, T. J., and Miller, R. J. (2004). Chemokine receptors are expressed widely by embryonic and adult neural progenitor cells. *J. Neurosci. Res.* 6, 20–34. doi: 10.1002/jnr.20001

Vizuete, M. L., Merino, M., Venero, J. L., Santiago, M., Cano, J., and Machado, A. (2000). Histamine infusion induces a selective dopaminergic neuronal death along with an inflammatory reaction in rat substantia nigra. *J. Neurochem.* 75, 540–552. doi: 10.1046/j.1471-4159.2000.0750540.x

Yanai, K., and Tashiro, M. (2007). The physiological and pathophysiological roles of neuronal histamine: an insight from human positron emission tomography studies. *Pharmacol. Ther.* 113, 1–15. doi: 10.1016/j.pharmthera.2006.06.008

Yoshitake, T., Yamaguchi, M., Nohta, H., Ichinose, F., Yoshida, H., Yoshitake, S., et al. (2003). Determination of histamine in microdialysis samples from rat brain by microbore column liquid chromatography following intramolecular excimer-forming derivatization with pyrene-labeling reagent. *J. Neurosci. Methods* 127, 11–17. doi: 10.1016/S0165-0270(03)00097-9

Electrode impedance analysis of chronic tungsten microwire neural implants: understanding abiotic vs. biotic contributions

***Viswanath Sankar*[1]*, Erin Patrick*[1]*, Robert Dieme*[1]*, Justin C. Sanchez*[2]*, Abhishek Prasad*[2]* and Toshikazu Nishida*[1]**

[1] *Electrical and Computer Engineering Department, University of Florida, Gainesville, FL, USA*
[2] *Biomedical Engineering Department, University of Miami, Coral Gables, FL, USA*

Edited by:
Ulrich G. Hofmann, Albert-Ludwigs-University Freiburg, Germany

Reviewed by:
Thilo Bernhard Krueger, inomed Medizintechnik GmbH, Germany
David Krapohl, Mid Sweden University, Sweden

***Correspondence:**
Abhishek Prasad, Department of Biomedical Engineering, University of Miami, 1251 Memorial Drive, Rm#203, Coral Gables, FL 33146, USA
e-mail: a.prasad@miami.edu

Changes in biotic and abiotic factors can be reflected in the complex impedance spectrum of the microelectrodes chronically implanted into the neural tissue. The recording surface of the tungsten electrode *in vivo* undergoes abiotic changes due to recording site corrosion and insulation delamination as well as biotic changes due to tissue encapsulation as a result of the foreign body immune response. We reported earlier that large changes in electrode impedance measured at 1 kHz were correlated with poor electrode functional performance, quantified through electrophysiological recordings during the chronic lifetime of the electrode. There is a need to identity the factors that contribute to the chronic impedance variation. In this work, we use numerical simulation and regression to equivalent circuit models to evaluate both the abiotic and biotic contributions to the impedance response over chronic implant duration. COMSOL® simulation of abiotic electrode morphology changes provide a possible explanation for the decrease in the electrode impedance at long implant duration while biotic changes play an important role in the large increase in impedance observed initially.

Keywords: chronic neural implants, electrode impedance, corrosion, insulation delamination, finite element modeling

INTRODUCTION

Tungsten micro-wire electrode arrays continue to be used as chronic implants for single-unit neuronal recording (Williams et al., 1999a,b; Rennaker et al., 2005; Rizk et al., 2009; Freire et al., 2011). Implanted electrodes in general suffer recording performance degradation over time (Williams et al., 1999a; Ward et al., 2009). Understanding the reasons for poor recording performance over time is integral for the adaptive design of future electrode arrays. For tungsten micro-wire electrodes, structural modification of the recording site by corrosion and insulation delamination (Sanchez et al., 2006; Patrick et al., 2011; Prasad et al., 2012; Streit et al., 2012) as well as tissue encapsulation due to the foreign-body immune response (Szarowski et al., 2003; Biran et al., 2005, 2007; McConnell et al., 2009) are known to occur. Although it is known that both abiotic and biotic effects contribute to changes at the electrode recording site, it is still unclear to what extent each effect has on the chronic recording performance of the electrode.

Impedance is a metric commonly used to assess electrode performance. Chronic *in-vivo* studies (Prasad and Sanchez, 2012) have confirmed a functional correlation between the electrode impedance value at 1 kHz and the overall neuronal yield during the implanted duration. It was observed in that study that low array yields were associated with very low impedance values or very high impedance values, and the best array yield was observed for an impedance range of 40–150 kΩ at 1 kHz for the implanted 50 μm diameter blunt-cut tungsten micro-wires. The electrode impedance also varied over time increasing during the first few weeks of implantation followed by a drop in the impedance value in the latter phase of the implant duration. Though these observations suggest that the electrode impedance is affected by some short-term and long-term factors, the underlying driving mechanisms are not fully understood. Furthermore, the impedance variation for tungsten microwires itself varied across different implanted animals.

The working model is that network analysis of the complex impedance spectra of implanted electrode arrays may yield useful information about the changes occurring in the vicinity of the electrode recording sites in the neural tissue. This is supported by the results of Williams et al. who showed a distinction between severe and nominal inflammatory response to tungsten electrodes implanted in an animal model for 19 days by comparing the complex impedance spectra (Williams et al., 2007). Nyquist plots were used to show the progression of the inflammatory response over time. However, the effect of corrosion or insulation delamination was not considered in their paper.

In this paper, we analyze the complex impedance spectra of tungsten micro-wire electrodes that were previously implanted for 9-months into the rat somatosensory cortex. We show progress toward decoupling the abiotic (e.g., recording-surface structural modification) effects from the biotic (e.g., tissue encapsulation) effects with the analysis of the complex impedance spectra of the implanted electrodes. Graphical comparisons as well as regression to an equivalent circuit model provide qualitative and quantitative results. Finite element analysis package COMSOL® Multiphysics® (Burlington, MA) is used to simulate abiotic effects of different electrode surface variations on the impedance. We used pre-implant and post-explant SEM imaging and surface roughness analysis to provide evidence of abiotic structural changes.

MATERIALS AND METHODS

ANALYSIS OF *IN-VIVO* ELECTRODE ARRAY DATA

Electrode array

Sixteen-channel micro-wire arrays [Tucker-Davis Technologies (TDT), Alachua FL] were used for this study. The microwires were 50 μm in diameter, 5 mm long, and blunt cut using a laser beam. The tungsten wires were plated with a thin film of gold of thickness ~2–5 μm and insulated with a layer of polyimide of approximate thickness 10 μm. The wires were positioned in a 2 × 8 configuration with spacing of 250 μm between two adjacent microwires.

Implantation and recording

The electrode array was implanted in the somatosensory cortex of an adult male Sprague-Dawley rat. Aseptic surgical techniques were used for the implantation procedure. All procedures were approved by the Institutional Animal Care and Use Committee, University of Miami, FL. Electrophysiological recordings were made on the animal three to four times a week and each recording session lasted approximately 20 min. A custom testbed was developed that allowed the animal to move freely during the recording session. Impedance was measured before every recording session on all 16 microwires using a small current (maximum 1.4 nA) that did not affect the electrode properties. The surgical and recording procedures are described in detail in Prasad and Sanchez (2012). The structural changes were investigated by imaging the electrodes surfaces before and after the implant.

Characterization of structural changes

The structural changes in the implanted electrodes were studied by characterizing the microwire arrays through qualitative methods using scanning electron microscope (SEM) imaging and quantitative methods via laser scanning microscope surface roughness measurements. Tungsten microwires were imaged before and after explantation using SEMs (CarryScope SEM, JEOL, Inc., and FEI XL-40 field emission gun SEM). The imaging procedure is described in detail in Prasad et al. (2012).

The pre- and post-implant SEM images of the electrode provided only a qualitative idea of the variation in the surface morphology. In order to quantitatively assess the surface roughness and corrosion depth of the implanted electrodes, some of the arrays were analyzed for surface roughness using a laser scanning microscope (Keyence VK-9700 Color 3D Laser Scanning Microscope) at the Materials Evaluation and Testing Laboratory, South Dakota State University. The depth profile of the wires in the array was measured and the average height with respect to the reference line was calculated.

Impedance measurement and analysis of magnitude at 1 kHz

The NanoZ® impedance tester (TDT, FL) was used to measure the daily *in-vivo* impedance values. The NanoZ applies a constant voltage of 4 mVpp sinusoidal waveform which results in a maximum test current of 1.4 nA. Compared to an estimated corrosion current on the order of 100 nA at equilibrium from results in Patrick et al. (2011), the 1.4 nA current used for the impedance measurements will negligibly affect the normal corrosion processes. The impedance measurement process involved 40 cycles of measurement on each microwire and an average value was calculated to minimize measurement errors. The impedances were recorded at 1, 2, 5, 10, 20, 50, 100, 200, 500 Hz, 1 and 2 kHz. Prior to implantation, the impedance of each microelectrode was characterized in 0.9% phosphate buffered saline (PBS) that served as a baseline for the *in vivo* measurements. In the case of *in vitro* pre-implant testing, the reference was made to a stainless steel ground wire connected to the MEA assembly and dipped in the same saline solution, whereas for *in vivo* chronic testing, the reference was made to the same stainless steel ground wire connected to a stainless steel bone screw drilled into the skull.

From the measured *in vivo* impedance data, the percentage change in impedance was calculated for each individual wire and averaged for all wires for the implanted duration. The impedance value measured on the surgery day was considered as the reference value and the percentage change was calculated for this reference. Since the temporal variation of the *in vivo* impedance approximately follows a Gaussian profile, the calculated percentage change in impedance values were fitted with a Gaussian curve using the built-in curve fitting tool in OriginPro® (OriginLab Corporation, Northampton, MA) given by

$$y = y_0 + \frac{A}{w\sqrt{\pi/2}} e^{-2\frac{(x-x_c)^2}{w^2}} \tag{1}$$

where, w is the standard deviation, x is the individual calculated value, x_c is the average, and A and y_0 are constants. Percentage change higher than 600% were treated as outliers and were not included in the calculations.

GRAPHICAL ANALYSIS AND REGRESSION OF COMPLEX IMPEDANCE DATA

The real and imaginary parts of the complex impedance data as a function of frequency were plotted with logarithmic scales on both axes to capture both low as well as high frequency data. These complex-plane impedance plots, compared to Nyquist or Bode plots, can better identify physical processes (Orazem et al., 2006) and make trends in the temporal changes more apparent. Eight timestamps were chosen to adequately capture the temporal impedance trend, day 1 of implant and days 7, 15, 31, 60, 106, 149, and 205 post implant.

Regression of the complex impedance data was performed using the non-linear least squares regression function in Matlab. The real and imaginary parts of the impedance spectrum were fit to one of two equivalent circuits shown in **Figure 1**. The circuit in **Figure 1A**, commonly known as the "Randles circuit," models the electrochemical interface of a bare metal electrode in an electrolyte neglecting the diffusion related Warburg impedance

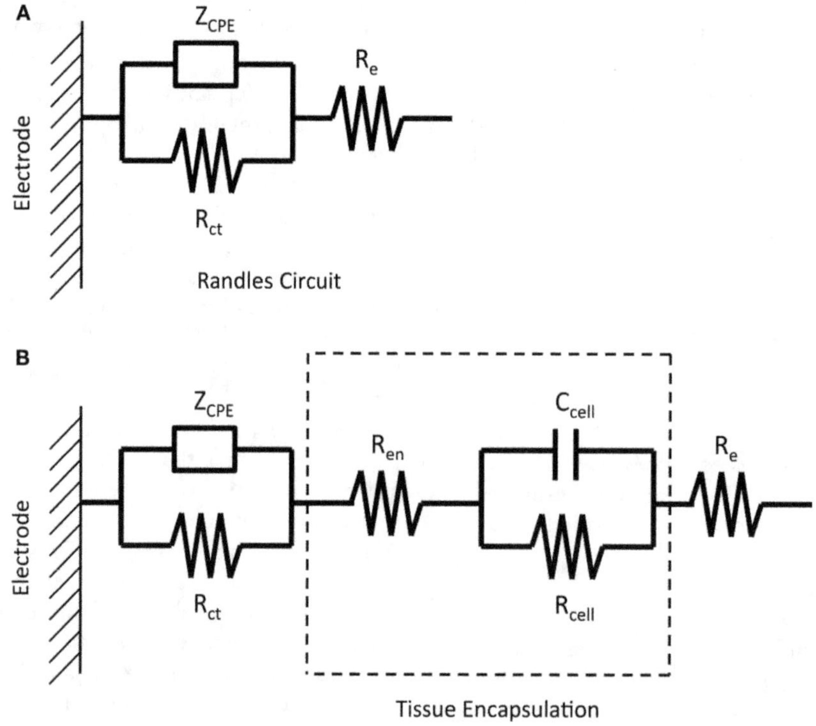

FIGURE 1 | Equivalent circuits representing the impedance of a micro-wire without the presence of tissue encapsulation due to the inflammatory response (A) and with the presence of tissue encapsulation (B).

(Brug et al., 1984; McAdams et al., 1995). R_{ct} is the charge transfer resistance, which models the resistive pathway due to electrochemical reactions (i.e., tungsten corrosion), and Z_{CPE} is the constant phase element impedance given by

$$Z_{CPE} = \frac{1}{(j\omega)^{\alpha} Q} \tag{2}$$

where ω is the frequency, α is a number from 0 to 1, and Q is the constant phase element (CPE) coefficient with units $s^{\alpha}/\Omega cm^2$. The CPE element is used to model the capacitive double layer at the electrode interface. The CPE, rather than an ideal capacitor, better accounts for non-idealities due to surface inhomogeneity (Brug et al., 1984) and is commonly used in electrode/electrolyte equivalent circuit models (McAdams et al., 1995; Johnson et al., 2005; Otto et al., 2006; Williams et al., 2007; Lempka et al., 2011). R_e models the resistance of the electrolyte seen by the electrode and is also referred to as the spreading resistance to a distant ground. **Figure 1B** adds a simplified circuit that models the tissue encapsulation layers through a series resistor R_{en} and parallel combination of a resistor R_{cell} and capacitor C_{cell}. (Johnson et al., 2005; Otto et al., 2006; Williams et al., 2007; Lempka et al., 2011). The tissue encapsulating the electrode due to the immune response consists of layers of extracellular matrix proteins (e.g., collagen, fibronectin, and laminin) and reactive glial cells and macrophages (Grill and Mortimer, 1994; Kim et al., 2004). R_{en} models encapsulation by extracellular matrix proteins, and C_{cell} and R_{cell} model the resistive and capacitive pathways through the cellular layer, respectively.

Figure 2 shows generic complex-plane impedance plots calculated using the two equivalent circuits in **Figure 1**. One distinguishing feature of the imaginary impedance as a function of frequency is the presence of only one peak for the Randles circuit and the presence of two peaks in the circuit that adds tissue encapsulation components to the Randles circuit. These peaks occur at the frequencies given by the reciprocal of the RC time-constants in the circuit. R_{ct} and Z_{CPE} determine the low-frequency peak and the high-frequency peak is determined by the adherent cellular components, C_{cell} and R_{cell}. Thus, the presence of a cellular biotic layer at the electrode surface may be inferred by examining the imaginary impedance data. The real impedance as a function of frequency provides information on the electrolyte and encapsulation resistance, R_e and R_{en}, at high frequencies where the impedance of CPE and C_{cell} are small compared to the parallel resistive components. The high-frequency asymptotic value converges to the electrolyte resistance R_e in the Randles circuit and the addition of R_e and R_{en}, for the circuit that includes encapsulation components. We use these graphical impedance analysis techniques to assess the factors causing temporal variation of impedance for our chronically implanted electrode array.

COMSOL® FINITE ELEMENT ANALYSIS (FEA)

Finite element analysis of the electrode-electrolyte interface was made in COMSOL® Multiphysics software package to investigate how the electrolyte resistance, R_e, changes over time due to

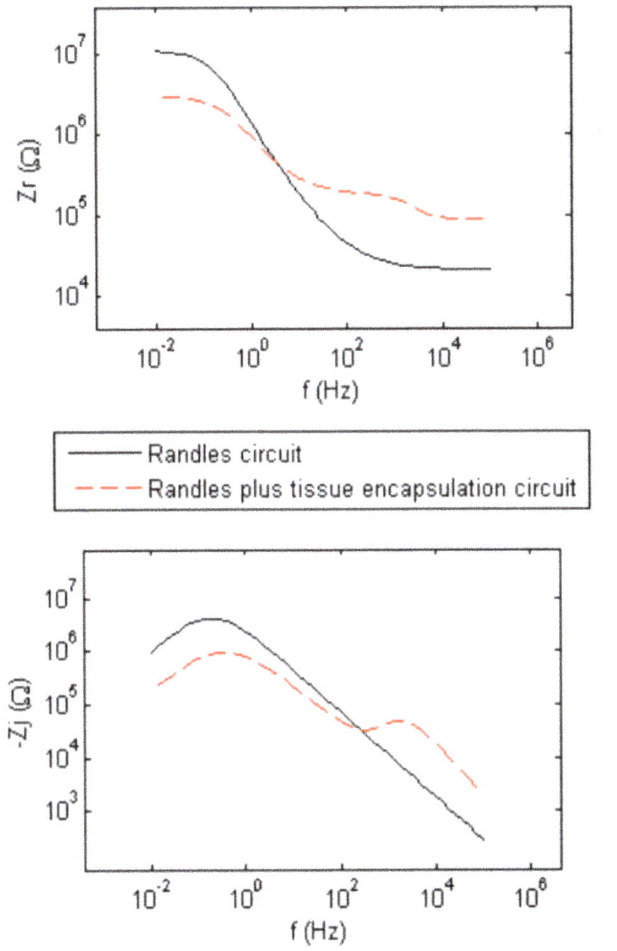

FIGURE 2 | Generic calculated real (Z_r) and imaginary (Z_j) parts of the complex impedance as a function of frequency representing the two equivalent circuits in Figure 1 having abiotic only and abiotic and biotic components which illustrate the presence of one peak for the Randles circuit and two peaks for the Randles combined with Tissue Encapsulation circuits for the imaginary impedance.

simulated structural modifications. The tungsten electrode was modeled using a three-dimensional (3-D) geometry consisting of a 50 μm thick tungsten microwire surrounded by 1 μm thick gold layer and insulated with 5 μm thick polyimide insulation surrounded by a region of cerebrospinal fluid (CSF) electrolyte. The COMSOL® AC/DC module (or electric current physics) was selected to numerically solve the governing physics. The electrolyte boundaries were extended up to 1 × 1 cm to satisfy the semi-infinite boundary condition. A point current source of 1 μA was placed at the center of the top (cortex boundary) surface of the electrode. **Figure 3** shows an illustration of the COMSOL® finite element 3-D model of the electrode-electrolyte interface. The electrode was assumed to be a uniform conductor; hence the potential distribution across the electrode is constant. A Dirichlet boundary condition of $V = 0$ was assumed at the electrolyte boundaries since the boundaries are supposed to be semi-infinite, while a von Neumann boundary condition of $\vec{n} \cdot \vec{j} = 0$

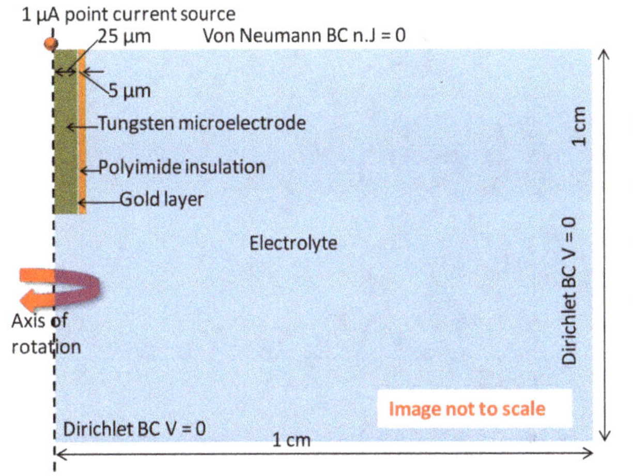

FIGURE 3 | Illustration of the electrode-electrolyte interface and the boundary conditions used in the COMSOL® finite element model.

Table 1 | Conductivity values used for the COMSOL® finite element model.

Material/layer	Conductivity (S/m)	References
Tungsten	18.94×10^6	Serway, 1998
Gold	40.98×10^6	Serway, 1998
Polyimide	1×10^{-16}	HD Microsystems, 2001
Cerebrospinal fluid	1.8	Baumann et al., 1997

was assumed at the cortex boundary, which ensured electrical insulation at the boundaries. The conductivities of the different materials used for the model are given in **Table 1**. Tetrahedral elements with size ranging from 1 to 400 μm were used for meshing the domains.

RESULTS

IN VIVO EXPERIMENTAL RESULTS

As described previously (Prasad et al., 2012), the electrode array under study was deemed a functionally optimal performing array having 50–70% of the wires functional during the extent of the implant (216 days). Also, the *in vivo* impedance magnitude measured at 1 kHz stayed within the 40–150 kΩ range determined optimal for functional electrophysiological recordings for this array type. The average temporal variation, averaged over 16 electrodes, is shown in **Figure 4**. The average change in impedance at 1 kHz follows a Gaussian profile. However since averaging can mask individual variation, it is also instructive to look at specific electrodes that highlight the variation between electrodes implanted at the same time in the same animal. Detailed data of the percent change in impedance magnitude at 1 kHz, complex-plane impedance plots over time, and neuronal yield data over time for one representative wire out of the array (wire 12) are shown in **Figure 5**. Data for all wires in the array are given in the supplemental materials.

Corrosion of the tungsten and delamination and cracking of the polyimide insulation are abiotic factors that contribute

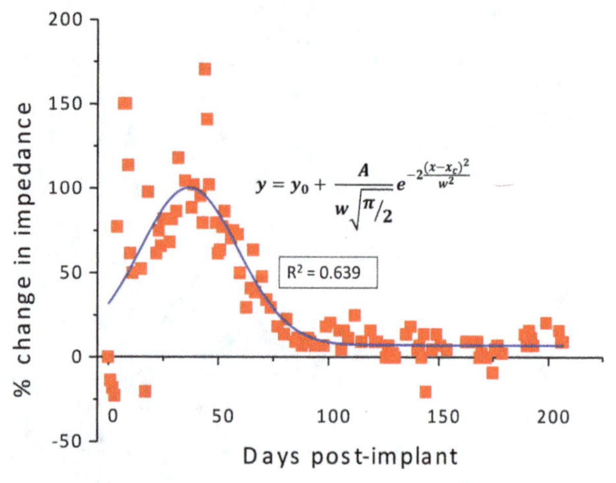

FIGURE 4 | Average percentage change in the *in-vivo* impedance averaged for all wires of electrode array R9 plotted against the implanted duration and fitted with a Gaussian curve.

to morphological changes at the electrode/tissue interface. SEM images of the recording site pre- and post-implant, and relief images of the surface showing a calculated corrosion depth for one wire out of the array (wire 12) are shown in **Figure 6**. Comparison between the pre-implant and the post-implant SEM images of the electrodes revealed similar amounts of tungsten corrosion in all the 16 wires. The tungsten core was recessed within the outer layers of gold and polymer insulation. The measured average corrosion depth for all of the wires was 38.8 μm with a standard deviation of 9.4 μm. Moreover, all wires had some variation of visible insulation damage including delamination and cracks. The majority of the damage was delamination at the electrode surface. In two electrodes out of the array, there were noticeable cracks in the insulation that reached, at maximum, 30 μm below the recording surface.

In all wires in the array, there were large variations in the impedance magnitude over time, with the largest variability occurring within the first few weeks. This large variability happens to occur when the abiotic and biotic factors are most in flux. For example, the rate of tungsten corrosion is larger within the first few weeks of implantation (Prasad et al., 2012), and the inflammatory response does not achieve its chronic stage until after 4–6 weeks (Turner et al., 1999). Thus it is unclear which factor, abiotic or biotic, contributes most to this trend.

We attempt to uncover the mechanisms for the temporal variations by examining the complex-plane impedance data for select days using the graphical analysis described in Graphical Analysis and Regression of Complex Impedance Data. **Figure 5** shows a trend in the complex impedance seen in all wires of the array. The imaginary impedance as a function of frequency (subfigure D) shows two peaks instead of one on every day except for the first day suggesting the presence of a second RC time-constant after day one. These observations suggest a definite biotic component to the impedance magnitude at 1 kHz after day one, since the peak due to a cellular component in the complex impedance vs. frequency is apparent. Our hypothesis that these temporal variations in the electrode impedance have a stronger biotic contribution in the days following implant surgery is supported by the large cellular changes that occur around the microelectrodes due to initial foreign body response. Also the peak occurring at higher frequencies (>400 Hz) is more pronounced primarily on days 7, 15, and 31 after implantation, which is usually the period during which the tissue encapsulation layer due to the inflammatory response is forming (Turner et al., 1999). The second peak is less pronounced in the later days and the impedance values at the higher frequencies decrease. The real part of the impedance as a function of frequency (subfigure C) shows a similar trend in all of the wires of the array in which the impedance value at higher frequencies (>50 Hz) increases to a maximum in the beginning (days 7–31) and then decreases and remains more constant over time. These results are also consistent with our previously reported results where we observed the tissue inflammatory response to be reducing for long-term animals such as the one examined here (Prasad et al., 2012). Further, an abiotic factor such as insulation deterioration is also one of the likely causes of the reduction of impedance in the chronic phase. Circuit elements R_e, and R_{en} are important factors in this trend and will shed more light on the influence of biotic and abiotic effects.

REGRESSION OF COMPLEX IMPEDANCE DATA

The goal of the regression is to quantify each circuit parameter such that the abiotic and biotic contributions to the impedance magnitude at 1 kHz may be identified. One electrode in the array, wire 12 (complex impedance shown in **Figures 5C,D**), was chosen as a representative sample for regression analysis. The impedance for day 1, since it only has one time constant, was fit to the Randles circuit and the remaining data sets were fit to the circuit that includes the encapsulation components. In the regression, one resistor encompassing R_e and R_{en} was used in the equivalent circuit that incorporated encapsulation components. **Figure 7** shows the regression results with fits to the limited data points.

Further analysis is needed to decouple the electrolyte resistance and the encapsulation resistance for all days after the first. The electrolyte impedance R_e is dependent on the surface morphology of the electrode. With corrosion and insulation deterioration occurring at the electrode surface, R_e will likely change over the implant time; however, the extent is not well understood. For example, what effect does a recessing electrode surface have on the electrolyte resistance? This question has not been addressed in the literature to the best of our knowledge. We rely on COMSOL numerical simulation to estimate the changes to R_e over time which is used to estimate a value for R_{en} (Discussion section).

COMSOL® FEA RESULTS

The response of structural changes to the electrolyte resistance is analyzed in COMSOL®. Our model for electrode surface morphology was developed based on our knowledge obtained from prior *in vitro* (Patrick et al., 2011) and *in vivo* (Prasad and Sanchez, 2012) impedance studies. It comprises morphological changes to the metal, tungsten, via corrosion and to the polymer insulation via crack formation and delamination.

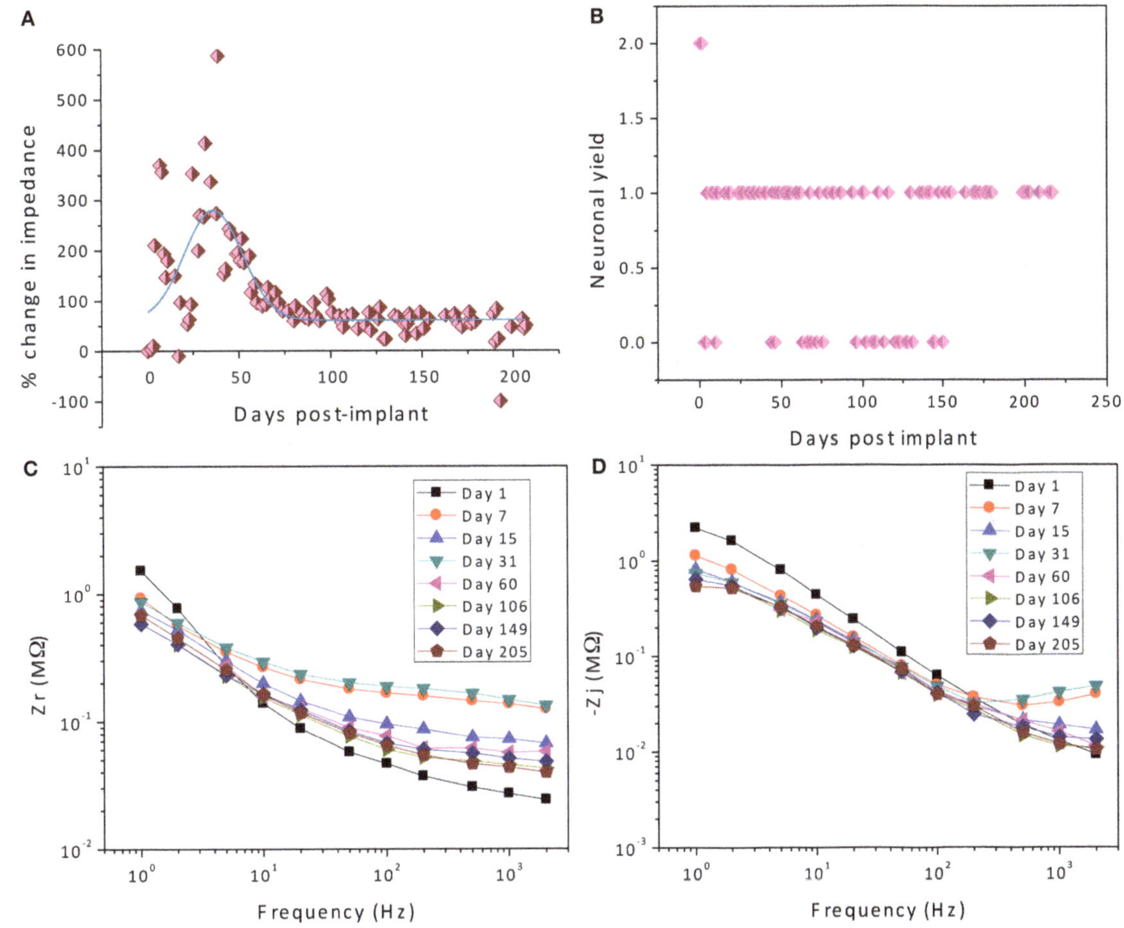

FIGURE 5 | Detailed data of the percent change in impedance magnitude at 1 kHz (A), neuronal yield data over time (B), complex-plane impedance plots over time (C,D) for wire 12.

The results from the *in vitro* and *in vivo* studies suggest that the electrode will undergo continuous corrosion during the implantation period. However, the corrosion rate may be highly dynamic. The rate of corrosion is influenced by the presence of chemical species such as hydrogen peroxide (H_2O_2) (Patrick et al., 2011), which is produced by reactive microglia that surround the implanted microwire. The *in-vitro* corrosion study showed that gold plated tungsten wires corrode at the rate of 10,000–20,000 μm/year in PBS in the presence of millimolar concentrations of H_2O_2, while the rate drops to 300–700 μm/year in the absence of H_2O_2 (Patrick et al., 2011).

In the *in vivo* setting, the immune response gives an indication for how corrosion may evolve. We have shown the corrosion to be present in all microwires but the rate of corrosion was found to be accelerated in the first few weeks following electrode implant compared to chronic periods (Prasad et al., 2012). Coincidentally, there are larger changes that occur in the vicinity of the electrode recording tips due to the inflammatory response in the early hours to weeks following implant. The inflammatory response activates the microglial cells, which produce superoxides and add unknown concentrations of H_2O_2 to the CSF (Burke and Lewis, 2000). During the first few weeks of implantation, we assume there is a higher concentration of H_2O_2, which leads to a higher rate of tungsten corrosion. When the inflammation response progresses to the gliosis phase, the number of surrounding glial cells decreases, and the glial sheath becomes more compact (Polikov et al., 2005). Hence, we assume the rate of corrosion decreases because there is a smaller amount of H_2O_2 being produced by the remaining glial cells, and the dense glial sheath may impede diffusion of reacting species, thereby making the corrosion rate mass-transfer limited. Thus far, our model for temporal tungsten morphology is that the exposed tungsten will uniformly corrode (as compared to pitting corrosion) as soon at it is implanted with a rate that will increase with time up to formation of the compact glial sheath and then decrease to a constant value. These assumptions were made after close observation of electrode recording sites for these arrays for varying implant durations (acute to up to 9 months).

The effect of two cases of electrode surface variations on the electrolyte impedance R_e were studied in detail. In both cases, corrosion is assumed to occur while in Case 1, the added variation due to insulation delamination/peeling is modeled and in Case 2, the added variation of insulation cracking is considered. **Figure 8** illustrates the model geometry for electrode surface

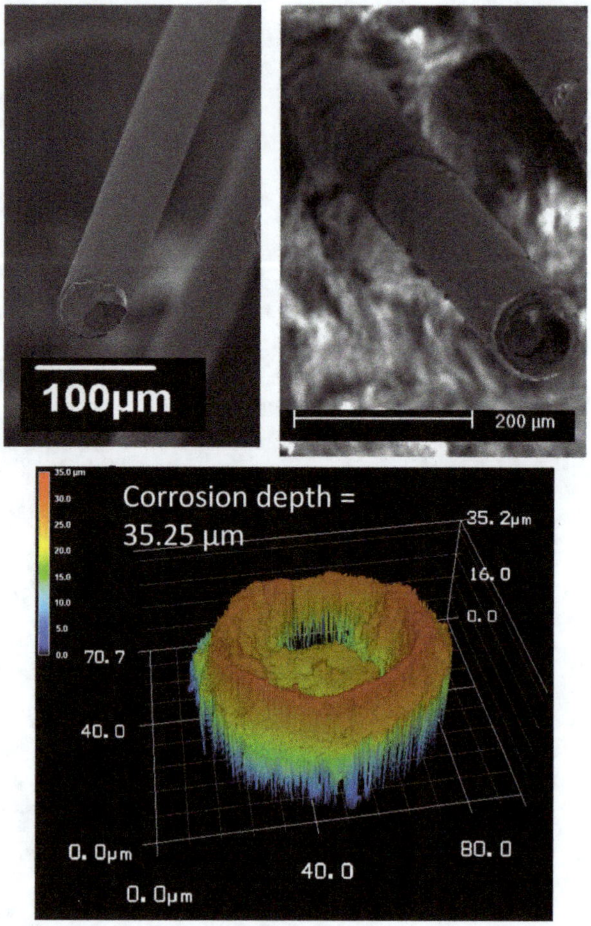

FIGURE 6 | SEM images of the recording site pre- and post-implant (top), and relief images of the surface showing a calculated corrosion depth (bottom) for wire 12.

modification over implant duration involving both corrosion and insulation delamination (Case 1) and both corrosion and insulation cracking (Case 2), respectively.

In Case 1, the insulation delamination was modeled as a gap between the electrode and the insulation (**Figure 8A**). Impedance was calculated at seven different instances with each instance representing a different surface. The first instance was a pristine wire with no corrosion or insulation delamination. Impedance calculated at this instance served as the baseline reference for the successive instances. The next two instances model the high corrosion phase of the electrode. No modification in insulation was included in these two instances. The final four instances model the simultaneous corrosion and insulation delamination phase. A rate of 15 μm per instance was assumed for modeling the high corrosion rate, while a rate of 0.5 μm per instance was assumed for the low corrosion rate. This ratio of 15:0.5 was chosen in accordance with the experimentally measured tungsten corrosion rate ratio of 10,000–20,000:300–700 in the presence and absence of hydrogen peroxide. A constant rate of 2 μm per instance was assumed for the increase in insulation gap width and length.

In Case 2, the insulation crack was modeled as a slit with a width that is proportional to the arc angle and a varying crack length (**Figure 8B**). Similar to Case 1, the impedance for Case 2 was calculated at seven different instances for the insulation-cracked case. As before, the first instance was a pristine wire serving as the baseline reference for the successive instances, and the next two instances model the high corrosion phase of the electrode, and the final four instances model the simultaneous corrosion and cracking in insulation phase. The same rate of 15 μm per instance was assumed for modeling the high corrosion rate, while a rate of 0.5 μm per instance was assumed for low corrosion rate. A constant rate of 2.5 μm per instance was assumed for the increase in insulation crack length and the width of the crack was set by fixing the arc angle at 15°, 30°, 60°, and 90° for each instance.

The COMSOL® simulated percentage changes in resistance for corrosion and (Case 1) insulation delamination and (Case 2) insulation cracking at different instances are given in **Figure 9**. Also the dimensions of the metal recession modeling corrosion and insulation delamination and cracks are also shown. It can be observed in **Figure 9** that the percent change in the electrode resistance increases steadily during the initial high corrosion-rate phase and decreases during the low corrosion and insulation damage phase, modeled either by insulation delamination or by insulation cracking, giving rise to a bell shape or Gaussian profile for both cases. The increase of resistance as a result of the tungsten recessing into its insulation is an interesting finding. However, it can be observed that the increase in resistance is only up to 14% and the decrease in resistance is up to −7% which is nearly one order of magnitude less than the observed *in-vivo* impedance changes.

DISCUSSION

ABIOTIC vs. BIOTIC CONTRIBUTIONS TO IMPEDANCE MAGNITUDE AT 1 kHz

Abiotic and biotic factors

Before estimating values for elements in the time-varying equivalent circuits, it is important to identify which factor, biotic or abiotic, will most affect the individual circuit elements. The biotic changes at the electrode/tissue interface are encapsulation by extracellular matrix proteins and glial cells brought on by the foreign-body immune response. The abiotic factors that lead to electrode surface morphology are corrosion and insulation deterioration.

The surface area of the recording electrode is constantly changing due to corrosion and insulation delamination. Hence, it is possible that the circuit elements that comprise the neural electrode equivalent circuit model will change over time due to the changing surface area. As seen from the COMSOL® results, the corrosion and subsequent recession of tungsten will cause an increase in the electrolyte resistance, R_e, while insulation delamination and cracking will decrease the resistance. Similarly, the Randles circuit parameters, charge transfer resistance (R_{ct}) and CPE coefficient Q, are also expected to vary with changes in the surface area. R_{ct} is inversely proportional to the surface area while Q (similar to a capacitance) is directly proportional to area.

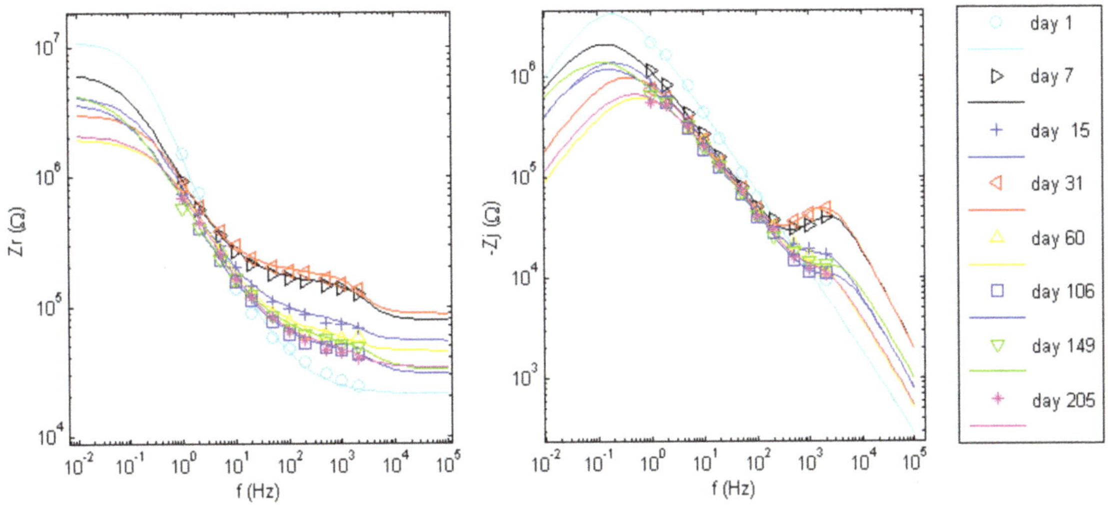

FIGURE 7 | Impedance data points and the regressed fit lines of complex impedance for wire 12 to the circuits shown in Figure 1. Day 1 was fit to the Randles circuit, only. The equivalent circuit with added tissue encapsulation components are used to fit the data for all other days post implant.

The key remaining question is whether the tissue encapsulation circuit will be affected, i.e., will abiotic changes affect biotic changes of the neural electrode? For a first order approximation, one would expect that the encapsulation components R_{cell} and C_{cell} will be unaffected by changes in surface area since they represent an independent cellular layer. However, it is possible that dynamic changes in abiotic factors such as the surface roughness and area compound the biotic changes due to re-engaging the immune response as fresh electrode surfaces are newly exposed over time. The biotic factors, encapsulation by extracellular matrix proteins and glial cells, will obviously control the circuit elements R_{en}, C_{cell}, and R_{cell}. However, R_{en} will be coupled with abiotic changes since it is also dependent on the surface morphology of the electrode. Moreover, the time-varying void left by the corroding tungsten and/or delaminating/cracking insulation might encourage ingrowth of extracellular matrix proteins and result in a larger encapsulation resistance than would be present for an ideal, non-corroded recording surface. Analysis of the regression suggests a multitude of factors contributing to the magnitude of the impedance change at 1 kHz for the array under study.

Analysis of regression

Using the results from the regression and the COMSOL® analysis, we can estimate the circuit elements in the equivalent circuits used to represent the electrode/tissue interface over the chronic implant time for wire 12. According to the COMSOL® results, R_e will initially increase a maximum of 14% from its day one value and decrease to only 7% below this value over time. These changes are small compared to the magnitude of the change of the combined regressed value for series resistance; thus for purposes of the regression analysis, R_e is assumed to be roughly constant and R_{en} is simply calculated to be the regressed value minus R_e for the Randles, day-one circuit. Nonetheless, the shape of the total impedance change (**Figure 4**) follows the shape of the electrolyte resistance change (**Figure 9**).

The real and imaginary parts of the complex impedance contribute to the overall magnitude of the impedance as described in Equation 3

$$Z_{mag} = \sqrt{Z_r^2 + Z_j^2}, \tag{3}$$

where Z_r and Z_j are the real and imaginary parts of the impedance, respectively. Thus it is useful to compare the real and imaginary parts of the different components in the equivalent circuits calculated at 1 kHz. The real and imaginary parts of the parallel combination of R_{ct} and Z_{CPE} are termed $Z_{r,j\text{-interface}}$ and given in **Table 2**. The estimated impedance for the parallel combination of R_{cell} and C_{cell} is termed $Z_{r,j\text{-cell}}$ and also given in **Table 2** along with estimated values for R_e and R_{en} from the regression analysis.

The contribution of the impedance at 1 kHz for components in the Randles circuit is $Z_{r\text{-interface}} + R_e$ and $Z_{j\text{-interface}}$ for the real and imaginary parts, respectively. The tissue encapsulation contribution is $Z_{r\text{-cell}} + R_{en}$ and $Z_{j\text{-cell}}$ for the real and imaginary parts, respectively. Since the real and imaginary parts have a non-linear relationship with the impedance magnitude, both are plotted separately and compared against the magnitude of the impedance in **Figure 10**. Here, key observations can be made. The real part of the impedance is much larger than the imaginary part at 1 kHz. Thus, the magnitude of the complex impedance is dominated by trends in the real part of the impedance as seen in **Figure 10A**.

There is no *a priori* assumed model for the time dependence of the tissue encapsulation process while the COMSOL® simulation of abiotic changes due to corrosion and insulation delamination/cracking indicate a Gaussian temporal dependence. There are several possible scenarios. Though regression analysis was

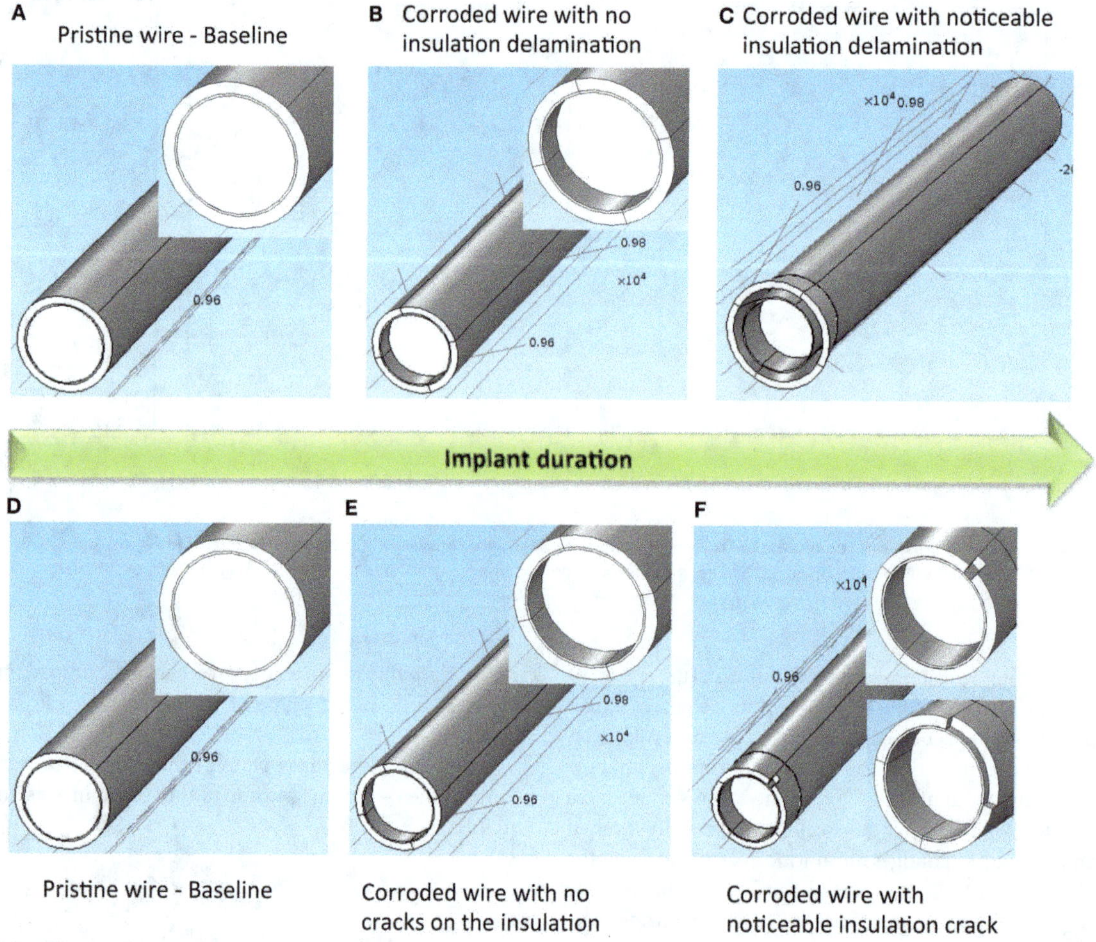

FIGURE 8 | Case 1 for modeled electrode surface modification over implant duration involving both corrosion and insulation delamination. **(A)** Pristine electrode with intact metal and insulation, **(B)** electrode with corroded metal and no insulation delamination, and **(C)** electrode with corroded metal and noticeable insulation delamination. Inset on the left and middle images shows a closer view of the gold layer around the tungsten. Case 2 for modeled electrode surface modification over implant duration involving both corrosion and insulation cracking. **(D)** Pristine electrode with intact metal and insulation, **(E)** electrode with corroded metal and no insulation crack, and **(F)** electrode with corroded metal and noticeable insulation crack. Inset on the left, middle and right images shows a closer view of the gold layer around the tungsten.

performed for only one electrode out of the array, because of the similarity of the trends in the complex impedance spectra for the remaining electrodes, the impedance changes are expected to be similar. We surmise that the rise in impedance magnitude, which resulted in an average increase of 100% is dominated by biotic tissue encapsulation factors; however, the coupling or acceleration of the biotic factors by the prolonged foreign body response due to corrosion is unknown. The subsequent fall in the impedance magnitude could be due to both biotic and abiotic factors. Since the tissue encapsulation layer is known to swell in the beginning and then decrease to a more compact layer in the chronic stage, a rise and fall in the impedance magnitude is possible. However, it should not decrease to a value that is lower than the initial value. In at least half of the electrodes in the array under study, the impedance magnitude decreased to a value that was 25–50% lower than the initial value. Therefore, abiotic effects that increased the surface area and perhaps greatly reduced the encapsulation R_{en} and electrolyte resistance R_e may be significant.

LIMITATIONS TO THE MODEL

The major source of error in our analysis is the assumption of the equivalent circuit for the *in vivo* electrode/tissue interface. Similar circuit elements were used previously to model the tissue encapsulation (Johnson et al., 2005; Otto et al., 2006; Williams et al., 2007; Lempka et al., 2011). The Randles circuit may not be a good model for an electrode undergoing corrosion where the microstructure contains numerous pores and other surface variations. Incorporation of porous electrode equivalent circuit models could provide a better fit to the experimental data. However, the dominance of the impedance due to tissue encapsulation at 1 kHz makes our estimation appropriate. The uncertainty in the regression was not calculated since a Monte Carlo approach would have been needed to calculate the error in the regressed

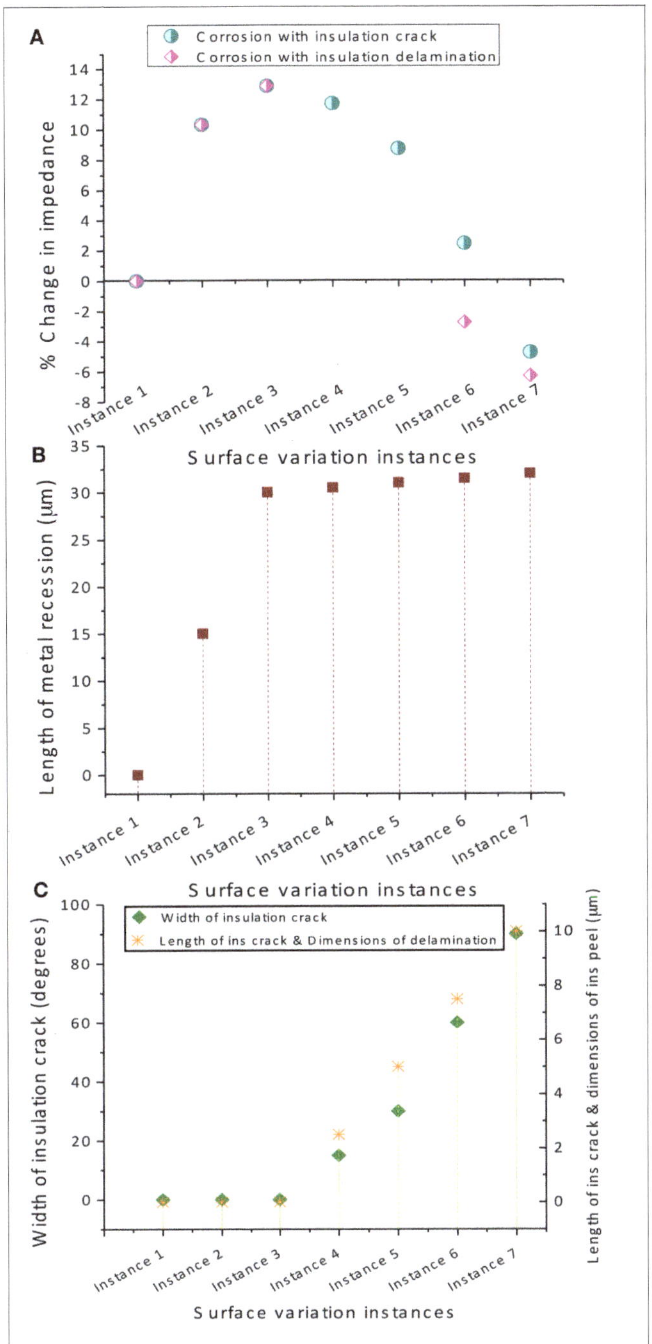

FIGURE 9 | COMSOL® 3D simulated results. (A) Percentage change in electrode impedance for corrosion and (Case 1) insulation delamination and (Case 2) insulation cracking at different instances, **(B)** variation in the metal recession length at different instances to model corrosion, and **(C)** variation of insulation crack width and length and delamination dimensions at different instances. Note that a converged solution could not be obtained for instances 4 and 5 for the insulation delamination case since the FEA solver could not generate a mesh for very small variations in geometry.

Table 2 | Real and imaginary parts of impedance of equivalent circuit parameters for wire 12.

	Impedance (kΩ) at 1 kHz					
Day	$Z_{r\text{-interface}}$	$Z_{j\text{-interface}}$	$Z_{r\text{-cell}}$	$Z_{j\text{-cell}}$	R_{en}	R_e
1	3.7	−11.4	0	0	0	21
7	4.2	−9.2	60.0	−24.8	57.4	21
15	3.2	−7.8	22.1	−9.8	32.6	21
31	3.8	−8.3	65.3	−30.1	77	21
60	4.2	−8.6	9.0	−5.8	24.0	21
106	4.4	−8.4	12.2	−3.4	9.0	21
149	5.1	−9.1	16.0	−4.7	11.4	21
205	4.4	−8.7	9.0	−4.7	12.7	21

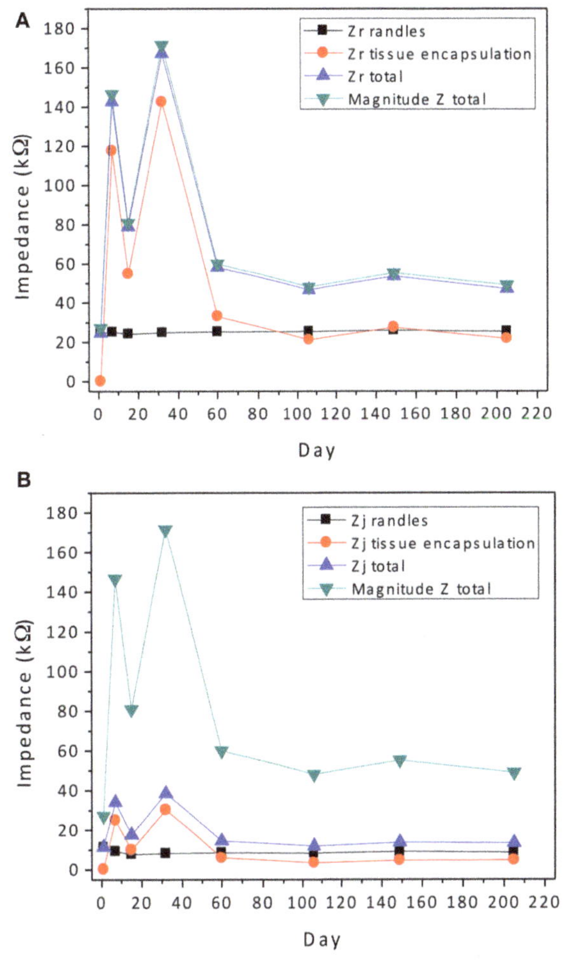

FIGURE 10 | Contribution of the abiotic and biotic components to the real (A) and imaginary (B) parts of the complex impedance compared to the magnitude of the total impedance. All impedance values were calculated at 1 kHz.

parameters. Finally, additional impedance data points at higher frequencies would improve the accuracy of the regression analysis. The maximum measurement frequency of 2 kHz was limited by the impedance tester used.

CONCLUSIONS

We examined the complex impedance trends of a 16 channel tungsten microwire array used in a chronic *in vivo* neural recording study. This array had good functional performance throughout the implant duration and its impedance magnitude at 1 kHz showed temporal variability in the first few weeks that on average was Gaussian in shape. Time varying equivalent circuits that model the varying surface morphology and tissue response were shown to exhibit different structure in the complex impedance. To better understand the origin of the temporal change in the real part of the complex impedance, the abiotic electrolyte resistance was modeled in COMSOL® using a time varying geometry that simulated changes in the recession depth of the electrode surface due to corrosion and insulation changes due to delamination and cracking. A similar Gaussian shape in the electrolyte resistance was observed due to the competing effects of recessed electrode surface and increased exposure of the electrode shank area. The latter abiotic mechanism of insulation delamination can result in a lower impedance than the original reference impedance while the biotic mechanisms of tissue encapsulation cannot. Conversely, tissue encapsulation could be responsible for the larger magnitude increase in the electrode impedance initially. It can be concluded that both biotic and abiotic factors play key roles in the observed electrode impedance change in chronically implanted recording electrodes.

To generalize the results of this study, a Gaussian temporal variation of the impedance magnitude at 1 kHz with a rise and fall that changes to upward of 500% represents the effect of the biotic inflammatory response at the electrode/tissue interface and abiotic corrosion and insulation deterioration at the electrode surface that does not necessarily hinder functional performance during the implant duration of 9 months. These results suggest that an electrode array whose impedance magnitude at 1 kHz has very dissimilar temporal variations than the electrodes in this study may indicate that an abnormal abiotic malfunction such as a mechanical failure in the array or severe insulation delamination may have occurred.

ACKNOWLEDGMENTS

We thank the staff at the Major Analytical Instrumentation Center (MAIC) at the University of Florida for their help with the SEM imaging of the electrodes and the staff at the Materials Evaluation and Testing Laboratory (METLAB) at the South Dakota State University for their help with analyzing the surface roughness and measuring the corrosion depth of the electrodes. This work was sponsored by the Defense Advanced Research Projects Agency (DARPA) Microsystems Technology Office under the auspices of Dr. Jack Judy (jack.judy@darpa.mil) through the Space and Naval Warfare Systems Center, Pacific grant no N66001-11-1-4009.

REFERENCES

Baumann, S. B., Wozny, D. R., Kelly, S. K., and Meno, F. M. (1997). The electrical conductivity of human cerebrospinal fluid at body temperature. *IEEE Trans. Biomed. Eng.* 44, 220–223. doi: 10.1109/10.554770

Biran, R., Martin, D., and Tresco, P. (2005). Neuronal cell loss accompanies the brain tissue response to chronically implanted silicon microelectrode arrays. *Exp. Neurol.* 195, 115–126. doi: 10.1016/j.expneurol.2005.04.020

Biran, R., Martin, D., and Tresco, P. (2007). The brain tissue response to implanted silicon microelectrode arrays is increased when the device is tethered to the skull. *J. Biomed. Mater Res. A* 82, 169–178. doi: 10.1002/jbm.a.31138

Brug, G., den Eeden, A. V., Sluyters-Rehbach, M., and Sluyters, J. (1984). The analysis of electrode impedances complicated by the presence of a constant phase element. *Electroanal. Chem.* 176, 275–295. doi: 10.1016/S0022-0728(84)80324-1

Burke, B., and Lewis, C. E. (2000). *The Macrophage.* New York, NY: Oxford University Press.

Freire, M. A. M., Morya, E., Faber, J., Santos, J. R., Guimaraes, J. S., Lemos, N. A. M., et al. (2011). Comprehensive analysis of tissue preservation and recording quality from chronic multielectrode implants. *PLoS ONE* 6:e27554. doi: 10.1371/journal.pone.0027554

Grill, W. M., and Mortimer, J. T. (1994). Electrical properties of implant encapsulation tissue. *Ann. Biomed. Eng.* 22, 23–33. doi: 10.1007/BF02368219

HD Microsystems. (2001). *Product Information: Pyralin PI2525, PI2555, PI-2575 & PI2556 I2525, PI2555, PI-2575 & PI2556.* Available online at: www.hdmicrosystems.com

Johnson, M. D., Otto, K. J., and Kipke, D. R. (2005). Repeated voltage biasing improves unit recordings by reducing resistive tissue impedances. *IEEE Trans. Neural Syst. Rehabil. Eng.* 13, 160–165. doi: 10.1109/TNSRE.2005.847373

Kim, Y. T., Hitchcock, R. W., Bridge, M. J., and Tresco, P. A. (2004). Chronic response of adult rat brain tissue to implants anchored to the skull. *Biomaterials* 25, 2229–2237. doi: 10.1016/j.biomaterials.2003.09.010

Lempka, S. F., Johnson, M. D., Moffitt, M. A., Otto, K. J., Kipke, D. R., and Mcintyre, C. C. (2011). Theoretical analysis of intracortical microelectrode recordings. *J. Neural Eng.* 8:045006. doi: 10.1088/1741-2560/8/4/045006

McAdams, E. T., Lackermeier, A., McLaughlin, J. A., Macken, D., and Jossinet, J. (1995). The linear and non-linear electrical properties of the electrode-electrolyte interface. *Biosens. Bioelectron.* 10, 67–74. doi: 10.1016/0956-5663(95)96795-Z

McConnell, G. C., Rees, H. D., Levey, A. I., Gutekunst, C. A., Gross, R. E., and Bellamkonda, R. V. (2009). Implanted neural electrodes cause chronic, local inflammation that is correlated with local neurodegeneration. *J. Neural Eng.* 6, 056003. doi: 10.1088/1741-2560/6/5/056003

Orazem, M. E., Pébère, N., and Tribollet, B. (2006). Enhanced graphical representation of electrochemical impedance data. *J. Electrochem. Soc.* 153, B129–B136. doi: 10.1149/1.2168377

Otto, K. J., Johnson, M. D., and Kipke, D. R. (2006). Voltage pulses change neural interface properties and improve unit recordings with chronically implanted microelectrodes. *IEEE Trans. Biomed. Eng.* 53, 333–340. doi: 10.1109/TBME.2005.862530

Patrick, E., Orazem, M., Sanchez, J., and Nishida, T. (2011). Corrosion of tungsten microelectrodes used in neural recording applications. *J. Neurosci. Methods* 198, 158–171. doi: 10.1016/j.jneumeth.2011.03.012

Polikov, V., Tresco, P., and Reichert, W. (2005). Response of brain tissue to chronically implanted neural electrodes. *J. Neurosci. Methods* 148, 1–18. doi: 10.1016/j.jneumeth.2005.08.015

Prasad, A., and Sanchez, J. (2012). Quantifying long-term microelectrode array functionality using chronic *in vivo* impedance testing. *J. Neural Eng.* 9, 026028. doi: 10.1088/1741-2560/9/2/026028

Prasad, A., Xue, Q.-S., Sankar, V., Nishida, T., Shaw, G., Streit, W. J., et al. (2012). Comprehensive characterization and failure modes of tungsten microwire arrays in chronic neural implants. *J. Neural Eng.* 9, 056015. doi: 10.1088/1741-2560/9/5/056015

Rennaker, R. L., Ruyle, A. M., Street, S. E., and Sloan, A. M. (2005). An economical multi-channel cortical electrode array for extended periods of recording during behavior. *J. Neurosci. Methods* 142, 97–105. doi: 10.1016/j.jneumeth.2004.07.018

Rizk, M., Bossetti, C., Jochum, T., Callender, S., Nicolelis, M., Turner, D., et al. (2009). A fully implantable 96-channel neural data acquisition system. *J. Neural Eng.* 6, 26002. doi: 10.1088/1741-2560/6/2/026002

Sanchez, J. S., Alba, N., Nishida, T., Batich, C., and Carney, P. (2006). Structural modifications in chronic microwire electrodes for cortical neuroprosthetics: a case study. *IEEE Trans. Neural Syst. Rehabil. Eng.* 14, 217–221. doi: 10.1109/TNSRE.2006.875581

Serway, R. A. (1998). *Principles of Physics.* 2nd Edn. Fort Worth, Texas; London: Saunders College Pub.

Streit, W., Xue, Q., Prasad, A., Sankar, V., Knott, E., Dyer, A., et al. (2012). Electrode failure: tissue, electrical, and material responses. *IEEE Pulse* 3, 30–33. doi: 10.1109/MPUL.2011.2175632

Szarowski, D. H., Andersen, M. D., Retterer, S., Spence, A. J., Isaacson, M., Craighead, H. G., et al. (2003). Brain responses to micro-machined silicon devices. *Brain Res.* 983, 23–35. doi: 10.1016/S0006-8993(03)03023-3

Turner, J. N., Shain, W., Szarowski, D. H., Andersen, M., Martins, S., Isaacson, M., et al. (1999). Cerebral astrocyte response to micromachined silicon implants. *Exp. Neurol.* 156, 33–49. doi: 10.1006/exnr.1998.6983

Ward, M., Rajdev, P., Ellison, C., and Irazoqui, P. (2009). Toward a comparison of microelectrodes for acute and chronic recordings. *Brain Res.* 1282, 183–200. doi: 10.1016/j.brainres.2009.05.052

Williams, J. C., Rennaker, R. L., and Kipke, D. R. (1999b). Stability of chronic multichannel neural recordings: implications for a long-term neural interface. *Neurocomputing* 26–27, 1069–1076. doi: 10.1016/S0925-2312(99)00106-X

Williams, J., Hippensteel, J., Dilgen, J., Shain, W., and Kipke, D. (2007). Complex impedance spectroscopy for monitoring tissue responses to inserted neural implants. *J. Neural Eng.* 4, 410–423. doi: 10.1088/1741-2560/4/4/007

Williams, J., Rennaker, R., and Kipke, D. (1999a). Long-term neural recording characteristics of wire microelectrode arrays implanted in cerebral cortex. *Brain Res. Brain Res. Protoc.* 4, 303–313. doi: 10.1016/S1385-299X(99)00034-3

9

Modeling physiological and pathological human neurogenesis in the dish

Vania Broccoli*, Serena G. Giannelli and Pietro G. Mazzara

Stem Cells and Neurogenesis Unit, Division of Neuroscience, San Raffaele Scientific Institute, Milan, Italy

Edited by:
Paolo Peretto, Università degli Studi di Torino, Italy

Reviewed by:
Harriet D. Baker, Cornell University Weill Medical College, USA
Gonzalo Alvarez-Bolado, University of Heidelberg, Germany

***Correspondence:**
Vania Broccoli, Stem Cells and Neurogenesis Unit, Division of Neuroscience, San Raffaele Scientific Institute, Via Olgettina 58, 20132 Milan, Italy
e-mail: broccoli.vania@hsr.it

New advances in directing the neuronal differentiation of human embryonic and induced pluripotent stem cells (hPSCs, abbreviation intended to convey both categories of pluripotent stem cells) have promoted the development of culture systems capable of modeling early neurogenesis and neural specification at some of their critical milestones. The hPSC-derived neural rosette can be considered the *in vitro* counterpart of the developing neural tube, since both structures share a virtually equivalent architecture and related functional properties. Epigenetic stimulation methods can modulate the identity of the rosette neural progenitors in order to generate authentic neuronal subtypes, as well as a full spectrum of neural crest derivatives. The intrinsic capacity of induced pluripotent cell-derived neural tissue to self-organize has become fully apparent with the emergence of innovative *in vitro* systems that are able to shape the neuronal differentiation of hPSCs into organized tissues that develop in three dimensions. However, significant hurdles remain that must be completely solved in order to facilitate the use of hPSCs in modeling (e.g., late-onset disorders) or in building therapeutic strategies for cell replacement. In this direction, new procedures have been established to promote the maturation and functionality of hPSC-derived neurons. Meanwhile, new methods to accelerate the aging of *in vitro* differentiating cells are still in development. hPSC-based technology has matured enough to offer a significant and reliable model system for early and late neurogenesis that could be extremely informative for the study of the physiological and pathological events that occur during this process. Thus, full exploitation of this cellular system can provide a better understanding of the physiological events that shape human brain structures, as well as a solid platform to investigate the pathological mechanisms at the root of human diseases.

Keywords: ESCs, iPSCs, neural tube, human neurogenesis, rosettes, neural crest, *in vitro* disease modeling, self-aggregation

USING hPSC-DERIVED ROSETTE FORMATION TO MODEL EARLY NEURULATION PROCESSES

The unique developmental potential and replicative capacity of hPSCs offers a nearly unlimited source of specific somatic cell types that can be exploited for *in vitro* mechanistic studies or cell transplantation therapies. Remarkably, neuronal cells were among the first lineages to be differentiated using hPSCs (Reubinoff et al., 2001; Zhang et al., 2001). Neuronal induction was first obtained by promoting the differentiation of hPSCs in aggregate-like embryoid bodies. Subsequently, aggregates were placed in stringent serum-free culture conditions, which selectively facilitate the survival and growth of neural cells. This transition toward the neural lineage is readily manifested in hPSCs (but not in their murine counterparts) because of the appearance of rosette-like structures within the differentiating hPSC colonies (Reubinoff et al., 2001; Zhang et al., 2001). These structures develop from progenitor cells, which line up close together to form a round, columnar epithelium that is reminiscent of blooming rosettes when viewed under bright light.

Further examination of these structures revealed that the rosettes are formed from neural progenitors. These neural progenitors are endowed with highly polarized morphology, as indicated by the presence of tight and adherence junctions at the side facing the internal lumen, while the external side is strongly enriched in laminin-rich extracellular matrix (Lazzari et al., 2006; Elkabetz et al., 2008; Colleoni et al., 2010). This architecture recapitulates the cellular organization of the neural tube, the embryonic primordium of the entire central nervous system (CNS), in both shape and function. In fact, within rosettes, the nuclei of neural progenitor cells undergo a stereotyped movement known as interkinetic nuclear migration, which is harmonized to the cell cycle stage and specific to authentic neural tube cells (Taverna and Huttner, 2010). Nuclei undergoing DNA synthesis localize at the outer edge of the neural tube, while mitotic divisions are confined to its innermost core, a pattern replicated in the same sequence by nuclei within the rosettes (Lazzari et al., 2006; Elkabetz et al., 2008; Colleoni et al., 2010). Therefore, rosettes share the same elementary organization of the developing neural tube; hence, they are equivalent to the developing neural tube with respect to structure and function (**Figure 1**). Rosette neural progenitors intertwine to create overlapping cellular layers; however, they remain constrained to the surface where they anchor. How rosettes can be adapted to the three-dimensional (3D) space, and which morphology and growth pattern they will follow in these culture conditions, have not yet been ascertained. This setting might enable the *in vitro* reproduction not only of neural tube organization, but also (and even more challenging) its organogenesis.

During development, the neural tube is highly patterned along the anterior-posterior and ventral-dorsal axes (Muñoz-Sanjuán and Brivanlou, 2002). In particular, its anterior portion is invariably committed to give rise to the different brain regions. It is worth noting that neural rosettes, when cultured in the mentioned culture conditions, acquire a specific regional code that coincides with the anterior-dorsal section of the developing neural tube, as demonstrated by the acquisition of a specific set of regional molecular markers (Elkabetz et al., 2008; Colleoni et al., 2010; Hu et al., 2010) (**Figure 1**). Considering that rosettes are induced in a medium that lacks any molecular inducer, these findings suggest that the commitment of the anterior-dorsal region represents the default state during neuronal induction, and only subsequent inductive clues, either cell or non-cell autonomous, might override this basal state, imposing other regional identities.

FROM NEURAL TUBE-LIKE ROSETTES TO NEURAL CREST CELL PROGENITORS

In serum-free neurobasal culture conditions, each differentiating hPSC rosette is scattered in an array of disorganized and unpatterned cells. Remarkably, the expression of two specific markers (p75 and HNK1) identified many of these cells as neural crest cells (Lazzari et al., 2006; Gossrau et al., 2007; Lee et al., 2007, 2010). Molecular analyses corroborated the acquisition of the neural crest identity, as shown by expression of the associated molecular determinants. Temporal analysis illustrated how neural crest cells originated by delaminating from rosette structures in a process similar to the epithelial-mesenchymal transition (EMT), which normally occurs during development when nascent neural crest cells arise from the neural tube (Curchoe et al., 2010). Spontaneous emergence of the neural crest component *in vitro* provides additional evidence that PSC-derived rosette structures acquire dorsal identity, since this is the side of the neural tube from which the neural crest is selectively induced during development (Le Douarin et al., 2004).

In agreement with this view, treatment of rosettes with Sonic hedgehog (Shh), a ventralizing morphogen expressed by the floor plate of the ventral neural tube, inhibits the expression of neural crest-specific genes while activating ventral neural tube markers (Colleoni et al., 2010). More importantly, subsequent culturing of neuralized hPSC colonies that had been exposed to epigenetic stimulation with the growth factors bFGF and EGF enabled the

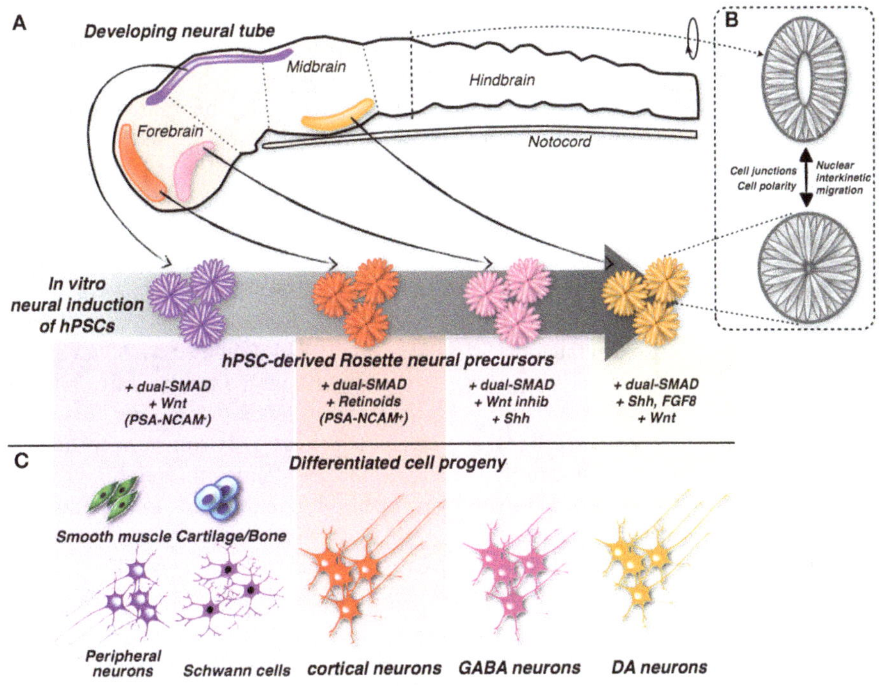

FIGURE 1 | Induction and differentiation of iPSC-derived rosette neural progenitors. (A) Modulation of neurodevelopmental molecular pathways by different combinations of small molecules can direct hPSCs into rosette neural progenitors with different positional identities along the developing neural tube. **(B)** The hPSCs-derived rosette and the neural tube share the same spatial organization showing cells with a remarkable polarization and cell-junction compartmentalization. In addition, relative nuclei position is depending by the cell-cycle stage in both systems. **(C)** According to their specific early commitment, hPSCs-derived rosette neural progenitors generate distinct neuronal sub-types and, in the case of hNCPCs, even non-neuronal somatic cells.

generation of stable cell lines of human neural crest progenitor cells (hNCPCs) (Lazzari et al., 2006; Lee et al., 2007, 2010; Colleoni et al., 2010). hPSC-derived hNCPCs exhibited a stable phenotype, even after sustained proliferation *in vitro* and multiple single cell disaggregation passages.

Notably, although hPSC colonies initially included CNS-like rosette progenitors, the rosette progenitors stopped multiplying and died out over few passages, giving rise to a population of pure hNCPCs (Colleoni et al., 2010). This probably occurred because rosette neural progenitors are extensively polarized epithelial cells, and therefore are susceptible to cell death upon single cell dissociation. Conversely, hNCPCs retained an intrinsic resilience to cell death that might have been gained with the EMT process and the acquirement of mesenchymal-like cell properties (Vega et al., 2004; Robson et al., 2006). Interestingly, the withdrawal of mitogens induced cell cycle exit and the differentiation of neural crest progenitors into an array of somatic cells, including sympathetic and sensory neurons, glial cells, melanocytes, myofibroblasts, cartilage, and bone cells (Lee et al., 2007; Colleoni et al., 2010). Although neural lineages are well represented, their *in vitro* maturation is a weeks-long process. In addition, glial cells progressed to a Schwann cell progenitor stage; these progenitors were positive for S100β and GFAP, although no sign of occurring myelination was ever detected (Lee et al., 2007; Colleoni et al., 2010). Therefore, it remains unknown whether hPSC-derived Schwann cells can be induced to differentiate, or whether they are able to generate functional myelin sheaths around axonal tracts. Clarification of this point will enable the establishment of a valuable model of human myelination.

Furthermore, taking into consideration other neural crest derivatives, an interesting study has recently determined the experimental conditions necessary for the maturation and enrichment of melanocytes from differentiating hNCPCs (Mica et al., 2013). Finally, mesodermal derivatives, including cartilage and bone, have been equally generated from hNCPCs (Lee et al., 2007; Colleoni et al., 2010). This finding may be of great interest for regenerative therapies, exploiting bone and cartilage replacement to treat, for example, trauma or osteoporosis. However, to continue along this direction, it is necessary to address the quality and type of cartilage that hNCPCs are able to generate, as well as (even more importantly) its stability, robustness, and longevity after *in vivo* transplantation.

The induction of both neural and mesenchymal cell lineages indicates that hPSC- derived NCPCs acquire a cranial identity in culture, because only head neural crest contributes to mesoderm-derived structures in the embryo (Le Douarin et al., 2004). Remarkably, clonal analysis identified hNCPCs with mesodermal and/or ectodermal potential similar to what has been described regarding hPSC-derived neural crest cells (Baroffio et al., 1991; Lee et al., 2007). However, different culture conditions or durations in culture can strongly drive hNCPCs from a neural to a mesenchymal phenotype (Lee et al., 2007; our unpublished results). Indeed, the exposure of hNCPCs to a serum-containing medium upregulated mesenchymal markers (e.g., CD73) and stimulated their differentiation into mesodermal derivatives (e.g., smooth muscle, cartilage, and bone cells) (Lee et al., 2007). Therefore, hNCPCs represent an ideal cellular system in which to investigate the molecular mechanisms that regulate this dual cell fate potential, as well as their subsequent final differentiation into a variety of distinct cell types.

LONG-LASTING NEURONAL PROGENITORS CELLS (hNPCs)

While isolating and expanding hNCPCs from hPSC-derived neural rosettes is a straightforward process, the generation of hNPCs is unfortunately hampered by their low survival rate upon rosette dissociation (Elkabetz et al., 2008; Koch et al., 2009). However, this hurdle has been significantly attenuated by the introduction of the Rho-associated protein kinase (ROCK) inhibitor Y-27632, which inhibits single-cell-induced death (Watanabe et al., 2007). hNPCs, which are capable of extensive self-renewal, clonogenicity, and multipotency, have been derived from rosettes by generating neurosphere-like floating aggregates or monolayer cultures (Zhang et al., 2001; Conti et al., 2005). The purity of hNPC cultures has yet to be convincingly assessed, and might be jeopardized by the presence of contaminating hNCPCs. This is an important caveat because many protocols rely on the manual isolation of rosettes, and therefore likely permit the incorporation of closely abutting hNCPCs, which can easily outnumber the hNPCs owing to their better survival and growth rate in the same culture conditions. Taking all of this into consideration, it is always worthwhile to test the presence of p75+ cells in hNPC cultures in order to verify neural crest cell contaminants. Kim et al. (2012) have conceived a valuable approach to prevent such contamination; they demonstrated that polysialylated-neural cell adhesion molecule is strongly enriched in rosette hNPCs, and thus cell sorting for this epitope enables the isolation of a pure population, devoid of any cellular contaminants.

The polysialylated-neural cell adhesion molecule-negative cell fraction is mainly comprised of hNCPCs, thus providing an approach to purify both cells types in a single-step procedure (Kim et al., 2012). Moreover, long-lasting proliferative hNPCs represent a renewable source of neurons and glia that, once established, is independent of hPSC culture. However, growth factor-dependent hNPC expansion might also lead to undesired effects. Indeed, Bilican et al. (2014) noted that chronic exposure to EGF might cause NPCs to lose their anterior identity while assuming a hindbrain regional code. Interestingly, the expansion of hNPCs in the presence of bFGF and physiological levels (3%) of O_2, is sufficient to enable long-term proliferation while maintaining the anterior character that is fundamental for stable differentiation of committed cortical neurons. How hNPCs are able to modify their competent state with respect to regional specification and give rise to different neuronal subtypes is still unclear. Some reports suggest that early hNPCs might still respond to inductive signals in order to acquire a different regional identity (Koch et al., 2009); however, they are unlikely to be able to maintain this capability without change over time and after extensive cell passaging. Given these last observations, several procedures have been established with the aim of generating a single neuronal subtype using direct differentiation of hPSC-derived neural rosettes, some of which are described in the next Section.

CORTICAL NEURONS

Although neural rosettes exhibit a default anterior regional code, their dissociation and subsequent neuronal differentiation in standard culture conditions (e.g., absence of morphogen supplementation) leads to a population of mature neurons that are representative of various brain regions. However, prolonged exposure to the BMP inhibitor Noggin is sufficient to efficiently induce differentiation mainly of cortical neurons (Espuny-Camacho et al., 2013) (**Figure 1**). In addition, the presence of retinoids (retinol-acetate and all-trans retinol) during neural induction and differentiation maximizes the conversion of cortical neurons (Shi et al., 2012). Both procedures converge on the progression of cortical neuronal differentiation with the initial generation of deep layer neurons; superficial layer neurons are generated later, during the development of the cerebral cortex. Therefore, the temporal sequence of neuronal subtype specification in this system mirrors the *in vivo* occurrence of the same process (Greig et al., 2013). Based on these data, one can envisage that this pattern of *in vitro* neurogenesis is mainly mediated by cell autonomous mechanisms, which might be intrinsically encoded within the neuronal progenitors. The generation of both deep and upper cortical neurons from hPSCs covers a very extensive timeframe, which might last for up to 3 months of culture, which dovetails with the delay in cortical neurogenesis that occurs in human embryos compared with mouse embryos (Shi et al., 2012; Espuny-Camacho et al., 2013). More importantly, hPSC-derived cortical neurons grafted into the frontal cortex of the neonatal brain were able to survive, mature, and extend their axons to the proper neuronal targets according to their layer specification (Espuny-Camacho et al., 2013). These data indicate that the use of this *in vitro* system enables the full acquisition of subtype identity, which is then fully elaborated after transplantation. Finally, the grafted human neurons developed functional properties and synaptic connectivity within 3 months after transplantation. It would be of great interest to challenge the transplantation of these neurons in healthy and injured adult brain, in order to verify whether they are able to mature and functionally integrate even in more prohibitive conditions.

GABAergic NEURONS

In contrast to excitatory (glutamatergic) cortical pyramidal neurons that project long distance, inhibitory (GABAergic) cortical interneurons make local synapses and are essential for the maintenance of balanced activity within neural circuits (Marín, 2013; Kepecs and Fishell, 2014). Interneuronal dysfunctions have been described in several disorders, including epilepsy, autism, schizophrenia, and Tourette's syndrome (Valiente and Marín, 2010; Alvarez Dolado and Broccoli, 2011; Marín, 2012). The direct differentiation of hPSCs into telencephalic GABAergic neurons has been achieved recently (Maroof et al., 2013; Nicholas et al., 2013). In both studies, early telencephalic GABAergic commitment of hPSCs was reported by the expression of green fluorescent protein (GFP) under the control of the Nkx2.1 promoter, which is fundamental for setting up the appropriate conditions for the specification of this neuronal subtype. In fact, optimal conditions were attained by combining exposure to BMP and Wnt inhibitors, which prime telencephalic identity, with Shh signaling stimulation, which induces ventral neuronal character, thus reaching up to 70% of Nkx2.1-GFP-positive, hPSC-derived, GABAergic neuronal precursors (**Figure 1**). Cortical interneurons include a different set of neuron types that have distinct roles in cortical development and function (Marín, 2013; Kepecs and Fishell, 2014). In these conditions, the prevalence of somatostatin-positive cells was observed, while many fewer interneurons expressing parvalbumin or VIP were detected. Thus, more work is needed to identify permissive conditions for the effective derivation of the later subtypes. Co-cultures with astrocytes or hippocampal neurons promoted hPSC-derived GABAergic neuronal maturation and functionality, including repetitive action potential firing, ionic channel currents, and synaptic currents. To directly prove their inhibitory synaptic activity, GABAergic neurons were excited by an optogenetic protocol that evoked robust postsynaptic currents in neighboring neurons, which were sensitive to the GABA antagonist bicuculline (Nicholas et al., 2013). Thus, hPSCs can be induced to differentiate into functional inhibitory GABAergic interneurons. It is interesting to point out that upon transplantation into neonatal brains, a fraction of the grafted neurons matured in the host neural tissue, gaining functional properties and synaptic connectivity, although several months of engraftment were required (Nicholas et al., 2013). These last results are particularly compelling in light of the fact that the transplantation of mouse native GABAergic precursors has proven therapeutic in treating animal models of epilepsy, schizophrenia, and Parkinson's disease (PD) (Southwell et al., 2014; Tyson and Anderson, 2014). All of these different pathological conditions have benefited from GABAergic neuronal transplantation, likely because it favors the re-organization of the neuronal circuit connections and the re-establishment of the correct balance between excitation and inhibition in cortical circuits (Southwell et al., 2014; Tyson and Anderson, 2014). In particular, this approach might have a straightforward application regarding the many forms of epilepsy that eventually reach an irreversible, drug-resistant stage.

DOPAMINERGIC NEURONS

Substantia nigra (A9) midbrain dopaminergic neurons are specifically lost during the initial phase of PD. The consequent loss of dopamine availability in striatal tissue is responsible for the troublesome motor impairments that severely affect PD patients. In fact, most of the drugs used to treat PD aim simply to restore sufficient levels of dopamine in the striatum, but cannot reverse or block the loss of dopaminergic neurons (Meissner et al., 2011). In this context, dopamine neuron replacement has been envisioned as a potential therapeutic strategy during the last decades (Dunnett et al., 2001; Lindvall and Björklund, 2011).

Transplantation of midbrain human fetal tissue provided a solid basis for a cellular approach to PD, confirming the ability of transplanted neurons to integrate into the host striatal tissues and sustain functional integration and a therapeutic effect (Barker et al., 2013). However, this approach had little clinical benefit, mainly because of the broad cell heterogeneity of the transplanted tissue, its minimal availability, and scarce immuno-compatibility (Lindvall and Björklund, 2004; Barker et al., 2013). Even worse, these issues were responsible for the development of the troubling side effect of graft-induced dyskinesia, which is experienced by some of the patients (Lane et al., 2010).

Given this context, hPSCs have long been considered a better renewable source of dopamine neurons that could potentially overcome these hurdles. To this purpose, many protocols have been developed for the *in vitro* differentiation of hPSCs into this particular class of neurons. Combined exposure to the morphogens Shh and FGF8, known to contribute to ventral midbrain neural commitment in the developing neural tube, was also found to instruct mouse and human PSCs to differentiate into tyrosine hydroxylase (TH)-positive dopamine neurons (Kim et al., 2002; Perrier et al., 2004; Lee et al., 2009) (**Figure 1**). However, the brain contains distinct dopamine neuronal clusters that differ with regard to function, connectivity, and molecular marker expression. This is a crucial issue because only transplantation of A9 [and not, for example, VTA (A10)] resident dopamine neurons can achieve maximal behavioral recovery in a mouse model of PD (Grealish et al., 2010). Reasonable graft-induced recovery depends on the correct innervation (and thereby the functional activation) of the striatum, which represents the physiological target structure of A9, but not A10, dopamine neurons (Grealish et al., 2010).

These results have far-reaching implications, indicating that the therapeutic benefits of cell transplantation approaches depend on the replacement of native neurons with cells that are close, if not identical, in nature and identity. Improvements in the differentiation of hPSCs into fully committed midbrain dopamine neurons have been attained by two recent studies (Kriks et al., 2011; Kirkeby et al., 2012). Both employed sustained stimulation of Wnt signaling (by inhibiting the enzyme glycogen synthase kinase 3β, GSK-3β) to robustly induce the differentiation of hPSCs into dopamine neurons (**Figure 1**). Neurons derived using this protocol exhibited midbrain character, as confirmed by the expression of the regional markers FoxA2 and Lmx1a (Kriks et al., 2011; Kirkeby et al., 2012). Remarkably, transplantation of these midbrain-specific dopamine neurons in the striatum resulted in significant behavioral recovery in both rodent and primate models of PD (Kriks et al., 2011; Kirkeby et al., 2012).

This transplantation strategy is designed to allocate transplanted dopamine neurons close to their physiological target (striatal neurons) in order to facilitate their functional connectivity, although grafted neurons would be ectopically located regarding their natural midbrain position. It is unknown whether this new neural circuit, its components necessarily re-organized, can fully restore physiological function without any concomitant behavioral alterations. To overcome this limitation, it would be interesting to test whether hPSC-derived neurons transplanted in the substantia nigra are able to re-establish nigro-striatal connections. Although the adult brain parenchyma is minimally permissive to axonal regrowth, grafted fetal dopaminergic neural precursors are surprisingly capable of generating a nigro-striatal pathway with an outgrowth pattern that matches the anatomy of the intrinsic system (Thompson et al., 2009). These results reveal some opportunities to reconstruct native neuronal circuits using a cell transplantation approach in the adult brain. Whether a similar approach can be envisioned using hPSC-derived dopamine neurons remains to be demonstrated.

IN VITRO NEURONAL MATURATION AND AGING

In vitro differentiation of hPSCs into neurons is a long and multistep process that matches all of the stages of embryonic neuronal commitment and differentiation. Therefore, the neurons that result from hPSC induction appear to be very immature soon after their specification; they acquire functional properties only after several weeks in culture. Mature functional and synaptic properties are observed in the majority of the hPSC-derived neurons after 8–12 weeks of culture (Ricciardi et al., 2012; Verpelli et al., 2013). Thus, this delay in functional maturation of the hPSC-derived neurons *in vitro* certainly hampers the conduct of functional studies using this system.

Supplementation of the culture medium with neurotrophins and cAMP can enhance neuronal differentiation and restrain cell death events (Soldner et al., 2009). However, a major differentiating stimulus is provided when hPSC-derived neurons are co-cultured on a primary astrocyte feeder layer. In fact, neuronal differentiation, dendrite development, excitability, and synaptic activity are all accelerated from 8- to 20-fold when hPSC-derived neurons are cultured on astrocytes rather than on laminin (Tang et al., 2013). Zhang et al. (2013) recently devised an interesting alternative. They have shown that hPSC differentiation can yield a high level of functional glutamatergic neuronal cells in less than 2 weeks through the forced expression of only one transcription factor, Neurogenin 2. This is an attractive procedure because neurons are generated directly from naïve hPSCs in a single manipulation step, thereby skipping all of the intermediate steps and saving time and labor. A similar approach has been employed recently to accelerate the generation of functional dopamine neurons by expressing the Ascl1, Nurr1, and Lmx1a genes in naïve hPSCs (Theka et al., 2013).

As mentioned above, neurons derived from hPSCs require time to mature fully and are comparable to cells at the immature fetal stage (Marchetto and Gage, 2012). This is particularly troublesome when one aims to study the mechanisms of neuronal aging and associated neurodegenerative disorders. In fact, neuronal aging is a major contributor to late-onset neurodegenerative disorders and must be taken into account when modeling such disorders. In order to model late-onset diseases, recent studies have employed hPSC-derived neuronal *in vitro* cultures that have been grown for up to 200 days (Dimos et al., 2008; Ebert et al., 2009). hPSCs represent an interesting system with which to follow changes in the morphological and functional properties of neurons over a long period of time *in vitro*, possibly mimicking some of the processes that occur during aging. However, new solutions are needed to accelerate the aging process of these neurons *in vitro*. Notably, a new approach has been recently proposed that involves the expression of progerin, a truncated form of lamin-A that is associated with premature aging (Miller et al., 2013). In fact, the expression of progerin in hPSC-derived fibroblasts and neurons induced multiple aging-related markers and characteristics, including the appearance of neuromelanin in dopamine neurons (Miller et al., 2013). It remains to be established which features of late-onset disease can be authentically recapitulated by the progerin-induced model *in vitro*. Similar to this study, other known age-specific molecular pathways might be explored to promote neuronal aging *in vitro* (Newgard and Sharpless, 2013).

PATHOLOGICAL NEUROGENESIS: MODELING HUMAN DISEASES USING NEURONS GENERATED *IN VITRO*

The advent of reprogramming adult human cells to become human induced pluripotent stem cells (hiPSCs) has revealed new opportunities to model disorders linked to a genetic cause. hiPSCs are able to self-renew and give rise to the affected somatic cells, providing an unlimited source of informative material to investigate diseases of interest. To date, a number of studies have validated this approach, modeling both neurological and neuropsychiatric disorders (Tiscornia et al., 2011; Zhu et al., 2011; Sandoe and Eggan, 2013). Monogenic diseases in which the mutated gene is known are particularly suitable for this approach. In this scenario, the function of the gene of interest can be restored, thus proving that the original mutation was indeed the causative factor of the disease-specific phenotype (Soldner et al., 2011; Liu et al., 2012). The approach is particularly relevant because the individual genetic variability of human sample often hampers any comparison between patient and healthy donor cells, disabling the detection of phenotype differences (Saha and Jaenisch, 2009). In fact, it would be necessary to analyze a large cohort of control and patient cells in parallel in order to address this matter, which would require a huge effort to generate and analyze a large range of hiPSC lines. Some compelling studies have been reported recently that illustrate the power of this approach in helping to identify new cellular and molecular mechanisms of disease; we report a few notable examples here.

Lee et al. (2010) developed an hiPSC model of familial dysautonomia, a disorder that causes depletion of the autonomic and sensory neurons, induced by mutations in the IKBKAP gene. In the hiPSC system, they were able to correlate the loss of IKBKAP gene expression with defects in neurogenesis and diminished cell motility in hiPSC-derived neural crest cells. Similarly, Marchetto et al. (2010) used neurons derived from the hiPSCs of individuals affected by Rett syndrome (RTT), an autism-like disorder caused by mutations in the methyl CpG binding protein MECP2. Lack of MeCP2 protein in hiPSC-derived neurons was associated with decreases in dendritic spines, synapses, and calcium oscillation frequency, as well as a concurrent reduction in nuclear size compared with control cells. A more recent study used an isogenic human embryonic stem cell model of RTT to identify a significant reduction in nascent protein synthesis (Li et al., 2013). Moreover, cells manifested a severe defect in AKT/mTOR pathway activity that resulted from the lack of MECP2 expression (Ricciardi et al., 2011; Li et al., 2013). More interestingly, the activation of AKT/mTOR signaling was sufficient to ameliorate the disease phenotypes in mutant hiPSC-derived neurons, by boosting protein synthesis. These data clearly show how the hiPSC modeling system is a convenient platform for the development of pharmacologic and genetic approaches that aim to revert a mutant phenotype using either a hypothesis-driven procedure or a more systematic solution.

A relevant question is whether hiPSC-based modeling can be fruitful for studying late-onset neurodegenerative diseases. In a recent study, hiPSC-derived neurons from patients with genetic or sporadic forms of Alzheimer disease (AD) did not exhibit enhanced susceptibility to cell death or changes in activity compared with controls (Israel et al., 2012). However, they did exhibit significantly higher levels of the pathological markers amyloid-β, phospho-Tau, and active GSK-3β than control cells. These hiPSC-derived neurons from AD patients also accumulated large RAB5-positive early endosomes compared with controls. Importantly, treatment of purified neurons with β-secretase inhibitors, but not γ-secretase inhibitors, caused significant reductions in phospho-Tau and GSK-3β levels (Israel et al., 2012). Therefore, a direct relationship can be drawn between the proteolytic processing of amyloid precursor protein, but not that of amyloid-β, in GSK-3β activation and Tau phosphorylation in hiPSC-derived neurons. These data suggest that hiPSC technology can be used to observe early pathological changes, possibly associated with the prodromal phase of AD, even if it does not faithfully recapitulate the phenotypes that characterize the late-onset phase.

NEURAL INDUCTION FROM A SINGLE LAYER TO THREE DIMENSIONS

The employment of cutting-edge culture procedures has recently elevated the potential of neural rosettes to recapitulate the events and mechanisms that underlie neural tube development to another dimension (Eiraku et al., 2008; Lancaster et al., 2013). Studies have recently reported the generation of *in vitro* 3D cell aggregates (organoids) that not only reproduce an organ's structure, but also recapitulate its function and development (Sato et al., 2009; Suga et al., 2011; Kadoshima et al., 2013). The applications of this technology to the investigation of still-unapproached aspects of organogenesis promise to bear relevant knowledge that is instrumental to a full understanding of tissue formation and pathogenesis.

The possibility of modeling human brain disease in a Petri dish (Eiraku et al., 2008) is certainly the most attractive, but innumerable implications can be imagined. Two different approaches have attempted to reproduce corticogenesis (and, even more surprisingly, brain morphogenesis) using hPSCs: quick re-aggregation of cells was determinant in the first case (Eiraku et al., 2008; Kadoshima et al., 2013), while larger and more complex structures (cerebral organoids) were achieved in the second case using a spinning bioreactor (Lancaster et al., 2013). Each approach generated a complex, multilayered structure that was able to self-organize and possessed morphogenetic features highly reminiscent of brain development. Among the most impressive: formation of an apical and basal membrane and specification of the anterior-posterior axis. Nonetheless, the specification of a larger number of brain areas (e.g., sub-pallial structures) was only detectable within cerebral organoids. This finding is particularly relevant because it has permitted the recapitulation of a key process of brain development that is highly correlated with numerous cortical deficits, such as the invasion of the neocortex by migrating GABAergic neurons originating in the sub-palladium.

Corticogenesis itself was also partially recapitulated in both cellular systems. Cortical development is a highly dynamic and complex process in which an internal layer of neuroepithelial progenitors (the ventricular zone) generates post-mitotic neurons that migrate and stratify in an inside-first outside-last fashion depending on their birth date (Molyneaux et al., 2007). As expected, the cardinal features of the neuroepithelial progenitors, already identified in neural rosettes, were also observed in the apical or luminal side of 3D structures, where progenitors reside. Further characterization of these cells revealed features typical of radial glial cells (RGCs, late progenitors of the neocortex), such as apical and basal processes. Moreover, a population of transient Tbr2-positive amplifying cells (which normally occupy the sub-ventricular zone of the developing cortex) was also identified adjacent to RGC-like cells. It is worth noting the description of a third type of progenitors predominantly derived from human cultures. The appearance of these cells (mainly characterized by the absence of the apical process) is highly reminiscent of outer-radial glial (oRG), an important hallmark of human neurogenesis in contrast to murine neurogenesis. The abundance of these cells in the developing human cortex has been associated with more complex structural features, such as cortical gyrification; thus, the presence of oRG-like cells indicates the faithful reproduction of human corticogenesis in 3D culture.

The identification of a progeny of post-mitotic neurons that form layers that are positioned basally over proliferative areas according to their time of birth has further confirmed the identity of the progenitor niche. The distribution and specification of post-mitotic neurons in quickly re-aggregated cells and in cerebral organoids has managed to recapitulate the early events of corticogenesis, although the realization of a fully layered cortex still remains to be established. Nonetheless, a simpler but equally laminated neuroepithelial structure, the retina (Eiraku et al., 2011; Nakano et al., 2012), was reproduced *in vitro* in similar culture conditions, once again confirming the ability of neuroepithelial cells to self-organize. The importance of this cardinal feature might lie in the ability of these cells to polarize (and consequently, to form rosettes). It was recently suggested that the same processes, polarization and rosette formation, are fundamentally involved in epiblast specification and self-organization, which emphasizes the intriguing hypothesis of a possible common mechanism in tissue morphogenesis.

The advent of 3D cultures can significantly change the way we see not only regenerative medicine, but also cell research en bloc. Although this system can provide unique information, great effort will have to be deployed to shepherd these expectations into solid reality.

ACKNOWLEDGMENTS

Work in Broccoli's laboratory is supported by funding from the European Research Council (AdERC), Italian Ministry of Health, IIT/SEED, CoEN, ERA-Net, and EC-FP7 program.

REFERENCES

Alvarez Dolado, M., and Broccoli, V. (2011). GABAergic neuronal precursor grafting: implications in brain regeneration and plasticity. *Neural Plast.* 2011:384216. doi: 10.1155/2011/384216

Barker, R. A., Barrett, J., Mason, S. L., and Björklund, A. (2013). Fetal dopaminergic transplantation trials and the future of neural grafting in Parkinson's disease. *Lancet Neurol.* 12, 84–91. doi: 10.1016/S1474-4422(12)70295-8

Baroffio, A., Dupin, E., and Le Dourin, N. M. (1991). Common precursors for neural and mesectodermal derivatives in the cephalic neural crest. *Development* 112, 301–305.

Bilican, B., Livesey, M. R., Haghi, G., Qiu, J., Burr, K., Siller, R., et al. (2014). Physiological normoxia and absence of EGF is required for the long-term propagation of anterior neural precursors from human pluripotent cells. *PLoS ONE.* 9:e85932. doi: 10.1371/journal.pone.0085932

Colleoni, S., Galli, C., Giannelli, S. G., Armentero, M. T., Blandini, F., Broccoli, V., et al. (2010). Long-term culture and differentiation of CNS precursors derived from anterior human neural rosettes following exposure to ventralizing factors. *Exp. Cell Res.* 316, 1148–1158. doi: 10.1016/j.yexcr.2010.02.013

Conti, L., Pollard, S. M., Gorba, T., Reitano, E., Toselli, M., Biella, G., et al. (2005). Niche-independent symmetrical self-renewal of a mammalian tissue stem cell. *PLoS Biol.* 3:e283. doi: 10.1371/journal.pbio.0030283

Curchoe, C. L., Maurer, J., McKeown, S. J., Cattarossi, G., Cimadamore, F., Nilbratt, M., et al. (2010). Early acquisition of neural crest competence during hESCs neuralization. *PLoS ONE.* 5:e13890. doi: 10.1371/journal.pone.0013890

Dimos, J. T., Rodolfa, K. T., Niakan, K. K., Weisenthal, L. M., Mitsumoto, H., Chung, W., et al. (2008). Induced pluripotent stem cells generated from patients with ALS can be differentiated into motor neurons. *Science* 321, 1218–1221. doi: 10.1126/science.1158799

Dunnett, S. B., Björklund, A., and Lindvall, O. (2001). Cell therapy in Parkinson's disease—stop or go? *Nat. Rev. Neurosci.* 2, 365–369. doi: 10.1038/35072572

Ebert, A. D., Yu, J., Rose, F. F. Jr., Mattis, V. B., Lorson, C. L., Thomson, J. A., et al. (2009). Induced pluripotent stem cells from a spinal muscular atrophy patient. *Nature* 457, 277–280. doi: 10.1038/nature07677

Eiraku, M., Takata, N., Ishibashi, H., Kawada, M., Sakakura, E., Okuda, S., et al. (2011). Self-organizing optic-cup morphogenesis in three-dimensional culture. *Nature* 472, 51–56. doi: 10.1038/nature09941

Eiraku, M., Watanabe, K., Matsuo-Takasaki, M., Kawada, M., Yonemura, S., Matsumura, M., et al. (2008). Self-organized formation of polarized cortical tissues from ESCs and its active manipulation by extrinsic signals. *Cell Stem Cell* 3, 519–532. doi: 10.1016/j.stem.2008.09.002

Elkabetz, Y., Panagiotakos, G., Al Shamy, G., Socci, N. D., Tabar, V., and Studer, L. (2008). Human, E. S. cell-derived neural rosettes reveal a functionally distinct early neural stem cell stage. *Genes Dev.* 22, 152–165. doi: 10.1101/gad.1616208

Espuny-Camacho, I., Michelsen, K. A., Gall, D., Linaro, D., Hasche, A., Bonnefont, J., et al. (2013). Pyramidal neurons derived from human pluripotent stem cells integrate efficiently into mouse brain circuits *in vivo*. *Neuron* 77, 440–456. doi: 10.1016/j.neuron.2012.12.011

Gossrau, G., Thiele, J., Konang, R., Schmandt, T., and Brüstle, O. (2007). Bone morphogenetic protein-mediated modulation of lineage diversification during neural differentiation of embryonic stem cells. *Stem Cells* 25, 939–949. doi: 10.1634/stemcells.2006-0299

Grealish, S., Jönsson, M. E., Li, M., Kirik, D., Björklund, A., and Thompson, L. H. (2010). The A9 dopamine neuron component in grafts of ventral mesencephalon is an important determinant for recovery of motor function in a rat model of Parkinson's disease. *Brain.* 133(pt 2), 482–495. doi: 10.1093/brain/awp328

Greig, L. C., Woodworth, M. B., Galazo, M. J., Padmanabhan, H., and Macklis, J. D. (2013). Molecular logic of neocortical projection neuron specification, development and diversity. *Nat. Rev. Neurosci.* 14, 755–769. doi: 10.1038/nrn3586

Hu, B. Y., Weick, J. P., Yu, J., Ma, L. X., Zhang, X. Q., Thomson, J. A., et al. (2010). Neural differentiation of human induced pluripotent stem cells follows developmental principles but with variable potency. *Proc. Natl. Acad. Sci. U.S.A.* 107, 4335–4340. doi: 10.1073/pnas.0910012107

Israel, M. A., Yuan, S. H., Bardy, C., Reyna, S. M., Mu, Y., Herrera, C., et al. (2012). Probing sporadic and familial Alzheimer's disease using induced pluripotent stem cells. *Nature* 482, 216–220. doi: 10.1038/nature10821

Kadoshima, T., Sakaguchi, H., Nakano, T., Soen, M., Ando, S., Eiraku, M., et al. (2013). Self-organization of axial polarity, inside-out layer pattern, and species-specific progenitor dynamics in human ES cell-derived neocortex. *Proc. Natl. Acad. Sci. U.S.A.* 110, 20284–20289. doi: 10.1073/pnas.1315710110

Kepecs, A., and Fishell, G. (2014). Interneuron cell types are fit to function. *Nature* 505, 318–326. doi: 10.1038/nature12983

Kim, D. S., Lee, D. R., Kim, H. S., Yoo, J. E., Jung, S. J., Lim, B. Y., et al. (2012). Highly pure and expandable PSA-NCAM-positive neural precursors from human ESC and iPSC-derived neural rosettes. *PLoS ONE.* 7:e39715. doi: 10.1371/journal.pone.0039715

Kim, J. H., Auerbach, J. M., Rodriguez-Gomez, J. A., Velasco, I., Gavin, D., Lumelsky, N., et al. (2002). Dopamine neurons derived from embryonic stem cells function in an animal model of Parkinson's disease. *Nature* 418, 50–56. doi: 10.1038/nature00900

Kirkeby, A., Grealish, S., Wolf, D. A., Nelander, J., Wood, J., Lundblad, M., et al. (2012). Generation of regionally specified neural progenitors and functional neurons from human embryonic stem cells under defined conditions. *Cell Rep.* 1, 703–714. doi: 10.1016/j.celrep.2012.04.009

Koch, P., Opitz, T., Steinbeck, J. A., and Brustle, O. (2009). A rosette-type, self-renewing human ES cell-derived neural stem cell with potential for *in vitro* instruction and synaptic integration. *Proc. Natl. Acad. Sci. U.S.A.* 106, 3225–3230. doi: 10.1073/pnas.0808387106

Kriks, S., Shim, J. W., Piao, J., Ganat, Y. M., Wakeman, D. R., Xie, Z., et al. (2011). Dopamine neurons derived from human ES cells efficiently engraft in animal models of Parkinson's disease. *Nature* 480, 547–551. doi: 10.1038/nature10648

Lancaster, M. A., Renner, M., Martin, C. A., Wenzel, D., Bicknell, L. S., Hurles, M. E., et al. (2013). Cerebral organoids model human brain development and microcephaly. *Nature* 501, 373–379. doi: 10.1038/nature12517

Lane, E. L., Björklund, A., Dunnett, S. B., and Winkler, C. (2010). Neural grafting in Parkinson's disease unraveling the mechanisms underlying graft-induced dyskinesia. *Prog. Brain Res.* 184, 295–309. doi: 10.1016/S0079-6123(10)84015-4

Lazzari, G., Colleoni, S., Giannelli, S. G., Brunetti, D., Colombo, E., Lagutina, I., et al. (2006). Direct derivation of neural rosettes from cloned bovine blastocysts: a model of early neurulation events and neural crest specification *in vitro*. *Stem Cells.* 24, 2514–2521. doi: 10.1634/stemcells.2006-0149

Le Douarin, N. M., Creuzet, S., Couly, G., and Dupin, E. (2004). Neural crest cell plasticity and its limits. *Development* 131, 4637–4650. doi: 10.1242/dev.01350

Lee, G., Chambers, S. M., Tomishima, M. J., and Studer, L. (2010). Derivation of neural crest cells from human pluripotent stem cells. *Nat. Protoc.* 5, 688–701. doi: 10.1038/nprot.2010.35

Lee, G., Kim, H., Elkabetz, Y., Al Shamy, G., Panagiotakos, G., Barberi, T., et al. (2007). Isolation and directed differentiation of neural crest stem cells derived from human embryonic stem cells. *Nat. Biotechnol.* 25, 1468–1475. doi: 10.1038/nbt1365

Lee, G., Papapetrou, E. P., Kim, H., Chambers, S. M., Tomishima, M. J., Fasano, C. A., et al. (2009). Modelling pathogenesis and treatment of familial dysautonomia using patient-specific iPSCs. *Nature* 461, 402–406. doi: 10.1038/nature08320

Li, Y., Wang, H., Muffat, J., Cheng, A. W., Orlando, D. A., Lovén, J., et al. (2013). Global transcriptional and translational repression in human-embryonic-stem-cell-derived Rett syndrome neurons. *Cell Stem Cell* 13, 446–458. doi: 10.1016/j.stem.2013.09.001

Lindvall, O., and Björklund, A. (2004). Cell therapy in Parkinson's disease. *NeuroRx* 1, 382–393. doi: 10.1602/neurorx.1.4.382

Lindvall, O., and Björklund, A. (2011). Cell therapeutics in Parkinson's disease. *Neurotherapeutics* 8, 539–548. doi: 10.1007/s13311-011-0069-6

Liu, G. H., Qu, J., Suzuki, K., Nivet, E., Li, M., Montserrat, N., et al. (2012). Progressive degeneration of human neural stem cells caused by pathogenic LRRK2. *Nature* 491, 603–607. doi: 10.1038/nature11557

Marchetto, M. C., Carromeu, C., Acab, A., Yu, D., Yeo, G. W., Mu, Y., et al. (2010). A model for neural development and treatment of Rett syndrome using human induced pluripotent stem cells. *Cell* 143, 527–539. doi: 10.1016/j.cell.2010.10.016

Marchetto, M. C., and Gage, F. H. (2012). Modeling brain disease in a dish: really? *Cell Stem Cell* 10, 642–645. doi: 10.1016/j.stem.2012.05.008

Marín, O. (2012). Interneuron dysfunction in psychiatric disorders. *Nat. Rev. Neurosci.* 13, 107–120. doi: 10.1038/nrn3155

Marín, O. (2013). Cellular and molecular mechanisms controlling the migration of neocortical interneurons. *Eur. J. Neurosci.* 38, 2019–2029. doi: 10.1111/ejn.12225

Maroof, A. M., Keros, S., Tyson, J. A., Ying, S. W., Ganat, Y. M., Merkle, F. T., et al. (2013). Directed differentiation and functional maturation of cortical interneurons from human embryonic stem cells. *Cell Stem Cell* 12, 559–572. doi: 10.1016/j.stem.2013.04.008

Meissner, W. G., Frasier, M., Gasser, T., Goetz, C. G., Lozano, A., Piccini, P., et al. (2011). Priorities in Parkinson's disease research. *Nat. Rev. Drug Discov.* 10, 377–393. doi: 10.1038/nrd3430

Mica, Y., Lee, G., Chambers, S. M., Tomishima, M. J., and Studer, L. (2013). Modeling neural crest induction, melanocyte specification, and disease-related pigmentation defects in hESCs and patient-specific iPSCs. *Cell Rep.* 3, 1140–1152. doi: 10.1016/j.celrep.2013.03.025

Miller, J. D., Ganat, Y. M., Kishinevsky, S., Bowman, R. L., Liu, B., Tu, E. Y., et al. (2013). Human iPSC-based modeling of late-onset disease via progerin-induced aging. *Cell Stem Cell* 13, 691–705. doi: 10.1016/j.stem.2013.11.006

Molyneaux, B. J., Arlotta, P., Menezes, J. R., and Macklis, J. D. (2007). Neuronal subtype specification in the cerebral cortex. *Nat. Rev. Neurosci.* 8, 427–437. doi: 10.1038/nrn2151

Muñoz-Sanjuán, I., and Brivanlou, A. H. (2002). Neural induction, the default model and embryonic stem cells. *Nat. Rev. Neurosci.* 3, 271–280. doi: 10.1038/nrn786

Nakano, T., Ando, S., Takata, N., Kawada, M., Muguruma, K., Sekiguchi, K., et al. (2012). Self-formation of optic cups and storable stratified neural retina from human ESCs. *Cell Stem Cell* 10, 771–785. doi: 10.1016/j.stem.2012.05.009

Newgard, C. B., and Sharpless, N. E. (2013). Coming of age: molecular drivers of aging and therapeutic opportunities. *J. Clin. Invest.* 123, 946–950. doi: 10.1172/JCI68833

Nicholas, C. R., Chen, J., Tang, Y., Southwell, D. G., Chalmers, N., Vogt, D., et al. (2013). Functional maturation of hPSC-derived forebrain interneurons requires an extended timeline and mimics human neural development. *Cell Stem Cell* 12, 573–586. doi: 10.1016/j.stem.2013.04.005

Perrier, A. L., Tabar, V., Barberi, T., Rubio, M. E., Bruses, J., Topf, N., et al. (2004). Derivation of midbrain dopamine neurons from human embryonic stem cells. *Proc. Natl. Acad. Sci. U.S.A.* 101, 12543–12548. doi: 10.1073/pnas.0404700101

Reubinoff, B. E., Itsykson, P., Turetsky, T., Pera, M. F., Reinhartz, E., Itzik, A., et al. (2001). Neural progenitors from human embryonic stem cells. *Nat. Biotechnol.* 19, 1134–1140. doi: 10.1038/nbt1201-1134

Ricciardi, S., Boggio, E. M., Grosso, S., Lonetti, G., Forlani, G., Stefanelli, G., et al. (2011). Reduced AKT/mTOR signaling and protein synthesis dysregulation in a Rett syndrome animal model. *Hum. Mol. Genet.* 20, 1182–1196. doi: 10.1093/hmg/ddq563

Ricciardi, S., Ungaro, F., Hambrock, M., Rademacher, N., Stefanelli, G., Brambilla, D., et al. (2012). CDKL5 ensures excitatory synapse stability by reinforcing NGL-1-PSD95 interaction in the postsynaptic compartment and is impaired in patient iPSC-derived neurons. *Nat. Cell Biol.* 14, 911–923. doi: 10.1038/ncb2566

Robson, E. J., Khaled, W. T., Abell, K., and Watson, C. J. (2006). Epithelial-to-mesenchymal transition confers resistance to apoptosis in three murine mammary epithelial cell lines. *Differentiation* 74, 254–264. doi: 10.1111/j.1432-0436.2006.00075.x

Saha, K., and Jaenisch, R. (2009). Technical challenges in using human induced pluripotent stem cells to model disease. *Cell Stem Cell* 5, 584–595. doi: 10.1016/j.stem.2009.11.009

Sandoe, J., and Eggan, K. (2013). Opportunities and challenges of pluripotent stem cell neurodegenerative disease models. *Nat. Neurosci.* 16, 780–789. doi: 10.1038/nn.3425

Sato, T., Vries, R. G., Snippert, H. J., van de Wetering, M., Barker, N., Stange, D. E., et al. (2009). Single Lgr5 stem cells build crypt-villus structures *in vitro* without a mesenchymal niche. *Nature* 459, 262–265. doi: 10.1038/nature07935

Shi, Y., Kirwan, P., Smith, J., Robinson, H. P., and Livesey, F. J. (2012). Human cerebral cortex development from pluripotent stem cells to functional excitatory synapses. *Nat. Neurosci.* 15, 477–846, S1. doi: 10.1038/nn.3041

Soldner, F., Hockemeyer, D., Beard, C., Gao, Q., Bell, G. W., Cook, E. G., et al. (2009). Parkinson's disease patient-derived induced pluripotent stem cells free of viral reprogramming factors. *Cell* 136, 964–977. doi: 10.1016/j.cell.2009.02.013

Soldner, F., Laganière, J., Cheng, A. W., Hockemeyer, D., Gao, Q., Alagappan, R., et al. (2011). Generation of isogenic pluripotent stem cells differing exclusively at two early onset Parkinson point mutations. *Cell* 146, 318–331. doi: 10.1016/j.cell.2011.06.019

Southwell, D. G., Nicholas, C. R., Basbaum, A. I., Stryker, M. P., Kriegstein, A. R., Rubenstein, J. L., et al. (2014). Interneurons from embryonic development to cell-based therapy. *Science* 344:1240622. doi: 10.1126/science.1240622

Suga, H., Kadoshima, T., Minaguchi, M., Ohgushi, M., Soen, M., Nakano, T., et al. (2011). Self-formation of functional adenohypophysis in three-dimensional culture. *Nature* 480, 57–62. doi: 10.1038/nature10637

Tang, X., Zhou, L., Wagner, A. M., Marchetto, M. C., Muotri, A. R., Gage, F. H., et al. (2013). Astroglial cells regulate the developmental timeline of human neurons differentiated from induced pluripotent stem cells. *Stem Cell Res.*11, 743–757. doi: 10.1016/j.scr.2013.05.002

Taverna, E., and Huttner, W. B. (2010). Neural progenitor nuclei IN motion. *Neuron* 67, 906–914. doi: 10.1016/j.neuron.2010.08.027

Theka, I., Caiazzo, M., Dvoretskova, E., Leo, D., Ungaro, F., Curreli, S., et al. (2013). Rapid generation of functional dopaminergic neurons from human induced pluripotent stem cells through a single-step procedure using cell lineage transcription factors. *Stem Cells Transl. Med.* 2, 473–479. doi: 10.5966/sctm.2012-0133

Thompson, L. H., Grealish, S., Kirik, D., and Björklund, A. (2009). Reconstruction of the nigrostriatal dopamine pathway in the adult mouse brain. *Eur. J. Neurosci.* 30, 625–638. doi: 10.1111/j.1460-9568.2009.06878.x

Tiscornia, G., Vivas, E. L., and Izpisúa Belmonte, J. C. (2011). Diseases in a dish: modeling human genetic disorders using induced pluripotent cells. *Nat. Med.* 17, 1570–1576. doi: 10.1038/nm.2504

Tyson, J. A., and Anderson, S. A. (2014). GABAergic interneuron transplants to study development and treat disease. *Trends Neurosci.* 37, 169–177. doi: 10.1016/j.tins.2014.01.003

Valiente, M., and Marín, O. (2010). Neuronal migration mechanisms in development and disease. *Curr. Opin. Neurobiol.* 20, 68–78. doi: 10.1016/j.conb.2009.12.003

Vega, S., Morales, A. V., Ocaña, O. H., Valdés, F., Fabregat, I., and Nieto, M. A. (2004). Snail blocks the cell cycle and confers resistance to cell death. *Genes Dev.* 18, 1131–1143. doi: 10.1101/gad.294104

Verpelli, C., Carlessi, L., Bechi, G., Fusar Poli, E., Orellana, D., Heise, C., et al. (2013). Comparative neuronal differentiation of self-renewing neural progenitor cell lines obtained from human induced pluripotent stem cells. *Front. Cell. Neurosci.* 7:175. doi: 10.3389/fncel.2013.00175

Watanabe, K., Ueno, M., Kamiya, D., Nisgiyama, A., Matsumura, M., Wataya, T., et al. (2007). A ROCK inhibitor permits survival of dissociated human embryonic stem cells. *Nat. Biotechnol.* 25, 681–686. doi: 10.1038/nbt1310

Zhang, S. C., Wernig, M., Duncan, I. D., Brüstle, O., and Thomson, J. A. (2001). *In vitro* differentiation of transplantable neural precursors from human embryonic stem cells. *Nat. Biotechnol.* 19, 1129–1133. doi: 10.1038/nbt1201-1129

Zhang, Y., Pak, C., Han, Y., Ahlenius, H., Zhang, Z., Chanda, S., et al. (2013). Rapid single-step induction of functional neurons from human pluripotent stem cells. *Neuron* 78, 785–798. doi: 10.1016/j.neuron.2013.05.029

Zhu, H., Lensch, M. W., Cahan, P., and Daley, G. Q. (2011). Investigating monogenic and complex diseases with pluripotent stem cells. *Nat. Rev. Genet.* 12, 266–275. doi: 10.1038/nrg2951

10

Cocaine inhibition of nicotinic acetylcholine receptors influences dopamine release

Alexandra Acevedo-Rodriguez[1], Lifen Zhang[1], Fuwen Zhou[2], Suzhen Gong[2], Howard Gu[3], Mariella De Biasi[4], Fu-Ming Zhou[2] and John A. Dani[5]*

[1] *Department of Neuroscience, Baylor College of Medicine, Houston, TX, USA*
[2] *Department of Pharmacology, University of Tennessee College of Medicine, Memphis, TN, USA*
[3] *Department of Pharmacology, Ohio State University, Columbus, OH, USA*
[4] *Departments of Psychiatry, Perelman School of Medicine, University of Pennsylvania, Philadelphia, PA, USA*
[5] *Department of Neuroscience, Perelman School of Medicine, University of Pennsylvania, Philadelphia, PA, USA*

Edited by:
Sukumar Vijayaraghavan, University of Colorado Health Science Center, USA

Reviewed by:
Dan McGehee, University of Chicago, USA
Sukumar Vijayaraghavan, University of Colorado Health Science Center, USA
Hitoshi Morikawa, University of Texas at Austin, USA

****Correspondence:***
John A. Dani, Department of Neuroscience, Perelman School of Medicine, University of Pennsylvania, 415 Curie Boulevard, 211 Clinical Research Building, Philadelphia, PA 19104, USA
e-mail: johndani@upenn.edu

Nicotinic acetylcholine receptors (nAChRs) potently regulate dopamine (DA) release in the striatum and alter cocaine's ability to reinforce behaviors. Since cocaine is a weak nAChR inhibitor, we hypothesized that cocaine may alter DA release by inhibiting the nAChRs in DA terminals in the striatum and thus contribute to cocaine's reinforcing properties primarily associated with the inhibition of DA transporters. We found that biologically relevant concentrations of cocaine can mildly inhibit nAChR-mediated currents in midbrain DA neurons and consequently alter DA release in the dorsal and ventral striatum. At very high concentrations, cocaine also inhibits voltage-gated Na channels in DA neurons. Furthermore, our results show that partial inhibition of nAChRs by cocaine reduces evoked DA release. This diminution of DA release via nAChR inhibition more strongly influences release evoked at low or tonic stimulation frequencies than at higher (phasic) stimulation frequencies, particularly in the dorsolateral striatum. This cocaine-induced shift favoring phasic DA release may contribute to the enhanced saliency and motivational value of cocaine-associated memories and behaviors.

Keywords: substantia nigra, ventral tegmental area, addiction, mesolimbic, voltammetry, nAChRs

INTRODUCTION

Midbrain dopamine (DA) projections to the striatum comprise an important neuronal system mediating the initiation of drug addiction (Bonci et al., 2003; Wise, 2004; Hyman et al., 2006). The most well known action of the addictive drug cocaine is its inhibition of monoamine transporters, such as the DA transporter (DAT), with an affinity of about 500 nM (Ritz et al., 1987; Pristupa et al., 1994; Jones et al., 1995). In the brains of abusers, however, cocaine often reaches concentrations of 5–10 μM for considerable durations, and higher concentrations are achieved for shorter times depending on the route of administration and other factors (Mittleman and Wetli, 1984; Evans et al., 1996; Ward et al., 1997; Fowler et al., 1998). In addition, cocaine inhibits α4β2-containing (α4β2*) nicotinic acetylcholine receptors (nAChRs) with an IC_{50} in the range of 5–15 μM (Damaj et al., 1999; Francis et al., 2000). This inhibition may be significant because α4β2* nAChRs (often in combination with α6) are highly expressed in DA neuron somata and terminals (Mansvelder and McGehee, 2000; Jones et al., 2001; Champtiaux et al., 2003; Wooltorton et al., 2003; Quik and McIntosh, 2006; Zanetti et al., 2006), and nAChRs have been shown to regulate the frequency dependence of DA release (Zhou et al., 2001; Rice and Cragg, 2004; Zhang and Sulzer, 2004; Exley and Cragg, 2008; Zhang et al., 2009a). Intertwined with the DA neurons and their axons, cholinergic neurons in the midbrain and brainstem project to the substantia nigra and ventral tegmental area (VTA) (Woolf and Butcher, 1986; Gould et al., 1989; Oakman et al., 1995), while cholinergic interneurons in the striatum innervate locally (Woolf and Butcher, 1981; Zhou et al., 2001; Nelson et al., 2014), providing the endogenous neurotransmitter ACh to the nAChRs in these DA areas.

In the striatum, DA release is normally dependent on both afferent spikes along DA fibers and nAChR activity at axonal and presynaptic locations (Zhou et al., 2001; Grady et al., 2002; Salminen et al., 2004; Zhang et al., 2009a). The nAChRs normally increase the initial DA release probability, and regulate the frequency dependence of DA release (Rice and Cragg, 2004; Zhang and Sulzer, 2004; Exley and Cragg, 2008; Zhang et al., 2009a). Cholinergic interneuron activity may directly facilitate DA release from DA axon terminals in the dorsal and ventral striatum (Cachope et al., 2012; Threlfell et al., 2012). Inactivation of nAChRs on the DA fibers decreases the DA release probability and increases the phasic to tonic DA ratio (Rice and Cragg, 2004; Exley and Cragg, 2008; Zhang et al., 2009a). Based on those published findings, we hypothesized that cocaine acts via nAChRs to regulate DA signals beyond the expected inhibition of DATs.

MATERIALS AND METHODS

MICE

Male and female C57BL/6J mice from The Jackson Laboratory (Bar Harbor, Maine), β2-subunit knockout (KO) mice (Xu et al., 1999), DAT knockin mice having DATs that are insensitive to cocaine (Chen et al., 2006), and their wild-type (W-T) littermates were used in our present study. The mutant mice were generated, maintained, euthanized and genotyped according to established procedures (Xu et al., 1999; Chen et al., 2006) and in accordance with national and institutional guidelines. Experiments on the mutant mice and their W-T littermates were performed double blind.

FAST-SCAN CYCLIC VOLTAMMETRY (FCV) IN STRIATAL BRAIN SLICES

For these studies, horizontal brain slices (**Figure 1**) containing the striatum (400 μm in thickness) from mice 1–3 months old were cut on a Leica VT1000 or Leica VT1200s vibratome (Zhang et al., 2009a). Anesthesia, handling, and experimental procedures followed our established techniques at 30°C (Zhou et al., 2001).

FCV was performed with home-made carbon-fiber electrodes constructed from P55S carbon fibers of 10 μm diameter (Amoco Polymers, Greenville, SC). Axopatch 200B amplifier, pClamp 9 software, and Digidata 1320A interface (Axon Instruments) were used to acquire and analyze data. The holding potential was 0 mV between scans. Scans of 20 ms duration were applied at 10 or 20 Hz. The scans were from 0 mV to −400 to 1000 to −400 to 0 at a rate of 300 mV/ms and were sampled at 50 kHz. The peaks of the voltammograms were plotted over time and converted to concentrations by post-experiment calibration with 0.1–5 μM DA standards.

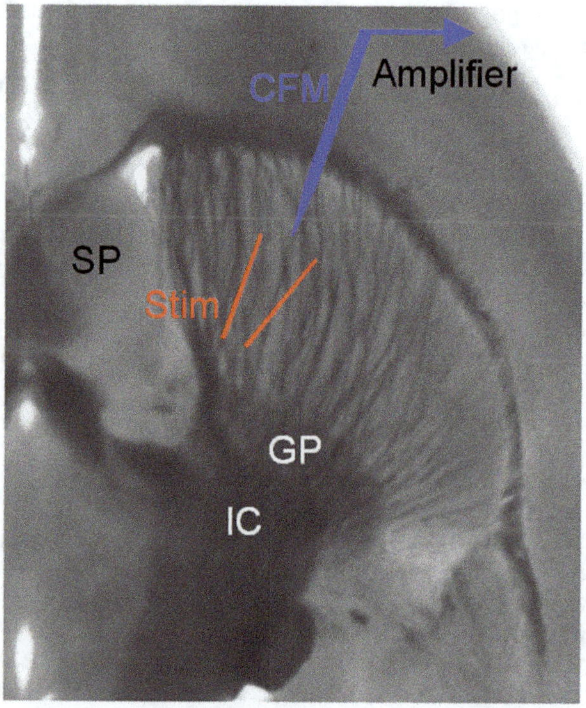

FIGURE 1 | Arrangement for electrical stimulation and FCV recording in striatal brain slices. The striatum is easily identified by its anatomical location and the distinct fiber bundles in horizontal brain slices. Local electrical stimulation in the striatum was delivered using a bipolar tungsten electrode. The two tips of the stimulating electrode were ~150 μm away from each other and from the carbon fiber microelectrode (CFM) tip. GP, globus pallidus; IC, internal capsule; SP, septum.

Local electrical stimulation in the striatum was delivered using a bipolar tungsten electrode (**Figure 1**). The two tips of the stimulating electrode were ~150 μm away from each other. The tip of the carbon-fiber recording electrode was 100–200 μm away from the two tips of the stimulating electrode. The stimuli were relatively weak (0.1–0.2 mA for 0.1 ms) helping to keep the recording stable and minimize local interactions. The interval between single pulses was usually 100 s. Additional types of stimulation were used: tonic stimulation of 4 pulses at 4 Hz, phasic stimulation of 4 pulses at 20 Hz, and paired pulses separated by 50 ms. Cocaine was bath-applied for 10 min and then was washed out.

PATCH CLAMP RECORDING OF MIDBRAIN DA NEURONS

Coronal or horizontal midbrain slices, 200–300 μm in thickness and containing the substantia nigra pars compacta (SNc) and/or the VTA, were prepared from 15 to 30 day old mice according to established procedures (Pidoplichko et al., 1997). Visualized recordings were made at 30°C using an Axopatch 200 and pClamp data acquisition and analysis software.

nAChR-mediated currents in putative DA neurons were induced by pressure application of 1 mM ACh using a Picospritzer (General Valve) attached to a puffer pipette (Pidoplichko and Dani, 2005). The puffer was ~30 μm from the neuron while ACh was applied (25 psi for 100 ms). Then, the puffer was retracted 100–200 μm between ACh applications by a computer-controlled manipulator to prevent leak-induced desensitization (Wooltorton et al., 2003; Pidoplichko and Dani, 2005). For this experiment, the brain slices were bathed in a normal extracellular solution containing (in mM): 125 NaCl, 2.5 KCl, 1.25 NaH_2PO_4, 25 $NaHCO_3$, 2.5 $CaCl_2$, 1.3 $MgCl_2$, and 10 D-glucose that were continuously bubbled with 95% O_2 and 5% CO_2. The intracellular solution contained (in mM): 135 KCl, 0.5 EGTA, 10 HEPES, 2 Mg-ATP, 0.2 Na-GTP, and 4 Na_2-phosphocreatine. pH 7.25, 280–290 mOsm. To record the fast voltage-activated sodium current (I_{Na}), the presumed nigral DA neuron (based on its slow firing rate at ~1 Hz in cell-attached mode, see Ding et al., 2011) was held at −90 mV and then stepped to 0 mV for 10 ms. For this experiment, 2.5 mM $CaCl_2$ were substituted by 2.5 mM $MgCl_2$, and extracellular NaCl was reduced to 25 mM, 20 mM TEA and 5 mM 4-AP were used to inhibit K currents; the following Cs-based intracellular solution was also used that contained (in mM): 135 CsCl, 0.5 EGTA, 10 HEPES, 2 Mg-ATP, 0.2 Na-GTP, 4 Na_2-phosphocreatine with pH was adjusted to 7.25 with CsOH.

Neurobiotin (0.2%) was included in the recording electrode and allowed to diffuse into the cell using approaches described previously (Pidoplichko et al., 1997). After recording, the brain slices were fixed in 4% paraformaldehyde in 0.1 M phosphate buffer. Double immunostaining was performed according to established procedures (Pidoplichko et al., 1997; Neuhoff et al., 2002). Tyrosine hydroxylase (TH, a marker for midbrain DA neurons) was detected with a sheep anti-TH primary antibody and rhodamine red-X-tagged donkey anti-sheep secondary antibodies (**Figure 2A2**). Neurobiotin was detected with red Cy2-tagged

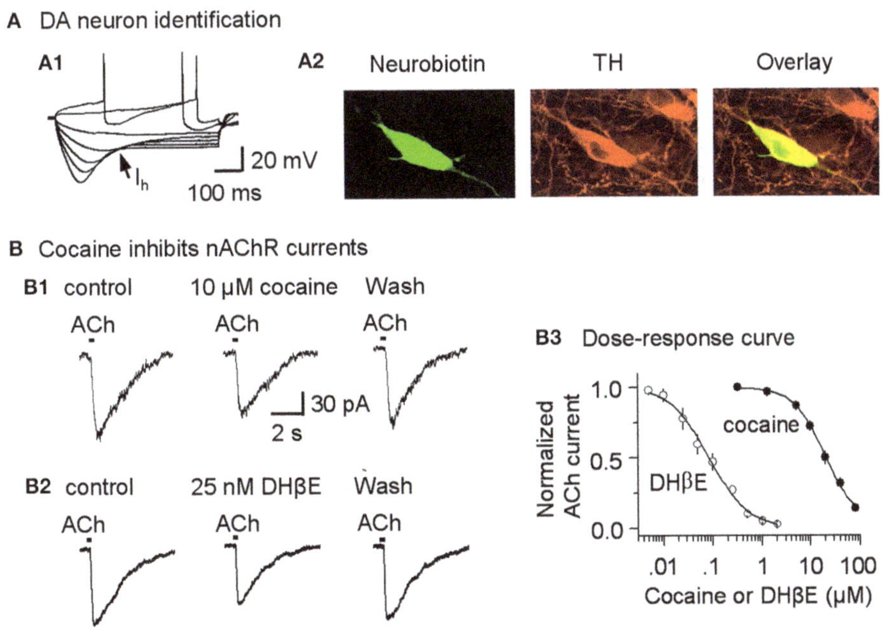

FIGURE 2 | Cocaine inhibits nicotinic currents in midbrain DA neurons from W-T mice. (A,A1) The membrane properties of presumed DA neurons from the lateral VTA or SNc were typical of DA neurons with a strong I_h sag (arrow). Injected current was 40 pA/step. Spikes were partially truncated for display. **(A,A2)** These midbrain DA neurons were backfilled with neurobiotin (green) and labeled for TH (red). The co-incidence of neurobiotin and TH is shown as yellow (Overlay), confirming the DA neuron identification. **(B,B1)** Three traces show nicotinic currents induced in a DA neuron by pressure application of ACh (1 mM, 100 ms pulse) under control conditions (left), with 10 μM cocaine present (middle), or with 25 nM DHβE present (right), which was applied after recovering from cocaine inhibition. The recordings were made in the presence of 1 μM atropine at a holding potential of −70 mV. **(B,B2)** Examples showing DHβE inhibits nicotinic currents in DA neurons. **(B,B3)** The dose-response relationships for inhibition of nAChR currents. The curves through the data were produced with $IC_{50} = 19.8\,\mu M$ and Hill coefficient = 1.3 for cocaine, and $IC_{50} = 82\,nM$ and Hill coefficient = 1.1 for DHβE with $n = 3–9$ per data point.

strepavidin antibody (**Figure 2A2**). Sections were examined on a Bio-Rad confocal laser-scanning microscope.

CHEMICALS

All chemicals including cocaine-HCl were purchased from Sigma Aldrich (St. Louis, MO) or Tocris (Ellisville, MO). Cocaine was also obtained from the NIH/NIDA's Drug Supply Program.

STATISTICS

The data are displayed as the mean and the standard error. Paired *t*-test was used to compare measurements before and during various pharmacological treatments. $P < 0.05$ was considered statistically significant. When applicable, the averaged data points in dose-response plots were fitted with the Hill equation to estimate IC_{50} and Hill coefficient. These and other computations were performed using the Origin analysis and plotting program (Northampton, MA).

RESULTS

COCAINE DIRECTLY INHIBITS nAChRs ON DA NEURONS

Because cocaine inhibits cloned neuronal nAChRs in heterologous expression systems (Damaj et al., 1999; Francis et al., 2000), we tested whether cocaine inhibits nAChRs expressed on DA neurons of the SNc and the lateral VTA (Picciotto et al., 1995; Pidoplichko et al., 1997; Mansvelder and McGehee, 2000; Wooltorton et al., 2003). DA neurons were initially identified by their characteristic membrane properties. The presumed DA neurons within the lateral midbrain fired spontaneously (2.1 ± 0.3 Hz, $n = 9$), displayed prominent I_h currents (**Figure 2A1**) and had relatively long spike durations (2.7 ± 0.3 ms at the base, $n = 9$). These membrane properties were consistent with commonly recognized DA neuron properties from this area (Neuhoff et al., 2002; Ford et al., 2006; Beckstead and Williams, 2007; Zhang et al., 2010; Ding et al., 2011; Li et al., 2011). These electrophysiologically identified DA neurons were further confirmed by back filling with neurobiotin and subsequently staining for TH (**Figure 2A2**).

In these DA neurons, pressure application of ACh (100 ms pulse of 1 mM ACh, 1 μM atropine was always present) induced currents (**Figure 2B1**, left trace) that have previously been characterized as predominantly β2* nAChR currents, and these currents can be inhibited by 1 μM dihydro-β-erythroidine (DHβE) (Alkondon and Albuquerque, 1993; Wooltorton et al., 2003). In the presence of a cocktail of antagonists to inhibit DA transporters (2 μM GBR12909), D_2-like autoreceptors (1 μM sulpiride), and muscarinic receptors (1 μM atropine), bath application of 10 μM cocaine inhibited the nAChR currents (**Figure 2B1**, middle trace). This concentration (10 μM cocaine) is within the range achieved by cocaine abusers and by animals during self-administration experiments (Mittleman and Wetli, 1984; Evans et al., 1996; Ward et al., 1997; Fowler et al., 1998; Nicola and Deadwyler, 2000). The dose-response curve for cocaine inhibition of nAChR currents from SNc DA neurons had an apparent IC_{50} of $19.8 \pm 1.5\,\mu M$ and Hill coefficient of 1.3 ± 0.3 ($n = 3$–9, **Figure 2B3**), and the results were statistically the same for nAChRs in the VTA (IC_{50} of $19.5 \pm 1.8\,\mu M$, Hill coefficient of 1.3 ± 0.2). To indicate the effectiveness of cocaine inhibition, the nicotinic antagonist, DHβE, was characterized with an apparent IC_{50} of 82.3 ± 4.3 nM and Hill coefficient of 1.1 ± 0.4 ($n = 3$–7, **Figures 2B2,B3**). These results suggest that cocaine directly inhibits nAChRs on DA neurons and, thus, acts as a weak nicotinic antagonist. Because the predominant β2-containing nAChRs on the cell body and axon terminals appear to be qualitatively similar (Champtiaux et al., 2003; Salminen et al., 2004; Quik and McIntosh, 2006), cocaine's nicotinic antagonism likely also occurs at DA axon terminals. Since the selective DAT inhibitor GBR12909 was also used in this study, we tested the potential effect of GBR12909 on nAChR-mediated currents as a separate control experiment. We found that GBR12909 (5 μM, the highest concentration we used) did not inhibit nAChR currents in 5 DA neurons tested. Since nAChRs facilitate DA release (Zhou et al., 2001; Rice and Cragg, 2004; Zhang and Sulzer, 2004; Zhang et al., 2009a; Threlfell et al., 2012), our result on cocaine inhibition of nAChRs leads to this question: can cocaine also affect DA release at DA axon terminals?

COCAINE INHIBITS DA RELEASE EVOKED BY A SINGLE PULSE

Cocaine is known to inhibit DA reuptake with a K_i of about 0.5 μM (Ritz et al., 1987). This effect is also well documented in the FCV literature (e.g., Jones et al., 1995) and readily observed under our current experimental conditions (see **Figures 6A1,B1**), but is not the focus of our present study. Our focus here is to determine if cocaine, at concentrations above what is needed to inhibit DATs, can affect DA release, because at the relatively high concentrations attained by abusers, the previous section suggests that cocaine inhibits nAChRs on DA fibers and terminals that normally regulate DA release. Therefore, we reasoned that cocaine at different concentrations alters the DA signal in qualitatively different manners via inhibition of DATs vs. nAChRs.

To examine cocaine's nAChR-mediated influence over DA signals, we electrically stimulated DA release and monitored the DA concentration using FCV in brain slices containing the striatum. The DA signal was evoked every 100 s in the dorsolateral striatum and was commonly stable for >2 h during our recordings (Zhou et al., 2001; Zhang et al., 2009a). Confounding mechanisms were minimized in all of the experiments by using pharmacological treatments. Sulpiride (1 μM) was used to inhibit DA autoinhibition by D_2-like receptors. SKF83566 (1 μM) was used to inhibit D_1-like receptors to prevent changes in cholinergic tone that affects DA release (Zhou et al., 2001). GBR12909 (1–5 μM), which has an IC_{50} ~10 nM vs. cocaine's IC_{50} ~0.5 μM, was used to minimize DA reuptake by DATs. Therefore, pretreatment with GBR12909 (1–5 μM) occludes cocaine's effect on DA reuptake by DATs.

Under these pharmacological conditions (with DATs inhibited), cocaine at concentrations that would normally inhibit DATs (0.1–1 μM) did not enhance the amplitude or duration of the already prolonged DA signal, as is indicated in the dose-response curve (**Figure 3B**, filled symbols). In other words, cocaine no longer enhanced the DA signal because DATs were already inhibited by GBR12909. However, at the same concentrations that inhibited nAChRs (**Figure 2B1**), cocaine (10 μM) and DHβE (25 nM) substantially inhibited DA release evoked by a single-pulse (1 p) stimulus (**Figures 3A,B**). Cocaine inhibited the DA signal with an estimated IC_{50} of $4.3 \pm 0.3\,\mu M$ ($n = 8$) and a Hill coefficient of 3 (**Figure 3B**, filled symbols). The high Hill coefficient is indicative of a cocaine effect on Ca^{2+}-triggered vesicular DA release, which has high cooperativity (Lou et al., 2005). Under the same pharmacological conditions, DA release evoked by 1 p also was inhibited by the nicotinic antagonist DHβE with an apparent IC_{50} of 22.3 ± 1.7 nM and Hill coefficient of 3 (**Figure 3B**, open symbols). The influence of cocaine over the DA release evoked by 1 p was comparable in the dorsolateral striatum (**Figures 3A,B**) and in the NAc shell of the ventral striatum (**Figures 3C,D**).

To verify that cocaine was not acting via DAT inhibition when GBR12909 was present in these experiments, we repeated the experiments using mutant mice possessing DATs that are insensitive to cocaine (Chen et al., 2006) instead of using GBR12909. A similar effect was seen when cocaine (10 μM) was applied while stimulating DA release in the presence of 1 μM sulpiride and 1 μM SKF83566 (**Figure 4A**, dorsolateral striatum; **Figure 4B**, NAc shell). The DA release to a 1 p stimulation was inhibited by cocaine (10 μM), and the dose-response relationships for cocaine inhibition of DA release is shown to the right in **Figure 4**. These results verify that cocaine inhibits DA release separately from its influence over DA reuptake or D2-like receptors.

COCAINE REDUCES DA RELEASE BY INHIBITING nAChRs

The results to this point show that cocaine can decrease DA release evoked by a 1 p stimulus. Cocaine's ability to inhibit nAChRs suggests that the mechanism of action is via nAChRs on DA fibers or terminals. The nAChRs that normally facilitate DA release contain the β2 subunit (Zhou et al., 2001; Salminen et al., 2004; Zhang et al., 2009a; Drenan et al., 2010; Exley et al., 2011). In nAChR β2-subunit KO mice, DA release does not depend on nAChR activation (Zhou et al., 2001; Zhang et al., 2009a). Therefore, if cocaine decreases DA release in response to a 1 p stimulus via nAChR inhibition, then β2-subunit KO mice should not show this cocaine-mediated effect.

In the dorsolateral striatum of β2-subunit KO mice, 1 p stimulation evoked nAChR-independent DA release that had an amplitude 70% smaller than that observed in W-T mice, as has been shown previously (Zhou et al., 2001). The smaller evoke DA signals are observable by comparing **Figure 3A** (left trace compared to the right trace after inhibition of nAChRs) to **Figure 5A** (left trace, note the change in scale). In the presence of GBR12909 (1–5 μM) to inhibit DATs, cocaine doses ranging from 50 nM to 5 μM did not affect the amplitude or duration of the evoked DA signal in β2-subunit KO mice (**Figure 5B**). A concentration of cocaine (10 μM) that caused a $74.9 \pm 7.8\%$ decrease in DA release in W-T mice (**Figures 3A,B**), produces only $7.6 \pm 2.4\%$ inhibition in nAChR β2 KO mice (**Figures 5A,B**). In W-T mice, cocaine reduced DA release with an IC_{50} of 4.3 μM (**Figure 5B**,

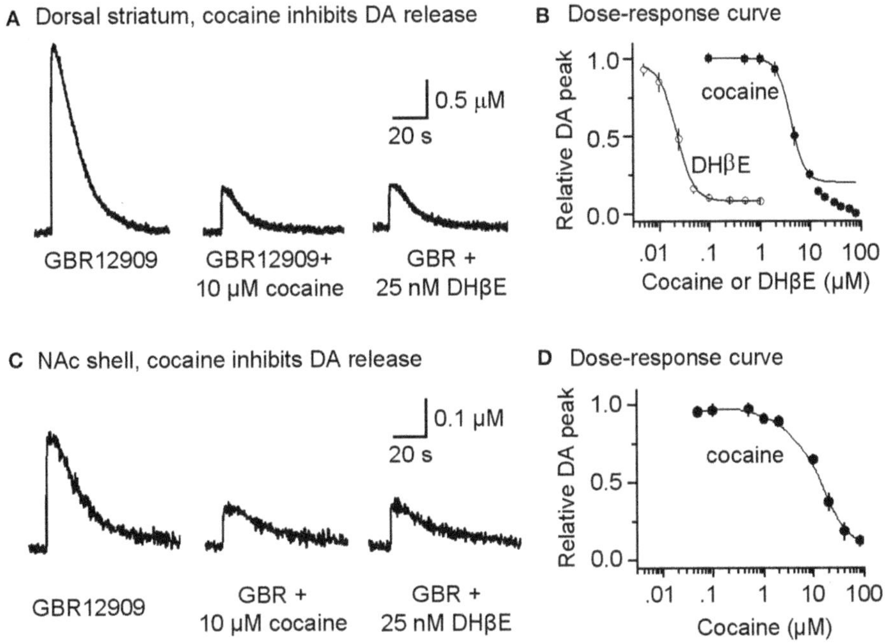

FIGURE 3 | Cocaine reduces DA release in the striatum from W-T mice. (A) Cocaine inhibits DA release from the dorsolateral striatum evoked by single-pulse (1 p) stimulation measured using fast-scan cyclic voltammetry. The recordings show the prolonged DA signal after DAT inhibition with 5 μM GBR12909 (left trace). DA release was substantially reduced by 10 μM cocaine (middle trace). After recovery from cocaine inhibition, 25 nM DHβE induced a similar inhibition of the DA signal (right trace). 1 μM sulpiride (D_2-like antagonist) and SKF83566 (D_1-like antagonist) were used to block local interactions in the striatum. **(B)** The dose-response relationships for inhibition of DA release. The curves through the data were produced with $IC_{50} = 4.3\,\mu M$ for cocaine and 22 nM for DHβE both with a Hill coefficient estimated to be 3 ($n = 4$–8 per data point). Data points with cocaine concentrations higher than 15 μM were not included in the fitting because a component arising from a local anesthetic effect was also present. **(C)** Likewise, cocaine inhibits DA release evoked by 1 p stimulation from the NAc shell measured using fast-scan cyclic voltammetry in the presence of 5 μM GBR12909, 1 μM sulpiride, and 1 μM SKF83566. **(D)** The dose-response relationship for inhibition of DA release in the NAc shell.

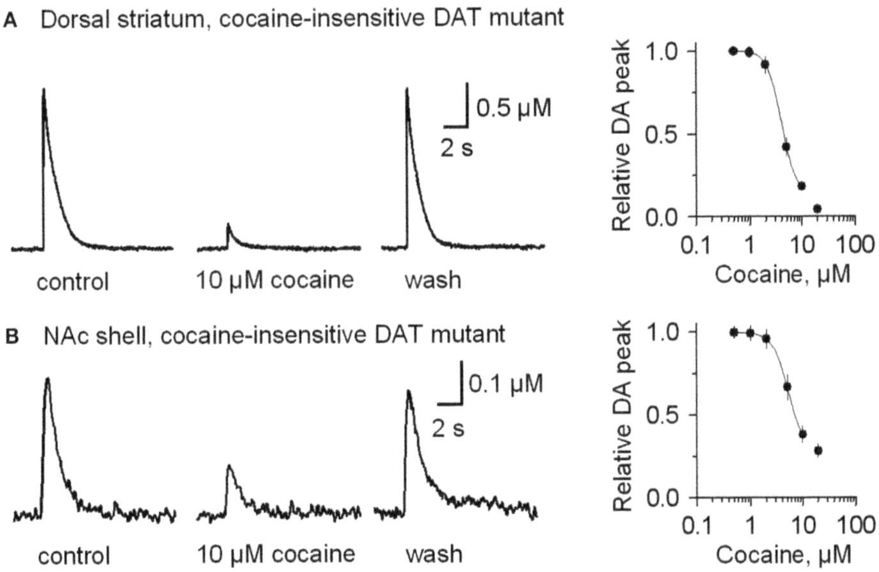

FIGURE 4 | In mutant mice having cocaine-insensitive DATs, DA release evoked by 1 p stimulation was still inhibited by cocaine (10 μM). (A) In 10 μM cocaine (middle trace) the DA signal was inhibited when compared to the control (left) or after washout of cocaine (right, wash). The dose-response relationship for cocaine inhibition (extreme right) was fitted with a curve through the data having $IC_{50} = 4\,\mu M$ and Hill coefficient = 3.2. **(B)** Likewise, cocaine (10 μM) inhibits DA release evoked by 1 p stimulation from the NAc shell. The dose-response relationship for inhibition of DA release in the NAc shell by cocaine (extreme right) was fitted by a curve with IC50 = 5.2 μM and the Hill coefficient = 3.0. The traces were collected in the presence of 1 μM sulpiride, and 1 μM SKF83566.

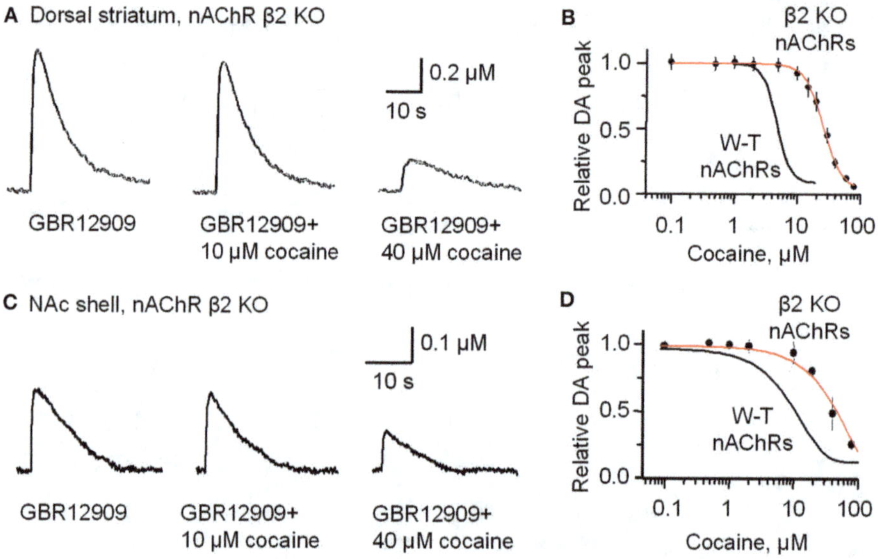

FIGURE 5 | In β2-subunit KO mice DA release evoked by 1 p stimulation was resistant to inhibition by cocaine (10 μM). (A) All the slices were bathed in 2 μM GBR12909 to block DATs and to remove complications arising from changes in DA reuptake. The control DA signal (left) evoked by 1 p stimulation shows a prolonged duration caused by inhibiting DA reuptake. In 10 μM cocaine (middle trace) there was slight inhibition of the DA signal. In 40 μM cocaine (right trace) there was a much greater inhibition of the DA signal. 1 μM sulpiride and SKF83566 were used to block local DA receptor influences within the striatum. **(B)** The dose-response relationship for cocaine inhibition of DA release in the dorsolateral striatum of β2-nAChR KO mice. The curve through the data was produced with $IC_{50} = 26\,\mu M$ and the Hill coefficient = 3 (red curve) (n = 4–6 slices). For comparison, the black curve from **Figure 1** obtained with W-T mice is given to show the substantial decrease in cocaine-mediated inhibition when β2* nAChRs were absent. **(C)** Likewise, cocaine (10 μM) did not, but cocaine (40 μM) did, inhibit DA release evoked by 1 p stimulation from the NAc shell again in the presence of 2 μM GBR12909, 1 μM sulpiride, and 1 μM SKF83566. **(D)** The dose-response relationships for inhibition of DA release in the NAc shell by cocaine in β2-subunit KO mice (red curve) (n = 4–5 slices) compared to the W-T mice (black curve).

smooth black curve), but in nAChR β2 KO mice the IC_{50} shifts to 26.4 ± 2.3 μM with a Hill coefficient of 3.0 (**Figure 5B**, red curve) (n = 4–6 slices for each data points). Comparable results (that may be similarly interpreted) were also obtained in the NAc shell (**Figures 5C,D**) from nAChR β2 KO mice.

For completeness, the whole range of cocaine's influence over the 1 p stimulated DA release is shown in the absence of GBR12909 in W-T mice normally expressing nAChRs in the dorsolateral striatum (**Figure 6A**) or the NAc shell (**Figure 6C**). At low cocaine concentrations, DATs are inhibited by cocaine, and the DA peak becomes larger (DAT effect, **Figures 6A,A1,C**). At cocaine concentrations above 1 μM, the DA peak decreases. As indicated by the earlier results, cocaine begins to inhibit nAChRs at this concentration (nAChR effect, **Figures 6A,C**). When nAChRs are absent (i.e., nAChR β2 KO mice), cocaine does not begin to inhibit the DA peak amplitude until ≥20 μM (**Figures 6B,B1,D**). The overall effect of cocaine acting via nAChRs is depicted in **Figure 6B**. The inhibition of the DA peak by ≥20 μM cocaine likely also involves the local anesthetic effect (Anesthetic effect, **Figure 6**), arising from cocaine inhibition of voltage-activated channels (e.g., sodium and/or calcium channels) and action potentials (O'Leary and Chahine, 2002). We verified that cocaine inhibited the fast sodium current in DA neuron somata in a dose-dependent manner (**Figures 7A,B**) that likely contributed to the decreased DA release seen at very high cocaine concentrations (Anesthetic effect, **Figure 6**). Because DA release depends of the 4th power of the intraterminal calcium concentration that arises from the depolarization caused by voltage-gated ion channels, cocaine's inhibition of voltage-gated channels (e.g., I_{Na} currents in **Figure 7**) is magnified when observing the effect over DA release (**Figure 6**).

COCAINE REDUCES PAIRED-PULSE DEPRESSION OF DA RELEASE DEPENDENT ON nAChRs

The results presented above indicate that cocaine acts as a nAChR antagonist at DA fibers and terminals in the striatum and via this mechanism reduces DA release evoked by a single pulse or low frequency stimulation. This reduction in DA release is, of course, relative to the release that would be seen if cocaine did not slightly inhibit nAChRs. Inhibition of nAChRs also has been shown to reduce paired-pulsed depression of DA release (Rice and Cragg, 2004; Zhang and Sulzer, 2004). Paired-pulse depression largely depends on the initial neurotransmitter release probability. The higher the initial release probability, the stronger the paired-pulse depression (Zucker and Regehr, 2002). Therefore, if cocaine is inhibiting nAChRs, it should decrease the initial DA release probability and reduce paired-pulse depression.

To test this idea, we performed paired-pulse experiments using two stimuli separated by 50 ms (i.e., 20 Hz). The experiments were conducted in the presence of sulpiride (1 μM) to block autoinhibition by D_2-like receptors and SKF83566 (1 μM) to block D_1-like receptors on cholinergic interneurons to prevent changes in cholinergic tone in the striatum. The DA signal was quantified by the area under the curve because the 2 pulse

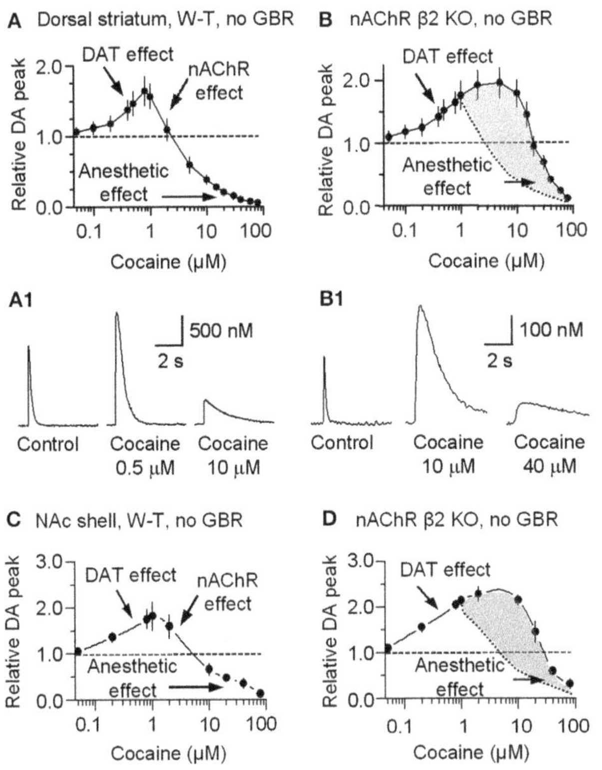

FIGURE 6 | Concentration-dependent multiple cocaine effects on the DA-release signal evoked by 1 p stimulation in the striatum measured by FCV. (A) In W-T mice DA signals were measured in the dorsolateral striatum while we bath applied cocaine ranging from 50 nM to 80 μM in the absence of GBR12909. At 50 nM to 1 μM, cocaine monotonically increased the amplitude and prolonged the duration of the evoked DA signal, as expected from cocaine's known inhibition of DATs (DAT effect). At cocaine concentrations above 1 μM, the DA peak decreased although the duration was further prolonged. This decrease is hypothesized to arise from cocaine inhibition of nAChRs (nAChR effect). **(B)** In β2-nAChR knockout (KO) mice in the absence of GBR12909, the DA signal is not dependent on nAChRs. Note that the mid-range cocaine inhibition of the DA amplitude is absent in these measurements (i.e., the nAChR effect is absent). The difference between cocaine's influences in the absence of β2-nAChRs is shaded in gray with the dotted curve representing the falling phase in **(A)**. **(A1,B1)** Examples of the multiple effects induced by different concentrations of cocaine in WT and in β2-nAChR KO mice. **(C)** In W-T mice, DA signaling in the NAc shell showed qualitatively similar cocaine effects as seen in the dorsal striatum. **(D)** In β2-nAChR KO mice, the DA signal is not dependent on nAChRs. The difference between cocaine's influences in the absence of β2-nAChRs is shaded in gray with the dotted curve representing the falling phase in **(C)**. In **(A–D)**, $n = 4$–7 slices for each data points.

protocol spreads the DA signal in time. The paired-pulse ratio (PPR) was defined as P_2/P_1. In the dorsolateral striatum of W-T mice, DA release displayed strong paired-pulse depression with a PPR of 0.12 ± 0.01, $n = 7$ (**Figures 8A1,A3**), consistent with published reports (Rice and Cragg, 2004; Zhang and Sulzer, 2004; Zhang et al., 2009a; Cachope et al., 2012; Threlfell et al., 2012). Although a high initial release probability is probably a key factor, the mechanism for this severe depletion of DA release is not established. In the presence of 10 μM cocaine, the PPR increased to 0.43 ± 0.06 ($n = 5$, $p < 0.05$; **Figures 8A1–A3**). Qualitatively similar results were obtained in the NAc shell: PPR was 0.47 ± 0.07, $n = 5$ in the control and 0.65 ± 0.08, $n = 5$ in 10 μM cocaine (not shown). These PPR numbers reflect the lower probability of release under control conditions in the NAc shell compared to the dorsal striatum, which was shown previously (Zhang et al., 2009a).

To examine further whether cocaine's mechanism of action on PPR was via nicotinic antagonism, we repeated the paired-pulse experiment in nAChR β2 KO mice. In the absence of the β2-containing nAChRs, the probability of release decreases especially for P_1 (Zhou et al., 2001). Thus, in β2 KO mice with no cocaine, the PPR was higher than in W-T mice, 0.38 ± 0.05, ($n = 5$, **Figures 8B1,B3**). More importantly, in the absence of functional β2-containing nAChRs, 10 μM cocaine did not significantly affect the PPR consistent with cocaine mechanistically acting via nAChR inhibition: 0.39 ± 0.06 ($n = 5$, **Figures 8B1–B3**). Qualitatively similar results were obtained in the NAc shell: PPR was 0.68 ± 0.06 ($n = 5$) in the β2 KO mice and 0.65 ± 0.06 ($n = 5$) when cocaine (10 μM) was applied (not shown). In the absence of β2-containing nAChRs, cocaine did not influence the PPR.

To further demonstrate that cocaine is altering the PPR via nAChRs not owing to its inhibition of DATs, we repeated the experiments in the presence of GBR12909 (5 μM) to inhibit DATs as a control for cocaine's inhibition of DATs. Just as seen in **Figures 8A,B**, cocaine caused an increase in the PPR when nAChRs are present (**Figures 8C1–C3**) but not in β2 KO mice (**Figures 8D1–D3**).

COCAINE ENHANCES PHASIC RELATIVE TO TONIC DA SIGNALS DEPENDENT ON nAChRs

The earlier results showed that cocaine decreases DA release evoked by a 1 p stimulus. A low release probability can be overcome by the residual Ca^{2+} in axon terminals produced by high frequency stimulation (Abbott and Regehr, 2004). Therefore, we tested whether cocaine favors phasic DA release evoked by high frequency stimulation.

Tonic DA release was evoked by 4 stimulation pulses given at 4 Hz, and phasic DA release was mimicked by 4 pulses given at 20 Hz because rodent DA neurons fire bursting spikes with an intraburst frequency of ~20 Hz and with 3–5 spikes per burst, and the averaged DA neuron firing rate is about 4 Hz (Hyland et al., 2002; Schultz, 2002; Zhang et al., 2009b). Under control conditions in the dorsolateral striatum, phasic and tonic DA release was very similar (Rice and Cragg, 2004; Zhang and Sulzer, 2004; Zhang et al., 2009a), with the ratio of phasic to tonic DA release being 1.10 ± 0.05, $n = 10$ (**Figures 9A1,C**). Inhibition of DATs by GBR12909 (up to 5 μM) did not affect the phasic to tonic ratio (**Figures 9A2,C**). In contrast, 10 μM cocaine reduced the tonic DA release more strongly than the phasic DA signal increasing the phasic to tonic DA ratio to 1.38 ± 0.15 ($n = 8$, $p < 0.05$, **Figures 9A3,C**). To test whether cocaine was acting via inhibition of nAChRs to influence the phasic to tonic ratio, we repeated the experiment in nAChR β2 KO mice. Under control conditions in β2 KO mice, the phasic to tonic DA release ratio was 1.58 ± 0.14 ($n = 6$, **Figures 9B1,C**), which is higher than in W-T mice. Equally important, cocaine (up to 10 μM) did not alter

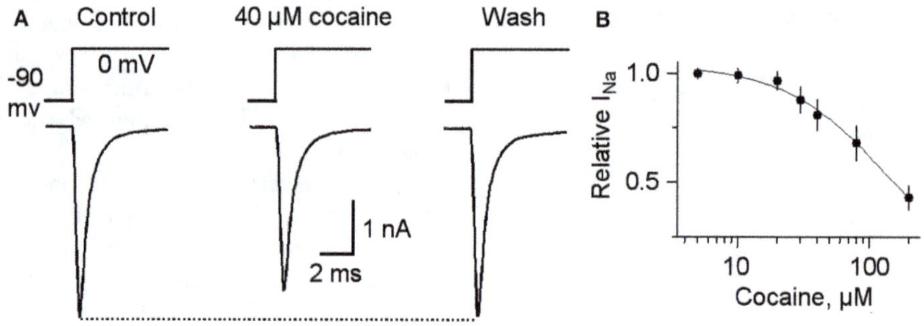

FIGURE 7 | Cocaine at high concentrations inhibits voltage-gated I_{Na}. (A) In 40 μM cocaine, I_{Na} was inhibited compared to the control or after cocaine washout. Holding potential was −90 mV and the testing potential was 0 mV for 10 ms given every 20 s. Extracellular and intracellular solutions are described in the Materials and Methods section. **(B)** The dose-response curve for cocaine inhibition of I_{Na} is shown on the right with a curve through the data with an $IC_{50} = 144$ and a Hill coefficient of 1.

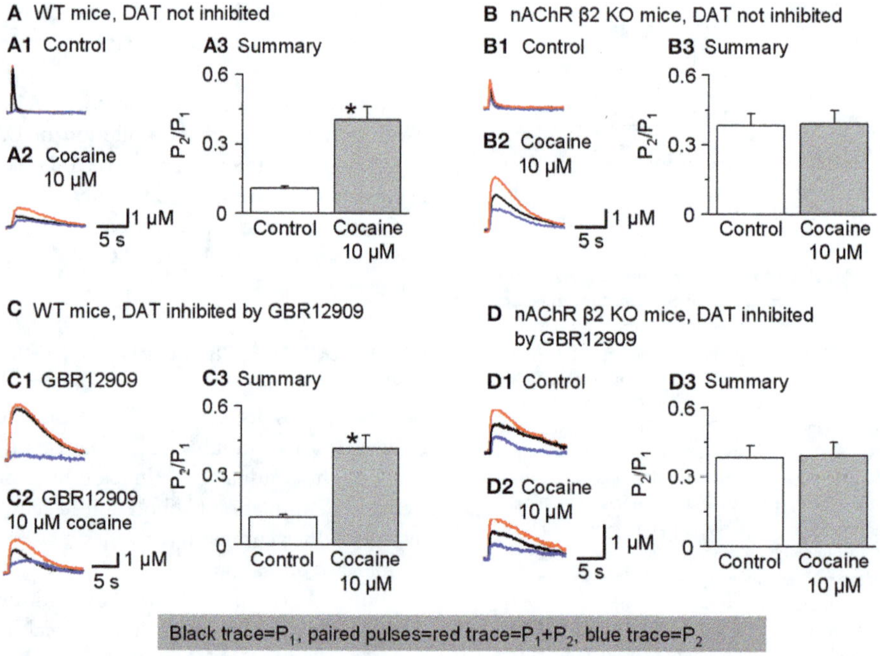

FIGURE 8 | Cocaine reduces paired-pulse depression of DA release in W-T but not in β2-nAChR KO mice. In this figure, P_1 was the 1 stimulus pulse-evoked DA signal shown in black and P_2 (shown in blue) was obtained by subtraction: the two paired pulses-evoked DA (red traces). **(A,A1–A3)** In W-T mice under control conditions (without inhibition of DATs), paired-pulse depression was strong, and the paired-pulse ratio (PPR, defined as P_2/P_1) was small. In 10 μM cocaine, the PPR significantly increased ($n = 6$). 1 μM sulpiride and SKF83566 were used in all these experiments to block local DA receptor interactions within the dorsolateral striatum. **(B,B1–B3)** In β2-nAChR KO mice (without inhibition of DATs), 10 μM cocaine did not affect the PPR ($n = 5$). **(C,C1–C3)** In W-T mice with DAT inhibition by GBR12909 (5 μM) cocaine (10 μM) still enhances the PPR ($n = 5$). **(D,D1–D3)** In β2-nAChR KO mice with inhibition of DATs, 10 μM cocaine did not affect the PPR ($n = 5$). $^*p < 0.01$.

the phasic to tonic DA ratio in β2 KO mice, 1.65 ± 0.17 ($n = 6$, **Figures 9B2,C**). These data support the hypothesis that cocaine acts via inhibition of nAChRs to increase the phasic to tonic DA ratio.

DISCUSSION

The results from our present study indicate that at concentrations achieved by cocaine abusers, cocaine inhibits nAChRs and increases the ratio of phasic to tonic DA release. For example, cocaine (10 μM) decreased DA release evoked by a single, isolated stimulation (1 p) by ~70%, but that DA signaling loss was partially recovered during a stimulus train (4 p at 20 Hz). Because this relative enhancement of phasic signaling is occurring while cocaine also inhibits DA reuptake (i.e., inhibits DATs), the phasic DA signals are larger during cocaine abuse. Salient, reward-related DA signals arising from phasic DA neuron firing (Grace, 2000) will be highly exaggerated in cocaine concentrations greater than about 2 μM, which are easily achieved by cocaine abusers

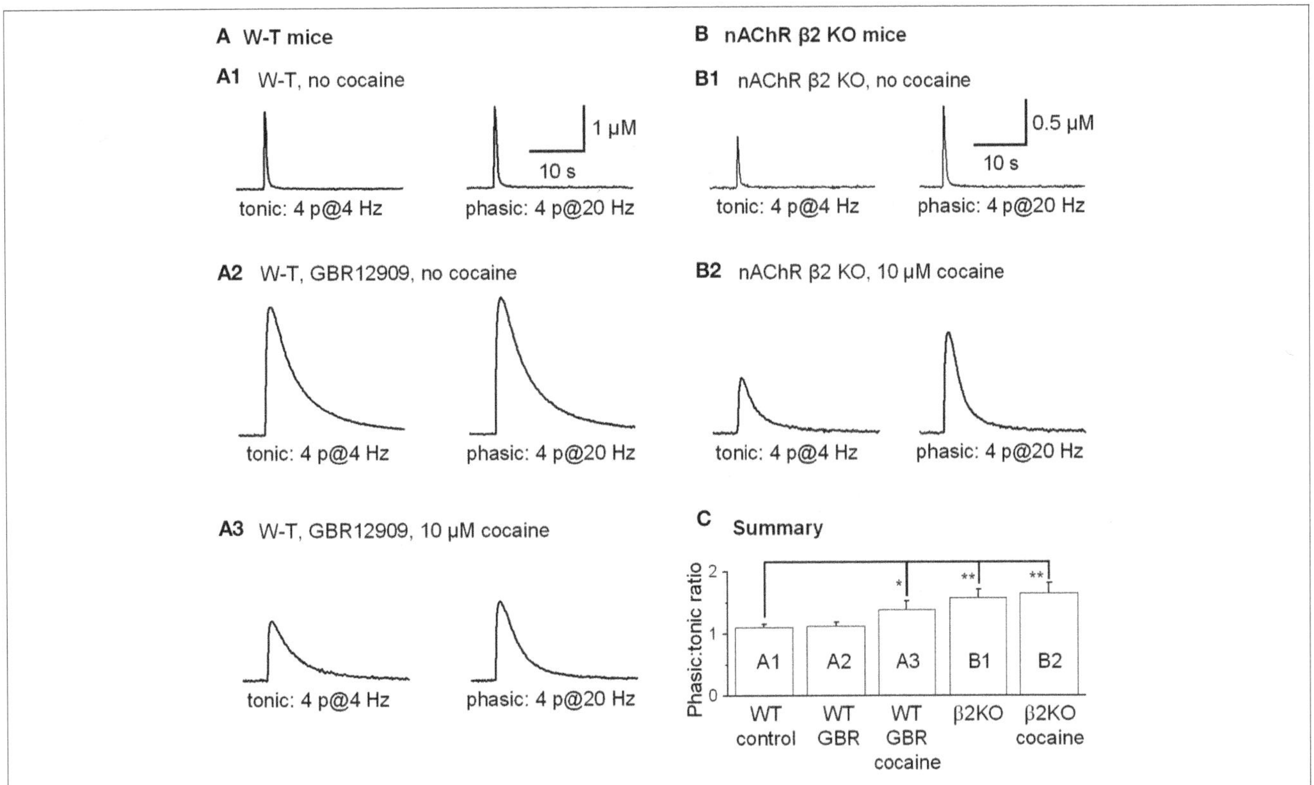

FIGURE 9 | Cocaine increased the phasic to tonic DA ratio in the dorsal striatum of W-T and nAChR KO mice. Sulpiride and SKF83566 both at 1 μM were used to block DA receptor interactions within the striatum. **(A,A1)** The FCV measurements of DA signals evoked by lower frequency tonic stimulation (4 Hz, 4-pulses, left trace) and by phasic stimulation (20 Hz, 4-pulses, right trace) under control conditions had a phasic to tonic DA signal ratio close to 1. **(A,A2)** In 5 μM GBR12909 to inhibit DATs selectively (no cocaine), the DA signals evoked by tonic stimulation (left trace) and by phasic stimulation (right trace) showed a phasic to tonic ratio near 1. GBR12909 prolonged the DA signal duration but did not enhance the phasic to tonic DA ratio. **(A,A3)** In 10 μM cocaine, the DA signals evoked by tonic stimulation (left trace) and phasic stimulation (right trace) showed a larger phasic to tonic ratio. The DA signals were broader because cocaine inhibited DATs and, thus, prolonged the DA signal duration. **(B,B1)** Cocaine did not increase the phasic to tonic DA ratio in the dorsal striatum in β2-nAChR KO Mice. The DA signal evoked by a tonic stimulation (4 Hz, 4-pulses, left trace) and phasic stimulation (20 Hz, 4-pulses, right trace) under control conditions. In β2-nAChR KO mice the phasic to tonic DA signal ratio was larger than 1 and larger than in W-T mice. **(B,B2)** In 10 μM cocaine, the DA signals evoked by a tonic stimulation (left trace) and by a phasic stimulation (right trace) were prolonged, but the ratio of phasic to tonic signal was unchanged compared to the no cocaine condition. Cocaine did not dose-dependently enhance the phasic to tonic DA ratio in β2-nAChR KO mice. Sulpiride and SKF83566 both at 1 μM were used to block DA receptor interactions within the striatum. **(C)** Summary graph showing the PPR under different conditions. $^{*}p < 0.05$, $^{**}p < 0.01$.

(Mittleman and Wetli, 1984; Evans et al., 1996; Ward et al., 1997; Fowler et al., 1998).

It must be kept in mind, however, that the striatal brain slice preparation and the exogenous electrical stimulation of the striatal tissue to evoke DA release is a reduced experimental model system that allows us to examine the different aspects of cocaine's effect on the DA signal in the striatum. As seen in **Figure 6B**, under these experimental conditions, cocaine's influence acting exclusively via nAChRs is mainly to diminish the DA release that would be even larger owing to cocaine's inhibition of DATs. By inhibiting nAChRs, the stimulus evoked DA release is not as large as would be achieved if the nAChRs were not partially inhibited by cocaine (Zhang et al., 2009a). In intact animals, cocaine's effects are more complex. For example, cocaine's inhibition of DA uptake increases the basal extracellular DA level that may activate the inhibitory D2 autoreceptors that in turn reduce DA release (Schmitz et al., 2002), complicating the determination of the physiological functions of the individual receptors and neurotransmitter systems.

NICOTINIC ANTAGONISM BY COCAINE REGULATES DA RELEASE IN THE STRIATUM

The results from this study indicate three different cocaine concentration ranges that induce different antagonist actions (best seen in **Figure 6**). At low concentrations, below 1 μM ($IC_{50} \cong$ 0.5 μM) (Ritz et al., 1987), cocaine inhibits DATs and elevates extracellular DA by reducing DA reuptake. This is probably cocaine's most common effect in cocaine abusers for the simple reason that low cocaine concentrations are more common and last longer than the high cocaine peak (Evans et al., 1996; Ward et al., 1997; Fowler et al., 1998). At intermediate concentrations above 2 μM (IC_{50} of 4.3 μM), also commonly achieved by cocaine abusers, cocaine begins to inhibit nAChRs (**Figure 3B**) and, thereby, alters DA signaling via nicotinic mechanisms (Zhou et al., 2001; Rice and Cragg, 2004; Zhang and Sulzer, 2004). At high concentrations above 10 μM ($IC_{50} \cong 26.4$ μM) that can be reached during a large cocaine dosing, local anesthetic-like effects begin (Mittleman and Wetli, 1984; O'Leary and Chahine, 2002). The mechanism for cocaine's stronger inhibition of DA release than that of voltage-gated Na current see in our data is not known; we speculate that the Na current at the DA axon fibers and terminals may be more sensitive to cocaine; the extensive DA axon fiber bifurcations may also increase the sensitivity of the action potential generation and propagation to cocaine inhibition (Matsuda et al., 2009; Debanne et al., 2011).

Our results show that in striatal slices from W-T mice, cocaine inhibited β2-containing nAChR-dependent DA release (from 1 p stimulation) with an IC_{50} of 4.3 μM (**Figure 3B**). In contrast, a six time greater cocaine concentration is needed to depress 1 p-stimulation DA release from β2-containing nAChR KO mice with an IC_{50} of 26.4 μM (**Figure 5B**). The data indicate that cocaine's inhibition of DA release is mediated by β2 nAChRs on DA fibers and terminals that normally regulate DA release (Zhou et al., 2001; Grady et al., 2002; Rice and Cragg, 2004; Salminen et al., 2004; Zhang and Sulzer, 2004; Zhang et al., 2009a). This conclusion is also supported by our finding that in DA neuron somata, cocaine inhibited the β2* nAChR current (**Figure 2B**), consistent with previous studies of cloned α4β2 nAChRs in expression systems (Damaj et al., 1999; Francis et al., 2000). The inhibition of nAChR currents and DA release was quantitatively mimicked by the selective nAChR antagonist DHβE (**Figure 2B2**). Because cocaine often reaches greater than 2 μM in the brains of abusers (Mittleman and Wetli, 1984; Evans et al., 1996; Ward et al., 1997; Fowler et al., 1998), our results indicate that biologically relevant cocaine levels directly alter DA release.

The observation that weak cocaine inhibition of nAChRs (**Figure 2B**) leads to a greatly amplified inhibition of DA release (**Figure 3A**) likely arises from the site of nAChR action. nAChRs on DA fibers and terminals regulate action potential propagation and presynaptic calcium signals. For example, nAChRs mediate direct and indirect Ca^{2+} elevation within axon terminals (Vernino et al., 1992, 1994; Lena et al., 1993; McGehee et al., 1995; Gray et al., 1996; Rathouz et al., 1996). Neurotransmitter release is related to a high power (≅4th) of intra-terminal Ca^{2+} (Zucker and Regehr, 2002; Lou et al., 2005). Consequently, even a small decrease in the nAChR-initiated presynaptic Ca^{2+} signal or depolarization would induce a larger decrease in DA release. This conclusion is supported by the quantitatively similar data obtained with the specific nAChR inhibitor, DHβE, which decreases nAChR-dependent DA release more strongly than nAChR-mediated currents (**Figures 2B, 3A**).

A number of recent studies have shown that nAChR activity on DA fibers and terminals regulates the relationship between afferent action potentials and DA release. The nAChRs on DA fibers and terminals increase the initial DA release probability, enhancing tonic DA signals (Grady et al., 2002; Rice and Cragg, 2004; Salminen et al., 2004; Zhang and Sulzer, 2004; Exley and Cragg, 2008; Zhang et al., 2009a). nAChR activation may also directly evoke action potentials in DA axon terminals and thus DA release (Cachope et al., 2012; Threlfell et al., 2012). Inhibiting or desensitizing striatal nAChRs decreases tonic DA release, but phasic DA release arising from stimulus trains is not inhibited. This nicotinic effect increases the ratio of phasic to tonic DA release arising from the biologically complex series of action potentials along DA fibers (Rice and Cragg, 2004; Zhang and Sulzer, 2004; Zhang et al., 2009a). By inhibiting nAChRs, cocaine influences this nicotinic mechanism that alters the frequency dependence of DA release favoring phasic signals.

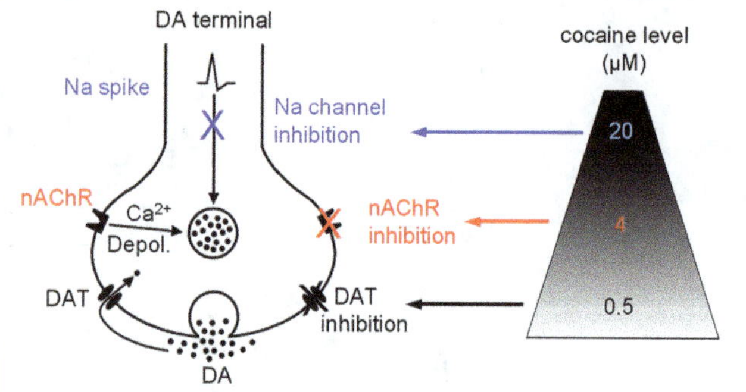

FIGURE 10 | Diagram showing that cocaine may inhibit DAT-mediated DA uptake and DA release via nAChRs and Na channels in a dose-dependent manner. Depol., depolarization.

BIOLOGICAL IMPLICATIONS

Our data indicate that besides inhibiting DAT, the most common effect on the DA system, cocaine, at concentrations (around 4 μM) readily achievable in cocaine abusers (Evans et al., 1996; Ward et al., 1997; Fowler et al., 1998), may also, via inhibiting nAChRs, alter DA release property. On rare occasions when the abuser uses very high doses of cocaine leading to a cocaine level ≥20 μM, cocaine's anesthetic effect may be triggered (**Figure 10**). The functional importance of our data obtained in brain slices is reflected in several behavioral studies showing that nicotinic agonism increases the abusive potential of cocaine whereas inhibition of nAChRs decreases cocaine reinforced behaviors (Reid et al., 1998; Zachariou et al., 2001; Schoffelmeer et al., 2002; Blokhina et al., 2005; Champtiaux et al., 2006; Zanetti et al., 2006). Particularly, pharmacological or genetic inactivation of nAChRs before exposure to cocaine was reported to disrupt place preference to cocaine, whereas low doses of nicotine were able to lower the threshold for cocaine induced place preference, and nAChR β2 KO mice showed decreased cocaine induced place preference (Zachariou et al., 2001). It was also reported that nAChR inhibition by mecamylamine dose dependently suppressed cocaine self-administration (Blokhina et al., 2005). These literature data clearly indicate that nAChRs are involved in cocaine's addictive processes, although the underlying neural mechanisms are likely to be complex. Therefore, it is reasonable to conclude that the mechanistic effects reported in this study contribute to those *in vivo* findings: acting via inhibition of nAChRs, cocaine increases the ratio of phasic to tonic DA release and thus potentially enhances its reinforcing abilities (Goto and Grace, 2005).

ACKNOWLEDGMENTS

We thank Martin Wessendorf (University of Minnesota) for advice on immunohistochemistry, and we thank Kechun Yang

(University of Pennsylvania) for his comments on the manuscript. This work was supported by grants from the National Institutes of Health DA021194, MH067119 (Fu-Ming Zhou), NS21229, DA09411 (John A. Dani), DA017173 (Mariella De Biasi).

REFERENCES

Abbott, L. F., and Regehr, W. G. (2004). Synaptic computation. *Nature* 431, 796–803. doi: 10.1038/nature03010

Alkondon, M., and Albuquerque, E. X. (1993). Diversity of nicotinic acetylcholine receptors in rat hippocampal neurons. I. Pharmacological and functional evidence for distinct structural subtypes. *J. Pharmacol. Exp. Ther.* 265, 1455–1473.

Beckstead, M. J., and Williams, J. T. (2007). Long-term depression of a dopamine IPSC. *J. Neurosci.* 27, 2074–2080. doi: 10.1523/JNEUROSCI.3251-06.2007

Blokhina, E. A., Kashkin, V. A., Zvartau, E. E., Danysz, W., and Bespalov, A. Y. (2005). Effects of nicotinic and NMDA receptor channel blockers on intravenous cocaine and nicotine self-administration in mice. *Eur. Neuropsychopharmacol.* 15, 219–225. doi: 10.1016/j.euroneuro.2004.07.005

Bonci, A., Bernardi, G., Grillner, P., and Mercuri, N. B. (2003). The dopamine-containing neuron: maestro or simple musician in the orchestra of addiction? *Trends Pharmacol. Sci.* 24, 172–177. doi: 10.1016/S0165-6147(03)00068-3

Cachope, R., Mateo, Y., Mathur, B. N., Irving, J., Wang, H. L., Morales, M., et al. (2012). Selective activation of cholinergic interneurons enhances accumbal phasic dopamine release: setting the tone for reward processing. *Cell Rep.* 2, 33–41. doi: 10.1016/j.celrep.2012.05.011

Champtiaux, N., Gotti, C., Cordero-Erausquin, M., David, D. J., Przybylski, C., Lena, C., et al. (2003). Subunit composition of functional nicotinic receptors in dopaminergic neurons investigated with knock-out mice. *J. Neurosci.* 23, 7820–7829.

Champtiaux, N., Kalivas, P. W., and Bardo, M. T. (2006). Contribution of dihydro-beta-erythroidine sensitive nicotinic acetylcholine receptors in the ventral tegmental area to cocaine-induced behavioral sensitization in rats. *Behav. Brain Res.* 168, 120–126. doi: 10.1016/j.bbr.2005.10.017

Chen, R., Tilley, M. R., Wei, H., Zhou, F., Zhou, F. M., Ching, S., et al. (2006). Abolished cocaine reward in mice with a cocaine-insensitive dopamine transporter. *Proc. Natl. Acad. Sci. U.S.A.* 103, 9333–9338. doi: 10.1073/pnas.0600905103

Damaj, M. I., Slemmer, J. E., Carroll, F. I., and Martin, B. R. (1999). Pharmacological characterization of nicotine's interaction with cocaine and cocaine analogs. *J. Pharmacol. Exp. Ther.* 289, 1229–1236.

Debanne, D., Campanac, E., Bialowas, A., Carlier, E., and Alcaraz, G. (2011). Axon physiology. *Physiol. Rev.* 91, 555–602. doi: 10.1152/physrev.00048.2009

Ding, S., Wei, W., and Zhou, F. M. (2011). Molecular and functional differences in voltage-activated sodium currents between GABA projection neurons and dopamine neurons in the substantia nigra. *J. Neurophysiol.* 106, 3019–3034. doi: 10.1152/jn.00305.2011

Drenan, R. M., Grady, S. R., Steele, A. D., McKinney, S., Patzlaff, N. E., McIntosh, J. M., et al. (2010). Cholinergic modulation of locomotion and striatal dopamine release is mediated by alpha6alpha4* nicotinic acetylcholine receptors. *J. Neurosci.* 30, 9877–9889. doi: 10.1523/JNEUROSCI.2056-10.2010

Evans, S. M., Cone, E. J., and Henningfield, J. E. (1996). Arterial and venous cocaine plasma concentrations in humans: relationship to route of administration, cardiovascular effects and subjective effects. *J. Pharmacol. Exp. Ther.* 279, 1345–1356.

Exley, R., and Cragg, S. J. (2008). Presynaptic nicotinic receptors: a dynamic and diverse cholinergic filter of striatal dopamine neurotransmission. *Br. J. Pharmacol.* 153(Suppl. 1), S283–S297. doi: 10.1038/sj.bjp.0707510

Exley, R., Maubourguet, N., David, V., Eddine, R., Evrard, A., Pons, S., et al. (2011). Distinct contributions of nicotinic acetylcholine receptor subunit {alpha}4 and subunit {alpha}6 to the reinforcing effects of nicotine. *Proc. Natl. Acad. Sci. U.S.A.* 108, 7577–7582. doi: 10.1073/pnas.1103000108

Ford, C. P., Mark, G. P., and Williams, J. T. (2006). Properties and opioid inhibition of mesolimbic dopamine neurons vary according to target location. *J. Neurosci.* 26, 2788–2797. doi: 10.1523/JNEUROSCI.4331-05.2006

Fowler, J. S., Volkow, N. D., Logan, J., Gatley, S. J., Pappas, N., King, P., et al. (1998). Measuring dopamine transporter occupancy by cocaine *in vivo*: radiotracer considerations. *Synapse* 28, 111–116. doi: 10.1002/(SICI)1098-2396(199802)28:2<111::AID-SYN1>3.0.CO;2-E

Francis, M. M., Vazquez, R. W., Papke, R. L., and Oswald, R. E. (2000). Subtype-selective inhibition of neuronal nicotinic acetylcholine receptors by cocaine is determined by the alpha4 and beta4 subunits. *Mol. Pharmacol.* 58, 109–119.

Goto, Y., and Grace, A. A. (2005). Dopaminergic modulation of limbic and cortical drive of nucleus accumbens in goal-directed behavior. *Nat. Neurosci.* 8, 805–812. doi: 10.1038/nn1471

Gould, E., Woolf, N. J., and Butcher, L. L. (1989). Cholinergic projections to the substantia nigra from the pedunculopontine and laterodorsal tegmental nuclei. *Neuroscience* 28, 611–623.

Grace, A. A. (2000). The tonic/phasic model of dopamine system regulation and its implications for understanding alcohol and psychostimulant craving. *Addiction* 95(Suppl. 2), S119–S128. doi: 10.1046/j.1360-0443.95.8s2.1.x

Grady, S. R., Murphy, K. L., Cao, J., Marks, M. J., McIntosh, J. M., and Collins, A. C. (2002). Characterization of nicotinic agonist-induced [(3)H]dopamine release from synaptosomes prepared from four mouse brain regions. *J. Pharmacol. Exp. Ther.* 301, 651–660. doi: 10.1124/jpet.301.2.651

Gray, R., Rajan, A. S., Radcliffe, K. A., Yakehiro, M., and Dani, J. A. (1996). Hippocampal synaptic transmission enhanced by low concentrations of nicotine. *Nature* 383, 713–716. doi: 10.1038/383713a0

Hyland, B. I., Reynolds, J. N., Hay, J., Perk, C. G., and Miller, R. (2002). Firing modes of midbrain dopamine cells in the freely moving rat. *Neuroscience* 114, 475–492. doi: 10.1016/S0306-4522(02)00267-1

Hyman, S. E., Malenka, R. C., and Nestler, E. J. (2006). Neural mechanisms of addiction: the role of reward-related learning and memory. *Annu. Rev. Neurosci.* 29, 565–598. doi: 10.1146/annurev.neuro.29.051605.113009

Jones, I. W., Bolam, J. P., and Wonnacott, S. (2001). Presynaptic localisation of the nicotinic acetylcholine receptor beta2 subunit immunoreactivity in rat nigrostriatal dopaminergic neurones. *J. Comp. Neurol.* 439, 235–247. doi: 10.1002/cne.1345

Jones, S. R., Garris, P. A., Kilts, C. D., and Wightman, R. M. (1995). Comparison of dopamine uptake in the basolateral amygdaloid nucleus, caudate-putamen, and nucleus accumbens of the rat. *J. Neurochem.* 64, 2581–2589. doi: 10.1046/j.1471-4159.1995.64062581.x

Lena, C., Changeux, J. P., and Mulle, C. (1993). Evidence for "preterminal" nicotinic receptors on GABAergic axons in the rat interpeduncular nucleus. *J. Neurosci.* 13, 2680–2688.

Li, W., Doyon, W. M., and Dani, J. A. (2011). Acute *in vivo* nicotine administration enhances synchrony among dopamine neurons. *Biochem. Pharmacol.* 82, 977–983. doi: 10.1016/j.bcp.2011.06.006

Lou, X., Scheuss, V., and Schneggenburger, R. (2005). Allosteric modulation of the presynaptic Ca^{2+} sensor for vesicle fusion. *Nature* 435, 497–501. doi: 10.1038/nature03568

Mansvelder, H. D., and McGehee, D. S. (2000). Long-term potentiation of excitatory inputs to brain reward areas by nicotine. *Neuron* 27, 349–357. doi: 10.1016/S0896-6273(00)00042-8

Matsuda, W., Furuta, T., Nakamura, K. C., Hioki, H., Fujiyama, F., Arai, R., et al. (2009). Single nigrostriatal dopaminergic neurons form widely spread and highly dense axonal arborizations in the neostriatum. *J. Neurosci.* 29, 444–453. doi: 10.1523/JNEUROSCI.4029-08.2009

McGehee, D. S., Heath, M. J., Gelber, S., Devay, P., and Role, L. W. (1995). Nicotine enhancement of fast excitatory synaptic transmission in CNS by presynaptic receptors. *Science* 269, 1692–1696. doi: 10.1126/science.7569895

Mittleman, R. E., and Wetli, C. V. (1984). Death caused by recreational cocaine use. An update. *JAMA* 252, 1889–1893.

Nelson, A. B., Hammack, N., Yang, C. F., Shah, N. M., Seal, R. P., and Kreitzer, A. C. (2014). Striatal cholinergic interneurons drive GABA release from dopamine terminals. *Neuron* 82, 63–70. doi: 10.1016/j.neuron.2014.01.023

Neuhoff, H., Neu, A., Liss, B., and Roeper, J. (2002). I(h) channels contribute to the different functional properties of identified dopaminergic subpopulations in the midbrain. *J. Neurosci.* 22, 1290–1302.

Nicola, S. M., and Deadwyler, S. A. (2000). Firing rate of nucleus accumbens neurons is dopamine-dependent and reflects the timing of cocaine-seeking behavior in rats on a progressive ratio schedule of reinforcement. *J. Neurosci.* 20, 5526–5537.

Oakman, S. A., Faris, P. L., Kerr, P. E., Cozzari, C., and Hartman, B. K. (1995). Distribution of pontomesencephalic cholinergic neurons projecting to substantia nigra differs significantly from those projecting to ventral tegmental area. *J. Neurosci.* 15, 5859–5869.

O'Leary, M. E., and Chahine, M. (2002). Cocaine binds to a common site on open and inactivated human heart (Na(v)1.5) sodium channels. *J. Physiol. (Lond.)* 541, 701–716. doi: 10.1113/jphysiol.2001.016139

Picciotto, M. R., Zoli, M., Lena, C., Bessis, A., Lallemand, Y., Le Novere, N., et al. (1995). Abnormal avoidance learning in mice lacking functional high-affinity nicotine receptor in the brain. *Nature* 374, 65–67. doi: 10.1038/374065a0

Pidoplichko, V. I., and Dani, J. A. (2005). Applying small quantities of multiple compounds to defined locations of *in vitro* brain slices. *J. Neurosci. Methods* 142, 55–66. doi: 10.1016/j.jneumeth.2004.07.012

Pidoplichko, V. I., De Biasi, M., Williams, J. T., and Dani, J. A. (1997). Nicotine activates and desensitizes midbrain dopamine neurons. *Nature* 390, 401–404. doi: 10.1038/37120

Pristupa, Z. B., Wilson, J. M., Hoffman, B. J., Kish, S. J., and Niznik, H. B. (1994). Pharmacological heterogeneity of the cloned and native human dopamine transporter: disassociation of [3H]WIN 35,428 and [3H]GBR 12,935 binding. *Mol. Pharmacol.* 45, 125–135.

Quik, M., and McIntosh, J. M. (2006). Striatal alpha6* nicotinic acetylcholine receptors: potential targets for parkinson's disease therapy. *J. Pharmacol. Exp. Ther.* 316, 481–489. doi: 10.1124/jpet.105.094375

Rathouz, M. M., Vijayaraghavan, S., and Berg, D. K. (1996). Elevation of intracellular calcium levels in neurons by nicotinic acetylcholine receptors. *Mol. Neurobiol.* 12, 117–131. doi: 10.1007/BF02740649

Reid, M. S., Mickalian, J. D., Delucchi, K. L., Hall, S. M., and Berger, S. P. (1998). An acute dose of nicotine enhances cue-induced cocaine craving. *Drug Alcohol Depend.* 49, 95–104. doi: 10.1016/S0376-8716(97)00144-0

Rice, M. E., and Cragg, S. J. (2004). Nicotine amplifies reward-related dopamine signals in striatum. *Nat. Neurosci.* 7, 583–584. doi: 10.1038/nn1244

Ritz, M. C., Lamb, R. J., Goldberg, S. R., and Kuhar, M. J. (1987). Cocaine receptors on dopamine transporters are related to self-administration of cocaine. *Science* 237, 1219–1223. doi: 10.1126/science.2820058

Salminen, O., Murphy, K. L., McIntosh, J. M., Drago, J., Marks, M. J., Collins, A. C., et al. (2004). Subunit composition and pharmacology of two classes of striatal presynaptic nicotinic acetylcholine receptors mediating dopamine release in mice. *Mol. Pharmacol.* 65, 1526–1535. doi: 10.1124/mol.65.6.1526

Schmitz, Y., Schmauss, C., and Sulzer, D. (2002). Altered dopamine release and uptake kinetics in mice lacking D2 receptors. *J. Neurosci.* 22, 8002–8009.

Schoffelmeer, A. N., De Vries, T. J., Wardeh, G., Van De Ven, H. W., and Vanderschuren, L. J. (2002). Psychostimulant-induced behavioral sensitization depends on nicotinic receptor activation. *J. Neurosci.* 22, 3269–3276.

Schultz, W. (2002). Getting formal with dopamine and reward. *Neuron* 36, 241–263. doi: 10.1016/S0896-6273(02)00967-4

Threlfell, S., Lalic, T., Platt, N. J., Jennings, K. A., Deisseroth, K., and Cragg, S. J. (2012). Striatal dopamine release is triggered by synchronized activity in cholinergic interneurons. *Neuron* 75, 58–64. doi: 10.1016/j.neuron.2012.04.038

Vernino, S., Amador, M., Luetje, C. W., Patrick, J., and Dani, J. A. (1992). Calcium modulation and high calcium permeability of neuronal nicotinic acetylcholine receptors. *Neuron* 8, 127–134. doi: 10.1016/0896-6273(92)90114-S

Vernino, S., Rogers, M., Radcliffe, K. A., and Dani, J. A. (1994). Quantitative measurement of calcium flux through muscle and neuronal nicotinic acetylcholine receptors. *J. Neurosci.* 14, 5514–5524.

Ward, A. S., Haney, M., Fischman, M. W., and Foltin, R. W. (1997). Binge cocaine self-administration in humans: intravenous cocaine. *Psychopharmacology (Berl.)* 132, 375–381. doi: 10.1007/s002130050358

Wise, R. A. (2004). Dopamine, learning and motivation. *Nat. Rev. Neurosci.* 5, 483–494. doi: 10.1038/nrn1406

Woolf, N. J., and Butcher, L. L. (1981). Cholinergic neurons in the caudate-putamen complex proper are intrinsically organized: a combined Evans blue and acetylcholinesterase analysis. *Brain Res. Bull.* 7, 487–507.

Woolf, N. J., and Butcher, L. L. (1986). Cholinergic systems in the rat brain: III. Projections from the pontomesencephalic tegmentum to the thalamus, tectum, basal ganglia, and basal forebrain. *Brain Res. Bull.* 16, 603–637.

Wooltorton, J. R., Pidoplichko, V. I., Broide, R. S., and Dani, J. A. (2003). Differential desensitization and distribution of nicotinic acetylcholine receptor subtypes in midbrain dopamine areas. *J. Neurosci.* 23, 3176–3185.

Xu, W., Orr-Urtreger, A., Nigro, F., Gelber, S., Sutcliffe, C. B., Armstrong, D., et al. (1999). Multiorgan autonomic dysfunction in mice lacking the beta2 and the beta4 subunits of neuronal nicotinic acetylcholine receptors. *J. Neurosci.* 19, 9298–9305.

Zachariou, V., Caldarone, B. J., Weathers-Lowin, A., George, T. P., Elsworth, J. D., Roth, R. H., et al. (2001). Nicotine receptor inactivation decreases sensitivity to cocaine. *Neuropsychopharmacology* 24, 576–589. doi: 10.1016/S0893-133X(00)00224-4

Zanetti, L., De Kerchove D'exaerde, A., Zanardi, A., Changeux, J. P., Picciotto, M. R., and Zoli, M. (2006). Inhibition of both alpha7* and beta2* nicotinic acetylcholine receptors is necessary to prevent development of sensitization to cocaine-elicited increases in extracellular dopamine levels in the ventral striatum. *Psychopharmacology (Berl.)* 187, 181–188. doi: 10.1007/s00213-006-0419-y

Zhang, H., and Sulzer, D. (2004). Frequency-dependent modulation of dopamine release by nicotine. *Nat. Neurosci.* 7, 581–582. doi: 10.1038/nn1243

Zhang, L., Doyon, W. M., Clark, J. J., Phillips, P. E., and Dani, J. A. (2009a). Controls of tonic and phasic dopamine transmission in the dorsal and ventral striatum. *Mol. Pharmacol.* 76, 396–404. doi: 10.1124/mol.109.056317

Zhang, T., Zhang, L., Liang, Y., Siapas, A. G., Zhou, F. M., and Dani, J. A. (2009b). Dopamine signaling differences in the nucleus accumbens and dorsal striatum exploited by nicotine. *J. Neurosci.* 29, 4035–4043. doi: 10.1523/JNEUROSCI.0261-09.2009

Zhang, T. A., Placzek, A. N., and Dani, J. A. (2010). *In vitro* identification and electrophysiological characterization of dopamine neurons in the ventral tegmental area. *Neuropharmacology* 59, 431–436. doi: 10.1016/j.neuropharm.2010.06.004

Zhou, F. M., Liang, Y., and Dani, J. A. (2001). Endogenous nicotinic cholinergic activity regulates dopamine release in the striatum. *Nat. Neurosci.* 4, 1224–1229. doi: 10.1038/nn769

Zucker, R. S., and Regehr, W. G. (2002). Short-term synaptic plasticity. *Annu. Rev. Physiol.* 64, 355–405. doi: 10.1146/annurev.physiol.64.092501.114547

11

Recent advancements in diffusion MRI for investigating cortical development after preterm birth—potential and pitfalls

J. Dudink[1]*†, K. Pieterman[1†], A. Leemans[2], M. Kleinnijenhuis[3], A. M. van Cappellen van Walsum[4] and F. E. Hoebeek[5]

[1] *Department of Neonatology, Pediatric Intensive Care and Pediatric Radiology, Erasmus Medical Center - Sophia Children's Hospital, Rotterdam, Netherlands*
[2] *Image Sciences Institute, University Medical Center Utrecht, Utrecht, Netherlands*
[3] *Oxford Centre for Functional Magnetic Resonance Imaging of the Brain, University of Oxford, Oxford, UK*
[4] *Department of Anatomy, Donders Institute for Brain, Cognition, and Behaviour, Radboud University Medical Center, Nijmegen, Netherlands*
[5] *Department of Neuroscience, Erasmus Medical Center Rotterdam, Rotterdam, Netherlands*

Edited by:
Silvia Comani, Università degli Studi G. d'Annunzio, Italy

Reviewed by:
Zoltan Nagy, University of Zurich, Switzerland
Jan Buijs, Maxima Medisch Centrum, Netherlands

***Correspondence:**
J. Dudink, Department of Neonatology, Pediatric Intensive Care and Pediatric Radiology, Erasmus Medical Center - Sophia Children's Hospital, Wytemaweg 80, 3015 CN Rotterdam, Netherlands
e-mail: j.dudink@erasmusmc.nl

† These authors have contributed equally to this work.

Preterm infants are born during a critical period of brain maturation, in which even subtle events can result in substantial behavioral, motor and cognitive deficits, as well as psychiatric diseases. Recent evidence shows that the main source for these devastating disabilities is not necessarily white matter (WM) damage but could also be disruptions of cortical microstructure. Animal studies showed how moderate hypoxic-ischemic conditions did not result in significant neuronal loss in the developing brain, but did cause significantly impaired dendritic growth and synapse formation alongside a disturbed development of neuronal connectivity as measured using diffusion magnetic resonance imaging (dMRI). When using more advanced acquisition settings such as high-angular resolution diffusion imaging (HARDI), more advanced reconstruction methods can be applied to investigate the cortical microstructure with higher levels of detail. Recent advances in dMRI acquisition and analysis have great potential to contribute to a better understanding of neuronal connectivity impairment in preterm birth. We will review the current understanding of abnormal preterm cortical development, novel approaches in dMRI, and the pitfalls in scanning vulnerable preterm infants.

Keywords: diffusion magnetic resonance imaging, DTI, cortical imaging technique, prematurity, cortical development, cortical development and plasticity, diffusion MRI

INTRODUCTION

During the final trimester of pregnancy, the human brain rapidly develops by a complex interplay of genetic, epigenetic and environmental factors. Preterm infants are born during this period that is critical for neuronal connectivity, brain growth and cortical maturation, which together puts them at risk for functional impairments that are likely to persist into later life (Saigal and Doyle, 2008; Volpe, 2009). In particular the development of the cerebral cortex is imperative for the social and emotional well-being (e.g., Salmaso et al., 2014). Histological studies in both animals and humans have demonstrated that white and gray matter develop in close relation, and that isolated white matter (WM) injury sparing the cerebral cortex is uncommon (Govaert et al., 2006; Pierson et al., 2007; Sizonenko et al., 2007; Volpe, 2009; Okabayashi et al., 2011). Diffusion-MRI (dMRI) is a valuable tool to study brain development *in vivo*, and is based on its ability to characterize diffusion patterns of water molecules within the brain (Basser et al., 1994). As these patterns are directly related to brain microstructure, different models have been developed to characterize the diffusion signal in detail. The diffusion tensor (DT) model has been commonly used for this purpose, and represents the diffusion characteristics within each voxel as an ellipsoid (Basser et al., 1994; Jones and Leemans, 2011). Using only six parameters, this model is able to provide a quantitative description of the diffusion characteristics representing neuroanatomy. The ellipsoidal shape is more elongated (cigar-shaped) in regions with highly aligned and densely packed tissue components, such as the corpus callosum, representing *anisotropic* diffusion. In contrast, the DT shape resembles a sphere in brain regions with less aligned fiber tissue, wherein the diffusion pattern is called *isotropic*. Several studies have pointed out that the DT model is less adequate in representing complex fiber orientations within a single voxel (Tournier et al., 2004, 2011; Jeurissen et al., 2013), which is furthermore reflected by the fact that diffusion tensor imaging (DTI) has been predominantly used to characterize large WM bundles such as the corpus callosum and pyramidal tract but hardly to study "complex" brain regions containing crossing fibers and more dispersedly organized microstructure such as gray matter (Martinussen et al., 2005; Pannek et al., 2014).

Present-day, neuroimaging studies resulted in the development of acquisition and processing pipelines designed to derive more detailed information about the precise diffusion characteristics within each voxel. These advances increase the applicability of dMRI to regions of more complex microstructure such as the cerebral cortex. Several higher-order models to fit the diffusion data have been developed recently, including models designed to study cortical microstructure, such as *neurite orientation dispersion and density imaging* (NODDI; Zhang et al., 2012). This mini-review will briefly outline these and other recent developments regarding cortical imaging and discuss related challenges and pitfalls.

INSIGHTS IN IMPAIRED CORTICAL DEVELOPMENT FROM HUMAN AND ANIMAL SPECIMEN STUDIES

For long, histological substrates of brain damage following preterm birth were most prominently characterized by large, focal WM lesions, adjacent to the ventricles, known as periventricular leukomalacia (PVL). Although cystic changes of WM are most prominent in PVL, several studies have outlined that relative sparing of the cerebral cortex is implausible in this type of WM injury. Andiman et al. (2010) histologically assessed the cortical microstructure in specimens of human tissue collected following focal periventricular WM injury possibly induced by preterm birth, and observed a significant reduction in pyramidal neuron density in layer V of the overlying cerebral cortex, indicating cell death of cortical neurons in focal WM injury (Andiman et al., 2010). A commonly used middle cerebral artery stroke model in mice showed comparable histological features, such as the histological abnormalities in layer V of the cortex. This included both morphological alterations of cell components and signs of neuronal necrosis (de Oliveira et al., 2014). In addition, subcortical nuclei were also affected in PVL cases, showing significant neuronal loss in thalamus, globus pallidus and the cerebellar dentate nucleus (Pierson et al., 2007). These findings exemplify that opposed to isolated WM injury, impaired neurodevelopment in preterm infants represents a complex interplay between gray and WM damage, leading to structural changes throughout the entire brain (Tymofiyeva et al., 2012; Ball et al., 2013a).

With the improved spatial resolution of state-of-the-art radiological techniques (e.g., ultra-high field MRI) the neonatal care specialists also encounter diffuse anatomical anomalies that affect both cortical and subcortical structures. Often these subtle aberrations are found in preterm children that suffered from hypoxia, ischemia or inflammation. Although the extent of such anatomical aberrations seems limited when visualized using conventional imaging, both human imaging and histology studies have demonstrated that these changes in the preterm brain can nevertheless significantly impact on long-term functional outcome (Ment et al., 2009). Moreover, using an experimental sheep model it was recently shown that the cortical development was severely affected following mild levels of ischemia, which evoked non-cystic and thus diffuse WM alteration (Dean et al., 2013). Using *ex vivo* high-field diffusion MRI it was also shown that normal cortical development was impeded, i.e., the physiological decrease in cortical anisotropy resulting from emerging cellular complexity during development was less pronounced in sheep exposed to moderate ischemia.

In contrast to focal WM changes such as PVL, the number of cortical neurons was not reduced in this type of WM damage, but Golgi-staining showed that ischemia induced a significant reduction of dendritic branching in the cerebral cortex, which could well explain the observed differences in anisotropy compared to age-matched controls. These results indicate that disrupted cortical development in moderate ischemia does not have to be linked to drastic effects like neuronal loss, but can also evoke "milder" effects like morphological aberrations (Dean et al., 2013).

Results of such translational studies of impaired cortical development are very useful, as they contribute to ensuring correct interpretation of *in vivo* human imaging results. By combining histology with MR-imaging in animal models and specimen studies, histological features of disrupted cortical development can be correlated to MR abnormalities seen in preterm born infants. Histology of the human cortex has been used as validation of normal brain cortical architecture (Kleinnijenhuis et al., 2013b; White et al., 2013), as well as to assess how histopathological findings correlate to cortical dMRI (Hulst and Geurts, 2011; Kolasinski et al., 2012; Gao et al., 2013; Leigland et al., 2013). These insights can be expected to help develop reliable, non-invasive, *in vivo* neuroimaging biomarkers for early prediction of impaired neurodevelopment.

MRI STUDIES OF IMPAIRED CORTICAL DEVELOPMENT IN HUMANS

The shift to more subtle radiologic abnormalities in both cortex and WM demands new ways to assess structure and development of the preterm brain. dMRI can provide additional insights in the characteristics of the preterm brain by mapping the diffusion pattern of water molecules. Because tissue components hinder the random motion of water molecules, dMRI measurements are directly related to underlying tissue microstructure (Basser and Jones, 2002; Mori and Van Zijl, 2002). Analysis of preterm brain damage using dMRI can thereby contribute to a better understanding of injury-mechanisms underlying impaired neurodevelopment, by revealing alterations in neuronal organization and extracellular matrix composition (Basser and Jones, 2002; Mori and Van Zijl, 2002).

Conventional T1 imaging has been used to assess the impact of preterm birth on cortical development. This sequence is particularly suitable for assessment of cortical volume and surface area, hence it provides good contrast between white and gray matter in combination with high spatial resolution. Studies making use of this have shown that cortical volume and surface area are substantially affected by preterm birth. Phillips et al. (2011) showed that in early childhood, cortical thickness was significantly higher and surface area significantly lower among preterm born infants than in term born controls (Phillips et al., 2011). This indicates that the normal pattern of cortical maturation—a combination of cortical thinning and surface area expansion—is substantially delayed or disrupted by preterm birth. The importance of these findings is highlighted by the fact that impaired cortical growth between 24 weeks and term-equivalent age is directly related to neurocognitive abilities in later life (Rathbone et al., 2011). The degree of cortical folding seems directly related to the extent of

WM connectivity (Melbourne et al., 2014), which is particularly relevant because studies in ex-preterm adolescents and adults show that characteristic changes in cortical folding, thickness and volume persist in later life (Martinussen et al., 2005; Nagy et al., 2011; Skranes et al., 2013).

ADVANCED DIFFUSION WEIGHTED IMAGING TECHNIQUES

Cortical diffusion MRI can help to determine *in vivo* how changes in cortical folding and thickness are related to cortical changes at a cellular level. Advances in dMRI, such as more widespread application of high-angular resolution diffusion imaging (HARDI), enable a more reliable assessment of cortical microstructure (Tuch et al., 2002). Benefits of HARDI acquisition arise from a substantial increase in number of diffusion-encoding directions, providing a more reliable and extensive characterization of the 3d diffusion profile. Next to an increase in angular resolution, increased spatial resolution is desirable, because it facilitates more reliable differentiation among cortical regions, underlying WM and surrounding cerebrospinal fluid. Higher-order processing algorithms of HARDI-data provide more detailed information than the tradition DT model, as these models aim at extracting the diffusion characteristics from each voxel more extensively.

The structure of the neocortex dramatically increases in complexity during development (McKinstry et al., 2002; Ball et al., 2013b). During developmental stages characterized by high densities of radial glial fibers, the DT model might be an adequate model for describing diffusion in the cortex (**Figure 1**). Furthermore, structural development of the cortex can be detected with the DT model (Neil et al., 1998; McKinstry et al., 2002), but the model's specificity is limited, because multiple features of the microstructure have similar effects on tensor characteristics (Vos et al., 2011, 2012). For example, the decrease in anisotropy observed over cortical development is thought to results from emerging dendritic arborization (Dean et al., 2013), but the same anisotropy decrease could also result from, for instance a reduction in radial glial fibers (Sizonenko et al., 2007). Most likely, these different changes happen concurrently and therefore it is essential to distinguish these contributions and other microstructural features, not only with postmortem techniques, but also with *in vivo* methods such as diffusion MRI.

As mentioned above, appealing alternatives to the DT model are available to capture more of the cortical complexity. The limitation of the DT model of describing diffusion behavior as an ellipsoid can be overcome by fitting models that allow more peaks in the modeled diffusion profile (Frank, 2002; Jansons and Alexander, 2003; Tuch et al., 2003; Tournier et al., 2004; Wedeen et al., 2005). By making use of high-angular resolution data, it is possible to fit more complex models which include multiple fibers. Such models have been widely adopted for resolving crossing fiber populations in WM tractography (Jeurissen et al., 2011, 2014; Pannek et al., 2014; Tax et al., 2014a). Likewise, complex cortical fiber arrangements emerging during gestation should also be reflected in the fiber orientation distributions derived from these data. Metrics specific to various cortical fiber populations might then be derived for application of this method in WM of the preterm brain (Raffelt et al., 2012; Dell'Acqua et al., 2013). Although radial and tangential components in the fiber orientation distribution have been *ex vivo* demonstrated (**Figure 2**) in adult human (Kleinnijenhuis et al., 2013a) and animal cortex (Dyrby et al., 2011), the performance of these models under such anisotropic conditions is uncertain (Parker et al., 2013). Furthermore, because scan time increases linearly with the number of directions, *in vivo* application of these elaborate sampling schemes in preterm newborns is particularly challenging.

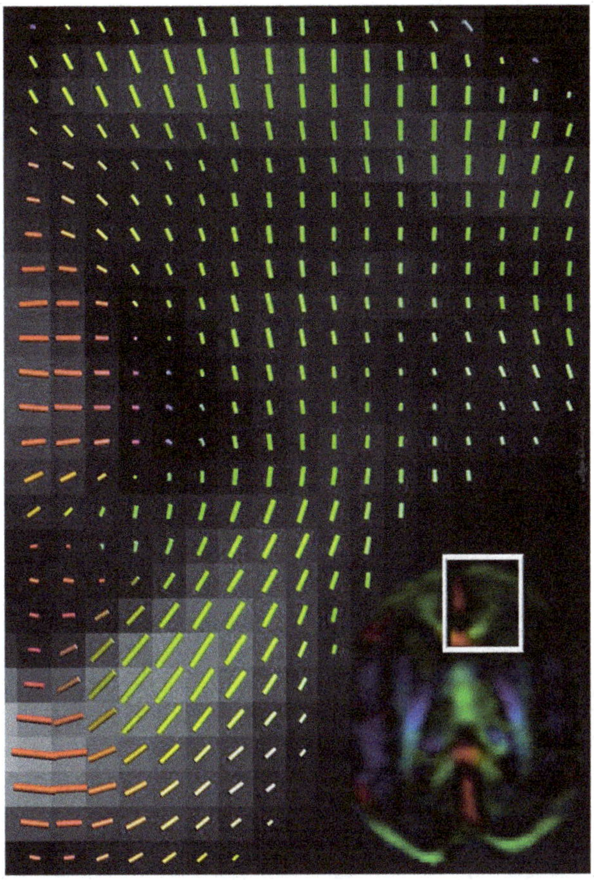

FIGURE 1 | Color-coded orientation map of a preterm infant's brain (born at 26 weeks of gestation and scanned at 30 weeks gestation at 1.5 Tesla MRI scanner) calculated from diffusion tensor imaging. Each pixel contains information about the eigenvector (Green color signifies preferential diffusion in the antero-posterior direction; Red in the latero-lateral direction; Blue in the superior-inferior direction) and extent of diffusion anisotropy (intensity of color) which summarizes the information obtained from each 3 × 3-matrix tensor. The cortex at 30 weeks gestation still has a clear radial organization (shown in close-up).

An innovation that could also be valuable for investigating the cortex in preterm infants is the estimation of quantitative measures of tissue microstructure. This approach surpasses the measures obtained from the DT model, as it can directly inform on the fraction, size and shape of various tissue compartments. Whereas extracellular water is—although hindered in its path—free to diffuse throughout the extracellular space, intracellular water is restricted within the bounds of the

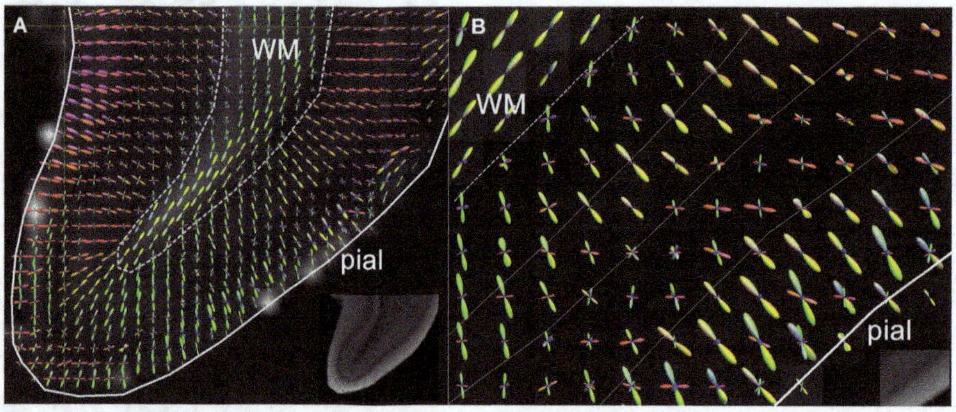

FIGURE 2 | (A) High resolution diffusion-MRI of sub-cortical white matter and cortical gray matter of the adult human primary visual cortex. High angular and spatial resolution data (768 directions at 300 micrometers isotropic resolution) was used to generate orientation distribution functions (ODF's) for each voxel. The spikes of the ODF are color-coded and represent the different directions of orientation within a single voxel. The ODF's in the cortex are mainly orientated perpendicular to the cortical surface, and represent its radial organization, whereas underlying white matter is arranged corticofugally. **(B)** Close-up of the cortex in a neighboring slice, showing that the ODF's are able to discern different layers of the cortex based on differences in microstructural characteristics between different laminae. The fractional anisotropy image is used as a backdrop image. Greyscale insets represent the anatomical GRE reference images showing cortical layers including the stria of Gennari. Adapted from Kleinnijenhuis et al. (2011).

cell. Sensitization to these different water pools is achieved by varying the b-value (or diffusion time), where higher b-values represent to some extent the intracellular signal, increasing the specificity to the tissue structures (e.g., Assaf and Basser, 2005). This simple principle has been used in several investigations of the preterm brain (Dudink et al., 2008; Ferizi et al., 2014; Pannek et al., 2014; Riffert et al., 2014). The diffusion kurtosis tensor (Jensen et al., 2005) is a somewhat more elaborate model that allows separation of the Gaussian and non-Gaussian contribution to the diffusion attenuation, assumed to represent the extracellular and intracellular spaces. A recent report demonstrates a marked decrease of radial kurtosis in the third trimester (Jeon, 2014), suggesting that it is a sensitive measure for disruption of radial glial fibers. Although the diffusion kurtosis isolates non-Gaussianity in the signal, it does not inform on the source of this non-Gaussianity. This is particularly relevant for the developing cortex, because non-Gaussianity can also result from fiber dispersion. The biophysical multi-compartment model NODDI (Zhang et al., 2012) is able to account for and inform on fiber dispersion, by explicitly including it in the signal model. The main parameters that can be estimated from the NODDI model are intracellular volume fraction and the orientation dispersion index. The first reports applying this model to the preterm brain (Eaton-Rosen, 2014; Kunz et al., 2014), suggest an increase in orientation dispersion during the third trimester, while the intracellular fiber volume fraction does not change.

DATA QUALITY AND PATIENT SAFETY

Although present-day and future innovations of dMRI offer new ways to increase understanding of disturbed cortical development in preterm infants, obtaining good quality images is particularly challenging in this patient group. For example, higher heart- and breathing rates in preterm infants and tendency of head movement during scanning can easily result in poor data quality, as dMRI sequences are motion-sensitive and artifact-prone. These matters are particularly relevant when studying cortical microstructure using these techniques, as certain types of distortions are more pronounced along the rim of brain tissue (Jones and Cercignani, 2010). Awareness of acquisition and processing steps determining data quality is therefore essential. To start with, fine-tuning of MR acquisition to the specific characteristic of the preterm brain and infant is desirable. Neonatal scanning hardware, such as neonatal coils, MR-compatible incubators, fixation pillows and noise-reducing earplugs have the potential to increase image quality and patient safety during scanning (Pannek et al., 2012). Furthermore, as neonatal dMRI data are highly sensitive to cardiac pulsation artifacts, the introduction of pulse triggering might benefit dMRI data quality considerably (Kozák et al., 2013). Still, extensive assessment of data quality is essential to ensure reliability of images. An approach combining visual inspection of raw diffusion data with software-based quality checks seems essential to ensure data reliability, as certain types of artifacts can hardly be seen on the diffusion data themselves (Tournier et al., 2011; Heemskerk et al., 2013). Dependent on the extent of quality loss, datasets need to be excluded from analysis or optimized using artifact and motion correction software in order to prevent inclusion of erroneous diffusion metrics in study results (Chang et al., 2005; Veraart et al., 2013; Collier et al., 2014; Plaisier et al., 2014; Tax et al., 2014b). This especially holds true for advanced neonatal diffusion MRI sequences, as complex acquisition and processing pipelines are accompanied with many pitfalls (Jones and Cercignani, 2010; Kersbergen et al., 2014).

CONCLUSION

High resolution dMRI has great potential to improve understanding of cortical neuronal connectivity impairment in children born preterm. During the fetal period, axons from and to the cortical plate also start to form, and tends to align in the early phase of development. This radial structure forms the basis for the columnar organization of the fetal cortex (Sidman and Rakic, 1973; Rakic, 2002). As advances in neonatal imaging hardware and software will reduce traditional limitations of dMRI, future neonatal dMRI studies could go as far as study normal and abnormal maturation of columnar organization of our neocortex (Mountcastle, 1997). Next to that, HARDI-based imaging studies in animals and adults have shown that it is possible to discern different cortical regions based on the unique diffusion-"fingerprint" of different cortical regions. Likely, these advances will eventually result in the development of microstructure-based atlases, which can be used to study developmental patterns and eventual plasticity of individual cortical regions that are defined using microstructure (Schnell et al., 2009; Nagy et al., 2013; Wu et al., 2014; Aggarwal et al., 2015). Validation of these new techniques using histology is essential to ensure good correlation between microstructure and imaging.

ACKNOWLEDGMENTS

The research of A. Leemans is supported by VIDI Grant 639.072.411 from the Netherlands Organisation for Scientific Research (NWO). The research of F. E. Hoebeek is supported by ZON-MW TOP-GO (10.066) and NWO-VIDI 864.11.016. The research of K. Pieterman is supported by a KNAW Ter Meulen Grant.

REFERENCES

Aggarwal, M., Nauen, D. W., Troncoso, J. C., and Mori, S. (2015). Probing region-specific microstructure of human cortical areas using high angular and spatial resolution diffusion MRI. *Neuroimage* 105, 198–207. doi: 10.1016/j.neuroimage.2014.10.053

Andiman, S. E., Haynes, R. L., Trachtenberg, F. L., Billiards, S. S., Folkerth, R. D., Volpe, J. J., et al. (2010). The cerebral cortex overlying periventricular leukomalacia: analysis of pyramidal neurons. *Brain Pathol.* 20, 803–814. doi: 10.1111/j.1750-3639.2010.00380.x

Assaf, Y., and Basser, P. J. (2005). Composite hindered and restricted model of diffusion (CHARMED) MR imaging of the human brain. *Neuroimage* 27, 48–58. doi: 10.1016/j.neuroimage.2005.03.042

Ball, G., Boardman, J. P., Aljabar, P., Pandit, A., Arichi, T., Merchant, N., et al. (2013a). The influence of preterm birth on the developing thalamocortical connectome. *Cortex* 49, 1711–1721. doi: 10.1016/j.cortex.2012.07.006

Ball, G., Srinivasan, L., Aljabar, P., Counsell, S. J., Durighel, G., Hajnal, J. V., et al. (2013b). Development of cortical microstructure in the preterm human brain. *Proc. Natl. Acad. Sci. U S A* 110, 9541–9546. doi: 10.1073/pnas.1301652110

Basser, P. J., and Jones, D. K. (2002). Diffusion-tensor MRI: theory, experimental design and data analysis—a technical review. *NMR Biomed.* 15, 456–467. doi: 10.1109/iembs.2002.1106328

Basser, P. J., Mattiello, J., and Lebihan, D. (1994). MR diffusion tensor spectroscopy and imaging. *Biophys. J.* 66, 259–267. doi: 10.1016/s0006-3495(94)80775-1

Chang, L. C., Jones, D. K., and Pierpaoli, C. (2005). RESTORE: robust estimation of tensors by outlier rejection. *Magn. Reson. Med.* 53, 1088–1095. doi: 10.1002/mrm.20426

Collier, Q., Veraart, J., Jeurissen, B., Den Dekker, A. J., and Sijbers, J. (2014). Iterative reweighted linear least squares for accurate, fast and robust estimation of diffusion magnetic resonance parameters. *Magn. Reson. Med.* doi: 10.1002/mrm.25351. [Epub ahead of print].

Dean, J. M., Mcclendon, E., Hansen, K., Azimi-Zonooz, A., Chen, K., Riddle, A., et al. (2013). Prenatal cerebral ischemia disrupts MRI-defined cortical microstructure through disturbances in neuronal arborization. *Sci. Transl. Med.* 5:168ra167. doi: 10.1126/scitranslmed.3004669

Dell'Acqua, F., Simmons, A., Williams, S. C., and Catani, M. (2013). Can spherical deconvolution provide more information than fiber orientations? Hindrance modulated orientational anisotropy, a true-tract specific index to characterize white matter diffusion. *Hum. Brain Mapp.* 34, 2464–2483. doi: 10.1002/hbm.22080

de Oliveira, J. L., Crispin, P., Duarte, E. C., Marloch, G. D., Gargioni, R., Trentin, A. G., et al. (2014). Histopathology of motor cortex in an experimental focal ischemic stroke in mouse model. *J. Chem. Neuroanat.* 57–58, 1–9. doi: 10.1016/j.jchemneu.2014.03.002

Dudink, J., Larkman, D. J., Kapellou, O., Boardman, J. P., Allsop, J. M., Cowan, F. M., et al. (2008). High b-value diffusion tensor imaging of the neonatal brain at 3T. *AJNR Am. J. Neuroradiol.* 29, 1966–1972. doi: 10.3174/ajnr.a1241

Dyrby, T. B., Baaré, W. F., Alexander, D. C., Jelsing, J., Garde, E., and Søgaard, L. V. (2011). An ex vivo imaging pipeline for producing high-quality and high-resolution diffusion-weighted imaging datasets. *Hum. Brain Mapp.* 32, 544–563. doi: 10.1002/hbm.21043

Eaton-Rosen, Z. (2014). "Cortical maturation in the preterm period revealed using a multi-component diffusion-weighted MR model," in *Proceedings of the International Society for Magnetic Resonance in Medice*, 0080.

Ferizi, U., Schneider, T., Panagiotaki, E., Nedjati-Gilani, G., Zhang, H., Wheeler-Kingshott, C. A., et al. (2014). A ranking of diffusion MRI compartment models with in vivo human brain data. *Magn. Reson. Med.* 72, 1785–1792. doi: 10.1002/mrm.25080

Frank, L. R. (2002). Characterization of anisotropy in high angular resolution diffusion-weighted MRI. *Magn. Reson. Med.* 47, 1083–1099. doi: 10.1002/mrm.10156

Gao, Y. R., Choe, A. S., Stepniewska, I., Li, X., Avison, M. J., and Anderson, A. W. (2013). Validation of DTI tractography-based measures of primary motor area connectivity in the squirrel monkey brain. *Plos One* 8:e75065. doi: 10.1371/journal.pone.0075065

Govaert, P., Lequin, M., Korsten, A., Swarte, R., Kroon, A., and Barkovich, A. J. (2006). Postnatal onset cortical dysplasia associated with infarction of white matter. *Brain Res.* 1121, 250–255. doi: 10.1016/j.brainres.2006.08.093

Heemskerk, A. M., Leemans, A., Plaisier, A., Pieterman, K., Lequin, M. H., and Dudink, J. (2013). Acquisition guidelines and quality assessment tools for analyzing neonatal diffusion tensor MRI data. *AJNR Am. J. Neuroradiol.* 34, 1496–1505. doi: 10.3174/ajnr.a3465

Hulst, H. E., and Geurts, J. J. G. (2011). Gray matter imaging in multiple sclerosis: what have we learned? *BMC Neurol.* 11:153. doi: 10.1186/1471-2377-11-153

Jansons, K. M., and Alexander, D. C. (2003). Persistent angular structure: new insights from diffusion MRI data. Dummy version. *Inf. Process. Med. Imaging.* 18, 672–683. doi: 10.1007/978-3-540-45087-0_56

Jensen, J. H., Helpern, J. A., Ramani, A., Lu, H., and Kaczynski, K. (2005). Diffusional kurtosis imaging: the quantification of non-gaussian water diffusion by means of magnetic resonance imaging. *Magn. Reson. Med.* 53, 1432–1440. doi: 10.1002/mrm.20508

Jeon, T. (2014). "Microstructural development of human brain cerebral cortex from early 3rd trimester to around the birth with diffusion kurtosis imaging," in *Proceedings of the International Society for Magnetic Resonance in Medice*, 1742.

Jeurissen, B., Leemans, A., Jones, D. K., Tournier, J. D., and Sijbers, J. (2011). Probabilistic fiber tracking using the residual bootstrap with constrained spherical deconvolution. *Hum. Brain Mapp.* 32, 461–479. doi: 10.1002/hbm.21032

Jeurissen, B., Leemans, A., Tournier, J. D., Jones, D. K., and Sijbers, J. (2013). Investigating the prevalence of complex fiber configurations in white matter tissue with diffusion magnetic resonance imaging. *Hum. Brain Mapp.* 34, 2747–2766. doi: 10.1002/hbm.22099

Jeurissen, B., Tournier, J. D., Dhollander, T., Connelly, A., and Sijbers, J. (2014). Multi-tissue constrained spherical deconvolution for improved analysis of multi-shell diffusion MRI data. *Neuroimage* 103, 411–426. doi: 10.1016/j.neuroimage.2014.07.061

Jones, D. K., and Cercignani, M. (2010). Twenty-five pitfalls in the analysis of diffusion MRI data. *NMR Biomed.* 23, 803–820. doi: 10.1002/nbm.1543

Jones, D. K., and Leemans, A. (2011). Diffusion tensor imaging. *Methods Mol. Biol.* 711, 127–144. doi: 10.1007/978-1-61737-992-5_6

Kersbergen, K. J., Leemans, A., Groenendaal, F., Van Der Aa, N. E., Viergever, M. A., De Vries, L. S., et al. (2014). Microstructural brain development between 30 and 40 weeks corrected age in a longitudinal cohort of extremely preterm infants. *Neuroimage* 103C, 214–224. doi: 10.1016/j.neuroimage.2014.09.039

Kleinnijenhuis, M., Barth, M., Zerbi, V., Sikma, K.-J., Küsters, B., Slump, C. H., et al. (2011). "Layer-specific diffusion weighted imaging in human primary visual cortex *in vitro*," in *Organization for Human Brain Mapping* (Quebec City, Canada), 2509.

Kleinnijenhuis, M., Zerbi, V., Küsters, B., Slump, C. H., Barth, M., and Van Cappellen Van Walsum, A. M. (2013a). Layer-specific diffusion weighted imaging in human primary visual cortex in vitro. *Cortex* 49, 2569–2582. doi: 10.1016/j.cortex.2012.11.015

Kleinnijenhuis, M., Zhang, H., Wiedermann, D., Küsters, B., Norris, D. G., and Van Cappellen Van Walsum, A.-M. (2013b). "Detailed laminar characteristics of the human neocortex revealed by NODDI and histology," in *Organization for Human Brain Mapping* (Seattle, WA), 3815.

Kolasinski, J., Stagg, C. J., Chance, S. A., Deluca, G. C., Esiri, M. M., Chang, E. H., et al. (2012). A combined post-mortem magnetic resonance imaging and quantitative histological study of multiple sclerosis pathology. *Brain* 135, 2938–2951. doi: 10.1093/brain/aws242

Kozák, L. R., Dávid, S., Rudas, G., Vidnyánszky, Z., Leemans, A., and Nagy, Z. (2013). Investigating the need of triggering the acquisition for infant diffusion MRI: a quantitative study including bootstrap statistics. *Neuroimage* 69, 198–205. doi: 10.1016/j.neuroimage.2012.11.063

Kunz, N., Zhang, H., Vasung, L., O'brien, K. R., Assaf, Y., Lazeyras, F., et al. (2014). Assessing white matter microstructure of the newborn with multi-shell diffusion MRI and biophysical compartment models. *Neuroimage* 96, 288–299. doi: 10.1016/j.neuroimage.2014.03.057

Leigland, L. A., Budde, M. D., Cornea, A., and Kroenke, C. D. (2013). Diffusion MRI of the developing cerebral cortical gray matter can be used to detect abnormalities in tissue microstructure associated with fetal ethanol exposure. *Neuroimage* 83, 1081–1087. doi: 10.1016/j.neuroimage.2013.07.068

Martinussen, M., Fischl, B., Larsson, H. B., Skranes, J., Kulseng, S., Vangberg, T. R., et al. (2005). Cerebral cortex thickness in 15-year-old adolescents with low birth weight measured by an automated MRI-based method. *Brain* 128, 2588–2596. doi: 10.1093/brain/awh610

McKinstry, R. C., Mathur, A., Miller, J. H., Ozcan, A., Snyder, A. Z., Schefft, G. L., et al. (2002). Radial organization of developing preterm human cerebral cortex revealed by non-invasive water diffusion anisotropy MRI. *Cereb. Cortex* 12, 1237–1243. doi: 10.1093/cercor/12.12.1237

Melbourne, A., Kendall, G. S., Cardoso, M. J., Gunny, R., Robertson, N. J., Marlow, N., et al. (2014). Preterm birth affects the developmental synergy between cortical folding and cortical connectivity observed on multimodal MRI. *Neuroimage* 89, 23–34. doi: 10.1016/j.neuroimage.2013.11.048

Ment, L. R., Hirtz, D., and Huppi, P. S. (2009). Imaging biomarkers of outcome in the developing preterm brain. *Lancet Neurol.* 8, 1042–1055. doi: 10.1016/s1474-4422(09)70257-1

Mori, S., and Van Zijl, P. C. (2002). Fiber tracking: principles and strategies—a technical review. *NMR Biomed.* 15, 468–480. doi: 10.1002/nbm.781

Mountcastle, V. B. (1997). The columnar organization of the neocortex. *Brain* 120(Pt. 4), 701–722. doi: 10.1093/brain/120.4.701

Nagy, Z., Alexander, D. C., Thomas, D. L., Weiskopf, N., and Sereno, M. I. (2013). Using high angular resolution diffusion imaging data to discriminate cortical regions. *PLoS One* 8:e63842. doi: 10.1371/journal.pone.0063842

Nagy, Z., Lagercrantz, H., and Hutton, C. (2011). Effects of preterm birth on cortical thickness measured in adolescence. *Cereb. Cortex* 21, 300–306. doi: 10.1093/cercor/bhq095

Neil, J. J., Shiran, S. I., McKinstry, R. C., Schefft, G. L., Snyder, A. Z., Almli, C. R., et al. (1998). Normal brain in human newborns: apparent diffusion coefficient and diffusion anisotropy measured by using diffusion tensor MR imaging. *Radiology* 209, 57–66. doi: 10.1148/radiology.209.1.9769812

Okabayashi, S., Uchida, K., Nakayama, H., Ohno, C., Hanari, K., Goto, I., et al. (2011). Periventricular leucomalacia (PVL)-like lesions in two neonatal cynomolgus monkeys (Macaca fascicularis). *J. Comp. Pathol.* 144, 204–211. doi: 10.1016/j.jcpa.2010.06.006

Pannek, K., Guzzetta, A., Colditz, P. B., and Rose, S. E. (2012). Diffusion MRI of the neonate brain: acquisition, processing and analysis techniques. *Pediatr. Radiol.* 42, 1169–1182. doi: 10.1007/s00247-012-2427-x

Pannek, K., Scheck, S. M., Colditz, P. B., Boyd, R. N., and Rose, S. E. (2014). Magnetic resonance diffusion tractography of the preterm infant brain: a systematic review. *Dev. Med. Child Neurol.* 56, 113–124. doi: 10.1111/dmcn.12250

Parker, G. D., Marshall, D., Rosin, P. L., Drage, N., Richmond, S., and Jones, D. K. (2013). A pitfall in the reconstruction of fibre ODFs using spherical deconvolution of diffusion MRI data. *Neuroimage* 65, 433–448. doi: 10.1016/j.neuroimage.2012.10.022

Phillips, J. P., Montague, E. Q., Aragon, M., Lowe, J. R., Schrader, R. M., Ohls, R. K., et al. (2011). Prematurity affects cortical maturation in early childhood. *Pediatr. Neurol.* 45, 213–219. doi: 10.1016/j.pediatrneurol.2011.06.001

Pierson, C. R., Folkerth, R. D., Billiards, S. S., Trachtenberg, F. L., Drinkwater, M. E., Volpe, J. J., et al. (2007). Gray matter injury associated with periventricular leukomalacia in the premature infant. *Acta Neuropathol.* 114, 619–631. doi: 10.1007/s00401-007-0295-5

Plaisier, A., Pieterman, K., Lequin, M. H., Govaert, P., Heemskerk, A. M., Reiss, I. K., et al. (2014). Choice of diffusion tensor estimation approach affects fiber tractography of the fornix in preterm brain. *AJNR Am. J. Neuroradiol.* 35, 1219–1225. doi: 10.3174/ajnr.A3830

Raffelt, D., Tournier, J. D., Rose, S., Ridgway, G. R., Henderson, R., Crozier, S., et al. (2012). Apparent fibre density: a novel measure for the analysis of diffusion-weighted magnetic resonance images. *Neuroimage* 59, 3976–3994. doi: 10.1016/j.neuroimage.2011.10.045

Rakic, P. (2002). Evolving concepts of cortical radial and areal specification. *Prog. Brain Res.* 136, 265–280. doi: 10.1016/s0079-6123(02)36023-0

Rathbone, R., Counsell, S. J., Kapellou, O., Dyet, L., Kennea, N., Hajnal, J., et al. (2011). Perinatal cortical growth and childhood neurocognitive abilities. *Neurology* 77, 1510–1517. doi: 10.1212/WNL.0b013e318233b215

Riffert, T. W., Schreiber, J., Anwander, A., and Knösche, T. R. (2014). Beyond fractional anisotropy: extraction of bundle-specific structural metrics from crossing fiber models. *Neuroimage* 100, 176–191. doi: 10.1016/j.neuroimage.2014.06.015

Saigal, S., and Doyle, L. W. (2008). An overview of mortality and sequelae of preterm birth from infancy to adulthood. *Lancet* 371, 261–269. doi: 10.1016/s0140-6736(08)60136-1

Salmaso, N., Jablonska, B., Scafidi, J., Vaccarino, F. M., and Gallo, V. (2014). Neurobiology of premature brain injury. *Nat. Neurosci.* 17, 341–346. doi: 10.1038/nn.3604

Schnell, S., Saur, D., Kreher, B. W., Hennig, J., Burkhardt, H., and Kiselev, V. G. (2009). Fully automated classification of HARDI in vivo data using a support vector machine. *Neuroimage* 46, 642–651. doi: 10.1016/j.neuroimage.2009.03.003

Sidman, R. L., and Rakic, P. (1973). Neuronal migration, with special reference to developing human brain: a review. *Brain Res.* 62, 1–35. doi: 10.1016/0006-8993(73)90617-3

Sizonenko, S. V., Camm, E. J., Garbow, J. R., Maier, S. E., Inder, T. E., Williams, C. E., et al. (2007). Developmental changes and injury induced disruption of the radial organization of the cortex in the immature rat brain revealed by in vivo diffusion tensor MRI. *Cereb. Cortex* 17, 2609–2617. doi: 10.1093/cercor/bhl168

Skranes, J., Løhaugen, G. C., Martinussen, M., Håberg, A., Brubakk, A. M., and Dale, A. M. (2013). Cortical surface area and IQ in very-low-birth-weight (VLBW) young adults. *Cortex* 49, 2264–2271. doi: 10.1016/j.cortex.2013.06.001

Tax, C. M., Jeurissen, B., Vos, S. B., Viergever, M. A., and Leemans, A. (2014a). Recursive calibration of the fiber response function for spherical deconvolution of diffusion MRI data. *Neuroimage* 86, 67–80. doi: 10.1016/j.neuroimage.2013.07.067

Tax, C. M., Otte, W. M., Viergever, M. A., Dijkhuizen, R. M., and Leemans, A. (2014b). REKINDLE: Robust extraction of kurtosis INDices with linear estimation. *Magn. Reson. Med.* doi: 10.1002/mrm.25165. [Epub ahead of print].

Tournier, J. D., Calamante, F., Gadian, D. G., and Connelly, A. (2004). Direct estimation of the fiber orientation density function from diffusion-weighted MRI data using spherical deconvolution. *Neuroimage* 23, 1176–1185. doi: 10.1016/j.neuroimage.2004.07.037

Tournier, J. D., Mori, S., and Leemans, A. (2011). Diffusion tensor imaging and beyond. *Magn. Reson. Med.* 65, 1532–1556. doi: 10.1002/mrm.22924

Tuch, D. S., Reese, T. G., Wiegell, M. R., Makris, N., Belliveau, J. W., and Wedeen, V. J. (2002). High angular resolution diffusion imaging reveals intravoxel white matter fiber heterogeneity. *Magn. Reson. Med.* 48, 577–582. doi: 10.1002/mrm.10268

Tuch, D. S., Reese, T. G., Wiegell, M. R., and Wedeen, V. J. (2003). Diffusion MRI of complex neural architecture. *Neuron* 40, 885–895. doi: 10.1016/s0896-6273(03)00758-x

Tymofiyeva, O., Hess, C. P., Ziv, E., Tian, N., Bonifacio, S. L., McQuillen, P. S., et al. (2012). Towards the "baby connectome": mapping the structural connectivity of the newborn brain. *PLoS One* 7:e31029. doi: 10.1371/journal.pone.0031029

Veraart, J., Sijbers, J., Sunaert, S., Leemans, A., and Jeurissen, B. (2013). Weighted linear least squares estimation of diffusion MRI parameters: strengths, limitations and pitfalls. *Neuroimage* 81, 335–346. doi: 10.1016/j.neuroimage.2013.05.028

Volpe, J. J. (2009). Brain injury in premature infants: a complex amalgam of destructive and developmental disturbances. *Lancet Neurol.* 8, 110–124. doi: 10.1016/s1474-4422(08)70294-1

Vos, S. B., Jones, D. K., Jeurissen, B., Viergever, M. A., and Leemans, A. (2012). The influence of complex white matter architecture on the mean diffusivity in diffusion tensor MRI of the human brain. *Neuroimage* 59, 2208–2216. doi: 10.1016/j.neuroimage.2011.09.086

Vos, S. B., Jones, D. K., Viergever, M. A., and Leemans, A. (2011). Partial volume effect as a hidden covariate in DTI analyses. *Neuroimage* 55, 1566–1576. doi: 10.1016/j.neuroimage.2011.01.048

Wedeen, V. J., Hagmann, P., Tseng, W. Y., Reese, T. G., and Weisskoff, R. M. (2005). Mapping complex tissue architecture with diffusion spectrum magnetic resonance imaging. *Magn. Reson. Med.* 54, 1377–1386. doi: 10.1002/mrm.20642

White, N. S., Leergaard, T. B., D'Arceuil, H., Bjaalie, J. G., and Dale, A. M. (2013). Probing tissue microstructure with restriction spectrum imaging: histological and theoretical validation. *Hum. Brain Mapp.* 34, 327–346. doi: 10.1002/hbm.21454

Wu, D., Reisinger, D., Xu, J., Fatemi, S. A., van Zijl, P. C., Mori, S., et al. (2014). Localized diffusion magnetic resonance micro-imaging of the live mouse brain. *Neuroimage* 91, 12–20. doi: 10.1016/j.neuroimage.2014.01.014

Zhang, H., Schneider, T., Wheeler-Kingshott, C. A., and Alexander, D. C. (2012). NODDI: practical in vivo neurite orientation dispersion and density imaging of the human brain. *Neuroimage* 61, 1000–1016. doi: 10.1016/j.neuroimage.2012.03.072

12

The intrahemispheric functional properties of the developing sensorimotor cortex are influenced by maturation

Marika Berchicci[1,2], Gabriella Tamburro[1,3] and Silvia Comani[1,4,5]*

[1] *BIND - Behavioral Imaging and Neural Dynamics Center, University "G. d'Annunzio" of Chieti-Pescara, Chieti, Italy*
[2] *Department of Movement, Human and Health Sciences, University of Rome "Foro Italico," Rome, Italy*
[3] *Department of Medicine and Aging Sciences, University "G. d'Annunzio" of Chieti-Pescara, Chieti, Italy*
[4] *Department of Neuroscience, Imaging and Clinical Sciences, University "G. d'Annunzio" of Chieti-Pescara, Chieti, Italy*
[5] *Casa di Cura Privata Villa Serena, Città Sant'Angelo, Italy*

Edited by:
Sophie Molholm, Albert Einstein College of Medicine, USA

Reviewed by:
Jin Fan, Queens College of The City University of New York and Icahn School of Medicine at Mount Sinai, USA
Julia Stephen, The Mind Research Network, USA
Urs Ribary, Simon Fraser University, Canada

****Correspondence:***
Silvia Comani, BIND - Behavioral Imaging and Neural Dynamics Center, Department of Neuroscience, Imaging and Clinical Sciences, University "G. d'Annunzio" of Chieti-Pescara, Via dei Vestini, 33, 66013 Chieti, Italy
e-mail: comani@unich.it

The investigation of the functional changes in the sensorimotor cortex has important clinical implications as deviations from normal development can anticipate developmental disorders. The functional properties of the sensorimotor cortex can be characterized through the rolandic mu rhythm, already present during infancy. However, how the sensorimotor network develops from early infancy to adulthood, and how sensorimotor processing contributes to the generation of perceptual-motor coupling remains largely unknown. Here, we analyzed magnetoencephalographic (MEG) data recorded in two groups of infants (11–24 and 26–47 weeks), two groups of children (24–34 and 36–60 months), and a control group of adults (20–39 years), during intermixed conditions of rest and prehension. The MEG sensor array was positioned over the sensorimotor cortex of the contralateral hemisphere. We characterized functional connectivity and topological properties of the sensorimotor network across ages and conditions through synchronization likelihood and segregation/integration measures in an individual mu rhythm frequency range. All functional measures remained almost unchanged during the first year of life, whereas they varied afterwards through childhood to reach adult values, demonstrating an increase of both segregation and integration properties. With age, the sensorimotor network evolved from a more random (infants) to a "small-world" organization (children and adults), more efficient both locally and globally. These findings are in line with prior studies on structural and functional brain development in infants, children and adults. We could not demonstrate any significant change in the functional properties of the sensorimotor cortex in the prehension condition with respect to rest. Our results support the view that, since early infancy, the functional properties of the developing sensorimotor cortex are modulated by maturation.

Keywords: sensorimotor cortex, functional organization, connectivity, synchronization likelihood, segregation, integration, rolandic mu rhythm

INTRODUCTION

In the cerebral cortex, functional domains such as visual, cognitive or sensorimotor control rely on the development of distinct and interconnected cortical and subcortical regions (Tau and Peterson, 2009). For instance, the transient loss of face orientation discrimination at 2 months of age may result from a conflict between subcortical and cortical pathways, also known as *transient functional deterioration* (Nakano and Nakatani, 2014). The subsequent recovery by 4–6 months of age can be interpreted as an establishment of coordination between the two systems. U-shaped changes in a given behavior have been observed in reaching (Butterworth, 1989) and cross-modal orientation (Taga et al., 2002). The developmental organization of these circuits is a complex process that begins at early gestational age (Kostovic et al., 1995) and continues until adulthood. The brain development begins with neuronal proliferation and proceeds with migration, apoptosis, synaptogenesis, pruning, myelination and cortical thinning (Giedd et al., 2009). These events are temporally overlapped and are genetically determined, epigenetically directed and environmentally influenced (Tau and Peterson, 2009) by sensorimotor and cognitive experiences.

Investigators working in the pediatric field have been particularly interested in the developmental properties of the mu rhythm, which reflects sensorimotor processing in the fronto-parietal network (Pineda, 2005). The adult mu rhythm, which falls within the alpha frequency range (8–13 Hz), is strongly

Abbreviations: SL_{MEAN}, mean synchronization likelihood; C, mean clustering coefficient; E_{loc}, local efficiency; L, characteristic path length; E_{glob}, global efficiency.

inhibited (i.e., desynchronized, suppressed) before and during the execution of a bodily movement (Cheyne et al., 2014), during the observation (Jarvelainen et al., 2004; Vogt et al., 2007) and the imagination (Grafton et al., 1996; Molnar-Szakacs et al., 2006) of a goal-directed action, and also during sensorimotor stimulation (Cheyne et al., 2003). The mu rhythm modulation is considered a neurophysiological measure of the mirror neuron system (MNS), which is a neuronal mechanism that matches perception and action, allowing goal-directed action understanding (Hari et al., 2000; Hummel et al., 2002; Muthukumaraswamy and Johnson, 2004; Depretto et al., 2006).

A growing body of literature indicates that action experience may also modulate the mu rhythm desynchronization (Calvo-Merino et al., 2006; van Elk et al., 2008; Cannon et al., 2013; Ruther et al., 2014). Recent work on the infant mu rhythm indicates that it is present in infancy (Stroganova et al., 1999; Marshall et al., 2002; Berchicci et al., 2011; Marshall and Meltzoff, 2011), although its peak activity occurs at lower frequency ranges as compared to older children and adults, as it occurs for other brain rhythms, such as the theta and delta rhythms (Orekhova et al., 2006; Cuevas et al., 2014). It has been observed that the infant mu rhythm desynchronizes during the execution of a goal-directed action as well as the observation of a previously learnt action, and that infants' self-experience has an influence on the expectations about others action. These findings support the notion that the action-perception coupling network appears early in life (Marshall and Meltzoff, 2014). However, no general agreement exists on the mechanisms leading to the onset of this network. One of the most popular views claims that perceptual-motor coupling is present at birth and is merely shaped by experience (Lepage and Theoret, 2007; Simpson et al., 2014). An alternative position suggests that sensorimotor experience plays a critical role in the generation of perceptual-motor coupling through general associative learning processes (Heyes, 2001; Cook et al., 2014). Support to this second view comes from studies (Southgate et al., 2009; de Klerk et al., 2014) where the authors showed how visual experience alone increased sensorimotor cortex engagement by activating the previously established visuomotor associations (Greenough et al., 1987; Stiles and Jernigan, 2010).

Indeed, the postnatal period represents a time of dramatic change in the brain structure and function. The brain grows to about 70% of its adult size by 1 year of age, to about 80% by age 2, and to 90% of its adult size between the age of 2 and 5 years, which is known as the "plateau" phase of development (Knickmeyer et al., 2008). With time, local connections within cortical circuits, especially in sensorimotor and visual cortices (Fransson et al., 2007), are fine-tuned, and long-range connections among circuits produce an increasingly unified and functionally organized neural network. Sets of regions that share temporally correlated activity are believed to represent and become functional networks (Damoiseaux et al., 2006), and some studies had provided advanced understanding of the functional architecture of the human brain during early development (Gao et al., 2009; Doria et al., 2010; Dosenbach et al., 2010).

Functional connectivity magnetic resonance imaging (fcMRI) has proved useful in newborn studies. Indeed, it offers insight into the earliest forms of cerebral connectivity in very young infants (Power et al., 2010; Smyser et al., 2011). Damaraju et al. (2014) recently characterized the development of intrinsic connectivity networks (ICNs) in infants aged between 4 and 9 months with resting state MRI (rsMRI) performed while sleeping without sedative medication. They observed that, with age, the connectivity strength decreased within local networks and increased between more distant networks. Other researchers (Gilmore et al., 2011) have shown that, from birth to 2 years of age, cortical thinning proceeds in a back to front direction and occurs first in the sensorimotor areas, followed by association areas and lastly by higher-order cortical areas, such as the prefrontal cortex and the posterior parietal cortex. Two types of age-related changes (from childhood to adulthood) in functional connectivity have been described so far: decreases in local connectivity among anatomically adjacent, but functionally distinct brain regions, because they are integrated in their own brain networks; increases in long-range connectivity among nodes that comprise each network (Fair et al., 2007; Kelly et al., 2009).

In contrast to the high spatial resolution but low temporal resolution of rsMRI and fcMRI, magnetoencephalography (MEG) and electroencephalography (EEG) enable the measurement of functional connectivity with high temporal resolution and medium level spatial resolution. Few studies (Ellingson, 1964; Vanhatalo and Kaile, 2006) have demonstrated the evolution of electro-cortical activity in the infant brain by means of EEG recording, with regional variability and increasingly synchronous activity between bilateral homologous regions. Event related potential (ERP) findings suggested that sensorimotor networks undergo rapid development during the first year of life (Bell and Fox, 1992; Lin et al., 2008). To estimate cortical functioning, Bell and Wolfe (2007) examined the developmental changes of electrical activity during a working memory task in infants and children by means of EEG power and coherence (a spectral measure of the functional coupling between neural generators), and observed similar changes in both measures: the widespread brain electrical activity typical in infancy (8 months of age) became more localized during early childhood (3 years of age). Righi et al. (2014) conducted a longitudinal study in infants at 6 and 12 months of age, and found that infants at risk of autism spectrum disorder had lower functional connectivity between frontal and parietal regions as indexed by linear coherence in gamma frequency band. Other very recent studies (Keehn et al., 2013; Imai et al., 2014) employed the near-infrared spectroscopy (NIRS) to look at the functional connectivity in term, pre-term, and Down syndrome infants, observing increased longer distance functional connectivity over the first year of life in normal developing infants as compared to pathological infants.

MEG was demonstrated to be a suitable method to investigate the function of the developing brain during infancy and childhood due to its non-invasive nature, its excellent temporal resolution and, with recent devices, also good spatial resolution. A technical and practical advantage of MEG systems in pediatric applications is that MEG signals are unaffected by the immature skull features such as fontanels, allowing for longitudinal neuro-developmental studies. In a recent study employing MEG recordings over the contra-lateral hemisphere during a prehension task and power spectrum analysis, Berchicci et al. (2011)

reported the presence of idling mu rhythm at rest and its suppression during prehension in infants (from 11 to 47 weeks of age) and pre-school children (from 2 to 5 years). In particular, they showed that mu rhythm peak frequency increases as a function of age (from 2.75 Hz at 11 weeks of age to 9.5 Hz at 3 years of age), and undergoes a rapid maturation during the first year of life. Based on the time-frequency analysis performed, the specific MEG signal waveform, and the position of the cluster of channels showing maximum mu rhythm desynchronization during prehension over the subject's head, Berchicci et al. (2011) also suggested a sensorimotor generator site for mu oscillatory activity.

Few studies using diffusion tensor imaging based fiber tractography or resting state fMRI have adopted a graph theoretical approach to characterize the developmental properties of the child brain. These studies have focused on the assessment of structural brain maturation (Lebel et al., 2008), on the analysis of intrinsic functional connectivity (Supekar et al., 2009), on the evolution of brain connectivity patterns (Yap et al., 2011), and on the development of neural systems underlying cognition (Fair et al., 2009). In general, they showed that the child brain develops with maturation from strong local connectivity toward a more distributed, predominantly functional based, connectivity pattern characterized by stronger integration.

However, little information is provided on the developmental trajectories of the functional properties of the sensorimotor cortex, and on how sensorimotor processing is modulated by sensorimotor experience. Here we analyzed the MEG data collected in our previous study (Berchicci et al., 2011) using a measure of functional connectivity and graph theoretical concepts to contribute to the understanding of the functional organization of the developing sensorimotor cortex from early infancy to adulthood. In an attempt to verify whether sensorimotor processing contributes to the generation of perceptual-motor coupling, we analyzed the MEG data recorded in two experimental conditions: at rest and during the execution of a prehension task.

We typified the functional organization over the sensorimotor cortex by means of functional connectivity and efficiency measures. Since the developmental properties of the mu rhythm reflect sensorimotor processing (Pineda, 2005), all measures were calculated within an individual mu rhythm frequency band to ensure that all findings referred to the sensorimotor network. Synchronization likelihood (Stam and van Djik, 2002), used in brain studies to quantify the probability for the functional interdependencies between neural signals, was used to reconstruct functional connectivity maps over the sensorimotor cortex. The type of functional efficiency over the sensorimotor network was estimated by means of segregation and integration measures (Stam, 2000) calculated on the functional connectivity maps. Functional segregation measures (i.e., mean clustering coefficient and local efficiency) quantify the specialized information processing occurring within densely interconnected groups of brain regions (Rubinov and Sporns, 2010), whereas functional integration measures (i.e., characteristic path length, Watts and Strogatz, 1998 and global efficiency, Latora and Marchiori, 2001) reckon the ability of a functional network to rapidly combine specialized information processing from distributed brain regions.

We also tried to explore whether any differences could be observed in the functional properties of the sensorimotor cortex during the execution of a prehension task, in order to provide information useful to understand the contribution of sensorimotor processing to the development of perceptual-motor coupling in infants and children. To this aim, we compared the global measures of functional connectivity and efficiency over the sensorimotor cortex at rest with those related to the execution of a prehension task. Prehension is one of the most remarkable examples of perception and action coupling in infants, since reaching for an object is guided by perceptual information on the relation between the self and the environment, which continuously changes as the posture (e.g., the motor system) is adjusted to that information (Hatwell, 1987). Therefore, prehension is a motor task suitable to explore whether sensorimotor processing contributes to the generation of perceptual-motor coupling.

Our investigation adds to prior studies that have considered either the rest condition or the observation of actions (Gilmore et al., 2011; Virji-Babul et al., 2012; Damaraju et al., 2014; Rotem-Kohavi et al., 2014), since we studied the functional properties over the developing sensorimotor cortex not only at rest but also during prehension. Moreover, by including infants below 6 months of age in our study population, we provided a valuable adjunct to studies on the developing brain.

Based on the knowledge that children and young-adults' brains have "small-world" organization at the global level (Supekar et al., 2009), and on the notion that fronto-temporal connections develop more slowly than other regions (Lebel et al., 2008), we expect that the functional properties over the sensorimotor network evolve, from infants to children and adults, toward a more efficient "small-world" organization. As well, based on the hypothesis that sensorimotor processing plays a role in the generation of perceptual-motor coupling, we expect to observe different functional organizations over the sensorimotor cortex for the rest and prehension conditions.

MATERIALS AND METHODS

PARTICIPANTS

Data collection was performed in infants, children and adults following a cross-sectional design. Participants were selected from a larger database of subjects (see Berchicci et al., 2011). Subjects experiencing any serious illnesses or developmental problems since birth (i.e., traumatic brain injury, seizures, and congenital conditions), or receiving any long-term medication were excluded from the study. Out of the 43 healthy infants enrolled (<12 months of age), 25 infants met all inclusion and exclusion criteria. Chronological age at entry in the study ranged between 11 and 47 weeks (mean $= 24.9$, $SD = 10.8$). The functional development of all infants was examined with the Kent Inventory of Developmental Skills (KIDS; Reuter et al., 1996). All infants were found to function within the normal range for age. Parent report was used to assess Apgar score (Apgar, 1953) at birth, which were all within normal limits (i.e., 8–10). However, due to poor signal quality that prevented a reliable calculation of the functional connectivity and efficiency measures, 11 infants had to be excluded from the study (see details in Section Statistical Analysis). Eighteen healthy children aged between 24 and 60 months were enrolled and met all inclusion and exclusion criteria, but, due to motion artifacts, only 12 children were included in the study population (mean = 37.3, *SD* = 12). Six right-handed adults (mean = 28.3, *SD* = 7.8) participated in the study as control group.

Based on the results of our prior study (see Berchicci et al., 2011), we knew that a large variation of the mu rhythm peak frequency occurred during the first year of life, indicating a rapid functional development. For this reason, we decided to split the group of infants in two age groups, one including the infants <6 months of age, and another including the infants <12 months of age. To have a similar number of subjects in all study groups, we split also the group of children in two age groups, one including the children with an age range of 24–34 months, and another including the children with an age range of 36–60 months. Details on the age groups can be found in Section Statistical Analysis.

The protocol was reviewed and approved by the Human Research Review Committee at the University of New Mexico Health Sciences Center and written informed consent was obtained from participant's guardians or adult participants after the description of the study protocol. Infants and children were recruited at day-care centers and from the community using word of mouth, brochures posted on campus, and social networks.

PROCEDURE AND TASK

The experimental setup is only briefly described herein; details can be found in our previous study (see Berchicci et al., 2011). Neuromagnetic activity was recorded using a multi-channel pediatric magnetoencephalography (MEG) system (Okada et al., 2006) for hemispheric recordings. The sensor array operated in a magnetically shielded room, consisted of 76 first-order axial gradiometers, and had a headrest with a smooth outer surface made of thick fiberglass. Inter-sensor distance was approximately 13 mm center-to-center. The headrest was based on a standard reference for the head size of babies. Since the thickness of the neonatal scalp and skull is about 3–4 mm, brain activity could be measured a few millimeters above the brain surface, providing excellent sensitivity.

Since participants performed the assigned tasks with their right hand, they were positioned on the MEG bed on their left side, and a pillow was used to support their back, if necessary. The left hemisphere of the head was positioned on the MEG headrest in order to cover the sensorimotor areas. To ensure child safety and to promote calmness during acquisition, a parent attended the child inside the magnetically shielded room. For each subject, two 5-min blocks of continuous MEG data were recorded. If the infant/child felt uncomfortable from lying still, or was getting drowsy and needed a break, data collection was stopped.

Two different experimental conditions were intermixed: *rest and prehension*. Under the *rest condition*, the participant remained motionless for about 10 s while the investigator stood in front of him/her at a distance of approximately 40 cm. Infants and children were visually engaged to prevent head motions. During the *prehension condition*, participants were invited (in case of adults and children) or directed (in case of infants) to squeeze a pipette placed at about 5 cm from their right hand. The pipette, small enough to be comfortably held and squeezed by infants and children, was connected to a pressure transducer to record the pressure exerted during prehension. Adults used a similar device with a button trigger. The pressure profile was synchronized with MEG data, hence permitting the identification of the time points at which squeezing started. This was necessary for MEG data post-processing purposes. The shielded room light was kept dim during all acquisition sessions to minimize distractions. The experimental sessions were recorded with a video camera synchronized with MEG recording to observe behavior and take note of any movement that might have occurred during acquisitions.

DATA ACQUISITION AND PRE-PROCESSING

MEG data were recorded with a sampling rate of 500 Hz. Although data acquisition was halted in cases of significant displacement of the child's head, residual artifacts, including small movements due to chewing/sucking and arm displacements, were rejected during MEG data pre-processing.

First, MEG channels not working properly were excluded from further analysis. Second, MEG data were band-pass filtered between 0.5 and 40 Hz using a forward-reverse Butterworth filter of the third order. Filtered MEG data were then processed with PCA for dimension reduction, and Independent Component Analysis (ICA, BinICA algorithm with open source toolbox, EEGlab, www.sccn.ucsd.edu/eeglab) was used to separate the independent components (ICs) of interest and to reject those related to artefactual sources. We allowed for a total of 20 ICs, and retained for further processing only those ICs that satisfied two conditions: a topological distribution compatible with the activation of the contralateral sensorimotor cortex, and a clear mu rhythm peak at the individual frequency of the subject, as identified in our previous study (see Berchicci et al., 2011). In general, we retained 2–4 ICs per subject, since the majority of ICs were related to noise, artifacts, MEG channels not working properly, or were seemingly related to brain activity but with a too high content of noise. An example of ICs separated for an infant at 36 weeks is provided in **Figure 1**, where one can see how ICs with a topological distribution that could be related to the activation of the sensorimotor cortex (e.g., IC6 or IC9), have a frequency content that is mainly due to noise. This type of ICs was not retained to reconstruct the brain signals. The retained ICs (ICs 7, 8, and 14 in the example of **Figure 1**) were re-projected on the sensors' positions to reconstruct the MEG source signals related to the true brain activity.

DATA ANALYSIS

Functional connectivity representations

For each subject, the pre-processed MEG signals were segmented according to the 4-s time intervals of rest and prehension identified in our previous study (see Berchicci et al., 2011) for both spontaneous mu rhythm (rest condition) and mu rhythm desynchronization (prehension condition). The rest time intervals were selected during the resting state far from prehension occurrences. The prehension time intervals were selected around prehension (as identified with the pressure transducer profile and the analysis of the video recordings) to include anticipatory cortical activity.

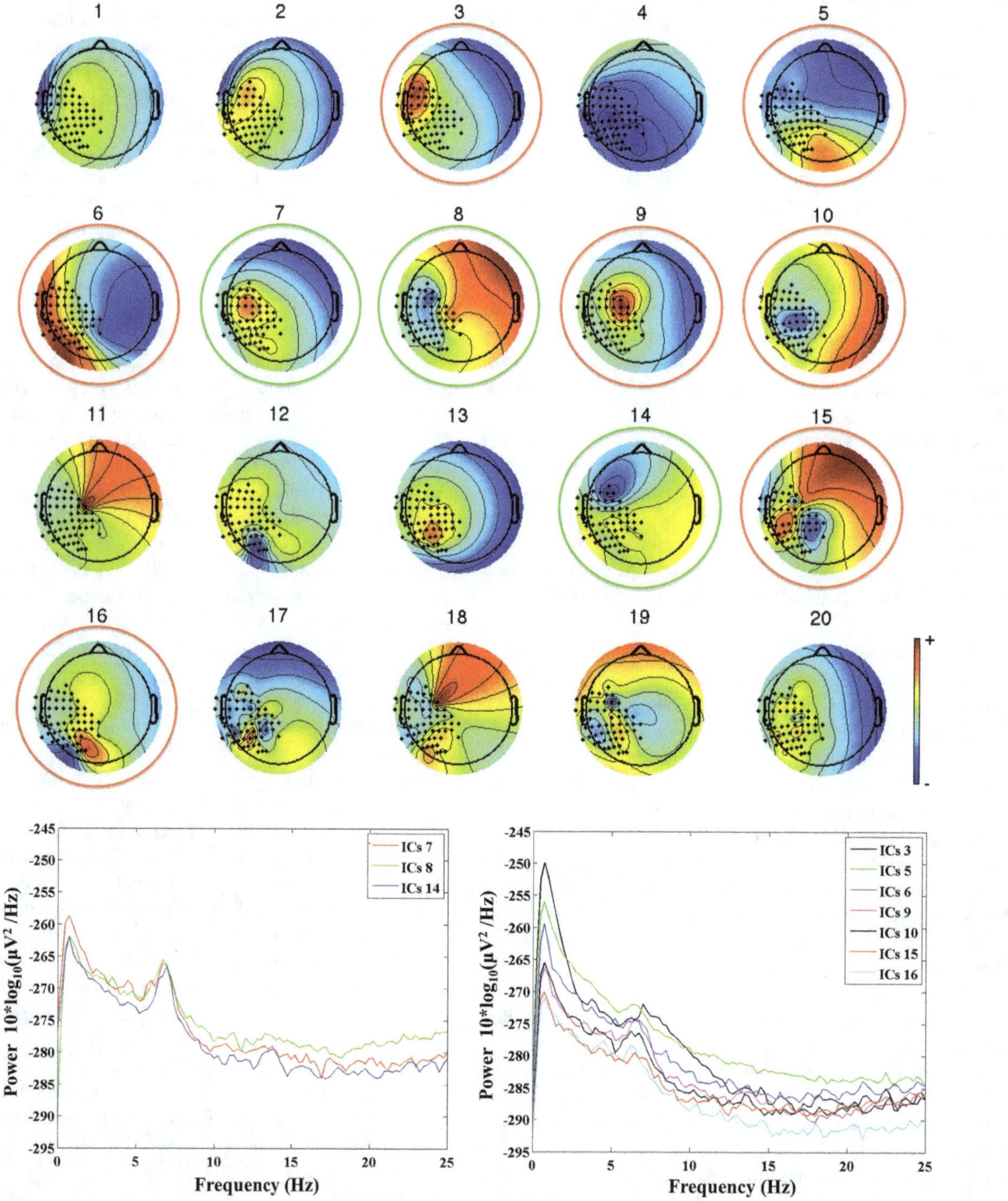

FIGURE 1 | Upper panel: the 20 ICs separated from the MEG recordings in an infant at 36 weeks (G2, mu peak frequency at 7.5 Hz). The ICs retained for further analysis are identified by a green circle, whereas the rejected ICs are identified by a red circle. **Lower panels:** power spectra of the retained ICs (on the left hand side), and of the rejected ICs (on the right hand side).

Hence, prehension time intervals started 1 s before movement onset.

The patterns of functional dependencies between the preprocessed MEG signals were estimated by means of the Synchronization Likelihood (SL) (data were analyzed using Brainwave v0.9.133.1, http://home.kpn.nl/stam7883/brainwave.html). This measure, introduced by Stam and van Djik (2002), gives a straightforward normalized estimate of the dynamical interdependencies between two or more simultaneously recorded time series. Differently from other connectivity measures such as coherence, this measure, closely related to the concept of generalized mutual information, overcomes the problems related to sub-systems dimensionality, and can be suitable for the analysis of non-stationary data, such as ours. In essence, SL describes how strongly the signal recorded by each channel is synchronized to the signals recorded by the other channels in the array at a given time instant or in a given time span.

For each subject and each experimental conditions (rest and prehension), we calculated one SL matrix for each 4-s time interval within a frequency band centered around the individual mu rhythm peak frequency (IMPF). The IMPF of each subject had been determined in our previous study (see Berchicci et al., 2011), and the frequency band used to calculate the SL matrices had high-pass and low-pass cut-off frequencies at (IMPF − 2 Hz) and (IMPF + 2 Hz) respectively. The SL matrices obtained for all time intervals in each condition were then averaged to obtain one average SL matrix. For each subject we then had two average SL matrices, one for the rest and one for the prehension condition.

To retain only significant functional connections across MEG signals, we thresholded each average SL matrix on the basis of its own SL values distribution, which is expected to be non-Gaussian. We calculated the Median and Median Absolute Deviation (MAD) of the distribution of SL values for each average SL matrix, and defined a new thresholded SL matrix (that we called SL_{MAD} matrix) where only the SL values > (Median + 1 MAD) were retained. All other SL values in the SL_{MAD} matrix were set equal to zero.

Since we analyzed the MEG signals in the sensor space, the SL_{MAD} matrices could still have a bias due to the spatial proximity of adjacent sensors. For this reason, we reconstructed the matrix of Euclidean inter-sensor distances M_{Eu} for all retained MEG channels, and calculated the coefficient of determination r^2 between M_{Eu} and the two SL_{MAD} matrices (one for rest and one for prehension) for each subject. We then retained for further analysis only the subjects for whom both SL_{MAD} matrices satisfied the condition $r^2 < 0.1$, hence ensuring that the SL values in the SL_{MAD} matrices do not depend on the Euclidean distances across neighboring MEG sensors.

To quantify the overall probability for functional connectivity over the sensorimotor areas at rest and during prehension, for each subject and each experimental condition we calculated the mean SL value in the SL_{MAD} matrix as:

$$SL_{MEAN} = \frac{1}{N}\sum_{i,j} SL_{MAD,i,j} \tag{1}$$

where N is the total number of SL values ≠ 0 in the SL_{MAD} matrix.

Measures of functional organization

We used graph theoretical concepts to study the topological features of the functional networks represented by the SL_{MAD} matrices. Within this framework, patterns of functional connections are represented as graphs where nodes (in our case the MEG sensors) are linked with edges (if connected). For each subject, we estimated the level of functional organization over the sensorimotor cortex at rest and during prehension by means of segregation and integration measures described below. To this aim, we calculated the segregation and integration measures on the SL_{MAD} matrices, where each SL value (when different from zero) represents the strength of the functional connection (edge) between two given MEG signals (nodes). As the comparison of graphs derived from brain networks requires a step of normalization, for instance by setting a fixed average degree (K) (van Wijk et al., 2010), prior to calculating segregation and integration measures we checked the degrees of the SL_{MAD} matrices of each subject included in the study population, and considered for further processing only those subjects whose SL_{MAD} matrices had the same degree in both rest and prehension (see also sub-Section Statistical Analysis).

Measures of functional segregation. Functional segregation in the brain refers to specialized information processing occurring within densely interconnected groups of brain regions (Rubinov and Sporns, 2010). In our case, functional connectivity was calculated by SL_{MAD} matrices in the sensor space, hence segregated neural processing will be suggested by statistical dependencies between clustered channels. We calculated two weighted measures of functional segregation:

(1) *Mean clustering coefficient C.* For a given node i (in our case, for a given MEG channel i), c_i is defined as the fraction of the node's neighbors (other MEG channels) that are directly connected with it (Watts and Strogatz, 1998). At the network level, the *mean clustering coefficient C* reflects the prevalence of clustered connectivity around individual nodes:

$$C = \frac{1}{n}\sum_{i \in N} c_i = \frac{1}{n}\sum_{i \in N}\frac{2t_i^w}{k_i\,(k_i - 1)} \tag{2}$$

where N is the set of all nodes in the network, and n is the number of nodes, k_i is the degree of node i (i.e., the number of links connected to node i), and t_i^w is the weighted geometric mean of triangles around i. High values of C indicate that a high number of connections exists among neighboring nodes.

(2) *Local efficiency E_{loc}.* The local efficiency is defined as the average efficiency of the local subgraphs. For weighted connectivity matrices, such as SL_{MAD} matrices, it is:

$$E_{loc} = \frac{1}{2}\sum_{i \in N}\frac{\sum_{j,h \in N, j \neq i}\left(w_{i,j}w_{i,h}\left[d_{j,h}^w\,(N_i)\right]^{-1}\right)^{1/3}}{k_i\,(k_i - 1)} \tag{3}$$

where, for a given triangle of vertices i,j,h, $w_{i,j}$, and $w_{i,h}$ are the weights between nodes i and j and nodes i and h respectively, and $d_{j,h}^w$ is the distance between nodes j and h, i.e., the minimum number of links connecting node j to node h. E_{loc} provides an information similar to the mean clustering coefficient C, but adds an indication on how much the system is *fault tolerant*, i.e., how efficient is the communication between the first neighbors of node i when it is removed. Local efficiency suggests a connection redundancy that protects the network from local errors and failures (Latora and Marchiori, 2001).

When high functional segregation is found in a functional connectivity matrix, the prevailing functional connections occur across neighboring brain areas (or, as in our case, across signals recorded by neighboring channels).

Measures of functional integration. In the brain, functional integration represents the ability to rapidly combine specialized information from distributed brain regions. Although our MEG recordings refer only to the hemisphere contra-lateral to the moving limb, we calculated two measures of functional integration to estimate how easily different brain regions communicate. The measures of functional integration are based on the concept of a path:

(1) *Characteristic path length L.* In a graph, the lengths of paths connecting two given nodes estimate the potential for functional integration in the network (Watts and Strogatz, 1998). The *characteristic path length L* is defined as the mean of the distances (i.e., the minimum path lengths) among all nodes pairs:

$$L = \frac{1}{n} \sum_{i \in N} \frac{\sum_{j \in N, j \neq i} d^{w}_{i,j}}{n-1} \quad (4)$$

where $d^{w}_{i,j}$ is the weighted distance between nodes i and j, i.e., the minimum number of links connecting node i to node j. Short paths, corresponding to low values of L, indicate a strong potential for integration within the network.

(2) *Global efficiency E_{glob}.* In functional connectivity data, such as the SL_{MAD} matrices, paths represent sequences of statistical associations between subsequent pairs of channels. The level of functional integration in the network can be represented by the *global efficiency E_{glob}*, which is the average inverse shortest path length (Latora and Marchiori, 2001; Achard and Bullmore, 2007). For weighted connectivity matrices:

$$E_{glob} = \frac{1}{n} \sum_{i \in N} \frac{\sum_{j \in N, j \neq i} (d^{w}_{i,j})^{-1}}{n-1} \quad (5)$$

When high functional integration is found in a functional connectivity matrix, the functional organization of the brain takes advantage of multiple specialized and densely connected areas that are linked with long distance functional connections for a more efficient information processing.

Statistical analysis

Linear regression analysis was performed on the individual measures to assess whether any linear correlation exists between age and/or mu rhythm peak frequency and the functional connectivity/efficiency measures.

Groups analysis was performed for each connectivity/efficiency measure on the age groups defined in Section Participants. In each age group, we retained only those subjects for whom the following two conditions were satisfied: (1) the determination coefficient r^2 between the individual SL_{MAD} matrices at rest and during prehension and the individual M_{Eu} matrix of the euclidean inter-sensor distances was smaller than 0.1, and (2) the degree of the individual SL_{MAD} matrices for rest and prehension was the same. The first condition guarantees that the SL_{MAD} matrices are independent on the inter-sensor distances, and the second condition satisfies the requirement for a reliable comparison of segregation and integration measures. Seven infants (age <6 months) and 4 infants (age <12 months) did not satisfy these conditions and were excluded from further analysis. The characteristics of the age groups are reported in **Table 1**.

Statistical analysis was performed using an ANOVA 5 (age groups) × 2 (conditions: rest, prehension) for each dependent variable, i.e., for the individual measure of functional connectivity (SL_{MEAN}), and for functional segregation (C and E_{loc}), and integration (L and E_{glob}) measures. Post-hoc comparisons were performed using Bonferroni corrections. Statistical significance was set at $p < 0.05$.

RESULTS

Linear regression analysis on the individual functional connectivity/efficiency measures did not show any significant linear dependence on age or mu rhythm peak frequency. In particular, the coefficient of determination r^2 between age and SL_{MEAN}, C, E_{loc}, L, and E_{glob} ranged between 0.197 and 0.465, and r^2 between mu rhythm peak frequency and SL_{MEAN}, C, E_{loc}, L, and E_{glob} ranged between 0.008 and 0.269, indicating no significant linear correlation between any connectivity/efficiency measure and age or mu rhythm peak frequency.

FUNCTIONAL CONNECTIVITY REPRESENTATIONS

The changes of the group-averaged SL_{MEAN} values with age in the two experimental conditions (rest and prehension) are summarized in **Figure 2**. ANOVA results on the individual measures of SL_{MEAN} showed significant differences across age groups [$F_{(4, 27)} = 4.546$ $p = 0.006$, $\eta^2_p = 0.402$, power $= 0.897$], no significant differences between conditions, and no interaction between groups and conditions. During the first year of life (groups G1 and G2), the average SL_{MEAN} values do not differ significantly, whereas around 2 years of age (group G3), SL_{MEAN} values start to increase toward the adult values (group G5). *Post-hoc* analysis showed significant differences only between the

Table 1 | Number of subjects included in each age group (N_{study}) out of those who met all inclusion and exclusion criteria ($N_{incl/excl}$).

Group	$N_{incl/excl}$	N_{study}	Age		Mu peak frequency (Hz) (Mean ± SD)
			Months	Years	
G1	14	7	2.75–6		4.46 ± 1.12
G2	11	7	6.5–11.75	<1	7.41 ± 0.61
G3	6	6	24–34	2–2.8	8.71 ± 0.64
G4	6	6	36–60	3–5	8.50 ± 0.52
G5	6	6		20–39	10.32 ± 1.20

For each age group, the age range and the mu rhythm peak frequency (Mean ± SD) are also reported.

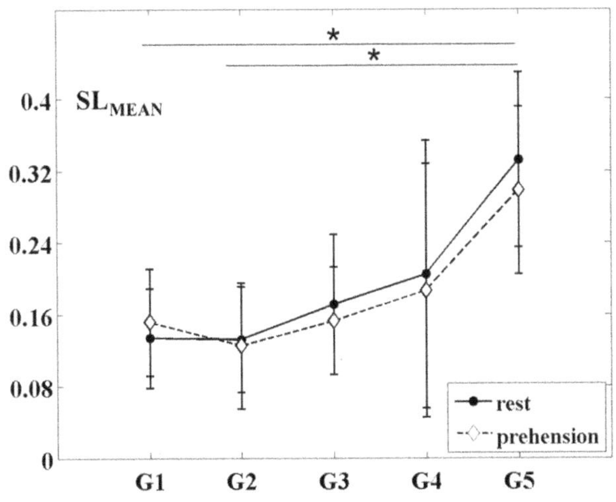

FIGURE 2 | Group-averaged SL_{MEAN} values (mean ± SD) for the five age groups (G1–G5) and the two experimental conditions (rest and prehension). $^*p < 0.05$.

group of adults G5 (0.315 ± 0.093) and the groups of infants G1 (0.143 ± 0.056; $p = 0.015$) and G2 (0.129 ± 0.062; $p = 0.007$).

These results indicate that, during infancy, the likelihood for functional connections over the sensorimotor cortex is much lower than in adulthood, and that it increases with age. Although no statistically significant difference was observed between conditions, it is interesting to observe that, in our group of very young infants (G1), the average SL_{MEAN} is slightly higher during prehension than at rest, whereas in the groups of children and in the group of adults the average SL_{MEAN} slightly decreases during prehension. This fact could deserve further investigation, possibly in larger populations of infants and children. Examples of SL_{MAD} matrices at rest and during prehension for each age group are provided in **Figure 3**. A typical layout of the MEG sensor array over the head is also shown. However, please consider that the same channels in different SL_{MAD} matrices could be positioned over different brain regions, as no information on the relative positions of the MEG channels with respect to the subject's head could be collected.

MEASURES OF FUNCTIONAL SEGREGATION

The changes of the group-averaged C and E_{loc} values with age in the two experimental conditions (rest and prehension) are summarized in **Figures 4A,B**. ANOVA results on the individual measures of C showed significant differences across age groups [$F_{(4, 27)} = 4.975$ $p = 0.004$, $\eta_p^2 = 0.424$, power = 0.924], no significant differences between conditions, and no interaction between groups and conditions. During the first year of life (groups G1 and G2), C remains almost unchanged, whereas around 2 years of age (group G3) it starts to increase toward the adult values (group G5). *Post-hoc* analysis showed significant differences between the group of adults G5 (0.231 ± 0.076) and the groups of infants G1 (0.094 ± 0.037; $p = 0.011$), G2 (0.083 ± 0.047; $p = 0.005$). A tendency toward significant difference was also observed between G5 and G3 (0.104 ± 0.041; $p = 0.030$).

Similarly, ANOVA results on the individual measures of E_{loc} showed significant differences across age groups [$F_{(4, 27)} = 5.223$ $p = 0.003$, $\eta_p^2 = 0.436$, power = 0.937], no significant differences between conditions, and no interaction between groups and conditions. During the first year of life (groups G1 and G2), E_{loc} remains almost unchanged, and around 2 years of age (group G3) it starts to increase toward the adult values (group G5). *Post-hoc* analysis showed significant differences between the group of adults G5 (0.266 ± 0.084) and the groups of infants G1 (0.112 ± 0.041; $p = 0.008$), G2 (0.100 ± 0.049; $p = 0.004$), whereas a tendency toward significant difference was observed between G5 and G3 (0.125 ± 0.045; $p = 0.026$).

These results indicate that, during infancy, global measures of functional segregation over the sensorimotor cortex are significantly lower than in adulthood, and that they increase with age. Although no statistically significant difference was observed between conditions, in the very young infants (G1), functional segregation seems to be higher during prehension than at rest, whereas in children and in adults it seems to decrease from rest to prehension. As for SL_{MEAN}, this aspect deserves further investigation in larger populations of infants and children.

MEASURES OF FUNCTIONAL INTEGRATION

The changes of the group-averaged L and E_{glob} values with age in the two experimental conditions (rest and prehension) are shown in **Figures 4C,D**. ANOVA results on the individual measures of L showed significant differences across age groups [$F_{(4, 27)} = 4.245$ $p = 0.009$, $\eta_p^2 = 0.386$, power = 0.873], no significant differences between conditions, and no interaction between groups and conditions. L tends to decrease with age, although discontinuously. *Post-hoc* analysis showed significant difference between the group of adults G5 (12.975 ± 3.034) and the group of older infants G2 (28.588 ± 7.575; $p = 0.007$), and a trend toward significant difference between G5 and the group of older children G4 (25.739 ± 10.494; $p = 0.047$).

ANOVA results on the individual measures of E_{glob} showed significant differences across age groups [$F_{(4, 27)} = 5.594$ $p = 0.002$, $\eta_p^2 = 0.453$, power = 0.952], no significant differences between conditions, and no interaction between groups and conditions. We can see that E_{glob} remains almost unchanged in infancy (groups G1 and G2), and that it increases with age. *Post-hoc* analysis showed significant differences between the group of adults G5 (0.158 ± 0.037) and the groups of infants G1 (0.071 ± 0.022; $p = 0.004$) and G2 (0.068 ± 0.029; $p = 0.003$). A tendency toward significant difference was observed between G5 and G3 (0.085 ± 0.027; $p = 0.030$).

Both measures indicate a significant difference of functional integration over the sensorimotor cortex between infancy and adulthood, and that functional integration over the sensorimotor cortex increases with age. Although no statistically difference was observed between conditions, both L and E_{glob} seem to indicate a higher functional integration during prehension in the very young infants (G1), whereas in children and in adults functional integration seems to decrease from rest to prehension. As for the other connectivity and segregation measures, this aspect deserves further investigation in larger populations of infants and children.

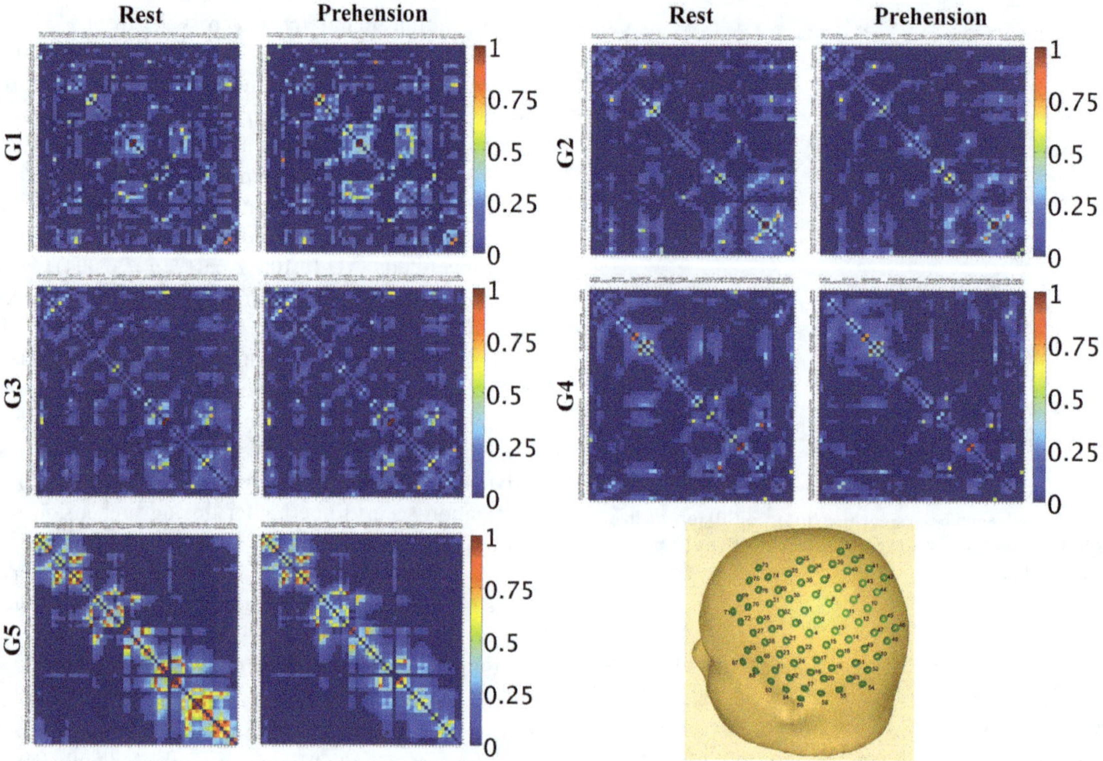

FIGURE 3 | Examples of SL_{MAD} matrices at rest and during prehension (one example per age group). G1: infant, 12 weeks; G2: infant, 36 weeks; G3: child, 34 months; G4: child, 41 months; G5: adult, 28 years. A schematic representation of the sensor array and its approximate placement over the left hemisphere is shown in the lower right hand panel. In the SL_{MAD} matrices, the MEG channels are displayed from the medial to the lateral areas.

DISCUSSION

Our goals were to contribute to the identification of the developmental trajectories of the functional properties over the sensorimotor cortex, and to explore whether any differences could be observed between the rest condition and the execution of a prehension task. To ensure that all findings were related to the sensorimotor cortex, all analyses were performed within a frequency band centered on the individual mu rhythm peak frequency of each subject, as defined in our previous study (Berchicci et al., 2011), since the mu rhythm is known to be the idling rhythm of the sensorimotor cortex. Furthermore, the use of a prehension task for the active condition permitted us to investigate the contribution of sensorimotor processing to the generation of perception and action coupling in infants.

We first observed that the probability of functional connectivity across the sensorimotor areas, estimated by means of SL_{MEAN}, remained almost unchanged during the first year of life, whereas it afterwards increased across groups to reach adult values, significantly different from the infant ones. This increase, occurring after 12 months of age, is in agreement with the suggested pattern of brain maturation in which areas with fronto-temporal connections develop more slowly than other regions (Lebel et al., 2008), and with the notion that motor experience increases the capacity of the whole network to work in an integrated way (Fair et al., 2009; Giedd et al., 2009; Boersma et al., 2011). Unfortunately, no information on the relative position of the MEG sensor array and the subject's head could be collected, therefore we could not precisely ascribe the observed functional connections across MEG signals to specific brain areas. Consequently, our observations on the probability of functional connectivity should be interpreted as global measures over the sensorimotor network.

To support the interpretation of these results, we used graph theoretical concepts to examine the changes occurring in the functional organization of the sensorimotor network across ages, and found that all segregation and integration measures showed a trend similar to SL_{MEAN}: during the first year of life these properties remained almost unchanged, whereas they increased significantly across groups afterwards, as assessed by a marked increase of both segregation parameters (C and E_{loc}), by a tendency of L to decrease, and by a clear increase of E_{glob} across age groups.

The age-related increase of the functional segregation parameters (C and E_{loc}) is compatible with the observation that the widespread brain electrical activity typical of infants (8 months of age) becomes more localized during early childhood (3 years of age) (Bell and Wolfe, 2007). We hypothesize that the increase of functional connections among adjacent cortical areas, which contributes to the functional specialization of the sensorimotor network and to the onset of a connection redundancy that protects the network from local errors and failures (Latora and Marchiori, 2001), is due to brain maturation, a process that involves both physical growth and the intellectual and/or emotional process of

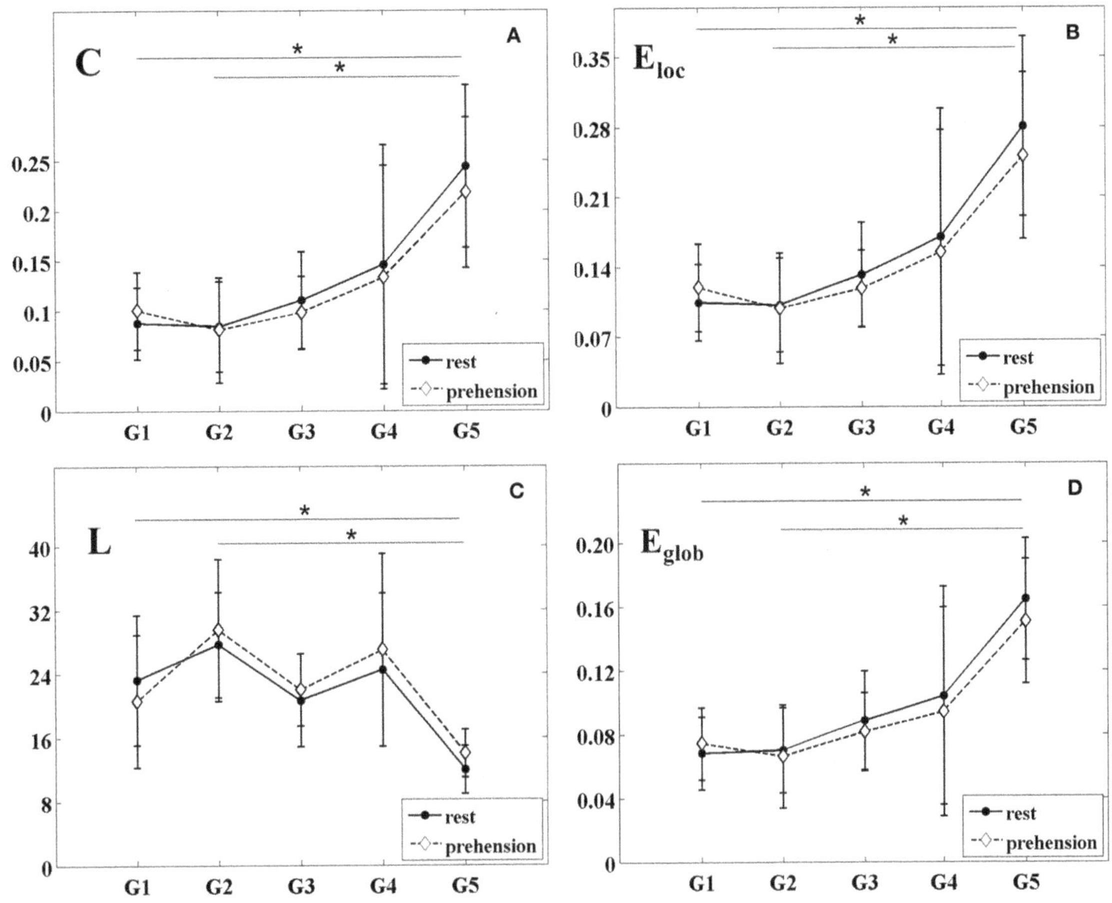

FIGURE 4 | Group-averaged values (mean ± SD) of the segregation and integration measures for the five age groups (G1–G5) and the two experimental conditions (rest and prehension). **(A)** mean clustering coefficient C; **(B)** local efficiency E_{loc}; **(C)** characteristic path length L; **(D)** global efficiency E_{glob}. $*p < 0.05$.

development. Also, the increase of local efficiency over the sensorimotor cortex is in line with the findings by Wu et al. (2013), who observed an age-related increase in the local efficiency of the whole functional networks, which may contribute to the development of modular information processing of functional systems.

Although the findings on the functional integration properties over the sensorimotor cortex should be taken with caution because the MEG sensor array covered only one hemisphere, it is interesting to observe that also these properties increased with age after the first year of life, and that the infant values were significantly different from the adult ones. The irregular trend of *L* is also worth noting, as it might be related to the occurrence of growth spurts that coincide with periods of discontinuous development in cognition (van Baal et al., 2001).

Overall, our findings on the functional segregation and integration properties over the sensorimotor cortex support the notion that maturation contributes to both the functional specialization of the sensorimotor network, and the wiring of more efficient long-range connections among different brain circuits. This interpretation is in agreement with the observations by Gao et al. (2011) on the increase of both local and global efficiency at rest from newborns to infants, and with the findings of Damaraju et al. (2014) that the connectivity strength between more distant networks increases with age in infants between 4 and 9 months. Conversely, our results are only partially compatible with the notion that strong local connectivity in the young brain gradually shifts toward stronger long-distance connectivity with maturation (van Baal et al., 2001; Lebel et al., 2008; Fair et al., 2009; Power et al., 2010; Yap et al., 2011).

Our results on the age-related increase of both local and global efficiency are consistent also with the outcome of other studies on the developing brain, which demonstrated a steady increase of global efficiency after 1 year of age (Fransson et al., 2007; Fan et al., 2011), a positive relationship between age and local efficiency throughout the life span (Supekar et al., 2009; Dennis et al., 2013; Wu et al., 2013), and the involvement of both segregation and integration in the development of the adult fronto-parietal network for adaptive online task control (Fair et al., 2007; Sepulcre et al., 2010). Our findings seem to support this interpretation of the functional evolution of the fronto-parietal network, known to host sensorimotor processing (Pineda, 2005). From this perspective, our results seem to fit well also with the suggestion that perceptual and cognitive developments involve the simultaneous segregation and integration of information-processing streams (Bunge and Wright, 2007), which in turn support the learning processing in infants and children (de Klerk et al., 2014).

Some authors have also suggested that the child brain has a small-world organization that combines the high clustering properties of an ordered network and the short path length of a random network (Fair et al., 2009; Supekar et al., 2009; Power et al., 2010; Boersma et al., 2011). Other authors have observed that, in school children, the brain functional networks evolve from more random toward a more ordered configuration (Smit et al., 2010, 2012; Boersma et al., 2011). Although our hemispheric recordings do not allow for general conclusions on the functional organization of the whole brain, nonetheless our results complement the above mentioned findings by suggesting that, during infancy, the functional properties over the sensorimotor network have a more random organization that, after 1 year of age, shifts toward a more efficient small-world configuration characterized by higher local and global efficiency. It is interesting to observe that this change toward a more efficient functional organization over the sensorimotor network continued throughout childhood until adulthood. The shift from a more random to a small-world configuration could be ascribed to brain maturation, which derives from changes at the structural level, with the thickening of long-range connections among distant brain regions starting during the first year of life (Yap et al., 2011) and with the emergence of inter-hemispheric connectivity earlier than longer-range antero-posterior connections (Bell and Fox, 1992), but is also shaped by experience, which can support the capacity of the network to create long-range connections that are functional to goal-directed actions (Wu et al., 2013; Rotem-Kohavi et al., 2014).

Unfortunately, we could not draw any conclusions on the contribution of sensorimotor processing to the generation of perceptual-motor coupling, since we did not find any significant difference in the functional properties over the sensorimotor cortex between rest and prehension. However, it is worth noting that the pattern of functional organization over the sensorimotor cortex seems to change around 1 year of age. All measures seem to suggest that, during infancy, prehension could be characterized, with respect to rest, by an increased probability of functional connectivity and by increased segregation and integration. This pattern seems to reverse after 1 year of age. These observations, if confirmed in future studies on larger populations of infants and children supported by measurements of motor experience, could indicate that, in young infants, perceptual-motor coupling is accompanied by an increased connectivity within the sensorimotor network to compensate for the lack of functional specialization to accomplish the given task (prehension). The evolution of this functional pattern could be due to the developmental timeline of the infant grasping or to the tight correlation between grasping recognition and execution, which are poor until 6 months of age (Del Giudice et al., 2009), hence requiring the recruitment of more functional resources in early infancy with respect to later ages. On the other hand, the pattern reversal that seems to occur after 1 year of age might indicate that maturation had fostered a more efficient execution of goal-directed actions, in line with the experience-dependent position on perceptual-motor coupling development of the sensorimotor cortex (Heyes, 2001; van Elk et al., 2008; Del Giudice et al., 2009; Cook et al., 2014), and with the concept that sensorimotor experience contributes to the development of more efficient functional networks to support sensorimotor development (Fransson et al., 2011).

We are aware that the impact of our study is limited by a number of factors. First, the shape and size of the MEG sensor array allowed the recording of brain activity originating only from one hemisphere. Consequently, our observations on the small-world topology of the child brain cannot be referred to the whole brain, and the interpretation of the integration measures needs to be cautious. Second, we employed a cross-sectional design for this study. Given that, during infancy and childhood, the brain undergoes a remarkable development at both structural and functional levels, the recorded brain activity could be influenced by the size of the scalp at different ages, which fits differently on the headrest covering the sensor array. Third, the measures of the topological features of the developing sensorimotor network were calculated in the sensor space rather than in the source space, because anatomical information on the baby's head and on its position with respect to the MEG sensor array could not be collected. This condition limits the interpretation of our results in terms of specific cortical areas. Fourth, we are aware of the small sample size of our age groups. However, study protocols like ours are difficult to perform in children and even more so in infants, and the analyses performed are extremely sensitive to noise and to other signal features that further reduced the number of retained subjects. Nonetheless, several research studies in adults and children have been considered reliable even when based on a small number of subjects (Nishitani and Hari, 2000; Simoes et al., 2004; Lepage and Theoret, 2006; van Schie et al., 2008).

In light of these limitations, further work is needed to validate our findings. However, we believe that our results add valuable information to the current knowledge on the functional development of the sensorimotor network during infancy and childhood. The human brain performs its sensory, cognitive and motor functions by dynamically employing highly complex and interwoven neuronal networks, with the first year of life being the most dynamic period of human postnatal brain development. Better understanding of the functional development of these networks during infancy may bring new insights on the pathophysiological mechanisms of neurological development, such as Down syndrome, autism spectrum disorders and cerebral palsy. Further studies employing whole head neuroimaging techniques during motor task execution and complemented with motor experience measurements are therefore needed to support the present findings, and to improve our understanding of the functional development of the sensorimotor network and its contribution to the generation of perceptual-motor coupling in infants.

AUTHOR CONTRIBUTIONS

The study presented here has been conceived and designed by Marika Berchicci and Silvia Comani. The experiments were performed by Marika Berchicci. Data were analyzed by Gabriella Tamburro, Silvia Comani, and Marika Berchicci. Data have been interpreted by Marika Berchicci, Gabriella Tamburro, and Silvia

Comani. The manuscript was written, revised and approved by Marika Berchicci, Gabriella Tamburro, and Silvia Comani.

REFERENCES

Achard, S., and Bullmore, E. (2007). Efficiency and cost of economical brain functional networks. *PLoS Comput. Biol.* 3:e17. doi: 10.1371/journal.pcbi.0030017

Apgar, V. (1953). A proposal for a new method of evaluation of the newborn infant. *Anesth. Analg.* 32, 260–267. doi: 10.1213/00000539-195301000-00041

Bell, M. A., and Fox, N. A. (1992). The relationship between frontal brain electrical activity and cognitive development during infancy. *Child Dev.* 63, 1142–1163. doi: 10.2307/1131523

Bell, M. A., and Wolfe, C. D. (2007). Changes in brain functioning from infancy to early childhood: evidence from EEG power and coherence working memory task. *Dev. Neuropsychol.* 31, 21–38. doi: 10.1207/s15326942dn3101_2

Berchicci, M., Zhang, T., Romero, L., Peters, A., Annett, R., Teuscher, U., et al. (2011). Development of mu rhythm in infants and preschool children. *Dev. Neurosci.* 33, 130–143. doi: 10.1159/000329095

Boersma, M., Smit, D. J. A., de Bie, H. M. A., Van Baal, G. C. M., Boomsma, D. I., de Geus, E. J. C., et al. (2011). Network analysis of resting state EEG in the developing young brain: structure comes with maturation. *Hum. Brain Mapp.* 32, 413–425. doi: 10.1002/hbm.21030

Bunge, S. A., and Wright, S. B. (2007). Neurodevelopmental changes in working memory and cognitive control. *Curr. Opin. Neurobiol.* 17, 243–250. doi: 10.1016/j.conb.2007.02.005

Butterworth, G. E. (1989). "On U-shaped and other transitions in sensorimotor development," in *Transition Mechanisms in Child Development,* ed A. de Ribaupierre (New York, NY: Cambridge University Press), 283–296.

Calvo-Merino, B., Grezes, J., Glaser, D. E., Passingham, R. E., and Haggard, P. (2006). Seeing or doing? Influence of visual and motor familiarity in action observation. *Curr. Biol.* 16, 1905–1910. doi: 10.1016/j.cub.2006.07.065

Cannon, E. N., Yoo, K. H., Vanderwert, R. E., Ferrari, P. F., Woodward, A. L., and Fox, N. A. (2013). Action experience, more than observation, influences mu rhythm desynchronization. *PLoS ONE* 9:e92002. doi: 10.1371/journal.pone.0092002

Cheyne, D., Gaetz, W., Garnero, L., Lachaux, J. P., Ducorps, A., Schwartz, D., et al. (2003). Neuromagnetic imaging of cortical oscillations accompanying tactile stimulation. *Cogn. Brain Res.* 17, 599–611. doi: 10.1016/S0926-6410(03)00173-3

Cheyne, D., Jobst, C., Tesan, G., Crain, S., and Johnson, B. (2014). Movement related neuromagnetic fields in preschool age children. *Hum. Brain. Mapp.* 35, 4858–4875. doi: 10.1002/hbm.22518

Cook, R., Bird, G., Catmur, C., Press, C., and Heyes, C. (2014). Mirror neurons: from origin to function. *Behav. Brain Sci.* 37, 177–192. doi: 10.1017/S0140525X13000903

Cuevas, K., Cannon, E. N., Yoo, K., and Fox, N. A. (2014). The infant EEG mu rhythm: methodological considerations and best practices. *Dev. Rev.* 34, 26–43. doi: 10.1016/j.dr.2013.12.001

Damaraju, E., Caprihan, A., Lowe, J. R., Allen, E. A., Calhoun, V. D., and Phillips, J. P. (2014). Functional connectivity in the developing brain: a longitudinal study from 4 to 9 months of age. *Neuroimage* 84, 169–180. doi: 10.1016/j.neuroimage.2013.08.038

Damoiseaux, J. S., Rombouts, S. A., Barkhof, F., Scheltens, P., Stam, C. J., Smith, S. M., et al. (2006). Consistent resting-state networks across healthy subjects. *Proc. Natl. Acad. Sci. U.S.A.* 103, 13848–13853. doi: 10.1073/pnas.0601417103

de Klerk, C. C. J. M., Johnson, M. H., Heyes, C. M., and Southgate, V. (2014). Baby steps: investigating the development of perceptual-motor couplings in infancy. *Dev. Sci.* 1, 1–11. doi: 10.1111/desc.12226

Del Giudice, M., Manera, V., and Keysers, C. (2009). Programmed to learn? the ontogeny of mirror neurons. *Dev. Sci.* 12, 350–363. doi: 10.1111/j.1467-7687.2008.00783.x

Dennis, E. L., Jahanshad, N., McMahon, K. L., de Zubicaray, G. I., Martin, N. G., Hickie, I. B., et al. (2013). Development of brain structural connectivity between ages 12 and 30: a 4-Tesla diffusion imaging study in 439 adolescents and adults. *Neuroimage* 64, 671–684. doi: 10.1016/j.neuroimage.2012.09.004

Depretto, M., Davies, M. S., Pfeifer, J. H., Scott, A. A., Sigman, M., Bookheimer, S. Y., et al. (2006). Understanding emotions in others: mirror neuron dysfunction in children with autism spectrum disorders. *Nat. Neurosci.* 9, 28–30. doi: 10.1038/nn1611

Doria, V., Beckmann, C. F., Arichi, T., Merchant, N., Groppo, M., Turkheimer, F. E., et al. (2010). Emergence of resting state networks in the preterm human brain. *Proc. Natl. Acad. Sci. U.S.A.* 107, 20015–20020. doi: 10.1073/pnas.1007921107

Dosenbach, N. U. F., Nardos, B., Cohen, A. L., Fair, D. A., Power, J. D., Church, J. A., et al. (2010). Prediction of individual brain maturity using fMRI. *Science* 329, 1358–1361. doi: 10.1126/science.1194144

Ellingson, R. J. (1964). Studies of the electrical activity of the developing human brain. *Prog. Brain Res.* 9, 26–53. doi: 10.1016/S0079-6123(08)63130-1

Fair, D. A., Cohen, A. L., Power, J. D., Dosenbach, N. U. F., Church, J. A., Miezin, F. M., et al. (2009). Functional brain networks develop from a "Local to Distributed" organization. *PLoS Comput. Biol.* 5:e1000381. doi: 10.1371/journal.pcbi.1000381

Fair, D. A., Dosenbach, N. U., Church, J. A., Cohen, A. L., Brahmbhatt, S., Miezin, F. M., et al. (2007). Development of distinct control networks through segregation and integration. *Proc. Natl. Acad. Sci. U.S.A.* 104, 13507–13512. doi: 10.1073/pnas.0705843104

Fan, Y., Shi, F., Smith, J. K., Lin, W., Gilmore, J. H., and Shen, D. (2011). Brain anatomical networks in early human brain development. *Neuroimage* 54, 1862–1871. doi: 10.1016/j.neuroimage.2010.07.025

Fransson, P., Aden, U., Blennow, M., and Lagercrantz, H. (2011). The functional architecture of the infant brain as revealed by resting-state fMRI. *Cereb. Cortex* 21, 145–154. doi: 10.1093/cercor/bhq071

Fransson, P., Skiold, B., Horsch, S., Nordell, A., Blennow, M., Lagercrantz, H., et al. (2007). Resting-state networks in the infant brain. *Proc. Natl. Acad. Sci. U.S.A.* 104, 15531–15536. doi: 10.1073/pnas.0704380104

Gao, W., Gilmore, J. H., Giovanello, K. S., Smith, J. K., Shen, D., Zhu, H., et al. (2011). Temporal and spatial evolution of brain network topology during the first two years of life. *PLoS ONE* 6:e25278. doi: 10.1371/journal.pone.0025278

Gao, W., Zhu, H., Giovanello, K. S., Smith, J. K., Shen, D., Gilmore, J. H., et al. (2009). Evidence on the emergence of the brain's default network from 2-week-old to 2-year-old healthy pediatric subjects. *Proc. Natl. Acad. Sci. U.S.A.* 106, 6790–6795. doi: 10.1073/pnas.0811221106

Giedd, J. N., Lalonde, F. M., Celano, M. J., White, S. L., Wallace, G. L., Lee, N. R., et al. (2009). Anatomical brain magnetic imaging of typically developing children and adolescence. *J. Am. Acad. Adolesc. Psychiatry* 48, 465–470. doi: 10.1097/CHI.0b013e31819f2715

Gilmore, J. H., Shi, F., Woolson, S. L., Knickmeyer, R. C., Short, S. J., Lin, W., et al. (2011). Longitudinal development of cortical and subcortical gray matter from birth to 2 years. *Cereb. Cortex* 22, 2478–2485. doi: 10.1093/cercor/bhr327

Grafton, S. T., Arbib, M. A., Fadiga, L., and Rizzolatti, G. (1996). Localization of action representations in humans by positron emission tomography. 2. Observation compared with imagination. *Exp. Brain Res.* 112, 103–111. doi: 10.1007/BF00227183

Greenough, W. T., Black, J. E., and Wallace, C. S. (1987). Experience and brain development. *Child Dev.* 58, 539–559. doi: 10.2307/1130197

Hari, R., Levanen, S., and Raij, T. (2000). Timing of human cortical functions during cognition: role of MEG. *Trends Cogn. Sci.* 4, 455–462. doi: 10.1016/S1364-6613(00)01549-7

Hatwell, Y. (1987). Motor and cognitive functions of the hand in infancy and childhood. *Int. J. Behav. Dev.* 10, 509–526. doi: 10.1177/016502548701000409

Heyes, C. M. (2001). Causes and consequences of imitation. *Trends Cogn. Sci.* 5, 253–261. doi: 10.1016/S1364-6613(00)01661-2

Hummel, F., Andres, F., Altenmuller, E., Dichgans, J., and Gerloff, C. (2002). Inhibitory control of acquired motor programs in the human brain. *Brain* 125, 404–420. doi: 10.1093/brain/awf030

Imai, M., Watanabe, H., Yasui, K., Kimura, Y., Shitara, Y., Tsuchida, S., et al. (2014). Functional connectivity of the cortex of term and preterm infants and infants with Down's syndrome. *Neuroimage* 85, 272–278. doi: 10.1016/j.neuroimage.2013.04.080

Jarvelainen, J., Schurmann, M., and Hari, R. (2004). Activation of the human primary motor cortex during observation of tool use. *Neuroimage* 23, 187–192. doi: 10.1016/j.neuroimage.2004.06.010

Keehn, B., Wagner, J. B., Tager-Flusberg, H., and Nelson, C. A. (2013). Functional connectivity in the first year of life in infants at-risk for autism: a preliminary near-infrared spectroscopy study. *Front. Hum. Neurosci.* 7:444. doi: 10.3389/fnhum.2013.00444

Kelly, A. M., Di Martino, A., Uddin, L. Q., Shehzad, Z., Gee, D. G., Riss, P. T., et al. (2009). Development of anterior cingulate functional connectivity from late childhood to early adulthood. *Cereb. Cortex* 19, 640–657. doi: 10.1093/cercor/bhn117

Knickmeyer, R. C., Gouttard, S., Kang, C., Evans, D.,Wilber, K., Smith, J. K., et al. (2008). A structural MRI study of human brain development from birth to 2 years. *J. Neurosci.* 28, 12176–12182. doi: 10.1523/JNEUROSCI.3479-08.2008

Kostovic, I., Judas, M., Petanjek, Z., and Sitlic, G. (1995). Ontogenesis of goal-directed behavior: anatomo-functional considerations. *Int. J. Psychophysiol.* 19, 517–527. doi: 10.1016/0167-8760(94)00081-O

Latora, V., and Marchiori, M. (2001). Efficient behavior of small-networks. *Phys. Rev. Lett.* 87:198701. doi: 10.1103/PhysRevLett.87.198701

Lebel, C., Walker, L., Leemans, A., Phillips, L., and Beaulieu, C. (2008). Microstructural maturation of the human brain from childhood to adulthood. *Neuroimage* 40, 1044–1055. doi: 10.1016/j.neuroimage.2007.12.053

Lepage, J. F., and Theoret, H. (2006). EEG evidence for the presence of an action observation-execution matching system in children. *Eur. J. Neurosci.* 23, 2505–2510. doi: 10.1111/j.1460-9568.2006.04769.x

Lepage, J. F., and Theoret, H. (2007). The mirror neuron system: grasping others' actions from birth? *Dev. Sci.* 10, 513–523. doi: 10.1111/j.1467-7687.2007.00631.x

Lin, W., Zhu, Q., Gao, W., Chen, Y., Toh, C. H., Styner, M., et al. (2008). Functional connectivity MR imaging reveals cortical functional connectivity in the developing brain. *Am. J. Neuroradiol.* 29, 1883–1889. doi: 10.3174/ajnr.A1256

Marshall, P. J., Bar-Haim, Y., and Fox, N. A. (2002). Development of the EEG from 5 months to 4 years of age. *Clin. Neurophysiol.* 113, 1199–1208. doi: 10.1016/S1388-2457(02)00163-3

Marshall, P. J., and Meltzoff, A. N. (2011). Neural mirroring systems: exploring the EEG mu rhythm in human infancy. *Dev. Cogn. Neurosci.* 1, 110–123. doi: 10.1016/j.dcn.2010.09.001

Marshall, P. J., and Meltzoff, A. N. (2014). Neural mirroring mechanisms and imitation in human infants. *Philos. Trans. R. Soc. Lond. B Biol. Sci.* 369:20130620. doi: 10.1098/rstb.2013.0620

Molnar-Szakacs, I., Kaplan, J., Greenfield, P. M., and Iacobini, M. (2006). Observing complex action sequences: the role of fronto-parietal mirror neuron system. *Neuroimage* 33, 923–935. doi: 10.1016/j.neuroimage.2006.07.035

Muthukumaraswamy, S. D., and Johnson, B. W. (2004). Changes in Rolandic mu-rhythm during observation of a precision grip. *Psychophysiol* 41, 152–156. doi: 10.1046/j.1469-8986.2003.00129.x

Nakano, T., and Nakatani, K. (2014). Cortical networks for face perception in two-month-old infants. *Proc. Biol. Soc.* 281:20141468. doi: 10.1098/rspb.2014.1468

Nishitani, N., and Hari, R. (2000). Temporal dynamics of cortical representation for action. *Proc. Natl. Acad. Sci. U.S.A.* 97, 913–918. doi: 10.1073/pnas.97.2.913

Okada, Y., Pratt, K., Atwood, C., Mascarenas, A., Reineman, R., Nurminen, J., et al. (2006). BabySQUID: a mobile, high-resolution multichannel magnetoencephalography system for neonatal brain assessment. *Rev. Sci. Instrum.* 77, 1–9. doi: 10.1063/1.2168672

Orekhova, E. V., Stroganova, T. A., Posikera, I. N., and Elam, M. (2006). EEG theta rhythm in infants and preschool children. *Clin. Neurophysiol.* 117, 1047–1062. doi: 10.1016/j.clinph.2005.12.027

Pineda, J. A. (2005). The functional significance of mu-rhythms: translating "seeing" and "hearing" into "doing." *Brain Res. Brain Res. Rev.* 50, 57–68. doi: 10.1016/j.brainresrev.2005.04.005

Power, J. D., Fair, D. A., Schlaggar, B. L., and Petersen, S. E. (2010). The development of human functional brain networks. *Neuron* 67, 735–748. doi: 10.1016/j.neuron.2010.08.017

Reuter, J., Katoff, L., and Gruber, C. (1996). *Kent Inventory of Developmental Skills (KIDS)*. Los Angeles, CA: Western Psychological Services.

Righi, G., Tierney, A. L., Tager-Flusberg, H., and Nelson, C. A. (2014). Functional connectivity in the first year of life in infants at risk for autism spectrum disorder: an EEG study. *PLoS ONE* 9:e105176. doi: 10.1371/journal.pone.0105176

Rotem-Kohavi, N., Hilderman, C. G. E., Liu, A., Makan, N., Wang, J. Z., and Virji-Babul, N. (2014). Network analysis of perception-action coupling in infants. *Front. Hum. Neurosci.* 8:209. doi: 10.3389/fnhum.2014.00209

Rubinov, M., and Sporns, O. (2010). Complex network measures of brain connectivity: uses and interpretations. *Neuroimage* 52, 1059–1069. doi: 10.1016/j.neuroimage.2009.10.003

Ruther, N. M., Brown, E. C., Klepp, A., and Bellebaum, C. (2014). Observed manipulation of novel tools leads to mu rhythm suppression over sensory-motor cortices. *Behav. Brain Res.* 261, 328–335. doi: 10.1016/j.bbr.2013.12.033

Sepulcre, J., Liu, H., Talukdar, T., Martincorena, I., Yeo, B. T. T., and Buckner, R. L. (2010). The organization of local and distant functional connectivity in the human brain. *PLoS Comput. Biol.* 6:e1000808. doi: 10.1371/journal.pcbi.1000808

Simoes, C., Salenius, S., and Curio, G. (2004). Short-term prediction of perturbation dynamics for 10- and 20-Hz MEG rhythms in human primary sensorimotor hand cortices. *Neuroimage* 22, 387–393. doi: 10.1016/j.neuroimage.2003.12.045

Simpson, E. A., Murray, L., Paukner, A., and Ferrari, P. F. (2014). The mirror neuron system as revealed through neonatal imitation: presence from birth, predictive power and evidence of plasticity. *Philos Trans. R. Soc. Lond. B Biol. Sci.* 369:20130289. doi: 10.1098/rstb.2013.0289

Smit, D. J., Boersma, M., Schnack, H. G., Micheloyannis, S., Boomsma, D. I., Hulshoff, P. H. E., et al. (2012). The brain matures with stronger functional connectivity and decreased randomness of its network. *PLoS ONE* 7:e36896. doi: 10.1371/journal.pone.0036896

Smit, D. J., Boersma, M., van Beijsterveldt, C. E., Posthuma, D., Boomsma, D. I., Stam, C. J., et al. (2010). Endophenotypes in a dynamically connected brain. *Behav. Genet.* 40, 167–177. doi: 10.1007/s10519-009-9330-8

Smyser, C. D., Snyder, A. Z., and Neil, J. J. (2011). Functional connectivity MRI in infants: exploration of the functional organization of the developing brain. *Neuroimage* 56, 1437–1452. doi: 10.1016/j.neuroimage.2011.02.073

Southgate, V., Johnson, M. H., Osborne, T., and Csibra, G. (2009). Predictive motor activation during action observation in human infants. *Biol. Lett.* 5, 769–772. doi: 10.1098/rsbl.2009.0474

Stam, C. J. (2000). Functional connectivity patterns of human magnetoencephalographic recordings: a 'small-world' network? *Neurosci. Lett.* 355, 25–28. doi: 10.1016/j.neulet.2003.10.063

Stam, C. J., and van Djik, B. W. (2002). Synchronization likelihood: an unbiased measure of generalized synchronization in multivariate data sets. *Physica D* 163, 236–251. doi: 10.1016/S0167-2789(01)00386-4

Stiles, J., and Jernigan, T. L. (2010). The basics of brain development. *Neuropsychol. Rev.* 20, 327–348. doi: 10.1007/s11065-010-9148-4

Stroganova, T. A., Orekhova, E. V., and Posikera, I. N. (1999). EEG alpha rhythm in infants. *Clin. Neurophysiol.* 110, 997–1012. doi: 10.1016/S1388-2457(98)00009-1

Supekar, K., Musen, M., and Menon, V. (2009). Development of large-scale functional brain networks in children. *PLoS Biol.* 7:e1000157. doi: 10.1371/journal.pbio.1000157

Taga, G., Ikejiri, T., Tachibana, T., Shimojo, S., Soeda, A., Takeuchi, K., et al. (2002). Visual feature binding in early infancy. *Perception* 31, 273–286. doi: 10.1068/p3167

Tau, G. Z., and Peterson, B. S. (2009). Normal development of brain circuits. *Neuropsychopharmacol* 35, 147–168. doi: 10.1038/npp.2009.115

van Baal, G. C., Boomsma, D. I., and de Geus, E. J. (2001). Longitudinal genetic analysis of EEG coherence in young twins. *Behav. Genet.* 31, 637–651. doi: 10.1023/A:1013357714500

van Elk, M., van Schie, H. T., Hunnius, S., Vesper, C., and Bekkering, H. (2008). You'll never crawl alone: neurophysiological evidence for experience-dependent motor resonance in infancy. *Neuroimage* 43, 808–814. doi: 10.1016/j.neuroimage.2008.07.057

Vanhatalo, S., and Kaile, K. (2006). Development of neonatal EEG activity: from phenomenology to physiology. *Semin. Fetal Neonatal Med.* 11, 471–478. doi: 10.1016/j.siny.2006.07.008

van Schie, H. T., Koelewijn, T., Jensen, O., Oostenveld, R., Maris, E., and Bekkering, H. (2008). Evidence for fast, low-level motor resonance to action observation: an MEG study. *Soc. Neurosci.* 3, 213–228. doi: 10.1080/17470910701414364

van Wijk, B. C., Stam, C. J., and Daffertshofer, A. (2010). Comparing brain networks of different size and connectivity density using graph theory. *PLoS ONE* 5:e13701. doi: 10.1371/journal.pone.0013701

Virji-Babul, N., Rose, A., Moiseeva, N., and Makan, N. (2012). Neural correlates of action understanding in infants: influence of motor experience. *Brain Behav.* 2, 237–242. doi: 10.1002/brb3.50

Vogt, S., Buccino, G., Wohlschlager, A. M., Canessa, N., Shah, N. J., Zilles, K., et al. (2007). Prefrontal involvement in imitation learning of hand actions: effects of practice and expertise. *Neuroimage* 37, 1371–1383. doi: 10.1016/j.neuroimage.2007.07.005

Watts, D. J., and Strogatz, S. H. (1998). Collective dynamics of 'small-world?' networks. *Nature* 393, 440–442. doi: 10.1038/30918

Wu, K., Taki, Y., Sato, K., Hashizume, H., Sassa, Y., Takeuchi, H., et al. (2013). Topological organization of functional brain networks in healthy children: differences in relation to age, sex, and intelligence. *PLoS ONE* 8:e55347. doi: 10.1371/journal.pone.0055347

Yap, P. T., Fan, Y., Chen, Y., Gilmore, J. H., Lin, W., and Shen, D. (2011). Development trends of white matter connectivity in the first years of life. *PLoS ONE* 6:e24678. doi: 10.1371/journal.pone.0024678

13

Hippocampal "cholinergic interneurons" visualized with the choline acetyltransferase promoter: anatomical distribution, intrinsic membrane properties, neurochemical characteristics, and capacity for cholinergic modulation

Feng Yi[1,2], Elizabeth Catudio-Garrett[1,2,3], Robert Gábriel[4,5], Marta Wilhelm[4,6], Ferenc Erdelyi[7], Gabor Szabo[7], Karl Deisseroth[8] and Josh Lawrence[1,2]*

[1] COBRE Center for Structural and Functional Neuroscience, The University of Montana, Missoula, MT, USA
[2] Department of Biomedical and Pharmaceutical Sciences, The University of Montana, Missoula, MT, USA
[3] Davidson's Honors College, The University of Montana, Missoula, MT, USA
[4] Department of Experimental Zoology and Neurobiology, University of Pécs, Pécs, Hungary
[5] János Szentágothai Research Center, Pécs, Hungary
[6] Department of Sport Biology, University of Pécs, Pécs, Hungary
[7] Laboratory of Molecular Biology and Genetics, Institute of Experimental Medicine, Hungarian Academy of Sciences, Budapest, Hungary
[8] Department of Bioengineering, Stanford University, Stanford, CA, USA

Edited by:
Sukumar Vijayaraghavan, University of Colorado Health Science Center, USA

Reviewed by:
Imre Vida, Charite, Germany
Jakob Von Engelhardt, German Center for Neurodegenerative Diseases (DZNE), Germany

***Correspondence:**
Josh Lawrence, Department of Biomedical and Pharmaceutical Sciences, COBRE Center for Structural and Functional Neuroscience, The University of Montana, 391 Skaggs Building, 32 Campus Drive, Missoula, MT 59812, USA
e-mail: josh.lawrence@umontana.edu

Release of acetylcholine (ACh) in the hippocampus (HC) occurs during exploration, arousal, and learning. Although the medial septum-diagonal band of Broca (MS-DBB) is the major extrinsic source of cholinergic input to the HC, cholinergic neurons intrinsic to the HC also exist but remain poorly understood. Here, ChAT-tauGFP and ChAT-CRE/Rosa26YFP (ChAT-Rosa) mice were examined in HC. The HC of ChAT-tauGFP mice was densely innervated with GFP-positive axons, often accompanied by large GFP-positive structures, some of which were Neurotrace/DAPI-negative and likely represent large axon terminals. In the HC of ChAT-Rosa mice, ChAT-YFP cells were Neurotrace-positive and more abundant in CA3 and dentate gyrus than CA1 with partial overlap with calretinin/VIP. Moreover, an anti-ChAT antibody consistently showed ChAT immunoreactivity in ChAT-YFP cells from MS-DBB but rarely from HC. Furthermore, ChAT-YFP cells from CA1 stratum radiatum/stratum lacunosum moleculare (SR/SLM) exhibited a stuttering firing phenotype but a delayed firing phenotype in stratum pyramidale (SP) of CA3. Input resistance and capacitance were also different between CA1 SR/LM and CA3 SP ChAT-YFP cells. Bath application of ACh increased firing frequency in all ChAT-YFP cells; however, cholinergic modulation was larger in CA1 SR/SLM than CA3 SP ChAT-YFP cells. Finally, CA3 SP ChAT-YFP cells exhibited a wider AP half-width and weaker cholinergic modulation than YFP-negative CA3 pyramidal cells. Consistent with CRE expression in a subpopulation of principal cells, optogenetic stimulation evoked glutamatergic postsynaptic currents in CA1 SR/SLM interneurons. In conclusion, the presence of fluorescently labeled hippocampal cells common to both ChAT-tauGFP and ChAT-Rosa mice are in good agreement with previous reports on the existence of cholinergic interneurons, but both transgenic mouse lines exhibited unexpected anatomical features that departed considerably from earlier observations.

Keywords: hippocampus, cholinergic modulation, glutamate transmission, optogenetics, transgenic mice

INTRODUCTION

Release of the neurotransmitter acetylcholine (ACh) in the HC is important for learning and memory (Micheau and Marighetto, 2011; Teles-Grilo Ruivo and Mellor, 2013). The major source of acetylcholine in the HC is extrinsic and supplied by the medial septum-diagonal band of Broca (MS-DBB) (Dutar et al., 1995). Lack of HC ACh is associated with cognitive deficits that are observed in Alzheimer's disease (Coyle et al., 1983).

In addition to the MS-DBB cholinergic projection, cholinergic interneurons intrinsic to the hippocampus have been found that may comprise an intrinsic source of ACh (Frotscher et al., 1986, 2000; Freund and Buzsáki, 1996; Romo-Parra et al., 2003). Although originally discovered almost 30 years ago using antibodies to the ACh synthesizing enzyme choline acetyltransferase (ChAT) (Frotscher et al., 1986), no information exists regarding their intrinsic membrane properties. Frotscher and colleagues demonstrated that this population does not contain mRNA for the GABA synthesizing enzymes GAD67 and GAD65 (Frotscher et al., 2000), consistent with the idea that cholinergic interneurons are not GABAergic in nature. With the visualization of these cells using transgenic mouse technology, interest in ChAT-positive cells has resurfaced (von Engelhardt et al., 2007). A recent study in which EGFP was expressed under the control of the ChAT promoter observed that cortical interneurons are highly colocalized with calretinin and/or VIP, implying that cholinergic interneurons are a specialized subpopulation of HC interneurons (Bayraktar et al., 1997; Tricoire and Cea-Del Rio, 2007; von Engelhardt et al., 2007; Chamberland et al., 2010; Chamberland and Topolnik, 2012). GFP-positive neurons have been observed in the HC of transgenic mice in which GFP is driven by the ChAT-promoter (von Engelhardt et al., 2007; Grybko et al., 2011), yet no study has systematically examined this population using transgenic mouse technology in the HC. Here, we investigated fluorescently labeled ChAT-tauGFP and ChAT-YFP neurons in the HC of ChAT-tauGFP and ChAT-Rosa mice, respectively. Consistent with earlier reports, both ChAT-tauGFP and ChAT-YFP neurons labeled a subpopulation of HC neurons in CA1 and CA3 stratum radiatum/stratum lacunosum moleculare. However, we also made several unexpected observations, including cell-sized en passant boutons in ChAT-tauGFP mice and an electrophysiologically distinct subpopulation of CA3 pyramidal cells in ChAT-Rosa mice.

MATERIAL AND METHODS

ETHICS STATEMENT

All procedures were performed in accordance with the University of Montana Institutional Animal Care and Use Committee (AUP 017-14).

GENERATION OF ChAT-Rosa AND GAD65-GFP/ChAT-CRE TRANSGENIC MICE

Rosa26EYFP$^{+/-}$ mice (Soriano, 1999; Srinivas et al., 2001; Madisen et al., 2009) were purchased from Jackson Laboratories (stock no. #007920, Bar Harbor, ME) and bred to homozygosity (Yi et al., 2014). ChAT-CRE mice (GM24 founder line, MMRRC 017269-UCD; Gong et al., 2007; Ivanova et al., 2010) were bred to homozygosity and maintained as a homozygous line. WT, heterozygosity, and homozygosity of ChAT-CRE mice were determined through qPCR similarly to previously established protocols in PV-CRE mice (Tesson et al., 2002; Yi et al., 2014). Heterozygous ChAT-Rosa26EYFP mice were then generated by crossing homozygous ChAT-CRE and homozygous Rosa26EYFP mice. In the present study, ChAT-Rosa was used to refer to ChAT-Rosa26EYFP mouse line, while ChAT-YFP was used to refer to EYFP-positive cells in ChAT-Rosa mice. ChAT-tauGFP mice, in which a tauGFP fusion protein was driven by the ChAT promoter (Grybko et al., 2011), were obtained from Sukumar Vijayaraghavan at University of Colorado-Denver. Homozygous ChAT-CRE mice were crossed with GAD65-GFP mice (López-Bendito et al., 2004; Cea-del Rio et al., 2010). Heterozygous neonates (P1-P3) from this cross were pre-screened for GFP expression using miner's lamp goggles (FHS/F01, Biological Laboratory Equipment Maintenance and Service, Ltd., Budapest, Hungary) equipped with 460-495 nm light source (FHS/LS-1B) and GFP/YFP emission filters (FHS/EF-3GY2) (Cea-del Rio et al., 2010, 2011). GAD65-GFP/ChAT-CRE mice were then bred to homozygosity through this pre-screening method, combined with the determination of CRE zygosity through qPCR (Tesson et al., 2002; Yi et al., 2014). After wean, mice were socially housed in shoebox-style ventilated cages in gender-specific groups (4–5 littermates per cage). Previous studies with ChAT-CRE or ChAT-Rosa mice have shown a high degree of specificity with endogenous ChAT expression in many brain regions, though not complete co-localization (Gong et al., 2007; Ivanova et al., 2010; Witten et al., 2010; Lopes et al., 2012).

IMMUNOCYTOCHEMISTRY (ICC) IN ChAT-Rosa AND ChAT-tauGFP MICE

Anti-GFP ICC was conducted to intensify the YFP or tauGFP signal, which reduced the laser power required to obtain high quality images, similarly to previously described in PV-GFP (Cea-del Rio et al., 2010) and PV-Rosa mice (Yi et al., 2014). After mice were deeply anesthetized and non-responsive to toe pinch, mice were first transcardially perfused with 50 ml ice cold 0.1 M phosphate buffered saline (PBS), followed by 40–50 ml of ice cold 4% paraformaldehyde (PFA) in PBS, at an approximate rate of 10 ml/min. After clearing of the liver, the mouse was then decapitated with scissors. The brain was carefully removed from the skull and immersed in 4% PFA overnight. In lateralization experiments, an incision was made on the right side of the cortex to preserve orientation in subsequent experiments. On the following day, the tissue block was mounted on a vibratome stage against a block of agarose (4% in dH_2O) in a PBS bath and sectioned (50 μm thickness) using a vibrating blade microtome (VT1000 S, Leica Microsystems Inc., Buffalo Grove, IL USA). Coronal sections, collected between −1.34 and −2.30 mm from bregma, were collected sequentially in a 24 well plate containing 1 ml PBS per well. For anti-GFP staining, every other slice was chosen, yielding approximately 9–12 slices (each containing a left and right hippocampus) per mouse. On Day 1, HC slices were washed 3 times for 10 min in PBS. Slices were placed in 1 ml of antibody diluent (1% BSA, 0.1% sodium azide, and 0.3% Triton-X in PBS; Gábriel et al., 1992). Primary chicken anti-GFP antibody (directed against YFP; 1:4000, cat# GFP-1020, Aves Labs, Tigard, OR) was then added and left overnight on a shaker at 16°C. In a subset of experiments, goat anti-calretinin antibody (1:200; cat# CG1, Swant, Switzerland) and rabbit anti-VIP antibody (1:200; cat# 9535-0204, AbD Serotec, NC, US) were added to the antibody diluent. On Day 2, slices were washed 3 times in PBS for 10 min each. Slices were then placed in PBS containing secondary antibodies for 2–4 h, followed by 3 washes in PBS for 10 min each. Secondary antibodies included donkey anti-chicken Alexa 488 (1:500; cat# 703-545-155, Jackson ImmunoResearch), donkey anti-goat 647 (1:250, cat# 705-605-143, Jackson ImmunoResearch, West Grove, PA, US), and donkey anti-rabbit Alexa 555 (1:250, cat# A-31572, Life Technologies).

For quantification experiments in ChAT-tauGFP and ChAT-Rosa mice, to define HC layers and label neurons, slices were counterstained with Neurotrace 435/455 Blue Fluorescent Nissl Stain (1:100, cat# N-21479, Life Technologies, Grand Island, NY) or Neurotrace 640/660 (1:100 cat# N-21483, Life Technologies,) for 30–45 min. Slices were then mounted on ColorFrost Plus microscope slides (cat# 9991011, Thermo Scientific) with VectaShield Hardset Mounting Medium (cat # H-1400, Vector Laboratories, Inc.) or Vectashiled Hardset Mounting Medium with DAPI (H-1200, Vector Laboratories, Inc.). Neurotrace 640/660 and DAPI staining exhibited consistent co-localization in all HC cells observed.

TYRAMIDE SIGNAL AMPLITIFCATION (TSA)

For anti-ChAT ICC, acute coronal MS-DBB and transverse HC slices at 300 μm were obtained (see Brain Slice Preparation section), incubated with colchicine (100 μg/mL, C9754-1G, Sigma-Aldrich, St. Louis, MO) in sucrose based cutting/storage (SBC) solution for 8 h, containing (in mM): 80 NaCl, 2.5 KCl, 24 $NaHCO_3$, 0.5 $CaCl_2$, 4 $MgCl_2$, 1.25 NaH_2 PO_4, 25 glucose, 75 sucrose, 1 ascorbic acid, 3 sodium pyruvate, saturated with 95% O_2/5% CO_2 (carbogen), pH 7.4. Slices were then fixed with 2% paraformaldehyde (PFA, cat# 15714-S, Electron Microscopy Sciences, Hatfield, PA) for 1 h (von Engelhardt et al., 2007). Slices were then crytoprotected in 30% sucrose solution in PBS overnight. Brain slices were re-sectioned at 60 μm using a freezing sliding microtome (HM430, Thermo Scientific, Waltham, MA, USA). After 2 hours incubation at room temperature in a gelatin-containing PBS solution (0.2% gelatin; PBS-GT) containing 0.25% Triton X-100 and 10% normal donkey serum, re-sectioned slices were incubated with a goat anti-ChAT primary antibody (1:500; cat# AB144P, EMD Millipore, 3 days) followed by overnight incubation with anti-GFP primary antibody (see previous section). Slices were then incubated with donkey anti-chicken Alexa 488 (1:500) and donkey anti-goat HRP (1:500; cat# AB180P, EMD Millipore) for 60 min. After 10 min incubation with a Tyramide Signal Amplification (TSA) Plus Cyanine Kit (cat# NEL745001KT, PerkinElmer, Waltham, MA) applied directly to the slices and 3xPBS washes, slices were stained with Neurotrace 435/455 Blue Fluorescent Nissl Stain for 30–45 min and mounted on slides. For negative controls, slices containing anti-ChAT primary antibody only or anti-goat HRP secondary antibody and TSA only were processed in parallel (**Figure S1**).

IMAGE ACQUISITION, CELL COUNTING, AND STATISTICAL ANALYSIS

A total of four ChAT-Rosa mice (11–12 weeks of age, 2 males and 2 females) and five ChAT-tauGFP mice (11–12 weeks of age, 2 males and 3 females) were used for quantification. Images were acquired with a Fluoview FV-1000 confocal imaging system equipped with 10× and 60× objectives (Olympus Center Valley, PA). Blue (405 nm), green (488 nm), and/or red (647 nm) channels were acquired sequentially. Tiles were acquired with ~10% overlap per field. Tiles were flat projected, saved as TIFF files, and either stitched automatically (as part of acquisition in Fluoview) or stitched manually (with Image J). HC ChAT-tauGFP or ChAT-YFP structures were scanned and marked with a color-coded symbol to ensure that they were not counted twice. Neurotrace-positive and Neurotrace-negative structures were distinguished in ChAT-tauGFP mice by toggling between channels in Fluoview or ImageJ. ChAT-tauGFP slices labeled with anti-GFP, DAPI, and Neurotrace 640/660 were selected for diameter measurements. In ImageJ, potential ChAT-tauGFP-positive cells were outlined with the polygon tool and added as objects to the ROI manager box. Feret's diameter (maximum caliper) was measured for each object and the results table was transferred to Excel.

Counting was performed in 11 areas: CA3 (SO, SP, SR, and SLM), CA1 (SO, SP, SR, and SLM), dentate gyrus (SM and SG), and hilus, comprising 11 groups. Each group (from 88 total hippocampi in ChAT-Rosa mice or 112 total hippocampi in ChAT-tauGFP mice) represented the total number of cells counted across all hippocampi. Groups were statistically compared on a per slice and per-layer basis using Prism 6 (Graphpad Software, Inc., La Jolla, CA). Most groups failed tests for normality (D'Agostino & Pearson omnibus normality test and Shapiro–Wilk normality test). Therefore, a Friedman test followed by Dunn's multiple comparisons test were used. The dentate granule cell layer and the hilus passed tests for normality; therefore, lateralization data were statistically compared with a One-Way ANOVA and Tukey's multiple comparison's test.

STEREOTAXIC INJECTION OF ChR2-mCHERRY AAV INTO DORSAL CA1 HC

AAV9 EF1.DIO.hChR2(H134R)-mCherry.WPRE.hGH (~10^{12} vc/ml) was strereotaxically injected into the ventral CA1 HC of adult GAD65-GFP/ChAT-CRE mice. Equipment and procedures for stereotaxic injection of AAV into dorsal CA1 HC of GAD65-GFP/ChAT-CRE mice were as previously described (Yi et al., 2014). Stereotaxic coordinates for AAV injection into ventral CA1 HC (1.5 μL at 0.25 μL/min per hemisphere) were: AP 2.9 mm, ML 3.3 mm, and DV 2.3 mm. Injected mice were used for imaging or electrophysiological recordings at least 2 weeks after survival surgery.

BRAIN SLICE PREPARATION

Both male and female ChAT-Rosa (24–45 day old) or adult GAD65-GFP/ChAT-CRE mice were used. Mice were anesthetized with 4% isoflurane and transcardially perfused with oxygenated, ice-cold, SBC solution. After decapitation, the brain was immediately placed in SBC solution saturated with carbogen. Transverse HC slices or coronal MS-DBB slices were cut at 300 μm on a Leica 1200S Vibratome, using the Leica Vibrocheck device to minimize vibration of the blade in the z-direction prior to use (Geiger et al., 2002). After sectioning, slices were placed in a storage chamber and incubated with carbogen-saturated SBC solution at 36–37°C until use.

WHOLE-CELL PATCH CLAMP RECORDINGS

After incubation for at least 30 min with SBC solution at 36–37°C, a single slice was gently placed on poly-D-lysine-coated glass coverslips (12 mm diameter, 0.09–0.12 thickness, cat# 633009, Carolina Biological Supply Company, Burlington, NC) and perfused at 34–35°C (TC-324B, Warner Instruments, Hamden, CT, USA) with extracellular solution (in mM): 125 NaCl, 2.5 KCl, 25 $NaHCO_3$, 2 $CaCl_2$, 1 $MgCl_2$, 1.25 NaH_2PO_4 and 20 glucose, saturated with carbogen, pH 7.4. Acute slices were then viewed using Infrapatch (Luigs and Neumann, Ratingen Germany) on an upright microscope (Axio Examiner D1, Carl Zeiss Microscopy, LLC, USA). Fluorescent YFP+ cells in slices from ChAT-Rosa mice or GAD65-GFP cells were identified using a Zeiss LED (505 nm for YFP; 470 nm for GFP; Colibri, Carl

Zeiss Microscopy, LLC, USA) and subsequently viewed under IR-Dodt contrast with a 63× water immersion objective (W Plan-Apo 63x/1.0 VIS-IR WD=2.1 M27, Carl Zeiss Microscopy, LLC, USA), similarly to previously described (Yi et al., 2014). Thin-wall glass capillaries (TW150F-3, World Precision Instruments; Sarasota, FL) were fabricated with a 2.5–4.5 MΩ tip resistance on a 2-step PC-10 Narishige vertical puller (East Meadow, NY, USA). Whole-cell recordings were obtained using a Multiclamp 700 B amplifier (Molecular Devices, Union City, CA), filtered at 4 kHz, and digitized at 20 kHz (Digidata 1440 A, Molecular Devices). Glass capillaries contained intracellular solution (IC; in mM): 110 potassium gluconate, 40 KCl, 10 HEPES, 0.1 EGTA, 4 MgATP, 0.3 Na_2GTP, 10 phosphocreatine and 0.2% biocytin, pH 7.2, osmolarity 290–300 mOsm. Seal resistances ranged from 1–2 GΩ and access resistance ranged from 4–20 MΩ. Bridge balance was used throughout current-clamp experiments and was monitored with a 100 ms long hyperpolarizing current step from −60 mV every 20 s. If access resistance changed by >20%, data were excluded from further analysis. For optogenetic stimulation, TTL-driven flashes from Zeiss LED were delivered to the whole slice to excite ChR2-mCherry-positive neurons. The AAV9-ChR2-mCherry infected ChAT-CRE cells in HC were reliably excited (9/9 cells) by delivery of 2 ms 470 nm light pulse at 5 Hz (**Figure S2**).

ANATOMICAL IDENTIFICATION OF RECORDED CELLS

Biocytin (0.2%) was included in the IC for *post-hoc* morphological identification of each recorded cell. Whole-cell mode was maintained for at least 15 min, the electrode was withdrawn slowly to allow cell membrane resealing to an outside-out patch, and the slice was perfused for an additional 10–15 min to allow biocytin to diffuse to distal intracellular compartments. Slices were fixed overnight at 4°C in PBS containing 4% PFA, transferred to PBS, and stored for up to 1 week at 4°C. After permeabilization with 0.3% Triton X-100 in PBS for 2 h at room temperature, slices were incubated in PBS overnight at 16°C with Alexa Fluor 633-conjugated streptavidin (cat # S-21375, final concentration 1 μg/ml; Life Technologies, Grand Island, NY) in PBS. Slices were cryopreserved in 30% sucrose containing PBS and resectioned at 100–150 μm thickness using a freezing sliding microtome. Resectioned slices underwent PBS washes, were incubated with Neurotrace 435/455 Blue Fluorescent Nissl Stain (1:100 in PBS) for 20 min, and were mounted on Colorfrost Plus slides (cat #99-910-11, Thermo Scientific) using Vectashield HardSet mounting medium (cat #H-1400, Vector Laboratories, Inc., Burlingame, CA). Sections were imaged with a Fluoview FV-1000 confocal imaging system (Olympus, Center Valley, PA) with a 25× objective (XLPL25XWMP, Olympus, Tokyo, Japan). Confocal stacks (800 × 800 pixels) of recorded cells were flat projected, rotated, and cropped in Photoshop 13.0 for display.

CHEMICAL REAGENTS

Acetylcholine chloride (A6625), DNQX (D0540), and gabazine (SR-95531; S106) were obtained from Sigma-Aldrich Inc. (St. Louis, MO). DL-APV was obtained from R&D Systems (Minneapolis, MN).

ANALYSIS OF ELECTROPHYSIOLOGICAL DATA

Electrophysiological data analysis was performed with Axograph X (Axograph Scientific, Sydney, Australia). All parameters, which included afterdeflection (ADF), input resistance (R_{in}) time constant (τ_m), cellular capacitance (C_m), action potential (AP) half width (measured from the first AP), and sag ratio (steady state (SS)/peak; in response to a 1 s long, −100 pA current step from −60 mV), were measured as described previously (Yi et al., 2014). A One-Way ANOVA and Tukey's multiple comparison test or a One-Way ANOVA and Dunn's multiple comparison test was used when appropriate.

RESULTS

REGION- AND LAMINA-SPECIFIC EXPRESSION IN THE HC OF ChAT-tauGFP AND ChAT-ROSA MICE

In ChAT-tauGFP mice, consistent with a previous study (Grybko et al., 2011), GFP labeling was highly visible as a dense plexus of axonal processes innervating every layer of the HC (**Figure 1A**). Occasionally, large, globular structures were observed among ChAT-tauGFP-positive fibers, suggestive of cholinergic interneurons (Grybko et al., 2011). To define HC layers and determine the cellular distribution of ChAT-tauGFP interneurons, sections were counterstained with DAPI and Neurotrace 640/660. As a positive control, ChAT-tauGFP cells were readily observed in the habenula (**Figures 1A–E**). In the HC, upon closer inspection, a subset of these cells were co-labeled with DAPI and Neurotrace (**Figures 1F–I**), consistent with a population of HC cholinergic interneurons (Frotscher et al., 1986, 2000; Grybko et al., 2011). Surprisingly, a subset of cell-sized ChAT-tauGFP-positive globular structures were negative for both DAPI and Neurotrace (**Figures 1J–M**). Axonal fibers were often observed leading into and out of these globular structures, suggesting that the were large, en passant boutons (see also **Figures S3E–J**).

We also examined ChAT-Rosa mice to visualize HC ChAT-YFP neurons. In contrast to the prominent axonal labeling in ChAT-tauGFP mice, YFP appeared to be localized predominantly to the somatodendritic domains, possibly due to the limited diffusion of cytosolic YFP into axon terminals. In ChAT-Rosa mice, ChAT-YFP structures in the HC were unambiguously neurons due to dendritic labeling and Neurotrace positivity (**Figure 2**). In accordance with previous studies (Frotscher et al., 1986, 2000), ChAT-YFP cells were distributed throughout the HC (**Figure 2A**). Consistent with expected expression of YFP in brain regions known to contain cholinergic neurons, ChAT-YFP cells were observed in the cortex (**Figure 2A**) (von Engelhardt et al., 2007) and medial habenula (**Figures 2A,B**) (Grybko et al., 2011; Ren et al., 2011). Within the HC, ChAT-YFP cells were found in the DG (**Figures 2A,C**), hilus (**Figures 2A,D**), CA3 (**Figures 2A,E,F**), and CA1 (**Figures 2A,G**). The diffuse YFP staining in the DG inner molecular layer, combined with the presence of YFP-positive cells in hilus (**Figures 2A,D**), suggests that mossy cells are labeled in ChAT-Rosa mice.

Theoretically, the distribution of ChAT-tauGFP and ChAT-YFP cells in the HC should be similar. However, due to the initial observation that some ChAT-tauGFP structures were negative for DAPI and Neurotrace (**Figures 1J–M**), we investigated

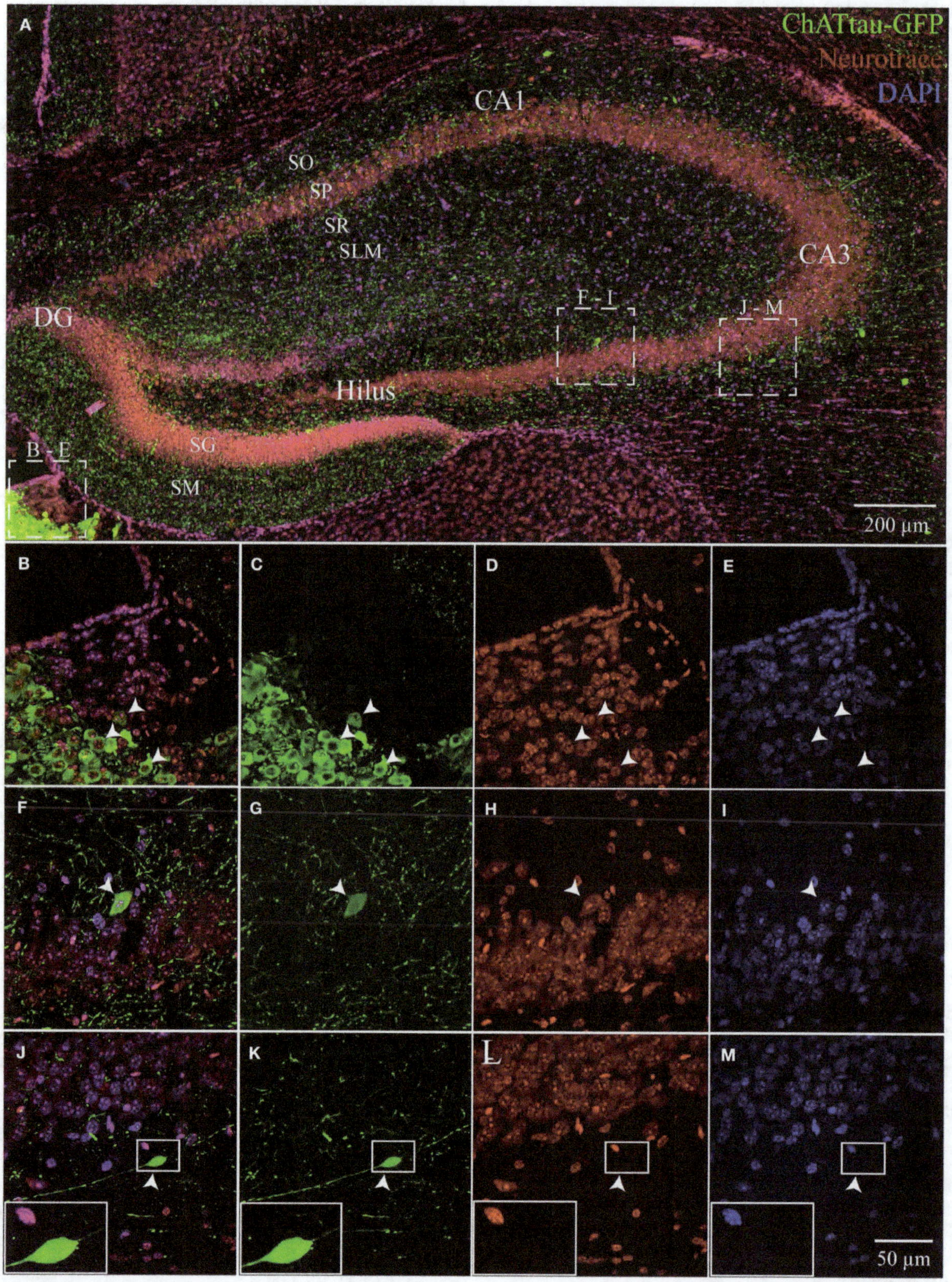

FIGURE 1 | Hippocampus and habenula in ChAT-tauGFP mice. (A) Flat-projected confocal image displaying (green) ChAT-tauGFP cells in the hippocampus. Cells and layers are counterstained with (red) Neurotrace 640/660 and DAPI (blue). Representative examples of Neurotrace/DAPI-positive ChAT-tauGFP cells in **(B–E)** habenula and **(F–I)** CA3 SP. **(J–M)** Representative example of a Neurotrace/DAPI-negative ChAT-tauGFP structure in the CA3 SO layer. (J-M, inset) Magnified view suggesting an en passant bouton. Dotted boxes in **(A)** show the relationship to **(B–M)**.

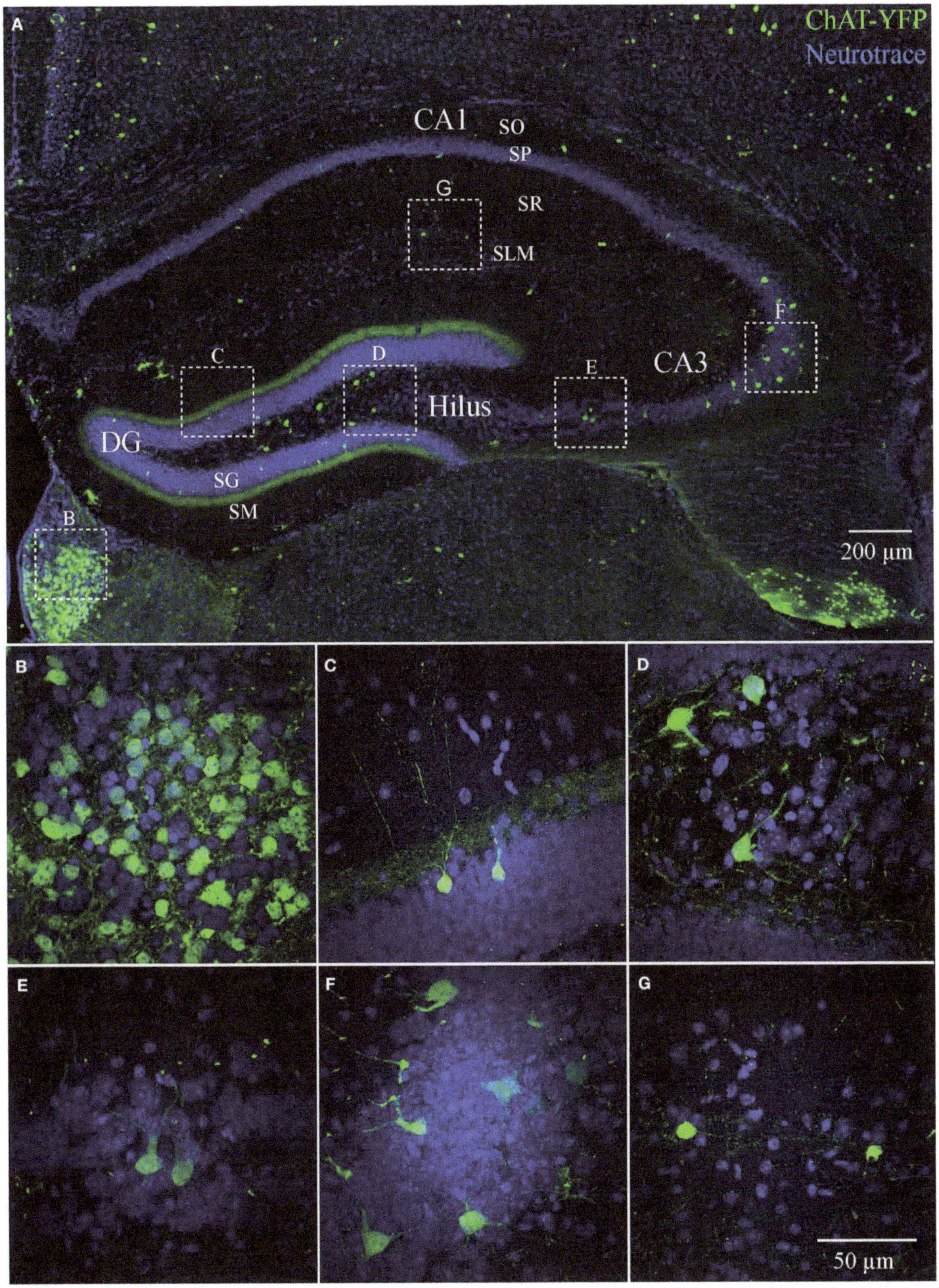

FIGURE 2 | Hippocampus and habenula in ChAT-Rosa mice. (A) Flat-projected confocal image displaying ChAT-YFP cells (green) in the hippocampus. Cells and layers are counterstained with Neurotrace 435/455 (blue). Magnified views of ChAT-YFP cells in **(B)** medial habenula and hippocampal subregions **(C)** DG, **(D)** hilus, **(E,F)** CA3, and **(G)** CA1. Dotted boxes in **(A)** show the relationship to **(B–G)**.

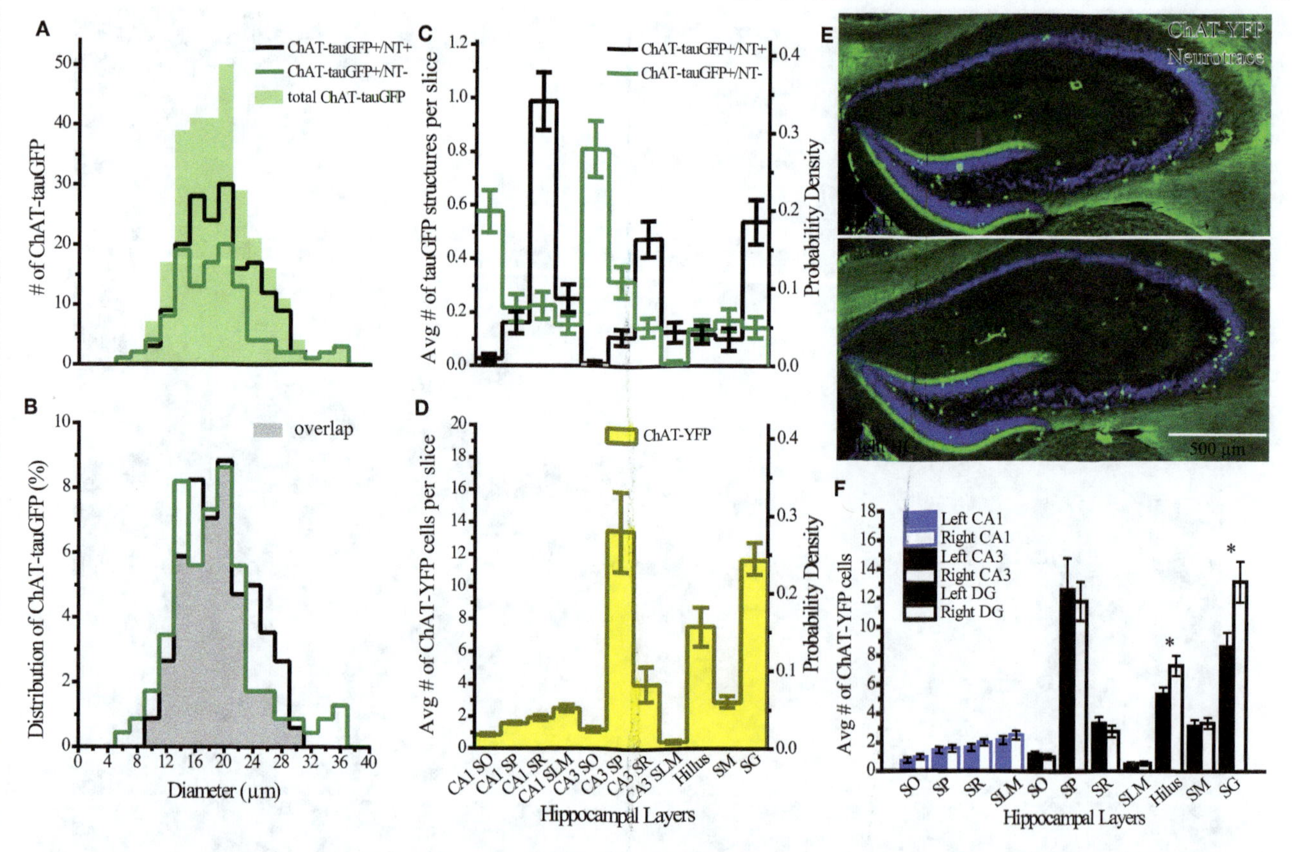

FIGURE 3 | Quantification of ChAT-tauGFP and ChAT-YFP cells. (A) Distribution of ChAT-tauGFP diameters (filled green; $n = 279$), categorized by presence (red, indicating true cells, $n = 167$) or absence (green, non-cells, $n = 116$) of Neurotrace 640/660 (2 µm bin). **(B)** Probability density; filled gray indicates the area of overlap. **(C)** Region and layer distribution for ChAT-GFP cells and non-cells. **(D)** Region and layer distribution of ChAT-YFP cells (all were Neurotrace-positive). Panels **(C,D)** are displayed both as average number per slice (left Y axis) and probability density function (right Y axis). **(E)** Flat-projected, confocal images of left (upper, horizontally flipped) and right (lower) HC from a ChAT-Rosa mouse, counterstained with (blue) Neurotrace 435/455. **(F)** Average number of cells in left (solid bars) or right (open bars) hippocampus (31 bilateral hippocampal sections across 3 ChAT-Rosa mice). *Denotes $p < 0.05$.

whether Neurotrace-negative and Neurotrace-positive ChAT-tauGFP structures could be differentiable based on size. Using the Ferret diameter as a measure (**Figures 3A,B**), size was not significantly different ($p = 0.16$, Mann–Whitney test; from 42 hippocampi of 2 mice) between of DAPI/Neurotrace-positive (18.4 ± 0.4 µm, $n = 163$) and DAPI/Neurotrace-negative structures (18.0 ± 0.6 µm; $n = 116$). These two groups had a similar distribution of diameters (**Figure 3A**). Moreover, the probability density function revealed a large region of overlap (80.6%; **Figure 3B**, gray), indicating that ChAT-tauGFP neuronal and non-neuronal structures could not readily be differentiated from each other based on size.

Because DAPI staining confirmed that Neurotrace was a reliable neuronal marker, we pooled quantification from 2 mice counterstained with DAPI/Neurotrace (**Figure 1**) and 3 mice counterstained with Neurotrace only (**Figure S3**). Consistent with the cellular distribution observed in ChAT-immunopositive cells in rat (Frotscher et al., 1986, 2000) and ChAT-EGFP cells in mouse (von Engelhardt and colleagues, unpublished observations), we found that the majority of Neurotrace-positive ChAT-tauGFP cells were observed in the stratum radiatum (SR) layer of CA1 ($34.1 \pm 3.7\%$, $p < 0.05$) and CA3 ($16.4 \pm 2.3\%$, $p < 0.05$), with fewer cells observed in other HC layers (**Figure 3C**, red; **Table 1**). Interestingly, the distribution of Neurotrace-negative structures was different, with a high percentage of these structures present in the stratum oriens of CA1 ($19.9 \pm 2.7\%$, $p < 0.05$) and CA3 ($28.0 \pm 4\%$, $p < 0.05$) (**Figure 3C**; **Table 1**). In summary, Neurotrace-positive ChAT-tauGFP cell counts are consistent with earlier work, but our results also reveal cell-sized Neurotrace-negative structures that resembled en passant boutons in ChAT-tauGFP mice.

We also quantified the distribution of ChAT-YFP cells in ChAT-Rosa mice. There was a larger number of ChAT-YFP cells in DG (22.3 ± 1.0, $p < 0.0001$) and CA3 (19.4 ± 1.2, $p < 0.0001$) than CA1 (6.9 ± 0.4, $n = 88$ hippocampi from 4 mice). Layer-specific differences were also observed within the HC of ChAT-Rosa mice ($p < 0.0001$, Friedman test; **Figure 3D**; **Table 2**). Within area HC CA1, there were more ChAT-YFP cells in stratum lacunosum moleculare (SLM; 2.5 ± 0.2, $p < 0.0001$) and SR (1.9 ± 1.4, $p = 0.017$) than in SO (0.9 ± 0.1). Within CA3, the region most densely populated with ChAT-YFP cells was in SP (13.7 ± 1.0), compared to SO (1.3 ± 0.1, $p < 0.0001$), SR

Table 1 | Regional and laminar distribution of ChAT-tauGFP counts.

Region	GFP+	layer	GFP+	GFP+/NT+	GFP+/NT−
CA1	289	SO	67	3 (0.9%)†	64 (19.9%)*
		SP	42	18 (5.6%)†	24 (7.5%)
		SR	135	110 (34.1%)	25 (7.8%)
		SLM	45	28 (8.7%)†	17 (5.3%)
CA3	222	SO	91	1 (0.3%)†	90 (28.0%)*
		SP	47	12 (3.7%)†	35 (10.9%)
		SR	69	53 (16.4%)§	16 (5.0%)
		SLM	15	14 (4.3%)†	1 (0.3%)
Hilus	28	Hilus	28	13 (4.0%)†	15 (4.7%)
DG	106	SM	30	11 (3.4%)†	19 (5.9%)
		SG	76	60 (18.6%)§	16 (5.0%)

*Values in the table were compiled from 56 hippocampal slices (112 hippocampi total) from 5 ChAT-tauGFP mice. †Denotes $p < 0.05$ compared to CA1 SR layer among GFP+/NT+ group. §Denotes $p < 0.05$ compared to CA3 SO layer among GFP+/NT+ group. *Denotes $p < 0.05$ compared to CA3 SLM layer among GFP+/NT− group. The percentage numbers are of the fraction of GFP+/NT+ or GFP/NT− within the their groups.*

Table 2 | Regional and laminar distribution of ChAT-tauGFP and ChAT-YFP cells.

Region	Layer	ChAT-tauGFP	ChAT-YFP
CA1	SO	0.03 ± 0.02	0.9 ± 0.1*
	SP	0.16 ± 0.04	1.6 ± 0.1*
	SR	0.98 ± 0.10	1.9 ± 1.4*
	SLM	0.25 ± 0.05	2.5 ± 0.2*
CA3	SO	0.01 ± 0.01	1.2 ± 0.1*
	SP	0.11 ± 0.03	13.7 ± 1.0*
	SR	0.47 ± 0.07	4.0 ± 0.3*
	SLM	0.13 ± 0.04	0.4 ± 0.1*
Hilus	Hilus	0.12 ± 0.03	7.6 ± 0.4*
DG	SM	0.98 ± 0.04	2.9 ± 0.2*
	SG	0.54 ± 0.08	11.8 ± 0.7*

*Data in the table are represented as mean cell number ± SEM per hippocampus, from a total of 44 hippocampal slices (88 hippocampi) from ChAT-Rosa mice and a total of 56 hippocampal slices (112 hippocampi) from ChAT-tauGFP mice. Asterisks denote multiple unpaired t-tests *$p < 0.05$.*

(4.0 ± 0.3, $p < 0.0001$), and SLM (0.4 ± 0.1, $p < 0.0001$). This high abundance of ChAT-YFP cells in SP was unique to CA3 and not observed in CA1 SP (1.6 ± 1.4, $p < 0.0001$). By contrast, there were more ChAT-YFP cells in CA1 SLM than CA3 SLM (0.4 ± 0.1, $p < 0.0001$). There were also layer-specific differences within DG. Similar to CA3, the highest density of ChAT-YFP cells was observed in the principal cell layer (11.8 ± 0.7) relative to the stratum moleculare layer of the dentate (2.9 ± 0.2, $p < 0.0001$). The hilus (7.6 ± 0.4) also had abundant ChAT-YFP cells comparable to the CA3 SP and granule cell layer of the DG ($p > 0.05$).

For every HC region, ChAT-YFP cells, which were invariably Neurotrace-positive, were more abundant than Neurotrace-positive ChAT-tauGFP cells ($p < 0.05$, multiple t-tests, **Table 2**). When normalized to total cell number, cellular distribution was different between ChAT-tauGFP and ChAT-Rosa mice. The majority of Neurotrace-positive ChAT-tauGFP cells were located in the in CA1 SR, CA3 SR, and DG SG layer (**Figure 3C**, red). In contrast, the majority of ChAT-YFP cells were present in CA3 SP, DG SG layer, and hilus (**Figure 3D**).

Finally, a lateralization difference was detected in the HC of ChAT-Rosa mice. The DG SG layer displayed higher abundance of ChAT-YFP cells in the right (13.2 ± 1.4) than left (8.6 ± 1.0) hemisphere ($p = 0.001$, paired t-test, **Figures 3E,F**). A right preference of ChAT-YFP cells was also observed in the hilus (R: 7.3 ± 0.7; L: 5.4 ± 0.5, $p = 0.009$, paired t-test, $n = 31$ HC slices from 3 mice). There was no lateralization bias in CA1 or CA3 ($p > 0.05$). On a per mouse basis, there are the same lateralization trends, although without significant difference, in DG SG layer (R: 136.0 ± 21.0; L: 89.3 ± 7.5, $n = 3$) and hilus (R: 75.7 ± 16.8; L: 55.3 ± 4.8, $n = 3$).

ANTI-ChAT IMMUNOREACTIVITY IS MORE READILY DETECTED IN ChAT-YFP CELLS FROM MS-DBB THAN HC

Although ChAT has been detected immunocytochemically in the HC, ChAT expression in rat was reported to be weaker in the HC than in the basal forebrain region (Frotscher et al., 1986, 2000). TSA amplification enabled us to achieve high signal-to-noise ratio of ChAT expression (see Material and Methods; **Figure S1**). In the MS-DBB (**Figures 4A–C**), ChAT expression was readily detected and co-localized strongly in ChAT-YFP cells (**Figures 4A–F**). In contrast, despite meticulously processing HC slices in parallel with positive controls in MS-DBB slices, ChAT labeling was observed in ChAT-YFP cells from only HC SR/LM layer (**Figures 5A–F**), but not in CA3 (**Figures 5G–I**) or DG (**Figures 5J–L**). Consistent with findings in ChAT-EGFP mice (von Engelhardt et al., 2007), ChAT expression was only partially overlapping in cortex and striatum (**Figures S4A–L**).

A SUBSET OF ChAT-YFP CELLS CO-LOCALIZE WITH CALRETININ AND VIP

Cortical ChAT-EGFP cells exhibit a high degree of co-localization with the calcium binding protein calretinin and neuropeptide VIP (Bayraktar et al., 1997; von Engelhardt et al., 2007). We sought to examine whether HC ChAT-YFP cells possess a similar degree of co-localization with calretinin and VIP. We found only partial co-localization (8.2%, 146/1785) of calretinin or VIP (2.0%, 22/1088) with ChAT-YFP (**Figure S5**), with the majority of calretinin-positive ChAT-YFP cells located in CA1 (50.7%, 74/146) and hilus (32.2%, 47/146), and populations sparsely localized to CA3 (15.1%, 22/146) and DG (2.1%, 3/146). In this experiment, some hilar ChAT-YFP neurons were observed to possess spiny proximal dendrites (**Figure S5D1**, open arrow), suggesting that the diffuse YFP labeling of the DG inner molecular layer (**Figure 2A**) could be accounted for by the axons of ChAT-YFP-positive mossy cells (Scharfman and Myers, 2012). VIP-positive ChAT-YFP cells were located in CA1 (81.8%, 18/22) and CA3 (18.2%, 4/22). Therefore, our data suggests that there is limited overlap of ChAT-YFP with calretinin and VIP.

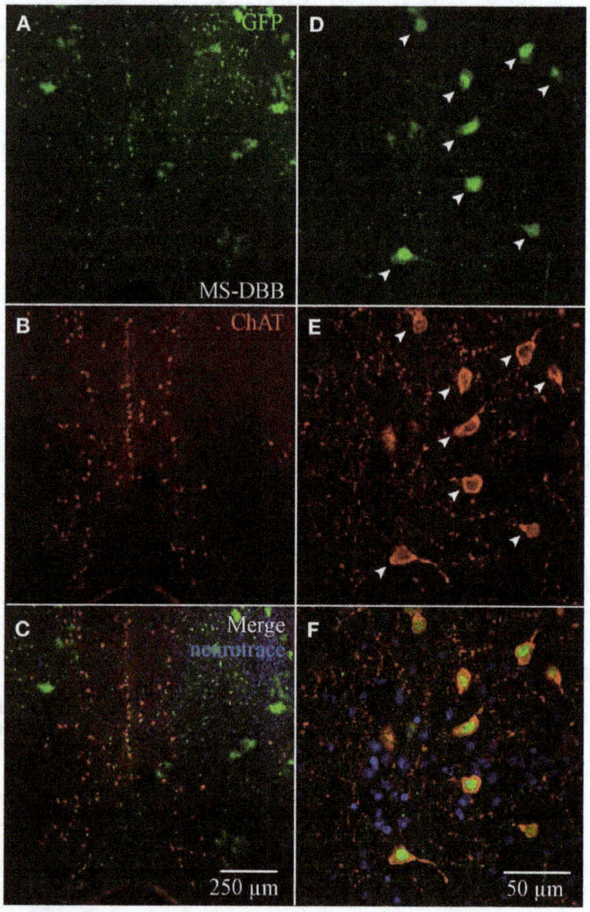

FIGURE 4 | Anti-ChAT labeling in MS-DBB ChAT-YFP cells. (A) YFP, **(B)** anti-ChAT, and **(C)** merged images from the MS-DBB. Higher magnification images **(D–F)** showing co-localization of anti-GFP and anti-ChAT labeling. MS-DBB showing co-localization of YFP and ChAT.

INTRINSIC MEMBRANE PROPERTIES OF HC ChAT-YFP CELLS

Using whole-cell patch clamp recording from ChAT-Rosa mice, we investigated the intrinsic membrane properties of two populations of HC ChAT-YFP cells in CA1 SR/LM and CA3 SP. Representative live images and morphologies of CA1 SR/LM (**Figure 6A**) and CA3 SP (**Figure 6B**) ChAT-YFP cells are shown. As a population, a subset of recorded HC CA1 SR/LM ChAT-YFP cells (5/11, **Table 3**) exhibited spontaneous firing, which was uncommon in CA3 SP ChAT-YFP cells (1/14). Upon injection of a 1 s long, +200 pA depolarizing current step, ChAT-YFP cells in CA1 SR/LM exhibited an irregular firing pattern (**Figure 6A4**), while CA3 SP ChAT-YFP cells exhibited a delayed firing phenotype (**Figure 6B4**). Although AP half-widths were comparable between CA1 SR/LM and CA3 SP ChAT-YFP cells (**Figures 6A5,B5, 7D**), CA1 SR/LM ChAT-YFP cells had higher R_{in} (**Figure 7A**) and smaller size (**Figure 7B**) than CA3 SP ChAT-YFP cells (**Table 3**). As expected from the differential R_{in} of these populations, CA1 SR/LM ChAT-YFP cells achieved a higher AP frequency than CA3 SP ChAT-YFP cells at small depolarizing current steps ($p < 0.05$ at +100 pA; **Table 3**), whereas CA3 SP ChAT-YFP cells tolerated larger current steps (**Figure 7C**). Therefore, the intrinsic membrane properties are distinct between CA1 SR/LM and CA3 SP ChAT-YFP populations, representing distinct ChAT-YFP subclasses.

The intrinsic membrane properties and appearance of thorny excrescences on the apical dendrites of CA3 ChAT-YFP cells (**Figure 6B3**) led us to compare ChAT-YFP cells to YFP-negative, presumably pyramidal cells, in the CA3 SP (**Figure 6C**). YFP-negative and ChAT-YFP cells in CA3 SP were not significantly different in C_m, R_{in}, and τ_m (**Table 3**). However, as a population, ChAT-YFP cells had a broader AP half-width than CA3 SP YFP-negative cells ($p = 0.013$; **Figures 6B5, 7D**). Therefore, on the basis of these findings, CA3 SP ChAT-YFP cells could be viewed as a distinct subclass of CA3 pyramidal cells.

Finally, we examined the intrinsic properties of MS-DBB and HC ChAT-YFP cells. MS-DBB ChAT-YFP cells (**Figure 6D**) were comparable to CA1 SR/LM cells in C_m, R_{in}, and τ_m (**Table 3**). In addition, MS-DBB ChAT-YFP cells had broad AP half-widths that were not significantly different than AP half-widths in HC ChAT-YFP cells (**Figures 6D, 7D; Table 3**).

HC ChAT-YFP CELLS UNDERGO CHOLINERGIC NEUROMODULATION

One intriguing hypothesis is that cholinergic interneurons themselves could be targets of cholinergic modulation (Tricoire and Cea-Del Rio, 2007). To investigate whether ChAT-YFP cells underwent cholinergic modulation, we applied ACh to HC ChAT-YFP cells (**Figure 8**). In the continuous presence of the AMPA receptor antagonist DNQX (25 µM), the NMDA receptor antagonist APV (50 µM) and the GABAA receptor antagonist gabazine (5 µM), we applied 1 s long depolarizing current to monitor the AP firing frequency of ChAT-YFP cells from CA1 SR/LM ChAT-YFP (**Figure 8A**) and CA3 SP ChAT-YFP cells (**Figure 8B**) while introducing bias current to maintain the membrane potential at −60 mV. Bath application of ACh (100 µM) increased AP frequency in CA1 SR/LM ChAT-YFP (100–200 pA step, **Figures 8A,B,I**) and CA3 SP ChAT-YFP (400–700 pA step, **Figures 8C,D,I**) cells. In CA1 SR/LM ChAT-YFP cells, the ACh-induced increase in AP frequency (from 13.2 ± 1.8 to 22.8 ± 2.6 Hz, $p = 0.0007$, $n = 11$, two-tailed paired t-test; **Figure 8I**) was accompanied by the elimination of the ADF (from -3.3 ± 0.4 to -0.7 mV $\pm$ 0.7 mV, $p = 0.0029$, Wilcoxon matched pairs-signed rank test; **Figure 8J**) and a modest increase in holding current (by -12.1 ± 6.6 pA, $p < 0.001$, Wilcoxon signed rank test; **Figure 8K**). In CA3 SP ChAT-YFP cells, the ACh-induced increase in AP frequency (from 10.1 ± 0.8 to 12.1 ± 1.4 Hz, $p = 0.020$, $n = 11$, Wilcoxon matched pairs signed rank test) was more modest and underwent a similar increase in holding current (by -13.0 ± 6.2 pA, $p < 0.001$, Wilcoxon signed rank test), but the AHP was converted to an ADP (from -2.1 ± 0.6 to 1.0 ± 0.5 mV, $p = 0.002$, Wilcoxon matched pairs signed rank test). Similar to previous studies in HC principal cells (Cole and Nicoll, 1983; Cobb and Davies, 2004), application of ACh increased AP frequency (from 12.1 ± 0.9 Hz to 26.1 ± 3.7 Hz, $p = 0.0044$, $n = 7$, paired t-test; **Figures 8F,I**), generated an ADP (-3.0 ± 1.4 to 0.6 ± 0.6 mV, $p = 0.0003$, paired t-test; **Figure 8J**), and increased holding current (-42.8 ± 9.0 pA, $p = 0.0032$, one sample t-test; **Figure 8K**) in CA3 pyramidal cells (PCs). However, the extent

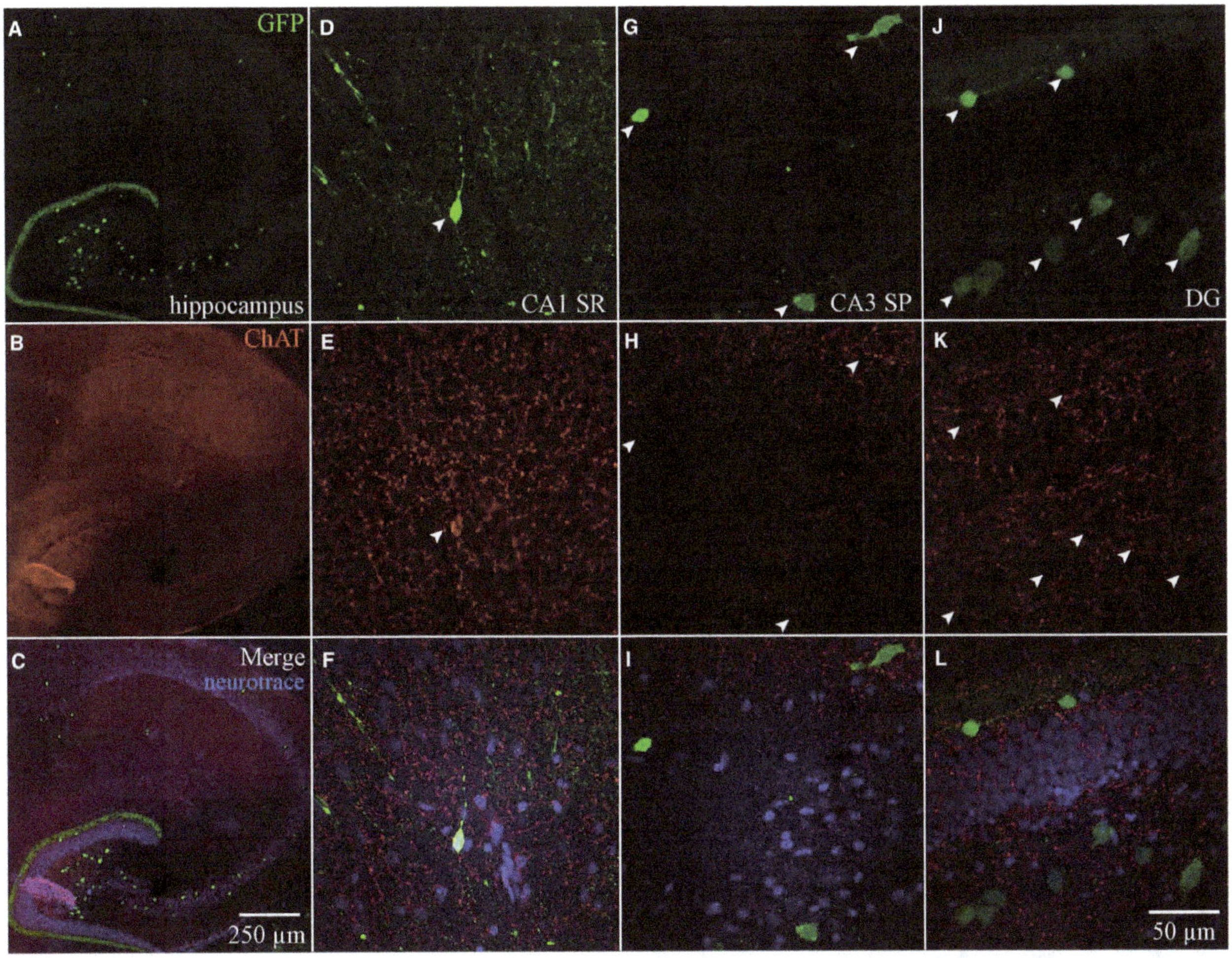

FIGURE 5 | Anti-ChAT labeling in HC ChAT-YFP cells. (A) YFP, **(B)** anti-ChAT, and **(C)** merged images from the HC. Higher magnification images in **(D–F)** CA1 SR, **(G–I)** CA3 SP, and **(J–L)** DG showing that anti-ChAT labeling is not detected in ChAT-YFP cells.

that ACh increased AP frequency was larger in CA1 SR/LM ChAT-YFP and CA3 PCs than CA3 SP ChAT-YFP cells ($p < 0.05$, One-Way ANOVA, **Figure 8L**). Finally, in contrast to HC ChAT-YFP cells, MS-DBB ChAT-YFP cells were not modulated by ACh ($p > 0.05$; **Figures 8D,H–L**). Taken together, ACh resulted in enhanced ChAT-YFP cells in both CA1 and CA3, but to different extents.

OPTOGENETIC STIMULATION OF HC ChAT-CRE NEURONS INDUCES GLUTAMATE RELEASE ONTO CA1 INTERNEURONS

To investigate the neurotransmitter phenotype of HC ChAT-CRE cells, we employed GAD65-GFP/ChAT-CRE mice (see Material and Methods), which enabled optogenetic stimulation of ChAT-CRE cells onto CA1 GAD65-GFP interneurons (López-Bendito et al., 2004; Cea-del Rio et al., 2010; Wierenga et al., 2010). Four weeks after the injection of floxed ChR2-mCherry AAV into HC of GAD65-GFP/ChAT-CRE mice, we performed whole cell recording on GAD65-GFP cells of CA1 SR/SLM (**Figures 9A–C**). In response to 470 nm light flashes (1–5 ms), EPSCs were evoked in 7/17 of recorded CA1 SR/SLM GAD65-GFP cells. Perfusion of AMPA and NMDA receptor blockers DNQX and APV fully blocked the light pulses induced EPSCs in 6/7 cells (**Figures 9D,E**). Consistent with monosynaptic stimulation, the onset of the glutamate EPSC occurred ~2 ms after onset of light stimulation. Post-hoc confocal analysis revealed colocalization points of ChR2-mCherry-positive presynaptic terminals with the somatodendritc region of recorded GAD65-GFP cells (**Figures 9H,I**), consistent with direct synaptic input from ChAT-CRE cells. In 1/7 cells, optogenetic stimulation elicited an inward polysynaptic current that was resistant to block by DNQX, APV, and mAChR antagonist atropine. Overall, these data indicate that optogenetic stimulation of intrinsic HC ChAT-CRE neurons results in glutamatergic excitation.

DISCUSSION

NEUROCHEMICAL IDENTITY AND CELLULAR DISTRIBUTION OF HC NEURONS VISUALIZED IN ChAT-tauGFP AND ChAT-ROSA MICE

HC cholinergic interneurons were described almost 30 years ago (Frotscher et al., 1986), and, in modern HC interneuron classification schemes, are recognized as one of over 21 distinct HC interneuron subtypes (Klausberger and Somogyi, 2008).

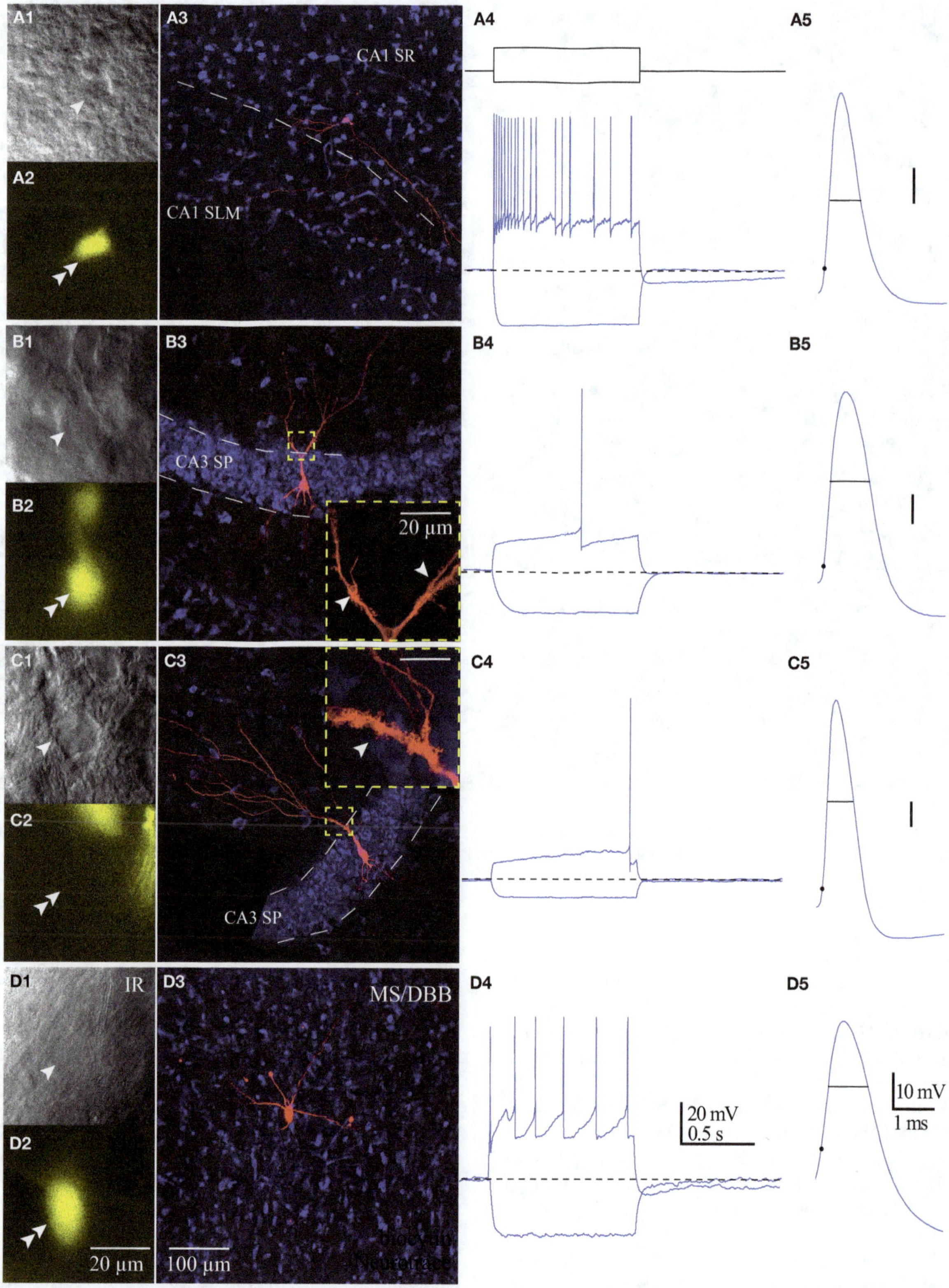

FIGURE 6 | Properties of HC ChAT-YFP cells. Morphology and intrinsic membrane properties of representative **(A)** CA1 SR/LM ChAT-YFP, **(B)** CA3 SP ChAT-YFP, **(C)** CA3 SP YFP-negative, and **(D)** MS/DBB ChAT-YFP cells. For each cell type, representative (1) live IR Dodt contrast images, (2) 505 nm fluorescent images, (3) flat-projected confocal image of the biocytin-filled cell, (4) voltage responses to 1 s long hyperpolarizing (−100 pA) or depolarizing (+200 pA) current steps, and (5) first AP half-width are displayed. Insets in panels **(B3,C3)**: thorny excrescences (white arrows) on the dendrites of **(B3)** CA3 SP ChAT-YFP and **(C3)** CA3 SP YFP-negative cells.

Table 3 | Properties of hippocampal ChAT-YFP neurons.

Property	CA1 ChAT-YFP	CA3 ChAT-YFP	CA3 PC	MS-DBB YFP
R_{in} (MΩ)	236.2 ± 13.8[†§*]	143.8 ± 12.9[§]	125.3 ± 11.3	369.8 ± 60.0[*]
τ_m (ms)	25.3 ± 1.8	38.3 ± 3.2	30.3 ± 2.3	25.4 ± 3.2
C_m (pF)	111.6 ± 7.6[†*]	267.0 ± 16.9[§]	243.2 ± 21.6	72.2 ± 4.8[*]
V_m (mV)	−57.9 ± 3.3	−67.9 ± 2.5	−75.0 ± 1.4	−46.9 ± 5.5
AP half width (μs)	969.6 ± 47.8[*]	1021.7 ± 38.0[*]	725.8 ± 26.5	1081.0 ± 42.0[*]
Sag (SS/peak)	0.95 ± 0.01	0.99 ± 0.01	1.00 ± 0.02	0.98 ± 0.01
Spontaneous firing	5/11	1/12	0/7	5/6
AP frequency (at 100 pA)	10.5 ± 1.9	0	0	4.3 ± 1.1

[†]Compared to CA3 SP ChAT-YFP cells; $p < 0.05$. [§]Compared to MSDBB ChAT-YFP cells; $p < 0.05$. [*]Compared to CA3 SP YFP-negative cells; $p < 0.05$.

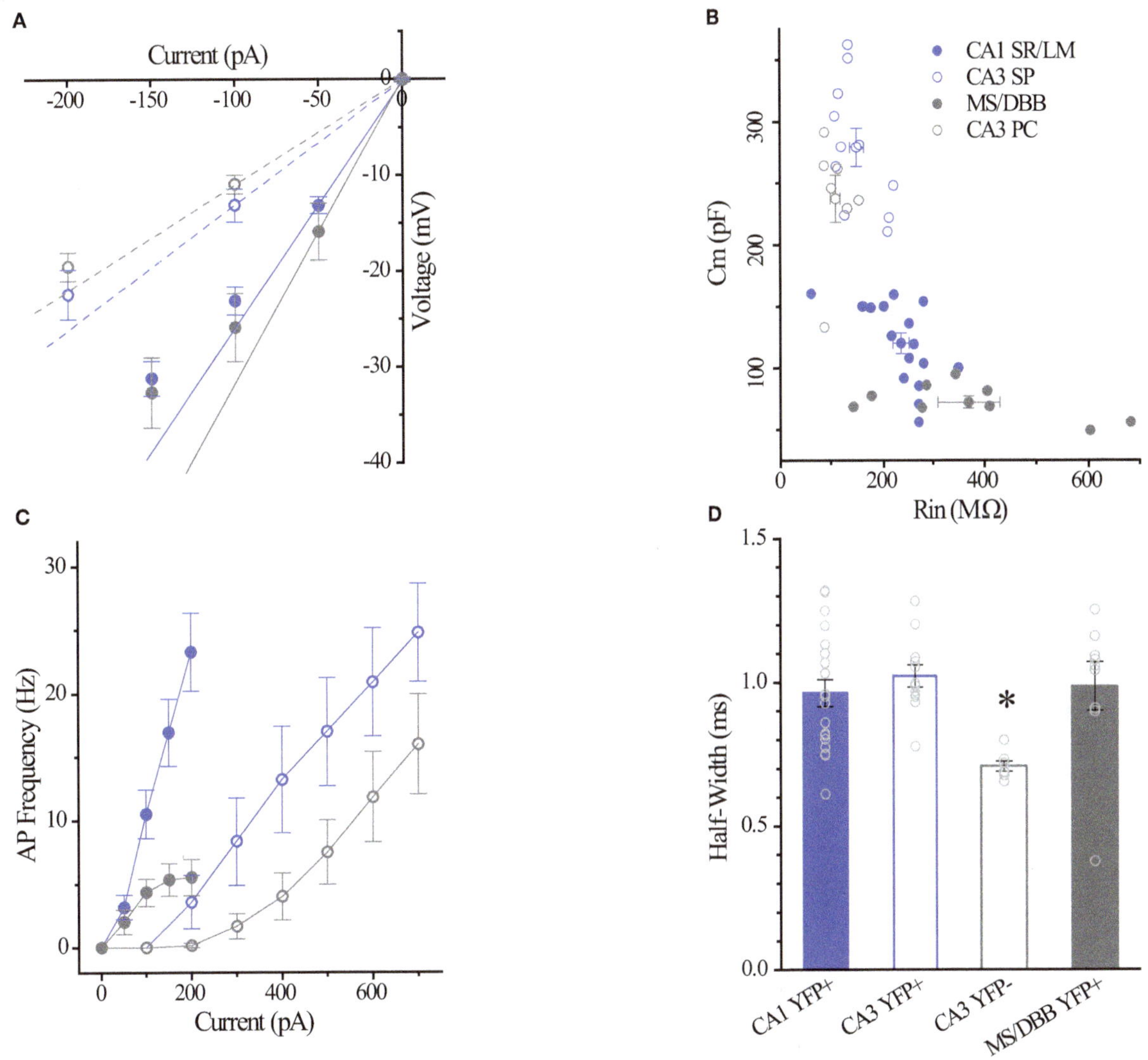

FIGURE 7 | Differences between CA1 and CA3 ChAT-YFP cells. (A) I–V relationship for CA1 ChAT-YFP ($n = 14$, blue filled circle), CA3 ChAT-YFP ($n = 9$, blue open circle), CA3 YFP-negative ($n = 7$, gray open circle), and MSDBB ChAT-YFP ($n = 6$, gray filled circle) cells. Lines denote slopes through 0 pA and (solid) −50 pA or (dotted) −100 pA points illustrating differences in R_{in}. **(B)** Plot of C_m vs. R_{in} for CA1 ChAT-YFP ($n = 20$), CA3 ChAT-YFP ($n = 12$), CA3 YFP-negative ($n = 7$), and MSDBB ChAT-YFP ($n = 9$) cells. **(C)** AP frequency vs. current step for the 4 cell types. **(D)** Bar graph showing narrower half width of CA3 YFP-negative cells than ChAT-YFP cells in CA1 SR/LM, CA3 SP, and MS/DBB (One-Way ANOVA). Asterisk (*) denotes $p < 0.05$ compared to CHAT-YFP cells in CA1, CA3 and MS-DBB.

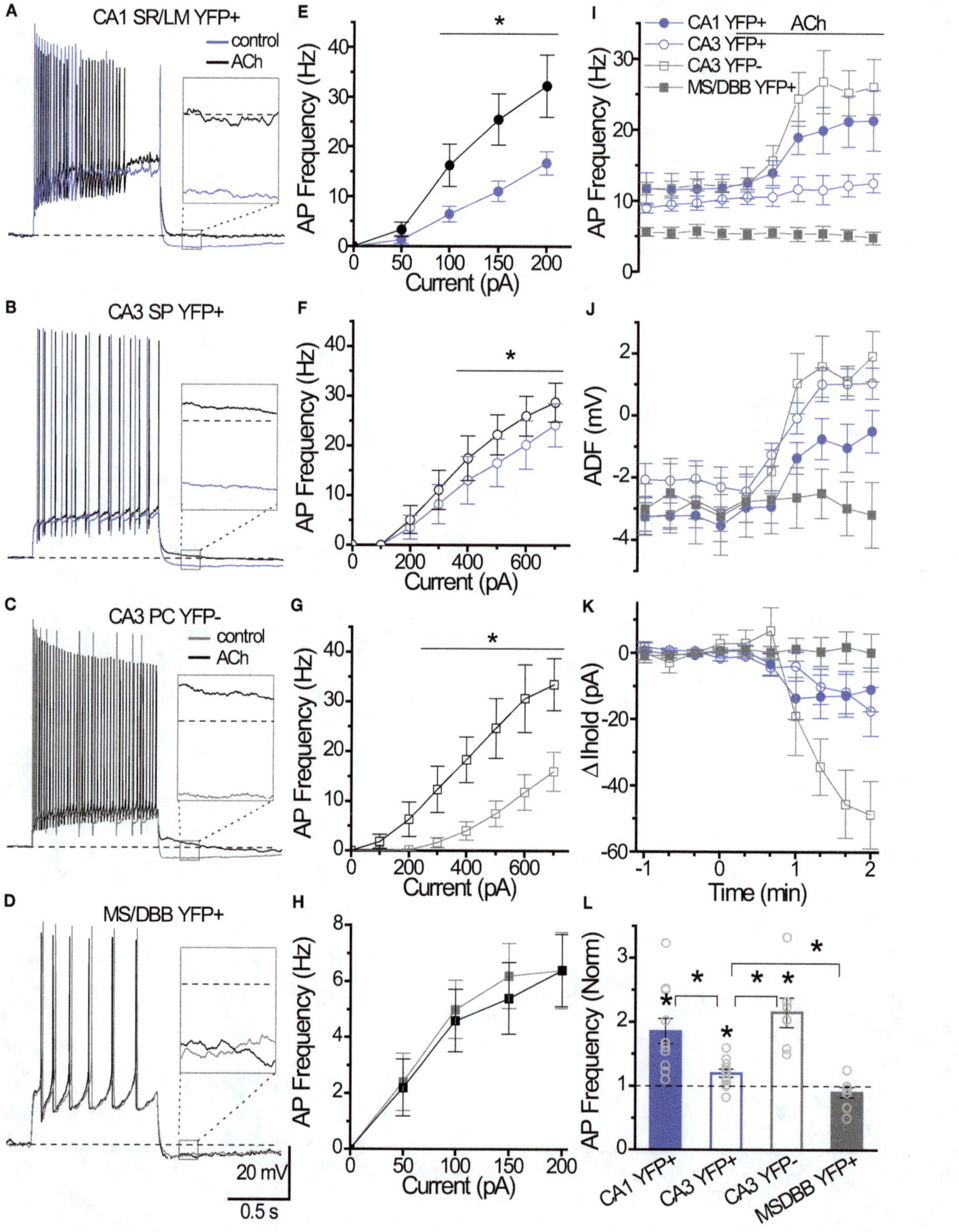

FIGURE 8 | Cholinergic modulation of Hippocampal ChAT-YFP cells. (A–D) Whole-cell voltage responses to the introduction of a 1 s long depolarizing current step from −60 mV in representative cells in (blue/gray) control and (red) 100 μM ACh. Inset, solid box expanded to illustrate the effect of ACh on afterdeflection (ADF) (dotted line indicates −60 mV baseline). **(E–H)** Input-output relationships from AP frequency vs. current step magnitude for CA1 YFP+ (E, close circle $n = 8$), and CA3 YFP+ (F, open circle, $n = 9$), CA3 YFP− (G, open square, $n = 6$) and MSDBB YFP+ (H, close square, $n = 5$) cells. *Denotes $p < 0.05$, Two-Way ANOVA. **(I–K)** Population data for the four group cells summarizing the time course of **(I)** AP frequency, **(J)** afterdeflection, **(K)** relative change in I_{hold} from (blue) control to (red; at time 0) ACh conditions. **(L)** Bar graph showing cholinergic modulation induced changed in normalized AP frequency. Black asterisks denote $p < 0.05$ compared to 1, one sample t-test. Red asterisks denote $p < 0.05$ between groups, One-Way ANOVA.

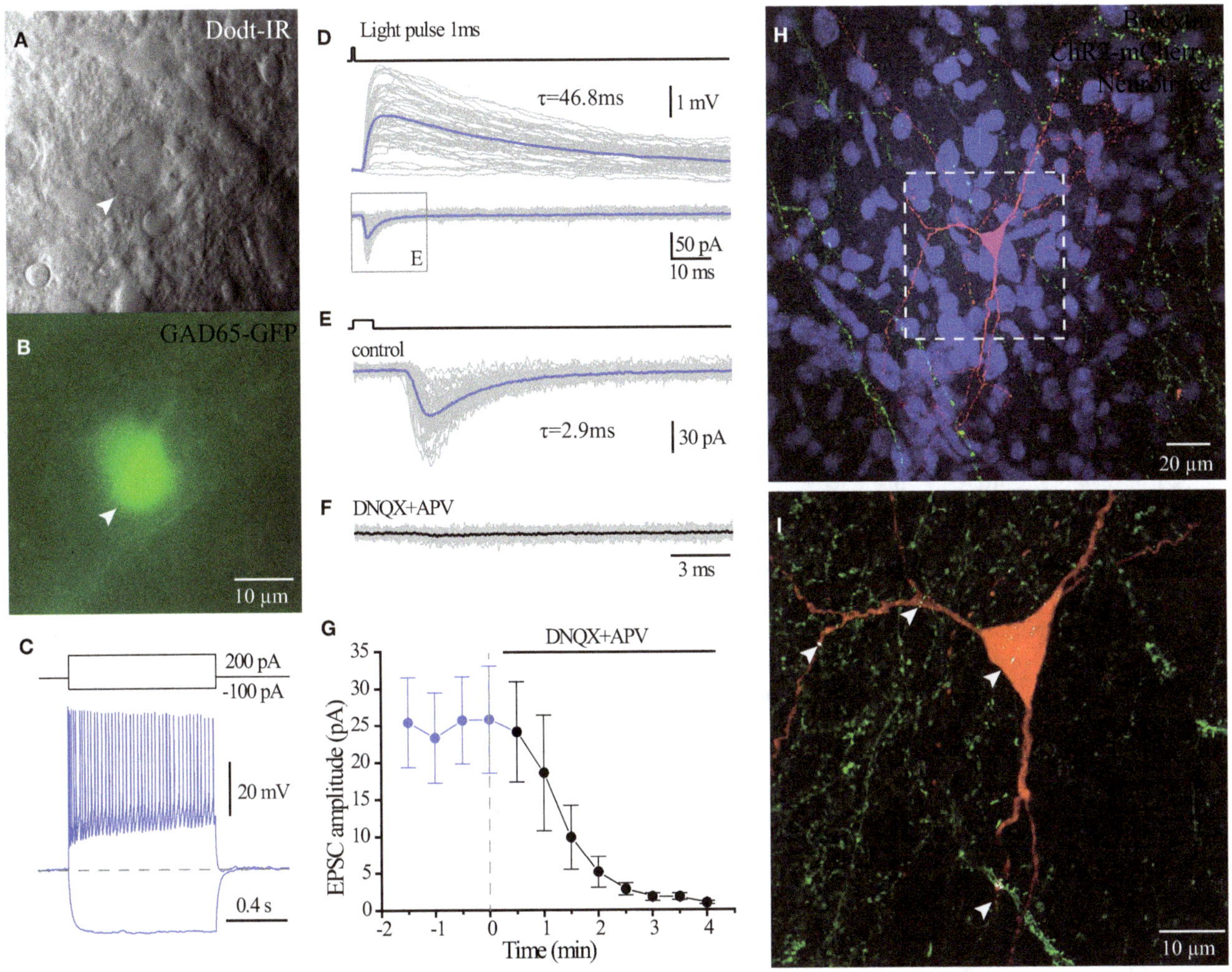

FIGURE 9 | Glutamate release from hippocampal ChAT-CRE cells. Live IR Dodt contrast image **(A)** and green fluorescent image **(B)** of a recorded GFP+ cell in hippocampal CA1 SR/LM layer. **(C)** Voltage responses to 1 s long hyperpolarizing (−100 pA) or depolarizing (200 pA) current steps. **(D)** Averaged light flashes (1 ms, 470 nm) induced EPSCs in acsf (blue) and DNQX+APV (red). **(E)** Population date showing the light induced EPSCs were blocked by ionotropic glutamate receptors blockers (Wilcoxon matched-pairs signed rank test, $n = 6$). **(F)** Flat-projection of a confocal image for the biocytin filled (red) cell with mCherry (green) and Neurotrace (blue). **(G)** White regions showing the co-localization of mCherry (ChAT-CRE-positive synaptic terminals) and biocytin (recorded GAD65-GFP cell).

In a previous study, ChAT-expressing neurons were shown to lack GAD65/67 mRNA (Frotscher et al., 2000). However, in cortex, ChAT-EGFP bipolar neurons immunoreactive for ChAT co-localize strongly with VIP and calretinin (von Engelhardt et al., 2007), which could overlap with GABAergic interneuron subtypes (Chamberland et al., 2010; Chamberland and Topolnik, 2012; Tyan et al., 2014). By contrast, cortical bipolar ChAT-EGFP cells lack GAD67 mRNA (von Engelhardt et al., 2007). Moreover, VIP/calretinin-positive interneurons tended to exhibit an irregular spiking, or stuttering phenotype (Porter et al., 1999; von Engelhardt et al., 2007).

In the present study, we investigated HC neurons that expressed fluorescent proteins under the control of the ChAT promoter (Gong et al., 2007; Grybko et al., 2011), enabling HC ChAT-positive cells to be revealed through transgenic mouse technology. In the initial examination of the HC of ChAT-tauGFP mice, GFP-containing fibers were found to densely innervate all layers of the hippocampus, most of which presumably arose from MS-DBB cholinergic projection neurons (Dutar et al., 1995). Although our use of Neurotrace was originally intended only to define HC layers, upon higher magnification, we noted that some tauGFP-positive structures that were originally counted as cells were actually negative for Neurotrace (**Figure S3**). We then used both Neurotrace and DAPI as cellular markers to unambiguously identify HC neurons in the ChAT-tauGFP population (**Figure 1**; **Table 1**). Consistent with HC ChAT-immunoreactive interneurons in rat (Frotscher et al., 1986, 2000) and ChAT-EGFP neurons in mice (von Engelhardt and colleagues, unpublished observations), we revealed that 59.4% of ChAT-tauGFP structures were labeled with both Neurotrace and DAPI (**Figure 3A**), particularly in CA1 and CA3 SR/SLM regions (**Figure 3C**). Interestingly, 40.6% of ChAT-tauGFP structures, which were comparable in diameter to the neuronal ChAT-tauGFP population (**Figures 3A,B**), lacked Neurotrace and DAPI (**Figure 3A**). These ChAT-tauGFP structures tended to be found in CA1 and CA3 stratum oriens, which may be a reflection of the density of MS-DBB cholinergic afferents in HC layers. Axon blebs, which can approach the size of ChAT-tauGFP globular structures measured here, are observed only after the axon is severed (Shu et al., 2006; Hu and Shu, 2012). However, the ChAT-tauGFP axon appears to be intact (**Figure 1K**, inset), resembling large, en passant boutons. These globular structures could result from the overexpression of tauGFP in cholinergic axons, and are therefore specific to ChAT-tauGFP mice. Supporting this hypothesis, cell sized ChAT-YFP-positive structures were invariably Neurotrace-positive neurons in ChAT-Rosa mice. In any case, the large diameter of many of these boutons provides a future opportunity to access cholinergic axons electrophysiologically and understand their intrinsic membrane properties, firing activity, and presynaptic modulatory capacity.

The GM24 line of ChAT-CRE mice generally has been used in combination with a ChR2 AAV or with a reporter line to optically stimulate (Witten et al., 2010) and/or visualize cholinergic neurons (Ivanova et al., 2010; Lopes et al., 2012) in various brain regions. However, no study has yet examined YFP-positive cells in the hippocampus of ChAT-Rosa mice. In examining the regional and laminar distribution of ChAT-YFP cells (**Figure 2**), there was some similarity to the original description of ChAT cells in the HC (Frotscher et al., 1986), especially in the location of small cells in the CA1 SR/SLM layer (**Figures 2A,G**). A majority (15/19) of CA1 SR/SLM neurons possessed a stuttering/irregular firing phenotype (**Figure 6**), which is reminiscent of the phenotypes of cortical ChAT-EGFP (von Engelhardt et al., 2007), cortical VIP/calretinin/ChAT (Porter et al., 1998, 1999), and HC VIP/calretinin (Tyan et al., 2014) interneuron subtypes.

In addition to similarities, we noted several differences when comparing the cellular distribution and neurochemical identity of ChAT-YFP cells with previous studies, as well as with the ChAT-tauGFP population also described here. Despite the strong co-localization of ChAT immunoreactivity in MS-DBB ChAT-YFP cells processed in parallel, ChAT immunoreactivity was rarely detected in HC ChAT-YFP cells. There are a number of possibilities that could explain this discrepancy. First, the discrepancy between YFP and anti-ChAT signals could be due to the ectopic expression of CRE in non-ChAT cells (Gong et al., 2007). Second, ChAT immunoreactivity is weaker in the hippocampus (Frotscher et al., 1986) and cortex (von Engelhardt et al., 2007) than in basal forebrain. Driving EGFP or EYFP expression under the control of the ChAT promoter may amplify the detection sensitivity of ChAT-expressing cells above the detection sensitivity of the anti-ChAT antibody. Third, access of the anti-ChAT antibody to the epitope binding site on ChAT may differ depending on the region and/or cell type. Fourth, CRE/loxP recombination may temporally dissociate YFP expression from ChAT expression. Unlike ChAT-EGFP (von Engelhardt et al., 2007) and ChAT-tauGFP (Grybko et al., 2011) mice, where ChAT and GFP expression are expected to be temporally correlated (Erickson et al., 2014), YFP expression in a ChAT-YFP neuron may only indicate that ChAT was transiently expressed during development of the ChAT-YFP neuron. Therefore, YFP may be expressed even if ChAT expression was strongly down-regulated during development.

In a recent study, fetal HC neurons immunopositive for vesicular glutamate transporter 1 (vGluT1) were observed to co-localize with ChAT (Bhargava et al., 2010), consistent with previous observations demonstrating glutamate and ACh co-release in some types of cholinergic neurons (Allen et al., 2006; Ren et al., 2011). However, ChAT immunoreactivity was absent from all but a small subpopulation of vGluT1-positive neonatal cells grown for 13 days in culture (Bhargava et al., 2010). Consistent with the idea that ChAT expression is downregulated in glutamatergic neurons, we found that a subset of CA3 SP neurons express ChAT-YFP (**Figures 2A,F**) but do not exhibit ChAT immunoreactivity (**Figures 5A–C, G–I**). Moreover, CA3 SP neurons were not well represented in ChAT-tauGFP mice (**Figure 3C**). However, optogenetic stimulation induced glutamatergic EPSCs in CA1 HC of ChAT-CRE mice (**Figures 9D–G**), indicating that CRE expression must persist in adult ChAT-CRE mice. ChR2-mCherry-expressing synaptic terminals were observed in CA1 (**Figures 9H,I**), most likely originating from CA3 SP ChAT-CRE cells. Although ChAT-YFP cells in the CA3 area that resemble pyramidal cells are distinct from non-fluorescent pyramidal cells (**Figure 7D**), these observations are consistent with conventional glutamatergic transmission from CA3 ChAT-CRE cells. CA3 ChAT-CRE cells most likely misexpress CRE-recombinase because they have no equivalent in the ChAT-tau GFP mice and exhibit no detectable ChAT immunoreactivity. In hilar ChAT-YFP cells, the presence of thorny excrescences (**Figure S5D**) and the diffuse YFP labeling in the DG inner molecular layer (**Figure S5A**) suggest that at least some of ChAT-YFP cells in hilus are mossy cells (Scharfman and Myers, 2012). Given the above observations, it will be of interest to examine other ChAT-CRE mouse lines for the presence of these cell populations.

Sparse ChAT immunoreactivity and some overlap with calretinin/VIP was observed in some CA1 cells, consistent with a population of Neurotrace-positive CA1 SR/SLM interneurons in ChAT-tauGFP mice (**Figure 3C**). These observations are consistent with the retention of ChAT, albeit at a lower level than in MS-DBB cholinergic neurons, in a small subset of the adult CA1 SR/SLM interneuron population (**Figures 4, 5**). A subset of CA1 VIP/calretinin interneurons are clearly GABAergic (Chamberland et al., 2010; Chamberland and Topolnik, 2012; Tyan et al., 2014), consistent with original observations made in cortex (Bayraktar et al., 1997; von Engelhardt et al., 2007). However, in situ hybridization data showed lack of GAD65/67 mRNA expression in rat ChAT immunopositive HC interneurons (Frotscher et al., 2000). We attempted to optogentically stimulate this CA1 interneuron population; however, it is likely that the glutamatergic output from CRE-expressing principal cells in CA3 or DG confounded this experimental design. Although it is possible that glutamate is also released (or co-released) from ChAT-CRE cells in CA1 or CA3 SR/SLM, future experiments that more narrowly focus on optogenetic stimulation of this population would unambiguously reveal neurotransmitter phenotype(s) of this interneuron subclass.

CHOLINERGIC MODULATION OF "CHOLINERGIC INTERNEURONS" DURING HC NETWORK OPERATIONS

ACh release is associated with HC-related behaviors (Pepeu and Giovannini, 2004). In the present study, we found that bath application of ACh enhanced the excitability of both HC CA1 SR/SLM and CA3 ChAT-YFP cells. Although we did not differentiate between nicotinic and muscarinic activation, our results clearly demonstrate that the cellular excitability of ChAT-YFP neurons is influenced by cholinergic neuromodulation. The ACh-induced increase in cellular excitability is most likely due to the activation of mAChRs, as suggested by similarities in mAChR-induced changes in intrinsic membrane properties similar to previous studies (Cole and Nicoll, 1983; Lawrence et al., 2006; Cea-del Rio et al., 2010; Dasari and Gulledge, 2011). However, it is possible that a subset of CA1 SR/SLM ChAT-YFP cells are enriched with a high density of nAChRs, as found in calretinin/VIP-positive cells in cortex (Porter et al., 1999). Indeed, a subset of ChAT-tauGFP axons arising from Neurotrace/DAPI-positive ChAT-tauGFP HC interneurons may contribute to the generation of α7 nAChR-mediated EPSCs in CA3 pyramidal cells (Grybko et al., 2011). Nevertheless, these observations raise the possibility that cholinergic interneurons could be excited by the endogenous release of ACh arising from either extrinsic or intrinsic sources.

What are the potential consequences of cholinergic modulation of ChAT-expressing neurons in the HC? Since ACh release from HC ChAT+ cells has not been definitively demonstrated, it remains an unresolved issue, but given the possible developmental downregulation of ChAT expression (Bhargava et al., 2010), ACh release from HC interneurons is likely to play a more prominent role during development than in the adult. Future studies investigating the expression of ChAT immunoreactivity during development of the HC are needed to clarify this issue. It is also possible that these same HC neurons may regress to an earlier stage of development under pathological conditions, and upregulate their synthesis and release of ACh. Evidence for cholinergic dysfunction occurs in epileptic tissue (Romo-Parra et al., 2003), and the abnormal release of ACh may account in part for such dysfunction. Finally, given the partial overlap with VIP and calretinin (**Figure S5**), we cannot rule out possible roles of ACh release from HC ChAT+ cells in neurovascular and/or neurometabolic coupling (Cauli et al., 2004, 2014).

Taken together, our efforts to investigate HC interneurons through transgenic mouse technology have improved our understanding of this heterogeneous class of neurons. However, many questions remain regarding their neurochemical identity, significance to HC function, and potential interaction with MS-DBB cholinergic networks. Next generation transgenic technology may provide additional tools that can be applied to examine distinct subpopulations of HC cholinergic interneurons.

ACKNOWLEDGMENTS

Support was from R01 NS069689 and P20RR015583 (JJL). COBRE grants P20RR015583, P20RR017670, and P20GM10356 supported core facilities. RG was a Fulbright Scholar. MW was a Scholar in Residence supported by a grant from the College of Health Professions and Biomedical Sciences, University of Montana. We thank Alison Hixon for preliminary examination of ChAT-Rosa mice, Sukumar Vijayaraghavan (UC Denver) for ChAT-tauGFP mice, Chris McBain (NIH) for GAD65-GFP mice, and Jerry Yakel (NIEHS) for AAV9 ChR2-mCherry. We thank Chris McBain, Ludovic Tricoire (CNRS, INSERM, Paris) and Christian Cea del Rio (UC-Denver) for critically evaluating an earlier version of the manuscript and Jakob von Engelhardt (DZNE, Heidelburg) for sharing unpublished data.

SUPPLEMENTARY MATERIAL

Figure S1 | Control experiments for anti-ChAT staining. Primary and secondary antibodies for GFP were added in all the experiments. **(A,B)** MS ChAT cells (red) were not revealed in goat anti-ChAT primary only slices. **(C,D)** MS ChAT cells were not revealed in non-primary incubated slices. **(E,F)** ChAT cells were detected in slices incubated with anti-ChAT primary, secondary and TSA.

Figure S2 | Optogenetic stimulation of HC ChAT-CRE cells. (A) Live ChR2-mCherry (590 nm) fluorescence and **(B)** live Dodt-IR contrast image of a ChAT-CRE cell in hippocampus CA1 SR layer. **(C)** Voltage responses upon introduction of (shift-option) ± 200 pA current steps. **(D)** Delivery of 470 nm flashes (blue, 2 ms duration) at 5 Hz for 5 s induced APs in the recorded ChR2-mCherry+ cell. Inset: overlaid AP waveforms.

Figure S3 | Presence of HC ChAT-tauGFP cells and structures in ChAT-tauGFP mice. (A) Flat-projected confocal image displaying (green) ChAT-tauGFP cells in the hippocampus. Cells and layers are counterstained with (blue) Neurotrace 435/455 Blue Fluorescent Nissl Stain. **(B–D)** Magnified views of a ChAT-tauGFP in CA1 SR region. **(E–J)** Large Neurotrace-negative ChAT-tauGFP structures resembling an en passant bouton.

Figure S4 | Detection of ChAT immunoreactivity in cortex and striatum. (A) YFP, **(B)** anti-ChAT, and **(C)** merged images from the cortex. Higher magnification images in **(D–F)**. **(G)** YFP, **(H)** anti-ChAT, and **(I)** merged images from the striatum. Higher magnification images in **(J–L)**. Arrows indicating GFP cells.

Figure S5 | A subset of HC ChAT-YFP cells co-localize with calretinin and VIP. (A) Flat-projected confocal image of the HC from a ChAT-Rosa mouse. Immunoreactivity for ChAT-YFP (green), calretinin (CR, blue), and VIP (red) are shown. **(B–E)** Magnified views of a ChAT-YFP cells in CA1 SR **(B)**, CA3 SP **(C)**, hilus **(D)**, and dentate gyrus **(E)**. Filled arrows denote co-localization of CR and/or VIP with ChAT-YFP cells; the open arrow denotes the thorny excrescences on one ChAT-YFP cell in hilus, suggestive of a mossy cell.

REFERENCES

Allen, T. G. J., Abogadie, F. C., and Brown, D. A. (2006). Simultaneous release of glutamate and acetylcholine from single magnocellular "cholinergic" basal forebrain neurons. *J. Neurosci.* 26, 1588–1595. doi: 10.1523/JNEUROSCI.3979-05.2006

Bayraktar, T., Staiger, J. F., Acsády, L., Cozzari, C., Freund, T. F., and Zilles, K. (1997). Co-localization of vasoactive intestinal polypeptide, gamma-aminobutyric acid and choline acetyltransferase in neocortical interneurons of the adult rat. *Brain Res.* 757, 209–217. doi: 10.1016/S0006-8993(97)00218-7

Bhargava, N., Das, M., Edwards, D., Stancescu, M., Kang, J.-F., and Hickman, J. J. (2010). Coexpression of glutamate vesicular transporter (VGLUT1) and choline acetyltransferase (ChAT) proteins in fetal rat hippocampal neurons in culture. *In Vitro Cell. Dev. Biol. Anim.* 46, 685–692. doi: 10.1007/s11626-010-9324-0

Cauli, B., Tong, X.-K., Rancillac, A., Serluca, N., Lambolez, B., Rossier, J., et al. (2004). Cortical GABA interneurons in neurovascular coupling: relays for subcortical vasoactive pathways. *J. Neurosci.* 24, 8940–8949. doi: 10.1523/JNEUROSCI.3065-04.2004

Cauli, B., Zhou, X., Tricoire, L., Toussay, X., and Staiger, J. F. (2014). Revisiting enigmatic cortical calretinin-expressing interneurons. *Front. Neuroanat.* 8:52. doi: 10.3389/fnana.2014.00052

Cea-del Rio, C. A., Lawrence, J. J., Erdelyi, F., Szabo, G., and McBain, C. J. (2011). Cholinergic modulation amplifies the intrinsic oscillatory properties of CA1 hippocampal cholecystokinin-positive interneurons. *J. Physiol.* 589, 609–627. doi: 10.1113/jphysiol.2010.199422

Cea-del Rio, C. A., Lawrence, J. J., Tricoire, L., Erdelyi, F., Szabo, G., and McBain, C. J. (2010). M3 muscarinic acetylcholine receptor expression confers differential cholinergic modulation to neurochemically distinct hippocampal basket cell subtypes. *J. Neurosci.* 30, 6011–6024. doi: 10.1523/JNEUROSCI.5040-09.2010

Chamberland, S., and Topolnik, L. (2012). Inhibitory control of hippocampal inhibitory neurons. *Front. Neurosci.* 6:165. doi: 10.3389/fnins.2012.00165

Chamberland, S., Salesse, C., Topolnik, D., and Topolnik, L. (2010). Synapse-specific inhibitory control of hippocampal feedback inhibitory circuit. *Front. Cell Neurosci.* 4:130. doi: 10.3389/fncel.2010.00130

Cobb, S. R., and Davies, C. H. (2004). Cholinergic modulation of hippocampal cells and circuits. *J. Physiol.* 562, 81–88. doi: 10.1113/jphysiol.2004.076539

Cole, A. E., and Nicoll, R. A. (1983). Acetylcholine mediates a slow synaptic potential in hippocampal pyramidal cells. *Science* 221, 1299–1301.

Coyle, J. T., Price, D. L., and DeLong, M. R. (1983). Alzheimer's disease: a disorder of cortical cholinergic innervation. *Science* 219, 1184–1190.

Dasari, S., and Gulledge, A. T. (2011). M1 and M4 receptors modulate hippocampal pyramidal neurons. *J. Neurophysiol.* 105, 779–792. doi: 10.1152/jn.00686.2010

Dutar, P., Bassant, M. H., Senut, M. C., and Lamour, Y. (1995). The septohippocampal pathway: structure and function of a central cholinergic system. *Physiol. Rev.* 75, 393–427.

Erickson, C. S., Lee, S. J., Barlow-Anacker, A. J., Druckenbrod, N. R., Epstein, M. L., and Gosain, A. (2014). Appearance of cholinergic myenteric neurons during enteric nervous system development: comparison of different ChAT fluorescent mouse reporter lines. *Neurogastroenterol. Motil.* 26, 874–884. doi: 10.1111/nmo.12343

Freund, T. F., and Buzsáki, G. Y. (1996). Interneurons of the hippocampus. *Hippocampus* 6, 347–470. doi: 10.1002/(SICI)1098-1063(1996)6:4<347::AID-HIPO1>3.0.CO;2-I

Frotscher, M., Schlander, M., and Leranth, C. (1986). Cholinergic neurons in the hippocampus. A combined light- and electron-microscopic immunocytochemical study in the rat. *Cell Tissue Res.* 246, 293–301.

Frotscher, M., Vida, I., and Bender, R. (2000). Evidence for the existence of non-GABAergic, cholinergic interneurons in the rodent hippocampus. *Neuroscience* 96, 27–31. doi: 10.1016/s0306-4522(99)00525-4

Gábriel, R., Wilhelm, M., and Straznicky, C. (1992). Microtubule-associated protein 2 (MAP2)-immunoreactive neurons in the retina of Bufo marinus: colocalisation with tyrosine hydroxylase and serotonin in amacrine cells. *Cell Tissue Res.* 269, 175–182.

Geiger, J. R. P., Bischofberger, J., Vida, I., Fröbe, U., Pfitzinger, S., Weber, H. J., et al. (2002). Patch-clamp recording in brain slices with improved slicer technology. *Pflugers Arch.* 443, 491–501. doi: 10.1007/s00424-001-0735-3

Gong, S., Doughty, M., Harbaugh, C. R., Cummins, A., Hatten, M. E., Heintz, N., et al. (2007). Targeting Cre recombinase to specific neuron populations with bacterial artificial chromosome constructs. *J. Neurosci.* 27, 9817–9823. doi: 10.1523/JNEUROSCI.2707-07.2007

Grybko, M. J., Hahm, E.-T., Perrine, W., Parnes, J. A., Chick, W. S., Sharma, G., et al. (2011). A transgenic mouse model reveals fast nicotinic transmission in hippocampal pyramidal neurons. *Eur. J. Neurosci.* 33, 1786–1798. doi: 10.1111/j.1460-9568.2011.07671.x

Hu, W., and Shu, Y. (2012). Axonal bleb recording. *Neurosci. Bull.* 28, 342–350. doi: 10.1007/s12264-012-1247-1

Ivanova, E., Hwang, G. S., and Pan, Z. H. (2010). Characterization of transgenic mouse lines expressing Cre recombinase in the retina. *Neuroscience* 165, 233–243. doi: 10.1016/j.neuroscience.2009.10.021

Klausberger, T., and Somogyi, P. (2008). Neuronal diversity and temporal dynamics: the unity of hippocampal circuit operations. *Science* 321, 53–57. doi: 10.1126/science.1149381

Lawrence, J. J., Statland, J. M., Grinspan, Z. M., and McBain, C. J. (2006). Cell type-specific dependence of muscarinic signalling in mouse hippocampal stratum oriens interneurones. *J. Physiol.* 570, 595–610. doi: 10.1113/jphysiol.2005.100875

Lopes, R., Verhey van Wijk, N., Neves, G., and Pachnis, V. (2012). Transcription factor LIM homeobox 7 (Lhx7) maintains subtype identity of cholinergic interneurons in the mammalian striatum. *Proc. Natl. Acad. Sci. U.S.A.* 109, 3119–3124. doi: 10.1073/pnas.1109251109

López-Bendito, G., Sturgess, K., Erdelyi, F., Szabo, G., Molnár, Z., and Paulsen, O. (2004). Preferential origin and layer destination of GAD65-GFP cortical interneurons. *Cereb. Cortex* 14, 1122–1133. doi: 10.1093/cercor/bhh072

Madisen, L., Zwingman, T. A., Sunkin, S. M., Oh, S. W., Zariwala, H. A., Gu, H., et al. (2009). A robust and high-throughput Cre reporting and characterization system for the whole mouse brain. *Nat. Neurosci.* 13, 133–140. doi: 10.1038/nn.2467

Micheau, J., and Marighetto, A. (2011). Acetylcholine and memory: a long, complex and chaotic but still living relationship. *Behav. Brain Res.* 221, 424–429. doi: 10.1016/j.bbr.2010.11.052

Pepeu, G., and Giovannini, M. G. (2004). Changes in acetylcholine extracellular levels during cognitive processes. *Learn. Mem.* 11, 21–27. doi: 10.1101/lm.68104

Porter, J. T., Cauli, B., Staiger, J. F., Lambolez, B., Rossier, J., and Audinat, E. (1998). Properties of bipolar VIPergic interneurons and their excitation by pyramidal neurons in the rat neocortex. *Eur. J. Neurosci.* 10, 3617–3628. doi: 10.1046/j.1460-9568.1998.00367.x

Porter, J. T., Cauli, B., Tsuzuki, K., Lambolez, B., Rossier, J., and Audinat, E. (1999). Selective excitation of subtypes of neocortical interneurons by nicotinic receptors. *J. Neurosci.* 19, 5228–5235.

Ren, J., Qin, C., Hu, F., Tan, J., Qiu, L., Zhao, S., et al. (2011). Habenula "cholinergic" neurons co-release glutamate and acetylcholine and activate postsynaptic neurons via distinct transmission modes. *Neuron* 69, 445–452. doi: 10.1016/j.neuron.2010.12.038

Romo-Parra, H., Vivar, C., Maqueda, J., Morales, M. A., and Gutiérrez, R. (2003). Activity-dependent induction of multitransmitter signaling onto pyramidal cells and interneurons of hippocampal area CA3. *J. Neurophysiol.* 89, 3155–3167. doi: 10.1152/jn.00985.2002

Scharfman, H. E., and Myers, C. E. (2012). Hilar mossy cells of the dentate gyrus: a historical perspective. *Front. Neural Circuits* 6:106. doi: 10.3389/fncir.2012.00106

Shu, Y., Hasenstaub, A., Duque, A., Yu, Y., and McCormick, D. A. (2006). Modulation of intracortical synaptic potentials by presynaptic somatic membrane potential. *Nature* 441, 761–765. doi: 10.1038/nature04720

Soriano, P. (1999). Generalized lacZ expression with the ROSA26 Cre reporter strain. *Nat. Genet.* 21, 70–71. doi: 10.1038/5007

Srinivas, S., Watanabe, T., Lin, C. S., William, C. M., Tanabe, Y., Jessell, T. M., et al. (2001). Cre reporter strains produced by targeted insertion of EYFP and ECFP into the ROSA26 locus. *BMC Dev. Biol.* 1:4. doi: 10.1186/1471-213X-1-4

Teles-Grilo Ruivo, L. M., and Mellor, J. R. (2013). Cholinergic modulation of hippocampal network function. *Front. Synaptic Neurosci.* 5:2. doi: 10.3389/fnsyn.2013.00002

Tesson, L., Heslan, J.-M., Ménoret, S., and Anegon, I. (2002). Rapid and accurate determination of zygosity in transgenic animals by real-time quantitative PCR. *Transgenic Res.* 11, 43–48. doi: 10.1023/A:1013928600442

Tricoire, L., and Cea-Del Rio, C. A. (2007). Illuminating cholinergic microcircuits in the neocortex. *J. Neurosci.* 27, 12119–12120. doi: 10.1523/JNEUROSCI.3856-07.2007

Tyan, L., Chamberland, S., Magnin, E., Camiré, O., Francavilla, R., David, L. S., et al. (2014). Dendritic inhibition provided by interneuron-specific cells controls the firing rate and timing of the hippocampal feedback inhibitory circuitry. *J. Neurosci.* 34, 4534–4547. doi: 10.1523/JNEUROSCI.3813-13.2014

von Engelhardt, J., Eliava, M., Meyer, A. H., Rozov, A., and Monyer, H. (2007). Functional characterization of intrinsic cholinergic interneurons in the cortex. *J. Neurosci.* 27, 5633–5642. doi: 10.1523/JNEUROSCI.4647-06.2007

Wierenga, C. J., Müllner, F. E., Rinke, I., Keck, T., Stein, V., and Bonhoeffer, T. (2010). Molecular and electrophysiological characterization of GFP-expressing

CA1 interneurons in GAD65-GFP mice. *PLoS ONE* 5:e15915. doi: 10.1371/journal.pone.0015915

Witten, I. B., Lin, S.-C., Brodsky, M., Prakash, R., Diester, I., Anikeeva, P., et al. (2010). Cholinergic interneurons control local circuit activity and cocaine conditioning. *Science* 330, 1677–1681. doi: 10.1126/science.1193771

Yi, F., Ball, J., Stoll, K. E., Satpute, V. C., Mitchell, S. M., Pauli, J. L., et al. (2014). Direct excitation of parvalbumin-positive interneurons by M1 muscarinic acetylcholine receptors: roles in cellular excitability, inhibitory transmission and cognition. *J. Physiol.* 592, 3463–3494. doi: 10.1113/jphysiol.2014.275453

14

Acute human brain responses to intracortical microelectrode arrays: challenges and future prospects

Eduardo Fernández[1,2]*, Bradley Greger[3], Paul A. House[4], Ignacio Aranda[5], Carlos Botella[6], Julio Albisua[7], Cristina Soto-Sánchez[1,2], Arantxa Alfaro[1,2] and Richard A. Normann[8]

[1] *Bioengineering Institute, Miguel Hernández University of Elche, Elche, Spain*
[2] *CIBER-BBN, Zaragoza, Spain*
[3] *School of Biological and Health Systems Engineering, Arizona State University, Tempe, AZ, USA*
[4] *Department of Neurosurgery, University of Utah, Salt Lake City, UT, USA*
[5] *Department of Pathology, Hospital General Universitario, Alicante, Spain*
[6] *Department of Neurosurgery, Hospital La Fe, Valencia, Spain*
[7] *Department of Neurosurgery, Fundación Jimenez Díaz and Hospital Rey Juan Carlos, Madrid, Spain*
[8] *Department of Bioengineering, University of Utah, Salt Lake City, UT, USA*

Edited by:
Ulrich G. Hofmann, University of Freiburg, Germany

Reviewed by:
Winnie Jensen, Aalborg University, Denmark
Tobias Holzhammer, ATLAS Neuroengineering, Belgium

Correspondence:
Eduardo Fernández, Bioengineering Institute, Miguel Hernández University of Elche, Avda. Universidad s/n, Elche 03202, Spain
e-mail: e.fernandez@umh.es

The emerging field of neuroprosthetics is focused on the development of new therapeutic interventions that will be able to restore some lost neural function by selective electrical stimulation or by harnessing activity recorded from populations of neurons. As more and more patients benefit from these approaches, the interest in neural interfaces has grown significantly and a new generation of penetrating microelectrode arrays are providing unprecedented access to the neurons of the central nervous system (CNS). These microelectrodes have active tip dimensions that are similar in size to neurons and because they penetrate the nervous system, they provide selective access to these cells (within a few microns). However, the very long-term viability of chronically implanted microelectrodes and the capability of recording the same spiking activity over long time periods still remain to be established and confirmed in human studies. Here we review the main responses to acute implantation of microelectrode arrays, and emphasize that it will become essential to control the neural tissue damage induced by these intracortical microelectrodes in order to achieve the high clinical potentials accompanying this technology.

Keywords: neural prosthesis, intracortical microelectrode, *in vivo* recording, biocompatibility, neurosurgery

INTRODUCTION

Since 1990, the field of neuroprosthetics has grown at an ever increasing rate. Although current research is also pursuing non-invasive techniques to acquire signals from the human brain, important scientific and clinical information has been gained from *in vivo* experiments with microelectrode arrays able to record or stimulate the nervous system with the aim of improving or replacing motor or sensory abilities that have been lost due to disease or injury. For example, auditory brainstem implants are being used to restore auditory function (Merkus et al., 2014); deep brain stimulators have been implanted successfully in patients for control of motor disorders, tremor, dystonia and chronic pain (Beitz, 2014; Nardone et al., 2014) and micro-array type devices have been implanted in artificial vision systems (Grill et al., 2009; Hatsopoulos and Donoghue, 2009; Normann et al., 2009; Fernandez and Hofmann, 2011). Moreover advances in prosthetic limbs and brain-machine interfaces are now providing hope of increased mobility and independence for amputees and paralyzed patients (Raspopovic et al., 2014) and intracortical micro-electrodes are being used to study epileptiform discharges in cases of intractable epilepsy (Weiss et al., 2013a,b). As more and more patients have benefited from this approach, the interest in neural interfaces has grown significantly and a new generation of penetrating microelectrode arrays are providing unprecedented access to the neurons of the central nervous system (CNS).

These studies have shown the utility of microelectrode recordings to resolve neural activity at the single neuron level and to interpret brain derived commands for fine-grained control of movements and translation of these signals into command signals that are able to control external devices (Hochberg et al., 2006; Andersen et al., 2010; Rao and Donoghue, 2014). However most penetrating microelectrode arrays currently have maximum *in vivo* lifetimes from several months to a few years (Suner et al., 2005; Prasad et al., 2012; Barrese et al., 2013). Therefore much work still needs to be done before these penetrating microelectrodes can be used for many clinical purposes. In this work we focused on the acute effects of implantation of penetrating microelectrode arrays in the human brain, emphasizing the relevance of surgical techniques and biocompatibility approaches to control the neural tissue damage induced by these intracortical probes in order to achieve the therapeutic benefits envisioned by these neural interfaces.

CURRENT MULTIELECTRODE-ARRAY TECHNOLOGIES

Technology partially achieved during the development of cardiac pacemakers has been successfully used in many other applications of implanted neural prostheses. During these years great efforts have been made to develop penetrating multi-electrode arrays with dimensions similar to the cortical neurons they target for recording or stimulation and that are able to maintain a stable signal in the CNS. The two main dominant approaches are multiple insulated metal microwires (Nicolelis and Lebedev, 2009; Freire et al., 2011; Carmena, 2013) and penetrating microelectrode arrays fabricated with micro-electro-mechanical-system technologies. These devices use various substrate materials that can either be flexible and based on polymers (Rousche et al., 2001; Chen et al., 2009; Kozai and Kipke, 2009; Hassler et al., 2011) or rigid such as the Utah Electrode Array (UEA; Normann, 2007), the Michigan array (Seymour and Kipke, 2007) or the NeuroProbes arrays (Neves, 2007; Calixto et al., 2013). However today, only a few of these devices are commercially available and do not yet exist as commercial, wireless, implantable, many-channel devices that can provide reliable recording and stimulation for many years.

An ideal neural interface would consist of an array containing many microelectrodes, which can "listen" and "talk" to still-functioning parts of the brain enabling bi-directional communication with ensembles of neurons. Each microelectrode would either record the electrical activity of a small population of neurons surrounding it or, when electrical current is passed through the electrode, activate small population of neurons. This approach has been difficult to realize because of the acute and chronic inflammatory reactions that can induce significant changes at the brain-electrode interface. Thus all neural probes need a stable electronic/neural interface that enables selective recording and/or activation of specific groups of neurons without deterioration of the electrodes or surrounding neural tissue. Consequently three areas have to be considered: the "*biosafety*", the "*biofunctionality*" and the "*biostability*" of the devices. Biosafety means that the microelectrodes do not harm the brain tissue in any significant way, biofunctionality is related to the ability of the microelectrodes to perform their intended function, and biostability means that the whole microelectrode array must not be susceptible to attack of biological fluids, proteases, macrophages or any metabolic byproducts (Marin and Fernandez, 2010). In addition successful devices should manifest "biotolerability" or the ability of the multielectrode-array to reside in the CNS for long periods of time. All these considerations impose extreme demands on stability and function of neural implants and place unique constraints on the architecture, materials, and surgical techniques used in the application of intracortical microelectrodes.

SURGICAL PROCEDURES FOR IMPLANTATION OF INTRACORTICAL MICROELECTRODES ARRAYS

Microelectrode arrays aimed to simultaneously record or stimulate neuronal populations have been successfully used in many animal models including non-human primates (Normann, 2007). However the only intracortical microelectrode array that has been FDA approved for long-term human studies is the UEA (Nordhausen et al., 1996). This microelectrode array consists of 100 small diameter silicon microneedles, built on a square grid with 400 μm spacing, that were designed to be inserted into the cerebral cortex to a depth of 1.5 mm, the level of thalamic input to the cerebral cortex (**Figure 1A**).

The UEA has been used in BrainGate clinical trials (Hochberg et al., 2006; Homer et al., 2013; Perge et al., 2013) and in research with epilepsy patients (Normann et al., 2009; Truccolo et al., 2011; Weiss et al., 2013a,b), and we have performed a number of preliminary experiments designed to establish the safety of the implantation procedures (House et al., 2006). These experiments were performed in persons suffering from epilepsy or brain tumors that had to undergo a surgical resection of a brain region. Briefly after exposure of the implantation site using standard neurosurgical equipment and procedures, the pia arachnoid was cut to allow access to the surface of the cerebral cortex. Even though the individual electrodes of the UEA are very sharp (with radius curvatures typically on the order of a few microns) we found that trying to push 100 electrodes into cortical tissues only depressed the surface of the tissue and resulted in only partial insertion of the electrode array. A pneumatically actuated precision instrument that allows the complete and safe insertion of the array in under 200 ms was developed to circumvent this difficulty (Rousche and Normann, 1992). Interestingly we found that it was necessary to fine adjust the parameters of the pneumatic inserter depending of the age of the patients, and that it was easier to get a complete insertion in young than in aged patients using low insertion pressures (around 15–20 psi).

HUMAN ACUTE REACTIVE RESPONSES AROUND IMPLANTED MICROELECTRODES

Implantation of any neural probe is always a traumatic procedure that implies some local damage of neurons, vasculature and other cells (**Figures 1C,D**). Thus, when a neural probe is inserted into the brain, some neurons and glial cells are killed or injured during insertion, blood vessels are disrupted, and the blood-brain barrier is compromised (**Figures 2A,B**). As a result, with most of our microelectrode array insertions in human cortex, we typically observed interstitial microhemorrhages emanating from the electrode tracks that extended in one or more directions. These microhemorrhages were limited to within a few millimeters of the microelectrode tracks although these were more evident around the edges of the arrays. This damage seemed to result from a combination of the numerous blood vessels encountered in the path of the penetrating electrodes plus some mechanical damage of small capillaries, especially at the borders of the array. Furthermore although the insertion of the UEA did not result in clinically relevant hemorrhages, some times we found petechial hemorrhages located below the tips of the electrodes (**Figures 2C,D**).

These microhemorrhages usually stopped spontaneously or after gentle irrigation with normal saline and we do not have any case where we had to remove the array due to the bleeding.

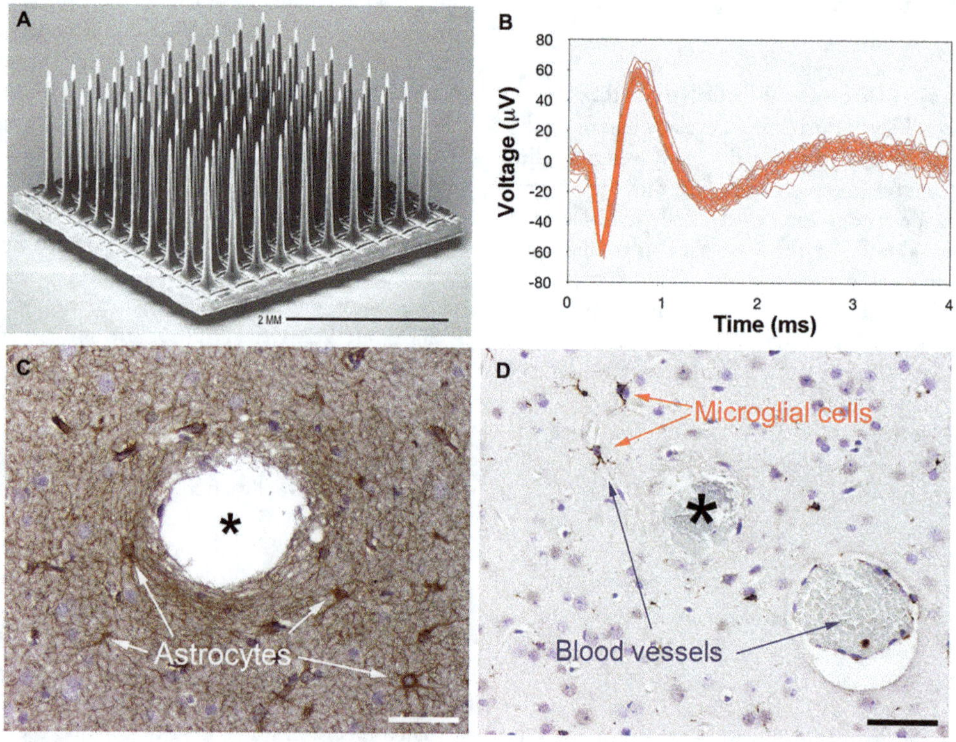

FIGURE 1 | Photographs showing the silicon-based Utah Electrode Array (UEA) and representative results of its implantation into human cortex. **(A)** Scanning electron micrograph of the UEA. **(B)** Single-unit responses recorded with the UEA from human temporal cortex (47 superimposed traces). **(C)** Astrocytes, labeled here with anti-glial fibrillary acidic protein antibody (GFAP) increase the thickness of their main processes, especially around electrode tracks (asterisk). **(D)** Resident microglial cells and blood-borne macrophages, labeled here with anti-CD45 antibody, become activated and migrate toward the electrodes. Note the electrode track filled with blood cells (asterisk) and a nearby blood vessel. Calibration bars = 50 μm.

However, due to this small bleeding various serum plasma proteins and blood cells stick on the surface of the electrodes and trigger complement system activation, platelet activation, clot formation and a large network of changes including the release of cytokines, invasion of blood-borne macrophages and edema. **Figure 2E** shows an example of the tip of an electrode after explantation. Many red blood cells are seen in close contact with electrode materials (see **Figure 2F**). Thus, microhemorrhaging is an important issue that should be taken into account to reduce the adverse nature of the reactions and maintain an ideal environment for the microelectrodes.

Array implantation also causes an early activation and migration of microglial cells towards the microelectrodes, which could reflect highly specific interactions mediated by selectins, integrins, cytokines and carbohydrate-binding receptors (Kaur et al., 2010; Linnartz et al., 2012). These microglial cells are very sensitive to pathological conditions, even if they respond only to variations in local extracellular ionic concentrations (Kreutzberg, 1996; Freire et al., 2011) and we have found that there is a rapid activation, in a matter of minutes, of these cells in human brain. **Figure 1D** shows an example in an experiment in which the UEA was kept in place for <10 min.

Usually these scavenger cells form a network of immune alert resident macrophages with a capacity for immune surveillance and control. Therefore the initial activation and migration of microglial cells are likely beneficial and include production of neurotrophic substances and cell adhesion molecules, which support injured neurons and appear necessary for restorative events to take place (Eddleston and Mucke, 1993). However, this largely beneficial initial phase can result in a more adverse long-term response that is dependent on the extent of the injury. Consequently more effort is needed to control these responses and ensure the function of the implant without eliciting either structural, cellular or metabolic changes that compromise the microelectrode array performance and/or that result in tissue degeneration around the implanted microelectrodes.

ELECTROPHYSIOLOGICAL RECORDINGS

As has been shown from experiments in rodents and non-human primates (Oliveira and Dimitrov, 2008), we found that the quality of the surgical implantation procedure plays a major role for tissue preservation and for the outcome of recordings. Our experimental results have demonstrated that high-quality microelectrode recordings from cerebral cortical neurons can be consistently obtained in both acute (intraoperative) and short term chronic (in an epilepsy monitoring unit) settings. An example of action potentials recorded with a UEA in the temporal cortex of a patient with medically intractable epilepsy is shown in **Figure 1B**. Single units are easily identifiable with a quality similar to that observed in rat, cat or non-human primate recordings. Furthermore,

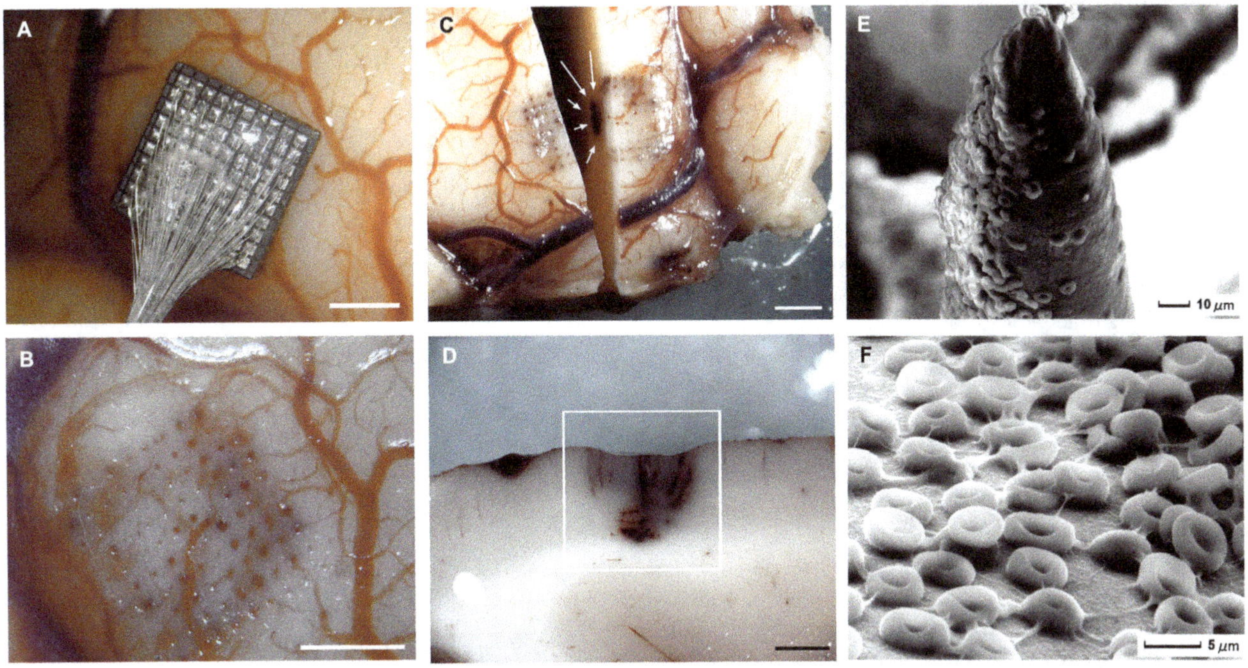

FIGURE 2 | Gross specimens of human temporal lobe implantations and scanning micrographs of the surface of the Utah Electrode Array after acute implantation in human brain. (A) Placement of an electrode array in temporal cortex. **(B)** Once the array has been removed there are some evident microhemorrhages. **(C)** Horizontal section showing blood in the outermost electrode tracks and petechial hemorrhages (white arrows) located below the tip of the electrodes. **(D)** Detail of the petechial hemorrhages. **(E)** Scanning electron micrograph of an electrode tip. Many red blood cells appear in close contact with electrode materials. **(F)** Detail of the red blood cells on the surface of the microelectrodes. Calibration bars A, B, C and D= 2 mm.

most of the presently available intracortical microelectrode arrays (including the UEA) allow recording of local field potentials that are very reliable and that can be used to detect changes in recording quality over time. Also, recording quality is affected by other surgical procedures: most drugs used for the induction and maintenance of general anesthesia decrease action potential firing rates and the information processing capacity in the neocortex (Hanrahan et al., 2013). In addition local fluctuation in K^+ and Ca^+ due to acute initial trauma can induce the silencing of neurons in the proximity of microelectrodes. Consequently recording sessions are usually initiated between 3–10 days after implantation.

The ability of intracortical microelectrodes arrays such as the UEA to record single units from human cortical neurons demonstrates that the implantation can be done without major complications, and emphasizes its potential role for studying encoding and processing of sensory and motor information by large neuronal ensembles. However significant variations in spike waveforms across time have been reported (Parker et al., 2011). These variations could reflect the initial acute response that can lead to chronic inflammatory reactions. Such reactions can negatively impact neurons and microelectrodes via induction of glial proliferation that produces a slow progressive decline in spike amplitude and in the number of viable channels. Furthermore recordings from individual neurons made with penetrating microelectrodes are often lost but then recover, possibly because of micro-motion of the device relative to the neural tissue (Parker et al., 2011). This problem can be mitigated with sophisticated action potential identification and daily recalibration.

CHALLENGES AND FUTURE WORK

Intracortical microelectrode arrays have several advantages over traditional macroelectrode brain electrophysiological techniques such as their ability to selectively access individual or small groups of cortical neurons and the possibility to deliver relevant spatio-temporal patterns of stimulation. This highlights their potential to restore some lost neural function through selective electrical stimulation or by recording activity from selected populations of neurons. Furthermore the procedures for the implantation of penetrating microelectrodes are straightforward and well within the reach of most well-trained neurosurgeons. Altogether these results suggest that intracortical microelectrodes could form the basis of new neuroprosthetic devices for treating many disorders of the nervous system. For example they are presently being used to obtain volitional command signals from primary motor cortex of people with high cervical spinal injuries or to provide a limited but useful sense of vision in profoundly blind. However the presence of acute inflammatory reactions that can lead to chronic inflammatory reactions affecting both the neural tissue and the surface of the microelectrodes must be better understood and new approaches pursued to mitigate these reactions. Controlling and reducing the neural tissue damage induced by these intracortical microelectrodes should aid in keeping these devices biologically and electrically viable for many years.

Factors affecting brain tissue reactions to intracortical microelectrodes include the mechanical trauma during insertion, implantation method, biological acute responses and the physical properties of the microelectrodes. Because the brain is so richly vascularized, we have observed that there is inevitable bleeding associated with electrode array insertion and this suggests that bleeding is an important issue that should be taken into account to reduce the neural tissue damage induced by the microelectrodes. Moreover the reliability of recording the same spiking activity over long time periods still remains an unresolved problem that must be solved in longer term human studies before these penetrating microelectrodes can be used for some clinical purposes.

In this framework, important criteria for clinical success are tissue and microelectrode preservation and the maintenance of a stable signal in the CNS for the longest time possible. Remarkable progress has been reported in the use of these penetrating microelectrode arrays, but the electrode-tissue interface remains one of the major obstacles. Intracortical microelectrodes need a stable electronic/neural interface that facilitates selective recording and/or activation of specific groups of neurons without damage to the electrodes or surrounding neural tissues. Consequently it is essential to better understand the signals that lead to neuroglial activation in human brain and to create a targeted intervention strategy to prevent or at least to control this response.

Progress in this area relies on scientists being able to integrate and utilize methodologies from disparate disciplines, such as biomedical engineering, biomaterials, neuroscience, neurology, neurosurgery, information and communication technologies, molecular biology, etc. We are optimistic that with an emphasis on collaboration and a concerted push for additional clinical trials, these technologies will form the basis of devices and therapies that will substantially reduce the burden of lost neurological functions. However progress will be incremental and researchers must avoid creating false expectations that could damage the credibility of these new technologies.

ACKNOWLEDGMENT

This work has been supported in part by grants MAT2012-39290-C02-01 from the Spanish Government, by the National Organization of the Spanish Blind (ONCE).

REFERENCES

Andersen, R. A., Hwang, E. J., and Mulliken, G. H. (2010). Cognitive neural prosthetics. *Annu. Rev. Psychol.* 61, 169–190, C1–C3. doi: 10.1146/annurev.psych.093008.100503

Barrese, J. C., Rao, N., Paroo, K., Triebwasser, C., Vargas-Irwin, C., Franquemont, L., et al. (2013). Failure mode analysis of silicon-based intracortical microelectrode arrays in non-human primates. *J. Neural Eng.* 10, 1–23. doi: 10.1088/1741-2560/10/6/066014

Beitz, J. M. (2014). Parkinson's disease: a review. *Front. Biosci. (Schol. Ed.)* 6, 65–74. doi: 10.2741/s415

Calixto, R., Salamat, B., Rode, T., Hartmann, T., Volckaerts, B., Ruther, P., et al. (2013). Investigation of a new electrode array technology for a central auditory prosthesis. *PLoS One* 8:e82148. doi: 10.1371/journal.pone.0082148

Carmena, J. M. (2013). Advances in neuroprosthetic learning and control. *PLoS Biol.* 11:e1001561. doi: 10.1371/journal.pbio.1001561

Chen, Y. Y., Lai, H. Y., Lin, S. H., Cho, C. W., Chao, W. H., Liao, C. H., et al. (2009). Design and fabrication of a polyimide-based microelectrode array: application in neural recording and repeatable electrolytic lesion in rat brain. *J. Neurosci. Methods* 182, 6–16. doi: 10.1016/j.jneumeth.2009.05.010

Eddleston, M., and Mucke, L. (1993). Molecular profile of reactive astrocytes–implications for their role in neurologic disease. *Neuroscience* 54, 15–36. doi: 10.1016/0306-4522(93)90380-x

Fernandez, E., and Hofmann, K. (2011). "Visual prosthesis," in *Handbook of Medical Technology*, eds R. Kramme, K.-P. Hoffmann and R. S. Pozos (Würburg: Springer), 821–834.

Freire, M. A., Morya, E., Faber, J., Santos, J. R., Guimaraes, J. S., Lemos, N. A., et al. (2011). Comprehensive analysis of tissue preservation and recording quality from chronic multielectrode implants. *PLoS One* 6:e27554. doi: 10.1371/journal.pone.0027554

Grill, W. M., Norman, S. E., and Bellamkonda, R. V. (2009). Implanted neural interfaces: biochallenges and engineered solutions. *Annu. Rev. Biomed. Eng.* 11, 1–24. doi: 10.1146/annurev-bioeng-061008-124927

Hanrahan, S. J., Greger, B., Parker, R. A., Ogura, T., Obara, S., Egan, T. D., et al. (2013). The effects of propofol on local field potential spectra, action potential firing rate and their temporal relationship in humans and felines. *Front. Hum. Neurosci.* 7:136. doi: 10.3389/fnhum.2013.00136

Hassler, C., Guy, J., Nietzschmann, M., Staiger, J. F., and Stieglitz, T. (2011). Chronic intracortical implantation of saccharose-coated flexible shaft electrodes into the cortex of rats. *Conf. Proc. IEEE Eng. Med. Biol. Soc.* 2011, 644–647. doi: 10.1109/IEMBS.2011.6090143

Hatsopoulos, N. G., and Donoghue, J. P. (2009). The science of neural interface systems. *Annu. Rev. Neurosci.* 32, 249–266. doi: 10.1146/annurev.neuro.051508.135241

Hochberg, L. R., Serruya, M. D., Friehs, G. M., Mukand, J. A., Saleh, M., Caplan, A. H., et al. (2006). Neuronal ensemble control of prosthetic devices by a human with tetraplegia. *Nature* 442, 164–171. doi: 10.1038/nature04970

Homer, M. L., Nurmikko, A. V., Donoghue, J. P., and Hochberg, L. R. (2013). Sensors and decoding for intracortical brain computer interfaces. *Annu. Rev. Biomed. Eng.* 15, 383–405. doi: 10.1146/annurev-bioeng-071910-124640

House, P. A., Macdonald, J. D., Tresco, P. A., and Normann, R. A. (2006). Acute microelectrode array implantation into human neocortex: preliminary technique and histological considerations. *Neurosurg. Focus* 20, 1–4. doi: 10.3171/foc.2006.20.5.5

Kaur, G., Han, S. J., Yang, I., and Crane, C. (2010). Microglia and central nervous system immunity. *Neurosurg. Clin. N. Am.* 21, 43–51. doi: 10.1016/j.nec.2009.08.009

Kozai, T. D., and Kipke, D. R. (2009). Insertion shuttle with carboxyl terminated self-assembled monolayer coatings for implanting flexible polymer neural probes in the brain. *J. Neurosci. Methods* 184, 199–205. doi: 10.1016/j.jneumeth.2009.08.002

Kreutzberg, G. W. (1996). Microglia: a sensor for pathological events in the CNS. *Trends Neurosci.* 19, 312–318. doi: 10.1016/0166-2236(96)10049-7

Linnartz, B., Bodea, L. G., and Neumann, H. (2012). Microglial carbohydrate-binding receptors for neural repair. *Cell Tissue Res.* 349, 215–227. doi: 10.1007/s00441-012-1342-7

Marin, C., and Fernandez, E. (2010). Biocompatibility of intracortical microelectrodes: current status and future prospects. *Front. Neuroeng.* 3:8. doi: 10.3389/fneng.2010.00008

Merkus, P., Di Lella, F., Di Trapani, G., Pasanisi, E., Beltrame, M. A., Zanetti, D., et al. (2014). Indications and contraindications of auditory brainstem implants: systematic review and illustrative cases. *Eur. Arch. Otorhinolaryngol.* 271, 3–13. doi: 10.1007/s00405-013-2378-3

Nardone, R., Holler, Y., Leis, S., Holler, P., Thon, N., Thomschewski, A., et al. (2014). Invasive and non-invasive brain stimulation for treatment of neuropathic pain in patients with spinal cord injury: a review. *J. Spinal Cord. Med.* 37, 19–31. doi: 10.1179/2045772313y.0000000140

Neves, H. (2007). Advances in cerebral probing using modular multifunctional probe arrays. *Med. Device Technol.* 18, 38–39.

Nicolelis, M. A., and Lebedev, M. A. (2009). Principles of neural ensemble physiology underlying the operation of brain-machine interfaces. *Nat. Rev. Neurosci.* 10, 530–540. doi: 10.1038/nrn2653

Nordhausen, C. T., Maynard, E. M., and Normann, R. A. (1996). Single unit recording capabilities of a 100 microelectrode array. *Brain Res.* 726, 129–140. doi: 10.1016/s0006-8993(96)00321-6

Normann, R. A. (2007). Technology insight: future neuroprosthetic therapies for disorders of the nervous system. *Nat. Clin. Pract. Neurol.* 3, 444–452. doi: 10.1038/ncpneuro0556

Normann, R. A., Greger, B., House, P., Romero, S. F., Pelayo, F., and Fernandez, E. (2009). Toward the development of a cortically based visual neuroprosthesis. *J. Neural Eng.* 6:035001. doi: 10.1088/1741-2560/6/3/035001

Oliveira, L. M. O., and Dimitrov, D. (2008). "Surgical techniques for chronic implantation of microwire arrays in rodents and primates," in *Methods for Neural Ensemble Recordings.* 2nd Edn., ed M. A. L. Nicolelis (Boca Raton, FL: CRC Press), 21–46.

Parker, R. A., Davis, T. S., House, P. A., Normann, R. A., and Greger, B. (2011). The functional consequences of chronic, physiologically effective intracortical microstimulation. *Prog. Brain Res.* 194, 145–165. doi: 10.1016/b978-0-444-53815-4.00010-8

Perge, J. A., Homer, M. L., Malik, W. Q., Cash, S., Eskandar, E., Friehs, G., et al. (2013). Intra-day signal instabilities affect decoding performance in an intracortical neural interface system. *J. Neural Eng.* 10:036004. doi: 10.1088/1741-2560/10/3/036004

Prasad, A., Xue, Q. S., Sankar, V., Nishida, T., Shaw, G., Streit, W. J., et al. (2012). Comprehensive characterization and failure modes of tungsten microwire arrays in chronic neural implants. *J. Neural Eng.* 9:056015. doi: 10.1088/1741-2560/9/5/056015

Rao, N. G., and Donoghue, J. P. (2014). Cue to action processing in motor cortex populations. *J. Neurophysiol.* 111, 441–453. doi: 10.1152/jn.00274.2013

Raspopovic, S., Capogrosso, M., Petrini, F. M., Bonizzato, M., Rigosa, J., Di Pino, G., et al. (2014). Restoring natural sensory feedback in real-time bidirectional hand prostheses. *Sci. Transl. Med.* 6:222ra219. doi: 10.1126/scitranslmed.3006820

Rousche, P. J., and Normann, R. A. (1992). A method for pneumatically inserting an array of penetrating electrodes into cortical tissue. *Ann. Biomed. Eng.* 20, 413–422. doi: 10.1007/bf02368133

Rousche, P. J., Pellinen, D. S., Pivin, D. P. Jr., Williams, J. C., Vetter, R. J., and Kipke, D. R. (2001). Flexible polyimide-based intracortical electrode arrays with bioactive capability. *IEEE Trans. Biomed. Eng.* 48, 361–371. doi: 10.1109/10.914800

Seymour, J. P., and Kipke, D. R. (2007). Neural probe design for reduced tissue encapsulation in CNS. *Biomaterials* 28, 3594–3607. doi: 10.1016/j.biomaterials.2007.03.024

Suner, S., Fellows, M. R., Vargas-Irwin, C., Nakata, G. K., and Donoghue, J. P. (2005). Reliability of signals from a chronically implanted, silicon-based electrode array in non-human primate primary motor cortex. *IEEE Trans. Neural Syst. Rehabil. Eng.* 13, 524–541. doi: 10.1109/tnsre.2005.857687

Truccolo, W., Donoghue, J. A., Hochberg, L. R., Eskandar, E. N., Madsen, J. R., Anderson, W. S., et al. (2011). Single-neuron dynamics in human focal epilepsy. *Nat. Neurosci.* 14, 635–641. doi: 10.1038/nn.2782

Weiss, S. A., Banks, G. P., Mckhann, G. M. Jr., Goodman, R. R., Emerson, R. G., Trevelyan, A. J., et al. (2013a). Ictal high frequency oscillations distinguish two types of seizure territories in humans. *Brain* 136, 3796–3808. doi: 10.1093/brain/awt276

Weiss, S. A., Mckhann, G. Jr., Goodman, R., Emerson, R. G., Trevelyan, A., Bikson, M., et al. (2013b). Field effects and ictal synchronization: insights from in homine observations. *Front. Hum. Neurosci.* 7:828. doi: 10.3389/fnhum.2013.00828

15

Anti-inflammatory polymer electrodes for glial scar treatment: bringing the conceptual idea to future results

Maria Asplund[1,2,3]*, Christian Boehler[1,2,3] and Thomas Stieglitz[1,3]

[1] Biomedical Microtechnology, IMTEK, Albert-Ludwigs Universität, Freiburg, Germany
[2] Freiburg Institute for Advanced Studies FRIAS, Albert-Ludwigs Universität, Freiburg, Germany
[3] BrainLinks-BrainTools Cluster of Excellence, Albert-Ludwigs Universität, Freiburg, Germany

Edited by:
Ulrich G. Hofmann, Albert-Ludwigs-University Freiburg, Germany

Reviewed by:
Pascal Darbon, Université de Strasbourg, France
Fabrice O. Morin, Fatronik-Tecnalia Foundation, Spain

***Correspondence:**
Maria Asplund, Biomedical Microtechnology, IMTEK, Albert-Ludwigs Universität, Georges-Köhler Allee 102, Freiburg 79108, Germany
e-mail: maria.asplund@imtek.de

Conducting polymer films offer a convenient route for the functionalization of implantable microelectrodes without compromising their performance as excellent recording units. A micron thick coating, deposited on the surface of a regular metallic electrode, can elute anti-inflammatory drugs for the treatment of glial scarring as well as growth factors for the support of surrounding neurons. Electro-activation of the polymer drives the release of the substance and should ideally provide a reliable method for controlling quantity and timing of release. Driving signals in the form of a constant potential (CP), a slow redox sweep or a fast pulse are all represented in literature. Few studies present such release *in vivo* from actual recording and stimulating microelectronic devices. It is essential to bridge the gap between studies based on release *in vitro,* and the intended application, which would mean release into living and highly delicate tissue. In the biological setting, signals are limited both by available electronics and by the biological safety. Driving signals must not be harmful to tissue and also not activate the tissue in an uncontrolled manner. This review aims at shedding more light on how to select appropriate driving parameters for the polymer electrodes for the *in vivo* setting. It brings together information regarding activation thresholds for neurons, as well as injury thresholds, and puts this into context with what is known about efficient driving of release from conducting polymer films.

Keywords: conducting polymer, dexamethasone, drug delivery, glial scarring, neural interfaces

INTRODUCTION

Recent advances in the field of conducting polymers point out their potential as drug delivery coatings from the surfaces of microelectrodes. This is of interest considering it comprises an opportunity to target cells in the close vicinity of an implant with high spatial and temporal control of release. Glial scarring is a physiological process that deteriorates electrode function by forming a substantial barrier for signal transduction. Persistent inflammation, following the scarring process, is believed to be the reason why neurons are lost at the site of the implant further complicating high resolution in recording and stimulation (Turner et al., 1999; Szarowski et al., 2003; Biran et al., 2005). Systemic treatment using anti-inflammatory drugs such as Dexamethasone (Dex) has been suggested as a possible strategy for facilitating close integration of the implant with neural tissue (Spataro et al., 2005). Conducting polymer electrodes designed to elute drugs upon electro-activation are an alternative to systemic treatment of glial scarring (Abidian et al., 2006; Wadhwa et al., 2006; Evans et al., 2009; Richardson et al., 2009; Luo and Cui, 2009a,b; Stevenson et al., 2010; Yue et al., 2013). Polymers in question are mainly Polypyrrole (PPy), poly(3,4-ethylene dioxythiophene) (PEDOT) but more recently also polyterthiophene (PTTh) has been suggested as a candidate (Stevenson et al., 2010). This functionality is until now almost exclusively studied *in vitro*. Here we discuss this intriguing possibility, its requirements in terms of electronic control of the implant, and the restrictions set by electrochemical safety limits, to form the basis for continued investigations *in vivo*.

Electro-activation is essential for triggering release but cannot be allowed to cause detrimental effects on the cellular microenvironment. The conducting polymer electrode is not analogous to a metallic electrode and direct currents can, and must, to some extent be tolerated to drive drugs out of the electrode. On the other hand, one must not overlook the possibility that by-products form in body fluids as a result of electro-activation, or that the neuronal circuitry is unintentionally activated, which means that potentials must be kept within strict boundaries. The solution that comes close at hand is to ensure that signals are maintained below the activation threshold. Then the question boils down to if this type of signal can be used to drive ionic drugs out of the electrode? The majority of studies focus on release by cyclic voltammetry (CV), a signal sufficiently slow to give room for diffusion limited processes to contribute, in contrast to fast stimulation pulses, generally designed to employ primarily capacitive effects.

Studies show that release can be precisely managed by the appropriate electrochemical driving signal. However, the means to keep exact control of charge and voltage are limited in an implant where three-electrode electrochemical systems are rarely implemented. Furthermore, the circuitry designed for stimulation *in vivo* cannot necessarily accommodate the same type of measurements and control as the electrochemical potentiostat.

Therefore, electronics and implantable reference electrodes that meet this requirement need to be developed. If glial scarring is really to be treated by the suggested method it cannot come at the cost of connecting lab animals to fully functional external potentiostats but the solution must come as a miniaturized implant.

Finally we intend to outline the possibilities in terms of quantities of drugs that can be delivered and, to some extent, the variety of drugs that could come in question. Most studies focus on delivery of the anti-inflammatory drug Dex but results point out that other drugs with similar size and charge could also be potential candidates.

In summary, we present the possibilities of conducting polymer based release for glial scar treatment. Benefits of the method will be put in perspective with design challenges that have to be met from the electronics side. This information is essential for enabling more studies to proceed to the implant stage, shedding light on how to make the best out of this novel and exciting concept.

ELECTRODEPOSITION OF CONDUCTING POLYMERS

Conducting polymers can be deposited on top of microelectrodes using an aqueous electrodeposition process. The reaction is driven in a supporting electrolyte in which the monomer (M) is dissolved or dispersed together with appropriate counter ions (CI). The monomers oxidized at the surface of the working electrode build up an insoluble layer of conducting polymer on its surface. To maintain charge neutrality, the negatively charged CI are at the same time electrostatically entrapped in the formed material according to the following reaction:

$$M + CI^{-} \xrightarrow{oxidize} (M)^{+}CI^{-} \tag{1}$$

The nature of the counter ion is decisive for the ionic exchange properties of the formed polymer (Bobacka et al., 2000; Jager et al., 2000). The CI can be small or large, inorganic or organic molecules, or a combination of several different negatively charged molecules can be included in the supporting electrolyte to form a more complex material. If a biologically relevant molecule is used as counter ion, the formed polymer can be biofunctionalized since the molecule is efficiently entrapped in the porous polymer matrix yet still available for reactions on the surface of the polymer material (Asplund et al., 2008). In addition it can be released from the polymer upon altering the polymer redox state.

There are some restrictions in the choice of biological ions that can come in question for the counter ion incorporation technique. The one step approach described above would work exclusively for negatively charged biomolecules. For the delivery functionality to be efficient, a further constraint is that the molecule must be sufficiently small to be able to diffuse through the polymer matrix. It is difficult to give a precise estimate on what could be considered as sufficiently small, since the porosity is not an absolute property but can be influenced by the electrodeposition process. To give some figure of merit, successful release has been shown for molecules up to the range of 0.5 kDa. Although some authors report release of substantially larger substances such as protein fragments, it is clear that this is more challenging and might primarily rely on actuation of the polymer material rather than electrostatic binding and release (Thompson et al., 2006; Evans et al., 2009; Richardson et al., 2009). This topic is discussed in detail in section Release Systems and Mechanisms.

As an alternative to the direct incorporation in Equation 1, an ion exchange approach can be used to drive ions into the already formed polymer film for subsequent release upon reversing the potential (Xiao et al., 2007). Furthermore, a carrier phase can be introduced into the material by allowing the polymer to form within a network of beads or fibers already containing the substance to be delivered (Abidian et al., 2006; Luo et al., 2011). A non-charged substance in the larger size range, which is made available in the supporting electrolyte, can be adsorbed to the surface in parallel with the deposition process and thereby also be mechanically entrapped although not electrostatically bound (Asplund et al., 2008). All these methods could in principle lead to a material with controlled delivery functionality similar to what is accomplished with the direct incorporation technique. The release dynamics can however be expected to differ. The focus of this review is primarily on controlled release based on direct incorporation according to Equation 1, although some results based on materials using other methods are also included.

Dex DELIVERY—QUANTITIES AND EFFICIENCY

The theoretically possible inclusion of Dex in a polymer film, based on the counter ion incorporation technique, can be estimated by Equation 2 (Skotheim and Reynolds, 2006):

$$m_{dopant} = \frac{Q_{dep}}{F} \cdot \frac{\gamma M_{dopant}}{2 + \gamma} \tag{2}$$

F stands for Faraday's constant and equals 96485 C/mol and Q_{dep} stands for deposition charge. With Dex as dopant, the commonly accepted assumption that the doping level $\gamma = 0.3$, and the molecular weight of Dex, $M_{Dex} = 392$ g/mol, Dex inclusion per charge consumed in the electrodeposition process would be approximately 700 μg/C. The deposition charge density that would be considered reasonable varies, depending on the stability of the polymer system, but 300 mC/cm^2 would clearly be within the realistic range. This would mean a total included Dex mass $m_{Dex} = 210$ μg/cm^2 according to Equation 2. Most likely higher deposition charges could be used (Li and Huang, 2007).

A handful of papers point out the Dex levels that would be required for efficient treatment of glial scarring. Based on the assumption that the volume of interest could be defined as a sphere of radius 500 μm enclosing the electrode (Wadhwa et al., 2006), and that an efficient concentration would be expected to lie within the range 0.2–1 μM (Golde et al., 2003; Shain et al., 2003; Zhong et al., 2005), further assuming a microelectrode radius of ~15 μm, the electrode would need to be able to deliver a concentration of 6–30 μg/cm^2 from its surface.

Considering various papers report delivery of Dex in the range 3–126 μg/cm^2 in total, several single efficient doses would be possible with the presented technology (Wadhwa et al., 2006; Moulton et al., 2008; Stevenson et al., 2010; Sirivisoot et al.,

2011; Xiao et al., 2012). In light of these values one might argue that optimizing control is even more important than maximizing output per pulse or sweep.

RELEASE SYSTEMS AND MECHANISMS

The drug delivery from a conducting polymer is a result of the interplay between electrostatic interaction with the surrounding electrolyte, mechanical actuation of the film as a response to the different swelling states upon redox, and conformational changes in the polymer structure. To which extent each of the mechanisms contributes varies depending on the film morphology, the triggering signal and the use of any additional CI and must therefore be evaluated separately for each case. Three types of triggering signals are considered here namely redox sweeping, constant potential (CP) and pulsing (**Figure 1**). Redox sweeping is mainly referred to as the electrochemical measurement term CV.

The most simple release system would be a one-layer deposition where an anionic drug is included as a counter ion directly in the deposition process. Assuming that the drug is thereby homogenously distributed within the polymer film, and electrostatic interaction is the only responsible mechanism, the quantity of drug that is released should be proportional to the applied charge. This simplified view would imply that it is only the absolute charge transfer over the interface that matters for the quantity of drug delivered, regardless of if the charge is delivered as a pulse or a sweep. However, this is a crude simplification for a vastly more complex process (Kontturi et al., 1998; Majumdar et al., 2008). In fact, experimental data shows that the dynamics of the release signal greatly matters for the outcome.

In **Table 1** a short compilation of release trigger signals and experienced results from different conducting polymer based release systems can be seen. Signals vary from steady potentials over slow CV sweeps to faster pulsed signals. From the experimental data reported in these studies it is evident that release is not solely ruled by charge transfer. Multiple ions contribute to charge transfer making the direct correlation of interfacial charge transfer to delivery of a specific species less trivial (Pyo et al., 1994; Jager et al., 2000; Pernaut and Reynolds, 2000; Li and Huang, 2007).

Some early work on PPy:ATP membranes gives important insight into the different mechanisms responsible for CP based drug delivery (Pyo et al., 1994; Pernaut and Reynolds, 2000). Based on parametric studies on inclusion and release of Adenosin Triphosphate (ATP), it was found that small, highly mobile cations are initially driven into the film and first after several minutes the release of ATP becomes the dominant process. Furthermore, even though the dissociation of the ionic drug from the polypyrrole chain may be fast, the actual release from the film is driven by diffusion and is therefore a slow process (Pernaut and Reynolds, 2000; Wadhwa et al., 2006; Li and Huang, 2007; Leprince et al., 2010). Fast signals would according to these findings mainly result in exchange of small anions/cations at the superficial layer of the polymer, for which the diffusion coefficients are low.

The majority of studies report that CV is vastly more efficient for driving release than CPs (Pyo et al., 1994; Pernaut and Reynolds, 2000; Wadhwa et al., 2006; Li and Huang, 2007). This underlines the complexity of the events involved in the release process far beyond what can be accounted for by the simplified electrostatic equation. The structural changes in the polymer upon redox are expected to play a major part. Most likely all the stored drug is not immediately accessible for release. Diffusion of ions within the film, and rearrangement of the polymer chains over time, exposes new deposits of drug that were not immediately accessible for the first release attempt.

Electro-actuation contributes to such conformational changes but in addition is expected to serve as a purely mechanical release mechanism for any substance entrapped within the film (Abidian et al., 2006; Thompson et al., 2006; Li and Huang, 2007). The polymer film can both shrink and swell upon reduction depending on the size of the counter ion (Jager et al., 2000). For CI in the intermediate size range such as Dex and ATP it is not straight forward to predict which mechanism would dominate. Nevertheless, repeated redox cycling will swell and shrink the film interchangeably. Actively reversing the potential at a slow rate, such as in CV, contributes to more efficient release for the anodic cycle both through inner rearrangement and through mechanical contraction of the matrix.

In summary, the efficiency with which interfacial charge transfer can contribute to release of the intended drug depends on the dynamics of the trigger signal. Furthermore, depending on diffusivity and thickness of the individual polymer film, the

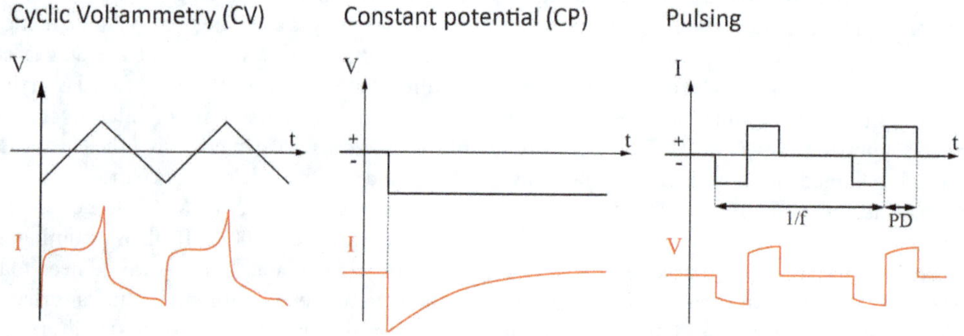

FIGURE 1 | The three different types of trigger signals for electrochemically controlled release that are discussed in the paper. The driving signal is outlined in black and the follower signal in red.

Table 1 | A compilation of experimental research concerning conducting polymer based drug delivery systems and the trigger signals used to control the release.

Study	Polymer:drug[a]	Delivery paradigm[b]	Detection scheme	Comment
Pyo et al., 1994	PPy:ATP	CV: −1 V to 0 V at 10 mV/s CP: −0.4 V; −0.5 V	Electrochemical Quartz Crystal Microbalance (EQCM)/UV	CV more efficient than CP, −0.5 V CP sufficient for release but not −0.4 V
Pernaut and Reynolds, 2000	PPy:ATP	CV CP, −0.4 V; 0.7 V; 0.8 V	UV	CV more efficient than CP. No release for −0.3 V and increase of release rate from −0.4 to −0.8 V
Abidian et al., 2006	PEDOT:Dex, nanofiber template technique	1 V with a scan rate of 0.1 V/s for 10 s Comment see ([c])	UV	–
Wadhwa et al., 2006	PPy:Dex	CV: −0.8 to 1.4 V at 100 mV/s	UV	CV more efficient than CP
Thompson et al., 2006	PPy:pTS:NT-3	Pulsed potential or current, −0.5 /+0.5 mA 5 Hz −20/+20 mA 5 Hz −0.6/+0.6 V 5 Hz CV: −0.8 to 1.0 V at 50 mV/s	Radiolabeling	–
Li and Huang, 2007	PPy:ATP	CV: 0 to −1.1 V at 10 mV/s Steps: −1.1 V, 60 s, 0 V, 60 s	Mass spectrometry	CV more efficient than a stepped potential
Evans et al., 2009	PPy:pTS:BDNF	Charged-balanced biphasic, 100 μs PD, 250 Hz, 60.2 mA, 25 μs open-circuit gap 3.78 ms short-circuit phase	Radio-labeling and ELISA	Comments see ([d])
Ge et al., 2009	PPy:ATP or PPy:SSA + PPy:Cl block layer	CP: −0.3 V; −0.5 V; −0.8 V; and −1.0 V	Fluorometer and bioluminescence	−0.3 V sufficient for ATP release. Higher potential −0.8/−1 V = faster release
Luo and Cui, 2009a	PPy:Dex nanosponge, direct incorporation + sponge	CP: −2.0 V; −0.5 V, 5 s + 5 s at 0 V	UV and fluorometer	−0.5 V gave linear and steady release
Richardson et al., 2009	PPy:pTS:NT3	Charge-balanced biphasic, PD 100 μs, 250 Hz, stimulation currents 350–825 mA	Radiolabeling	
Leprince et al., 2010	PPy:Dex	CV: −0.8 to 0.9 V at 100 mV/s	UV	Scan rate influences release rate
Stevenson et al., 2010	PTTh:Dex	CP: 0 V; 0.6 V pulsed potential 0 V to +0.6 V at 1 Hz	UV	0.6 V CP is used to suppress NOT activate release
Ru et al., 2011	PPy:ATP	CP: −0.8 V	UV	
Li et al., 2012	PPy:TCF	CP: −0.3 V; −0.4 V; and −0.5 V vs. SCE	Gas chromatography mass spectrometry	−0.4 V vs. SCE gave efficient release
Xiao et al., 2012	PEDOT:Dex and PEDOT:Dex CNTs	CV: −0.8 to 1.4V at 50 mV/s	UV	

Results were selected with regard to on if they presented a system based at least partially on direct incorporation of drug at electropolymerization.

[a] *Direct incorporation at electropolymerization unless otherwise stated.*

[b] *Potentials given are vs. Ag:AgCl unless otherwise stated.*

[c] *Not reported as CV, direct quote from paper "1V with a scan range of 0.1 Vs^{-1} for 10 s."*

[d] *Should be noted that there was no dramatic difference between active and passive release.*

Abbreviations: pTS, paratoluenesulphonate; NT-3, neurotrophin-3; BDNF, Brain Derived Neurotrophic Factor; SSA, sulfosalicylic acid; TCF, trichlorfon; CNTs, Carbon NanoTubes.

output of drug can be expected to vary. It is possible to alter the electrodeposition protocol to achieve higher diffusivity of the film, or even build layers with different properties to optimize the active vs. passive release behavior for matching a certain release protocol (Pernaut and Reynolds, 2000; Ge et al., 2009; Ru et al., 2011; Jiang et al., 2013). Moreover, the effect of the purely mechanical actuation can be further exploited by including pores in the film, for instance by a templated electrodeposition process (Abidian et al., 2006; Luo and Cui, 2009a; Luo et al., 2011). While in early work, the systems studied were single layers, advanced strategies to increase porosity of the films and boost their storage capacity are more frequently reported in recent times. In a system where entrapment is not solely based on electrostatic interaction, the mechanical actuation could be expected to be the dominant mechanism for release.

Despite the complexity of delivery mechanisms, one can make a few general assumptions on which type of signal that would be the most efficient for release from a polymer system regardless of its structure. It is clear that the theoretical arguments speak in favor for slow signals rather than fast pulsing, and especially for CV which would allow both mechanical actuation and electrostatics to contribute. There is a substantial risk that fast signals will not lead to efficient transfer of the intended ions. Furthermore, for a pulsed signal, the electrode will return to the open cell potential in between releases (mono-phasic pulsing) or even be actively reversed (bi-phasic pulsing). This means each delivery will be immediately followed by a signal actively driving the ionic flow in the opposite direction. This could in theory mean a reuptake of drug. However, the infiltration of small ions from solution to replace the larger ions delivered is more likely. One way to minimize the plausible reuptake of drug would be to allow the molecules additional time to diffuse away from the surface and be replaced by other ions at the reversed potential, speaking for the introduction of an interpulse delay time.

It should be noted that despite all these points speaking for active release with slow signals, release has been experimentally proven also for systems with fast pulsing (Evans et al., 2009; Richardson et al., 2009; Thompson et al., 2010). Thompson et al. do not specifically report pulse duration, only that they use biphasic stimulation delivered at a 5 Hz frequency. Granted that this means the full time was used for delivery of pulse trains this would however mean PDs in the range of 100 ms which is far from the PDs that would normally be used to trigger neural activity. The pulses reported by Evans et al. and also by Richardsson et al. come closer to real stimulation parameters with pulse widths of 100 μs delivered at 250 Hz (Evans et al., 2009; Richardson et al., 2009). It should be mentioned that there was no dramatic difference between active and passive release in the PPy/pTS/BDNF system but clearly an effect for the PPy:pTS:NT3 system. This would speak for a release controlled by conformational changes of the polymer rather than an electrostatic driving force. The authors in addition argue for that changes in hydrophobic properties of the polymer matrix would contribute to release in this case.

The CV ranges reported vary widely. The lowest vertex potential reported is at −1 V and the highest vertex potential at 1.4 V vs. Ag:AgCl. Commonly, only the anodic part of the sweep is used. It has also been pointed out that the scan rate further influences release efficiency of the single CV (Leprince et al., 2010). Sweep rates reported are in the range of 10–100 mV/s. For the constant potential driven systems, the potentials required to actively drive release are in the range of −0.3 to −0.5 V vs. Ag:AgCl. Clearly this will depend on the nature of the ionic drug, which conducting polymer that is used and the morphological properties of the individual polymer layer.

To some extent, a conducting polymer film that is physically degrading upon electrochemical stress can also act as a controlled delivery system. As the film falls apart, molecules that were immobilized in the structure are released at a rate that can be controlled by the level of stress. The weakest link is often the adhesion to the underlying substrate leading to complete or fragmental delamination, depending on the film cohesion. It might be difficult to judge whether a certain system performs delivery based on actuation, electrostatic interactions or simply by degradation, something that might be less favorable with an electrode intended for long term use, by only studying the release of the intended species. Ideally, one should therefore analyze if other molecules or particles are expelled from the film in parallel to the drug (Boehler and Asplund, in press). It should also be noted that conducting polymers degrade by over-oxidation meaning that the electronic structure is disrupted leading to a non-conducting material. PPy is more vulnerable to over-oxidation than PEDOT, and also the counter ion has an influence on the electronic stability (Yamato et al., 1995; Thaning et al., 2010). For this type of degradation the material itself remains at the electrode but progressive over-oxidation will influence the ion conducting properties and thereby the delivery mechanism over time.

RELEASE TRIGGER SIGNALS—FROM THE SIDE OF BIOLOGICAL SAFETY

In the previous section, the efficiency of the three release signals was discussed. However, other practical aspects such as the availability of devices capable of delivering these signals, as well as the safety for the biological environment, should naturally be taken into consideration. In the following section, the three trigger signals in **Figure 1** are therefore discussed with regard to the safety of neurons.

In general, the restrictions that would apply to a signal to be applied *in vivo* could be summarized as follows:

1. The signal transfer should take place through reversible processes which do not lead to the formation of electrochemical by-products in the tissue or corrosive reactions at the electrode.
2. The signal must not trigger undesired activity in the neural network.
3. The signal must not induce damage to neurons.

These conditions do not completely apply for the situation where the aim is to use the signal to drive controlled release. In this case, ideally the trigger signal should be designed to be practically invisible from the side of the neuron, yet still be efficient for pushing out drugs in a reasonable time frame and with good control of the delivered amount. While restriction 1 is of the utmost importance for metallic electrodes it is not directly transferrable to polymer electrodes. The aim is to exchange the ionic drug in the polymer for other ions naturally available in tissue so irreversibility is to some extent here a necessity. However, the limitation of the electrode potential to prevent redox reactions in proteins and water as well as pH-shifts is a must.

It is also highly desirable that the signal used for drug release does not result in undefined excitation of surrounding neurons as in restriction 2. Normally, when evaluating how to stimulate neural tissue, the ambition is to assemble signals that are efficient in precise activation of a defined population of cells at current/pulse durations chosen to induce minimal electrochemical stress on the electrode. For the drug release approach, the signal needs to be optimized from close to the opposite perspective. The ambition would be to use a release signal that does not substantially influence surrounding cells but is efficient in pushing drugs out of the electrode.

Last, but not least, it is well-known that electrical stimulation of neurons can induce cellular injury even when the delivered stimulation is well within the boundaries given by the electrochemical safety (Shannon, 1992; Veraart et al., 2004). Normally such effects do not occur below the levels which can trigger neural activity which would ensure that a signal that confines to condition 2 is a conservative limit also for restriction 3. However, these injury thresholds are most of the time given with consideration to the pulsing parameters that would be considered normal for neural excitation. It is therefore advisable to take a closer look at the safety boundaries from this perspective when more unconventional pulsing parameters might be put into use.

PULSING

A standard pulse for recruitment of intracortical neurons would be a biphasic train of rectangular pulses of constant current delivered at a frequency in the range of 100–400 Hz, commonly around 200 Hz (see **Figure 1**). The minimum current strength needed to excite neuronal tissue (threshold current, I_{th}) depends on the pulse duration (PD) as in the strength-duration relationship depicted in **Figure 2**. PD should as a rule of thumb be chosen close to the chronaxy of the intended target tissue which in practice means durations in the range of 100–300 μs for myelinated nerve fibers. Longer pulse durations would not be energy efficient for activation of neurons and in addition would increase the probability for non-reversible corrosive processes at the electrode site (Tehovnik, 1996).

When stimulating at PDs close to the chronaxy, typical threshold currents for neural activation would be estimated to be around 10 μA, but recent studies show that actual activation thresholds can be expected to be even lower than 4 μA (reported for 200 μs PD and 250 Hz) (Tehovnik et al., 2006; Histed et al., 2009). Since the objective of the PEDOT electrode is drug delivery rather than activation, stimulation should be kept below threshold not to evoke neural activity unintentionally. In practice and according to the generally accepted current-duration relationship, this leaves two alternatives (Tehovnik, 1996). Either shortening the pulses to increase the threshold current, or use longer pulses and stay well-below the rheobase. For a pulse substantially longer than the chronaxy this means at least below 2 μA, preferably even lower. The longer the pulse, the more charge would be expected to be required to activate neurons. This clearly rather speaks for maximizing charge and thereby possibilities for ionic delivery by driving longer pulses at lower currents.

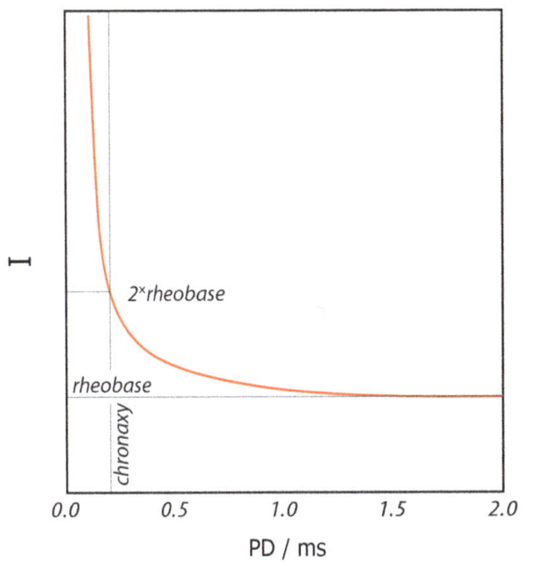

FIGURE 2 | Strength-duration relationship for excitable tissue. Red line shows the threshold current, I_{th}, at which neuronal tissue is excited for a rectangular stimulation pulse of duration PD.

If a small and highly local amount of activated neurons can be tolerated, currents can naturally be set higher. This is something that would have to be evaluated with respect to the exact placement of the particular electrode. With knowledge of the excitability constant, K, of the target tissue, efficient spread of stimulation can be estimated, over the radius r, for a given case according to $I = K{*}r^2$ (Tehovnik, 1996; Tehovnik et al., 2006). This would provide a reasonable estimate for the volume of cells affected by a pulse if exceeding the threshold in the given case.

Tissue damage can occur as a consequence of inappropriately chosen stimulation parameters, even though the given stimulation is within the electrochemical safety limits of the electrode material. It is broadly accepted that important factors to consider are charge per phase and charge density delivered from the electrode (McCreery et al., 1990; Shannon, 1992). The mechanisms behind such effects are not completely understood but it is believed that electroporation is a main contributor to this kind of tissue damage as well as mass action phenomena, for instance depletion of oxygen or glucose, or excessive release of glutamate, caused by local neural overactivity (Merrill et al., 2005). Since signals in the case discussed here should be chosen with the aim not to induce neural signaling, only electroporation would need to be considered.

Taking also restriction 3 into account, there is reason to ask if there is a risk for the occurrence of electroporation based on this type of pulsing? A detailed insight into how the threshold for electroporation can be expected to vary with other stimulation parameters is given by Butterwick et al. (2007). One conclusion of their work is that, for longer pulses (PDs in the range of ms), the threshold current density at which electroporation can be expected to occur is lower than for shorter pulses. The threshold current density scales with PD approximately as 1/sqrt(PD). It is also clear from their results that with pulsing frequencies exceeding 50 Hz repetition frequency thresholds are significantly lower than for single shots. For electrodes smaller than 300 μm it is further concluded that total current would be the main limitation, and injury thresholds would not to the same extent be influenced by current density as is seen with the larger electrodes. Their results are based on measurements in chicken retinas but correlate well to measurements in earlier work concerning injury thresholds in cortical tissue (McCreery et al., 1990; Shannon, 1992; Veraart et al., 2004). It is therefore assumed that the safe limits reported would be a reasonable figure of merit for stimulation of any target tissue in the central as well as in the peripheral nervous system.

The lowest threshold where stimulation induced damage was detected in their experiments was determined to be 61 mA/cm^2 at a pulse duration of 6 ms for repetitive pulsing (>50 Hz). Translated to a microelectrode of 50 μm that would correspond to a charge per pulse of 7.2 nC. However, for pulses shorter than the ms, threshold currents are substantially higher. Deduced from the data presented by Butterwick, for the 600 μs, expected thresholds would rather be in the range of 0.2 A/cm^2. Due to the shorter pulse length this would in fact mean a lower charge per phase threshold, for the 50 μm electrode 2.3 nC/phase. This would speak for that electroporation could occur even with a minor elevation of the stimulation current.

The study also presents results regarding the influence of the size of the electrode and the values cited above relate to a large electrode, not a microelectrode. If taking their results concerning microelectrodes into account, here smaller than 300 μm in diameter, the threshold charge per phase that could safely be delivered did in fact not depend on electrode size. The smallest electrode used in their experiment was ~100 μm in diameter and the threshold, when investigated on the retina cells using 600 μs single pulses, were found to be ~70 nC per phase. This threshold should, according to their theory of size independence, also be valid for smaller electrodes. Even though these particular results describe thresholds for one single pulse, there is substantial margin to the 1.2 nC given by the 2 μA and 600 μs suggested as suitable sub-threshold stimulation (second paragraph, section Pulsing).

In summary, also from the perspective of restriction 3, it would be recommendable to work with PDs longer than the chronaxy. It further appears as if PDs are on the longer side, and threshold current is estimated to be below the rheobase, there is no substantial risk for disruption of cellular membrane integrity as a consequence of the pulsed trigger signal.

In order to establish boundaries for safety it is of interest to glance at the field of deep brain stimulation (DBS), where intracortical stimulation has been therapeutically used over more than a decade. The technology is FDA approved and one could thereby argue that these stimulation protocols have already been proven safe for use in patients. Kern and Kumar (2007) report common values for the Sub Thalamic Nucleus (STN) DBS to be in the range 130–185 Hz with typical pulse durations of 60 μs. However, the extremely short pulse durations used for DBS are most likely not efficient for drug expulsion. Release relies to large extent on slower processes as has already been discussed in the previous section.

CYCLIC VOLTAMMETRY

It has already been pointed out that slow redox sweeping of the electrode has been found efficient for delivery of ionic drugs. The stimulation effects of CV in brain tissue are not specifically addressed in the literature. Theoretically, if the current-duration curves are extrapolated into infinitely long pulses, which would be a reasonable approximation for the smooth transitions of a CV curve, the suggestion would be that as long as the current is still below the rheobase the neurons would not be excited.

If the neuronal activity is not directly influenced, the restrictions would rather be set by the possibly detrimental electrochemical reactions that could occur as a by-product of any excessive voltage. The two parameters to consider are the vertex potentials and the sweep rate. The non-conservative constraints for the vertex potentials would be given by the water window (−0.6 V to 0.8 V vs. Ag:AgCl) since the evolution of hydrogen (−0.6 V) and oxygen (0.8 V), respectively, would occur at the electrode upon exceeding this window. Over-oxidation of PEDOT would not be expected to occur at voltages lower than 1.1 V and is therefore not a limiting factor in this case. This is however not sufficient to support that no other electrochemical reactions of importance take place within this window. Furthermore, appropriate reference electrodes are often not available in the implanted situation meaning that possible variations in applied voltages must be taken into account. Materials do either not deliver a stable potential in chronic implantations or biofouling clogs pores in ion-selective membranes.

One example on actual parameters used in a similar biological setting can be found in recent work monitoring electrochemical characteristics of implanted electrodes. Kane et al. (2011) employs the full water window at a sweep rate of 50 mV/s for their *in vivo* CV investigations and do not report any adverse tissue response as a consequence. In the sensor literature, fast CV is often suggested for instance for *in vivo* monitoring of neurotransmitters. It should be noted that so far sweep rates used are in the range of 300 V/s and thus far beyond what has been proposed for drug release (Pihel et al., 1996). The biological response was not the primary target for the analysis in either study and was therefore not carefully observed. Scans used for analytical purposes in an experiment with a sedated animal, and limited to a few occasions, are not necessarily suitable for repeated use in proximity of a population of highly sensitive cells. In both studies animals were anaesthetized which might not be possible to perform on a bi-weekly to weekly basis needed to support efficient drug release.

BIAS POTENTIAL

A bias potential of approximately −0.5 V vs. Ag:AgCl could be used to drive drug release. Cells are not expected to respond adversely to a steady potential if kept within reasonable boundaries. For instance, a positive interpulse bias potential of 0.6 V has been suggested as a method for boosting performance of iridium oxide electrodes and has been applied to SIROF coatings *in vivo* (Cogan et al., 2006; Kane et al., 2011). The authors comment that the long-term consequences of the low net current needed to maintain the bias potential has not yet been explored. However, for the drug release, the bias potential would only be applied at the specific occasions where drug release is requested which qualifies as a limited time frame and should be safe for use.

DISCUSSION

OTHER RELEASE STRATEGIES AND DRUGS

Apart from Dex, also various other anti-inflammatory drugs like α-MSH, IL-1-RA, or heparin have been proposed in literature for treatment of inflammatory reactions. These molecules target different receptor pathways in the inflammation cascade and can thus be interesting alternatives or complements to the Dex (Bridges and Garcia, 2008; Go et al., 2012). All of the listed molecules are typically delivered from passively eluting systems due to their chemical properties and overall size, which makes them incompatible with the ion-exchange principle provided by conducting polymers. In contrast, Dex is in the appropriate size range (392 Da) and features an anionic charge characteristic, which makes is eligible for both passive and actively controlled release systems. Furthermore, Dex is known to be the most potent glucocorticoid drug for anti-inflammatory treatment due to its effect in multiple receptor pathways, which reveals this drug as first choice for the realization of an anti-inflammatory drug eluting system for treatment of the glial scar. For a more detailed description of relevant molecules and their impact on the adverse host response to implanted biomedical devices the excellent review by Bridges et al. is strongly recommended (Bridges and Garcia, 2008). It should be mentioned that it would be possible to use a deposition technique not relying on direct incorporation to combine the active delivery approach also with these substances (Abidian et al., 2006; Luo et al., 2011).

It is a valid question to ask how the actively controlled release of Dex from a microelectrode would compare to a delivery coating passively leaking Dex into tissue, or systemic treatment (Shain et al., 2003; Spataro et al., 2005; Zhong and Bellamkonda, 2007). The latter has the clear downside of requiring much higher total doses distributed to reach an efficient concentration at the point of interest and side-effects would thus be a main concern. In situ delivery, avoiding the counterproductive neuroendocrine feedbacks, is from this perspective clearly beneficial regardless of if the system is based on a passive or active release approach.

The active release system offers controllability but for a limited quantity whereas the passive system can cover the complete surface of a probe, thereby storing a much larger quantity, but hold few options to influence release dynamics. From the data available in literature it is difficult to judge whether such a system would be more successful in mitigating inflammation than the actively triggered release approach. The answer to this question could only be given if the necessary time course of the treatment was known. It is still an open question whether the anti-inflammatory treatment over the time course of a month, which would be the critical period in which the scar forms, influences the state of the surrounding tissue also in the long term (Szarowski et al., 2003; Biran et al., 2005; Potter et al., 2012). If it does, the lower quantity delivered by the microelectrodes might still be sufficient, meaning higher drug load is not a substantial benefit but could be traded for more precise release control. On the other hand, treatment might be needed for a much longer time period which would make the opportunity to load a higher quantity of drug much more attractive. A certain control of release dynamics in the passive release system could still be accomplished by carefully tailoring the degradability properties of the release matrix. In theory, nothing speaks against that such a system in the future could include certain responsiveness to biological factors, for instance react to chemical factors present for a higher degree of inflammation, by increasing the release rate.

It should be noted that such a delivery matrix, which can act as the golden standard for passive release, does not yet exist. Thus, the passive release system relies on substantial development in this direction in the same way as the polymer electrodes hold room for future optimization. Recent result show that also surface immobilized Dex might have an effect for improving probe integration which illustrates the need for further work to elucidate the underlying mechanisms involved in the tissue response to Dex (Grand et al., 2010). In summary, the passive delivery approach should be pursued in parallel with the active delivery systems, as an interesting alternative or even additional approach, since the use of the one delivery system in fact does not exclude the use of the other as a complement.

RELEASE TRIGGER SIGNALS—CONCLUDING REMARKS

Taking all the considerations regarding efficiency and safety into account they all speak in favor for slow release signals. CV seems to be the most suitable from the efficiency perspective and most likely a moderate use of voltammetric sweeping will not be harmful to tissue or lead to undeliberate excitation of the neuronal network. This however needs to be confirmed in experiments.

In practice, the equipment needed to perform well-controlled CV at the implant site might however not always be available. Proper CV measurements require a three-electrode electrochemical control system and the technologies for on-probe integration of stable reference electrodes on implants are not yet established (Tolosa et al., 2013).

Considering this practical aspect, it might therefore still be the most convenient to use a pulsed signal for release rather than a sweep. In this case it would be advisable to aim for low currents and PDs significantly longer than the chronaxy. Furthermore, to present as little stress as possible to the tissue, low pulsing frequencies should be used. Lowering the pulsing frequency and compensating by extending the overall stimulation time should have little effect on the release itself but would allow higher currents before stimulation induced damage to neurons can be expected to occur (Butterwick et al., 2007). Charge balance is not a necessity for this kind of drug release. On one hand it might contribute to increased actuation, on the other hand it might be counterproductive if the Dex ions are immediately retrieved by the reversed pulse. An interpulse delay could mitigate the second effect.

One possibility to, with a simple device, imitate the effect of a CV is to exchange the sweep with interchangeable voltage steps, set to the upper and lower vertex potential. Microsized devices capable of maintaining a fixed voltage vs. a reference, and suitable for implantation, have been described by others (Islam et al., 2010). In **Figure 3**, the current response of a PEDOT:Dex electrode to a cyclic voltammogram can be seen as well as the current response to a rectangular pulse. It is clear that the current flow follows another scheme than in the carefully controlled slow CV. What this in practice would mean for the drug release should be further investigated experimentally.

Finally, not only efficiency of release but also controllability should be considered. For the application, it is desirable that a precise dose of Dex can be delivered at each attempt, which means the response to the trigger signal must be predictable. Taking the complexity of events involved in release into account, such one to one correlation is not trivial to accomplish. More likely, the response of the polymer will change over time and with each delivery attempt, something that must be carefully considered to ensure the trigger signal has the intended effect throughout the full experimental time frame. This needs to be further investigated before a specific polymer delivery system is put into use.

Since the drug delivery systems reviewed here are intended for local treatment targeting only the cells in the immediate vicinity of the electrode, it is highly desirable that the very same electrode used for delivery can still function as a neural interface. For recording this is not expected to be a problem since both PEDOT and PPy are known for their low impedance in this respect. Although the drug delivery electrodes in general are outperformed by the regular surfactant based conducting polymer materials in terms of impedance, it has repeatedly been shown that also drug containing conducting polymer electrodes still lower the impedance in comparison to a bare metallic surface (Wadhwa et al., 2006; Luo et al., 2011).

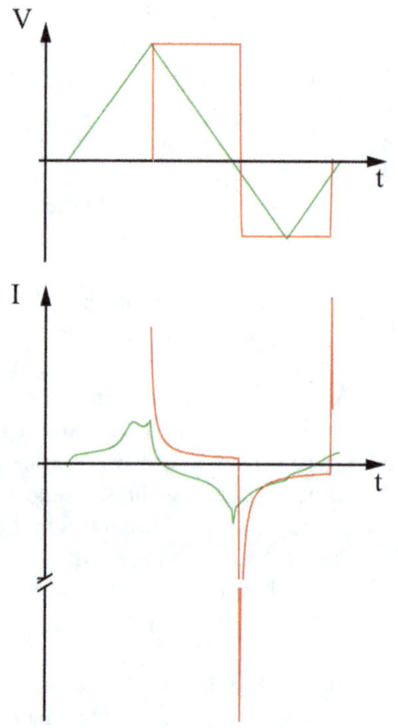

FIGURE 3 | A comparison between the current response to a swept voltage vs. a stepped voltage for a PEDOT:Dex delivery system. Measurement was performed in PBS and vs. an Ag:AgCl reference.

For stimulation the central question would be if stimulation can be performed without unintentionally triggering release? From the literature reviewed here it is not possible to make a conclusive statement on whether this would at all be possible. As discussed, some authors do indeed present release based on the type of fast pulsing that would be common to use for stimulation purposes (Evans et al., 2009; Richardson et al., 2009). However, it can be concluded that slow sweeps are vastly more effective for drug release (**Table 1**) and several authors report that they need to reach a certain voltage before actual release is triggered (e.g., Pyo et al., 1994; Pernaut and Reynolds, 2000). It is plausible that smart materials design can further exploit this effect making the release-free stimulation possible within certain boundaries.

REFERENCES

Abidian, M. R., Kim, D. H., and Martin, D. C. (2006). Conducting-polymer nanotubes for controlled drug release. *Adv. Mater.* 18, 405–409. doi: 10.1002/adma.200501726

Asplund, M., Von Holst, H., and Inganas, O. (2008). Composite biomolecule/PEDOT materials for neural electrodes. *Biointerphases* 3, 83–93. doi: 10.1116/1.2998407

Biran, R., Martin, D. C., and Tresco, P. A. (2005). Neuronal cell loss accompanies the brain tissue response to chronically implanted silicon microelectrode arrays. *Exp. Neurol.* 195, 115–126. doi: 10.1016/j.expneurol.2005.04.020

Bobacka, J., Lewenstam, A., and Ivaska, A. (2000). Electrochemical impedance spectroscopy of oxidized poly(3,4-ethylenedioxythiophene) film electrodes in aqueous solutions. *J. Electroanal. Chem.* 489, 17–27. doi: 10.1016/S0022-0728(00)00206-0

Boehler, C., and Asplund, M. (in press). A detailed insight into drug delivery from PEDOT based on analytical methods: effects and side-effects. *J. Biomed. Mater. Res. A.*

Bridges, A. W., and Garcia, A. J. (2008). Anti-inflammatory polymeric coatings for implantable biomaterials and devices. *J. Diabetes Sci. Technol.* 2, 984–994.

Butterwick, A., Vankov, A., Huie, P., Freyvert, Y., and Palanker, D. (2007). Tissue damage by pulsed electrical stimulation. *IEEE Trans. Biomed. Eng.* 54, 2261–2267. doi: 10.1109/TBME.2007.908310

Cogan, S. F., Troyk, P. R., Ehrlich, J., Plante, T. D., and Detlefsen, D. E. (2006). Potential-biased, asymmetric waveforms for charge-injection with activated iridium oxide (AIROF) neural stimulation electrodes. *IEEE Trans. Biomed. Eng.* 53, 327–332. doi: 10.1109/tbme.2005.862572

Evans, A. J., Thompson, B. C., Wallace, G. G., Millard, R., O'leary, S. J., Clark, G. M., et al. (2009). Promoting neurite outgrowth from spiral ganglion neuron explants using polypyrrole/BDNF-coated electrodes. *J. Biomed. Mater. Res. A* 91A, 241–250. doi: 10.1002/jbm.a.32228

Ge, D., Tian, X., Qi, R., Huang, S., Mu, J., Hong, S., et al. (2009). A polypyrrole-based microchip for controlled drug release. *Electrochim. Acta* 55, 271–275. doi: 10.1016/j.electacta.2009.08.049

Go, D. P., Palmer, J. A., Gras, S. L., and O'connor, A. J. (2012). Coating and release of an anti-inflammatory hormone from PLGA microspheres for tissue engineering. *J. Biomed. Mater. Res. A* 100A, 507–517. doi: 10.1002/jbm.a.33299

Golde, S., Coles, A., Lindquist, J. A., and Compston, A. (2003). Decreased iNOS synthesis mediates dexamethasone-induced protection of neurons from inflammatory injury *in vitro*. *Eur. J. Neurosci.* 18, 2527–2537. doi: 10.1046/j.1460-9568.2003.02917.x

Grand, L., Wittner, L., Herwik, S., Gothelid, E., Ruther, P., Oscarsson, S., et al. (2010). Short and long term biocompatibility of NeuroProbes silicon probes. *J. Neurosci. Methods* 189, 216–229. doi: 10.1016/j.jneumeth.2010.04.009

Histed, M. H., Bonin, V., and Reid, R. C. (2009). Direct activation of sparse, distributed populations of cortical neurons by electrical microstimulation. *Neuron* 63, 508–522. doi: 10.1016/j.neuron.2009.07.016

Islam, A. B., Haider, M. R., Atla, A., Islam, S. K., Croce, R., Vaddiraju, S., et al. (2010). "A potentiostat circuit for multiple implantable electrochemical sensors," in *Electrical and Computer Engineering (ICECE), 2010 International Conference*, (Wuhan), 314–317.

Jager, E. W. H., Smela, E., and Inganas, O. (2000). Microfabricating conjugated polymer actuators. *Science* 290, 1540–1545. doi: 10.1126/science.290.5496.1540

Jiang, S., Sun, Y., Cui, X., Huang, X., He, Y., Ji, S., et al. (2013). Enhanced drug loading capacity of polypyrrole nanowire network for controlled drug release. *Synth. Met.* 163, 19–23. doi: 10.1016/j.synthmet.2012.12.010

Kane, S. R., Cogan, S. F., Ehrlich, J., Plante, T. D., and McCreery, D. B. (2011). Electrical performance of penetrating microelectrodes chronically implanted in cat cortex. *Conf. Proc. IEEE Eng. Med. Biol. Soc.* 2011, 5416–5419. doi: 10.1109/iembs.2011.6091339

Kern, D. S., and Kumar, R. (2007). Deep brain stimulation. *Neurologist* 13, 237–252. doi: 10.1097/NRL.0b013e3181492c48

Kontturi, K., Pentti, P., and Sundholm, G. (1998). Polypyrrole as a model membrane for drug delivery. *J. Electroanal. Chem.* 453, 231–238. doi: 10.1016/s0022-0728(98)00246-0

Leprince, L., Dogimont, A., Magnin, D., and Demoustier-Champagne, S. (2010). Dexamethasone electrically controlled release from polypyrrole-coated nanostructured electrodes. *J. Mater. Sci. Mater. Med.* 21, 925–930. doi: 10.1007/s10856-010-4008-6

Li, L. D., and Huang, C. B. (2007). Electrochemical/electrospray mass spectrometric studies of electrochemically stimulated ATP release from PP/ATP films. *J. Am. Soc. Mass Spectrom.* 18, 919–926. doi: 10.1016/j.jasms.2007.01.015

Li, Y., Ewen, R. J., Campbell, S. A., and Smith, J. R. (2012). Electrochemically controlled release of antischistosomiasis agents from polypyrrole. *J. Mater. Chem.* 22, 2687–2694. doi: 10.1039/c2jm15298c

Luo, X., and Cui, X. T. (2009a). Sponge-like nanostructured conducting polymers for electrically controlled drug release. *Electrochem. commun.* 11, 1956–1959. doi: 10.1016/j.elecom.2009.08.027

Luo, X., Matranga, C., Tan, S., Alba, N., and Cui, X. T. (2011). Carbon nanotube nanoreservior for controlled release of anti-inflammatory dexamethasone. *Biomaterials* 32, 6316–6323. doi: 10.1016/j.biomaterials.2011.05.020

Luo, X. L., and Cui, X. T. (2009b). Electrochemically controlled release based on nanoporous conducting polymers. *Electrochem. Commun.* 11, 402–404. doi: 10.1016/j.elecom.2008.11.052

Majumdar, S., Kargupta, K., and Ganguly, S. (2008). Mathematical modeling for the ionic inclusion process inside conducting polymer-based thin-films. *Polym. Eng. Sci.* 48, 2229–2237. doi: 10.1002/pen.21170

McCreery, D. B., Agnew, W. F., Yuen, T. G., and Bullara, L. (1990). Charge density and charge per phase as cofactors in neural injury induced by electrical stimulation. *IEEE Trans. Biomed. Eng.* 37, 996–1001. doi: 10.1109/10.102812

Merrill, D. R., Bikson, M., and Jefferys, J. G. (2005). Electrical stimulation of excitable tissue: design of efficacious and safe protocols. *J. Neurosci. Methods* 141, 171–198. doi: 10.1016/j.jneumeth.2004.10.020

Moulton, S. E., Imisides, M. D., Shepherd, R. L., and Wallace, G. G. (2008). Galvanic coupling conducting polymers to biodegradable Mg initiates autonomously powered drug release. *J. Mater. Chem.* 18, 3608–3613. doi: 10.1039/B805481a

Pernaut, J. M., and Reynolds, J. R. (2000). Use of conducting electroactive polymers for drug delivery and sensing of bioactive molecules. A redox chemistry approach. *J. Phys. Chem. B* 104, 4080–4090. doi: 10.1021/jp994274o

Pihel, K., Walker, Q. D., and Wightman, R. M. (1996). Overoxidized polypyrrole-coated carbon fiber microelectrodes for dopamine measurements with fast-scan cyclic voltammetry. *Anal. Chem.* 68, 2084–2089. doi: 10.1021/ac960153y

Potter, K. A., Buck, A. C., Self, W. K., and Capadona, J. R. (2012). Stab injury and device implantation within the brain results in inversely multiphasic neuroinflammatory and neurodegenerative responses. *J. Neural Eng.* 9:046020. doi: 10.1088/1741-2560/9/4/046020

Pyo, M., Maeder, G., Kennedy, R. T., and Reynolds, J. R. (1994). Controlled release of biological molecules from conducting polymer modified electrodes: The potential dependent release of adenosine 5'-triphosphate from poly(pyrrole adenosine 5'-triphosphate) films. *J. Electroanal. Chem.* 368, 329–332. doi: 10.1016/0022-0728(93)03071-V

Richardson, R. T., Wise, A. K., Thompson, B. C., Flynn, B. O., Atkinson, P. J., Fretwell, N. J., et al. (2009). Polypyrrole-coated electrodes for the delivery of charge and neurotrophins to cochlear neurons. *Biomaterials* 30, 2614–2624. doi: 10.1016/j.biomaterials.2009.01.015

Ru, X. N., Shi, W., Huang, X., Cui, X., Ren, B., and Ge, D. T. (2011). Synthesis of polypyrrole nanowire network with high adenosine triphosphate release efficiency. *Electrochim. Acta* 56, 9887–9892. doi: 10.1016/j.electacta.2011.08.063

Shain, W., Spataro, L., Dilgen, J., Haverstick, K., Retterer, S., Isaacson, M., et al. (2003). Controlling cellular reactive responses around neural prosthetic devices using peripheral and local intervention strategies. *IEEE Trans. Neural Syst. Rehabil. Eng.* 11, 186–188. doi: 10.1109/TNSRE.2003.814800

Shannon, R. V. (1992). A model of safe levels for electrical stimulation. *IEEE Trans. Biomed. Eng.* 39, 424–426. doi: 10.1109/10.126616

Sirivisoot, S., Pareta, R., and Webster, T. J. (2011). Electrically controlled drug release from nanostructured polypyrrole coated on titanium. *Nanotechnology* 22:085101. doi: 10.1088/0957-4484/22/8/085101

Skotheim, T. A., and Reynolds, J. R. (2006). *Conjugated Polymers: Theory, Synthesis, Properties and Characterization.* Boca Raton: CRC Press.

Spataro, L., Dilgen, J., Retterer, S., Spence, A. J., Isaacson, M., Turner, J. N., et al. (2005). Dexamethasone treatment reduces astroglia responses to inserted neuroprosthetic devices in rat neocortex. *Exp. Neurol.* 194, 289–300. doi: 10.1016/j.expneurol.2004.08.037

Stevenson, G., Moulton, S. E., Innis, P. C., and Wallace, G. G. (2010). Polyterthiophene as an electrostimulated controlled drug release material of therapeutic levels of dexamethasone. *Synth. Met.* 160, 1107–1114. doi: 10.1016/j.synthmet.2010.02.035

Szarowski, D. H., Andersen, M. D., Retterer, S., Spence, A. J., Isaacson, M., Craighead, H. G., et al. (2003). Brain responses to micro-machined silicon devices. *Brain Res.* 983, 23–35. doi: 10.1016/S0006-8993(03)03023-3

Tehovnik, E. J. (1996). Electrical stimulation of neural tissue to evoke behavioral responses. *J. Neurosci. Methods* 65, 1–17. doi: 10.1016/0165-0270(95)00131-X

Tehovnik, E. J., Tolias, A. S., Sultan, F., Slocum, W. M., and Logothetis, N. K. (2006). Direct and indirect activation of cortical neurons by electrical microstimulation. *J. Neurophysiol.* 96, 512–521. doi: 10.1152/jn.00126.2006

Thaning, E. M., Asplund, M. L., Nyberg, T. A., Inganas, O. W., and von Holst, H. (2010). Stability of poly(3,4-ethylene dioxythiophene) materials intended for implants. *J. Biomed. Mater. Res. B Appl. Biomater.* 93, 407–415. doi: 10.1002/jbm.b.31597

Thompson, B. C., Chen, J., Moulton, S. E., and Wallace, G. G. (2010). Nanostructured aligned CNT platforms enhance the controlled release of a neurotrophic protein from polypyrrole. *Nanoscale* 2, 499–501. doi: 10.1039/b9nr00259f

Thompson, B. C., Moulton, S. E., Ding, J., Richardson, R., Cameron, A., O'leary, S., et al. (2006). Optimising the incorporation and release of a neurotrophic factor using conducting polypyrrole. *J. Control. Release* 116, 285–294. doi: 10.1016/j.jconrel.2006.09.004

Tolosa, V. M., Wassum, K. M., Maidment, N. T., and Monbouquette, H. G. (2013). Electrochemically deposited iridium oxide reference electrode integrated with an electroenzymatic glutamate sensor on a multi-electrode arraymicroprobe. *Biosensors Bioelectron.* 42, 256–260. doi: dx.doi.org/10.1016/j.bios.2012.10.061

Turner, J. N., Shain, W., Szarowski, D. H., Andersen, M., Martins, S., Isaacson, M., et al. (1999). Cerebral astrocyte response to micromachined silicon implants. *Exp. Neurol.* 156, 33–49. doi: 10.1006/exnr.1998.6983

Veraart, C., Duret, F., Brelén, M., Oozeer, M., and Delbeke, J. (2004). Vision rehabilitation in the case of blindness. *Expert Rev. Med. Devices* 1, 139–153. doi: 10.1586/17434440.1.1.139

Wadhwa, R., Lagenaur, C. F., and Cui, X. T. (2006). Electrochemically controlled release of dexamethasone from conducting polymer polypyrrole coated electrode. *J. Control. Release* 110, 531–541. doi: 10.1016/j.jconrel.2005.10.027

Xiao, Y., Che, J., Li, C. M., Sun, C. Q., Chua, Y. T., Lee, V. S., et al. (2007). Preparation of nano-tentacle polypyrrole with pseudo-molecular template for ATP incorporation. *J. Biomed. Mater. Res. A* 80, 925–931. doi: 10.1002/jbm.a.31001

Xiao, Y., Ye, X., He, L., and Che, J. (2012). New carbon nanotube-conducting polymer composite electrodes for drug delivery applications. *Polym. Int.* 61, 190–196. doi: 10.1002/pi.3168

Yamato, H., Ohwa, M., and Wernet, W. (1995). Stability of polypyrrole and poly(3,4-ethylene dioxythiophene) for biosensor application. *J. Electroanal. Chem.* 397, 163–170. doi: 10.1016/0022-0728(95)04156-8

Yue, Z., Moulton, S. E., Cook, M., O'leary, S., and Wallace, G. G. (2013). Controlled delivery for neuro-bionic devices. *Adv. Drug Deliv. Rev.* 65, 559–569. doi: 10.1016/j.addr.2012.06.002

Zhong, Y. H., and Bellamkonda, R. V. (2007). Dexamethasone-coated neural probes elicit attenuated inflammatory response and neuronal loss compared to uncoated neural probes. *Brain Res.* 1148, 15–27. doi: 10.1016/j.brainres.2007.02.024

Zhong, Y., McConnell, G. C., Ross, J. D., Deweerth, S. P., and Bellamkonda, R. V. (2005). "A novel dexamethasone-releasing, anti-inflammatory coating for neural implants," in *Neural Engineering, 2005. Conference Proceedings. 2nd International IEEE EMBS Conference* (Arlington), 522–525.

Organic electrode coatings for next-generation neural interfaces

Ulises A. Aregueta-Robles [1], Andrew J. Woolley [1,2], Laura A. Poole-Warren [1], Nigel H. Lovell [1] and Rylie A. Green [1] *

[1] Graduate School of Biomedical Engineering, University of New South Wales, Sydney, NSW, Australia
[2] School of Medicine, University of Western Sydney, Sydney, NSW, Australia

Edited by:
Ulrich G. Hofmann, Albert-Ludwigs-University Freiburg, Germany

Reviewed by:
Anja Kunze, University of California, Los Angeles, USA
Ulrich G. Hofmann, Albert-Ludwigs-University Freiburg, Germany

***Correspondence:**
Rylie A. Green, Graduate School of Biomedical Engineering, University of New South Wales, Sydney, NSW 2052, Australia
e-mail: r.green@unsw.edu.au

Traditional neuronal interfaces utilize metallic electrodes which in recent years have reached a plateau in terms of the ability to provide safe stimulation at high resolution or rather with high densities of microelectrodes with improved spatial selectivity. To achieve higher resolution it has become clear that reducing the size of electrodes is required to enable higher electrode counts from the implant device. The limitations of interfacing electrodes including low charge injection limits, mechanical mismatch and foreign body response can be addressed through the use of organic electrode coatings which typically provide a softer, more roughened surface to enable both improved charge transfer and lower mechanical mismatch with neural tissue. Coating electrodes with conductive polymers or carbon nanotubes offers a substantial increase in charge transfer area compared to conventional platinum electrodes. These organic conductors provide safe electrical stimulation of tissue while avoiding undesirable chemical reactions and cell damage. However, the mechanical properties of conductive polymers are not ideal, as they are quite brittle. Hydrogel polymers present a versatile coating option for electrodes as they can be chemically modified to provide a soft and conductive scaffold. However, the *in vivo* chronic inflammatory response of these conductive hydrogels remains unknown. A more recent approach proposes tissue engineering the electrode interface through the use of encapsulated neurons within hydrogel coatings. This approach may provide a method for activating tissue at the cellular scale, however, several technological challenges must be addressed to demonstrate feasibility of this innovative idea. The review focuses on the various organic coatings which have been investigated to improve neural interface electrodes.

Keywords: coatings, carbon nanotubes, conductive polymers, hydrogels, living electrodes, material properties

INTRODUCTION

Neurological injuries and disorders affect up to a billion people worldwide and this number is estimated to increase considerably as life expectancy continues to rise (World Health Organization, 2006). Neuroprosthetic intervention is an increasingly popular method for alleviating symptoms or returning function to patients suffering from these disorders. Despite the impressive results of some electrical therapies, such as auditory implants (McCreery, 2008; Shannon, 2012), deep brain stimulators (DBS; Andrade et al., 2006; Perlmutter and Mink, 2006; Lozano and Lipsman, 2013), functional electrical stimulation (FES) of the spinal cord (Collinger et al., 2013) and vision prostheses (Shepherd et al., 2013), considerable improvement in device technology is required to enable greater control of physiological outcomes (Normann, 2007). Current state-of-the-art neuroprostheses generate an electrical field in the target tissue using metallic electrodes to elicit or suppress neuronal action potentials (Perlmutter and Mink, 2006; Li and Mogul, 2007; Normann, 2007; Wilson and Dorman, 2008; Collinger et al., 2013; Shepherd et al., 2013). Many such devices also use the same metallic electrodes to record neural responses (Normann, 2007). Most metallic electrodes inject charge through the generation of electrons at the electrode surface, however in physiological systems charge is carried by electrolytes (ions). At the electrode–electrolyte interface, charge must be transferred from electrons to ions by either Faradic (electrochemical reactions) or capacitive (double-layer charging) mechanisms which are dependent on the material selected for the electrode (Merrill et al., 2005; Cogan, 2008). Typically platinum (Pt), gold and platinum-iridium (Pt-Ir) are used for fabricating biomedical electrodes (Brummer et al., 1983; Geddes and Roeder, 2003). Pt has historically been considered the preferred metal used for electrodes in neuroprostheses (Brummer et al., 1983; Cogan, 2008), with cochlear implants, DBS and retinal implants all using Pt for neural interfacing. This is due to the electrochemical stability and corrosion resistance of Pt (White and Gross, 1974) which has been demonstrated to have limited reactivity to biological environments compared to other metals (Merrill et al., 2005; Polikov et al., 2005). However, while technological advances have driven the miniaturization of electronics leading to smaller implant devices (Nakayama and Matsuda, 1995; Schuettler et al., 2005; Cheung, 2007; Wester et al., 2009), aspects of Pt electrical, mechanical, and biological performance remain as limiting factors which prevent the application of high-density microelectrode arrays for neural interfacing.

For every electrode there is an intrinsic charge injection limit, restricting the voltage that can be safely generated at the electrode's surface. Once this voltage is breached, purely capacitive charge transfer can no longer be maintained and irreversible faradaic reactions occur. Beyond this electrochemical limit, also known as the water window, irreversible electrolysis of water can result in tissue damage, electrode dissolution, pH changes and production of unwanted chemical species (McCreery et al., 1997; Zhong et al., 2001; Green et al., 2008a; Poole-Warren et al., 2010; Niina et al., 2011). Additionally, as an electrode is reduced in size the charge it must pass per unit area increases, directly increasing the voltage on the electrode and hence reducing the total charge which can be safely delivered. It has been shown that to stimulate light percepts by electrical stimulation of the retina in visually impaired patients, a charge density between 48 and 357 $\mu C/cm^2$ is required (Humayun et al., 2003; Mahadevappa et al., 2005), but the electrochemical injection limit of Pt has been reported as ranging from 20 to 150 $\mu C/cm^2$ (Rose and Robblee, 1990; Green et al., 2012c). This small range of overlap means that bare metal electrodes cannot be safely reduced in size and still maintain safe charge injection at a therapeutic level. With the increasing pressure to reduce the size of electrodes, driven by the need to make smaller but higher resolution implants, Pt electrical properties have become a challenging issue (Green et al., 2012c; Shepherd et al., 2013). New electrode geometries, materials, or coatings must be used to increase the charge transfer surface area such that the safety limits are preserved. Surface modifications, through electrode roughening or coating, have been reported to have great potential for increasing the charge injection capacity of microelectrodes, as detailed later in this review (Cogan et al., 2005; Schuettler et al., 2005; Abidian et al., 2010; Green et al., 2012b,c, 2013a).

Mechanically, Pt is significantly stiffer than the neural tissue with which it interfaces (Green et al., 2012b). The elastic modulus of Pt is about 164 GPa (Merker et al., 2001), but most neural tissue has a modulus of less than 100 kPa (Lacour et al., 2010). This mechanical disparity can exacerbate the chronic inflammatory response at the implant site, as the shear between a stiff electrode and the soft neural tissue continues to incite inflammation during tissue movement and device micromotion (Rousche et al., 2001; Leach et al., 2010). More flexible device designs move with the tissue, which can reduce damage at the neural interface (Richter et al., 2013), but require tethering which creates damage in adjacent tissue sites (Tyler and Durand, 2002). Electrode coatings, in particular polymeric films which utilize conductive polymers or hydrogels, have been shown to impart a softer electrode interface, around 1 MPa (Yang and Martin, 2006; Green et al., 2012b) and it is expected that these coatings can be used to dampen or mediate the mechanical difference between a metal electrode and the tissue with which it interfaces.

Chronic biological responses to metal electrodes have been reported to challenge the maintenance of an effective neural interface (Turner et al., 1999; Biran et al., 2005; Barrese et al., 2013). The implantation and chronic presence of a neural interfacing device in the central nervous system (CNS) induces a cascade of biological processes which can ultimately isolate the electrode and gradually decrease device performance. Reports and reviews on implantation trauma have detailed the cellular and molecular interactions involved in the acute inflammatory response which primarily includes immune cell activation and migration, and local ischemia (Fitch and Silver, 2008; Zhong and Bellamkonda, 2008; Whitney et al., 2009). The biological environment is further altered as the ongoing inflammatory response produces reactive astrocytosis in the damaged area (Banati et al., 1993; Fitch and Silver, 1997; Babcock et al., 2003). Over time, layers of activated microglia, invading macrophages, reactive astrocytes and migrating meningeal fibroblasts can encapsulate CNS implants (Turner et al., 1999; Cui et al., 2003). Extra layers of non-excitable cells will increase the neural interface impedance. For recording electrodes this reduces the possibility of recording and localizing single unit activity due to a diminished signal to noise ratio (SNR). As Pt is a relatively stable material which has limited interaction with the biological environment, immune cells are prevented from dissolving the electrodes. However, a persistent effort to disintegrate metal sites yields a constant environment of cytotoxic factors that may contribute to migration away from and cell death near the electrodes, including the target neurons (Weldon et al., 1998). Furthermore, Pt and other metallic electrodes are typically produced with smooth surfaces which do not encourage neural tissue integration, as a result immune cells can access the gap between the electrode and target cells. Several detailed studies have described the chronic biological response to implantable electrodes in animal models (Hascup et al., 2009; Ward et al., 2009; Leach et al., 2010; Woolley et al., 2011).

In the literature, the limitations associated with Pt electrode performance have been addressed through several varied approaches, which include passivation and surface texturing of electrodes to reduce impedance and enhance tissue integration (Cogan et al., 2005; Schuettler, 2007; Abidian et al., 2010; Green et al., 2012a,b). However, it is through the development of new coating technologies that improvement can be made more widely across the electrical, mechanical and biological properties of electrodes. In particular the use of carbon nanotubes (CNTs), CPs, hydrogels and conductive hydrogels (CHs), depicted in **Figure 1**, have shown that tailored approaches can be used to create multi-functional electrode arrays which not only improve the electrode material properties, but also provide biomolecules to aid in the establishment of a chronically stable neural interface. While substantial research has been conducted on CNTs, CPs, hydrogels and composite polymers, it is important to understand both the advantages and limitations of these materials and how they impact on the biological environment. Furthermore, as greater demands on electrode technologies drive the development of next-generation bionic devices, it is proposed that tissue engineered electrodes, such as that shown in **Figure 1** (bottom, right) may provide an avenue for directly interfacing with neural cells through synaptic communication. This review highlights the materials and emerging technologies that address some of the issues related to conventional smooth metallic electrodes including enhancing charge transfer, tissue integration and reducing mechanical mismatch. Furthermore it proposes an innovative approach to creating electrodes which use neural cells embedded within the electrode surface for a more natural approach to cell activation which may reduce scar tissue formation and aid in the establishment of a stable neural interface.

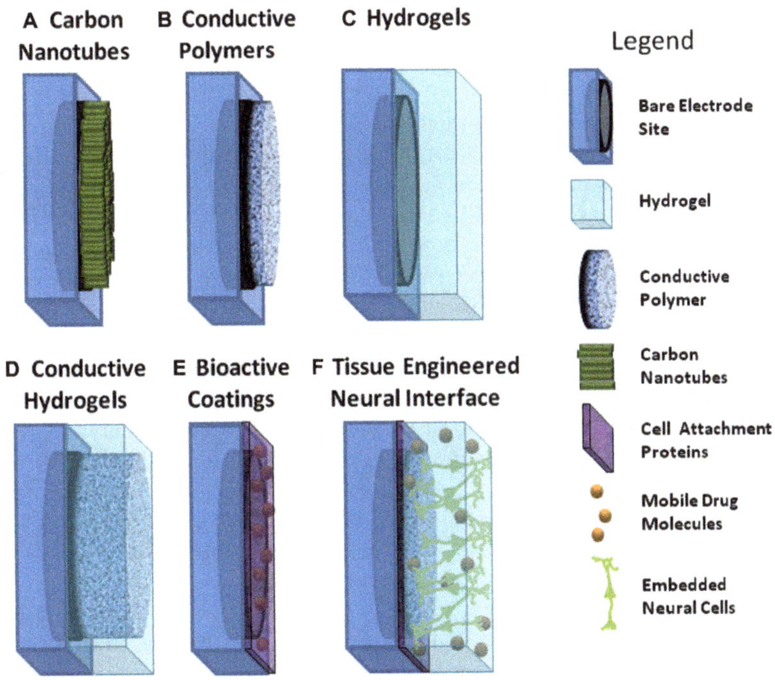

FIGURE 1 | Schematic of coating approaches used for addressing the limitations of metallic electrodes. **(A)** aligned carbon nanotubes on metallic electrodes; **(B)** conductive polymers electrodeposited on metallic electrodes; **(C)** hydrogels polymerised to coat electrode site and device; **(D)** interpenetrating network of conductive polymer grown through hydrogel coating to form conductive hydrogel over electrode sites; **(E)** electrode site coated with biologically active molecules; **(F)** schematic of ideal tissue engineered interface incorporating combined coating approaches of conductive polymers, hydrogels and attachment factors with neural cells.

COATINGS FOR NEURAL INTERFACES

A common objective of modifying an electrode surface is to impart roughening or rather an increased electrochemical surface area. Several roughened morphologies have been shown to enhance charge transfer to within safe stimulation limits (Rose and Robblee, 1990; Cogan et al., 2007; Green et al., 2013b) as well as providing a surface to improve neuronal attachment (Hallab et al., 2001; Fan et al., 2002). Roughening the surface can be achieved by altering the existing metallic surface or through coating with an alternate material. While direct modification of the metallic surface can impart roughness without significantly altering the electrode chemistry (Green et al., 2010c), the benefits are limited, in that the material stiffness and chemical compatibility with the biological system remains unchanged. Electrodes can be coated through a variety of methods including electrochemical deposition (Cui et al., 2003; Geddes and Roeder, 2003; Green et al., 2008a; Abidian et al., 2010; Hassler et al., 2011), physical vapor deposition (Geddes and Roeder, 2003; Gabay et al., 2007; Shoval et al., 2009; Chen et al., 2011) such as sputtering (Geddes and Roeder, 2003) or evaporation, spin-coating (Green et al., 2010c; Lacour et al., 2010) or dip-coating (Schuettler et al., 2005) from solutions which require curing (Fieberg and Reis, 2002; Chen et al., 2011; Rao et al., 2012) or cross-linking (Guimard et al., 2007). The method employed depends strongly on the type of material which is required for the coating. Electrochemical deposition is used to apply a material directly to an electrode site (Cui et al., 2001b; Bartlett et al., 2002; LaVan et al., 2003), but other methods coat the entire construct and often require post-processing to ensure the coating is applied only to the required areas of the electrode array (Kim et al., 2008; Abidian and Martin, 2009). Both organic coatings such as CNTs, CPs, and CHs, and inorganic coatings including Pt-Black, titanium nitride (TiN) and iridium oxide (IrOx) have been used to impart increased charge injection capacity to metallic electrodes (Cogan et al., 2005; Schuettler, 2007; Abidian et al., 2010; Green et al., 2012a,b). However, the organic coatings hold a significant benefit over the inorganic coatings as they can be easily modified to include functional molecules to influence the biological response. Organic polymers based on hydrogels present an alternate coating option. While hydrogels do not inherently impart a roughened surface area, they have been shown to provide mechanical and biological benefits to electrodes which, in turn improve the chronic electrical performance. Additionally, hydrogels have formed the basis of several composite coatings which utilize the combination of a conductive component embedded in a non-conductive polymer matrix.

CARBON NANOTUBES

Carbon nanotubes have remarkable mechanical and electrical properties that exhibit noted interaction with neural tissue. CNTs are cylinders formed from seamless sheets of graphene with a wall thickness of 1 atom. Single walled CNTs (SWCNTs) as the name suggests have only one sheet creating a single cylinder, but multi-walled CNTs (MWCNTs) have multiple concentric cylinders of graphene. Some of the methods used to apply CNTs to electrodes are chemical vapor deposition (CVD) (Heim et al., 2012), immersion drying (Haghighi and Bozorgzadeh, 2011) and electrodeposition (Yang et al., 2010; Suzuki et al., 2013). CVD presents some drawbacks as it yields secondary toxic chemicals that require further purification (De Volder et al., 2013), also this technique requires higher temperatures process and this limits the possible materials that can be coated. CNT coatings produced by immersion are limited in durability, as the nanotubes are not bonded to surface. Electrodeposition is considered a simpler method to coat films with controllable thickness yielding a mechanically stable coating (Yang et al., 2010). It is worth noting that CNTs do not simply adhere to metallic substrates and as a result must be chemically modified or embedded within a polymer matrix to remain adhered to an electrode. As such all of the coatings described are composites of CNTs.

Perhaps one of the most important properties of CNTs is their ability to enhance electrical properties of metallic electrodes. The addition of CNTs to both insulating and conductive materials results in electrodes with higher charge storage capacity (CSC) and lower impedance (Green et al., 2008b; Xiao et al., 2012; David-Pur et al., 2013). By increasing the thickness of a coating containing CNTs the CSC has been reported to be as high as 70 mC/cm^2 (Luo et al., 2011b), although in this study the CNTs were embedded in a CP which likely contributed to the high CSC. It has also been shown that the presence of CNTs in a CP composite can stabilize the electrochemical properties of the coating (Green et al., 2008b). Similarly, several studies on electrodes coated with CNTs report a substantial increase in SNR for recording electrodes (Gabay et al., 2007; Yu et al., 2007; Keefer et al., 2008; Lin et al., 2009; Shoval et al., 2009; Hsu et al., 2010; Suzuki et al., 2013) which is thought to be predominantly due to the low impedance CNTs impart to electrodes (Keefer et al., 2008). In particular, (Shoval et al., 2009) presents an evident increase in SNR when recording neuronal activity from retina tissue. In this work CNT coatings increased the ability to record voltage spikes, increasing the SNR by up to three times in comparison with titanium nitride electrodes.

The low volume, high surface area of nanotubes means that they can dramatically increase the charge transfer area of an electrode. Their nanoscale features which enable them to penetrate cellular membranes, are also expected to enhance electrical performance by promoting a more intimate interaction with tissue. (Suzuki et al., 2013) detected action potentials and field postsynaptic potentials employing a multi-electrode array (MEA) coated with planar CNTs. In stimulation electrodes, a low impedance and decreased activation threshold have been achieved by several groups who have embedded CNTs in flexible polymer substrates including parylene-C, poly(dimethyl siloxane) (PDMS) and the CP polypyrrole (Nguyen-Vu et al., 2006; Wang et al., 2006; David-Pur et al., 2013). The safe charge injection limit of CNT containing coatings have been reported to be between 1.6 and 2.5 mC/cm^2 (Wang et al., 2006; Luo et al., 2011b). This is more than 10 times the charge injection reported for Pt.

Carbon nanotubes are very stiff materials with a Young modulus of 1.25TPa (Krishnan et al., 1998). This is a significant drawback when interfacing with neural tissue where mechanical mismatch between the device and cells is one of the main factors contributing to chronic inflammation. However, it is arguable that the nanoscale dimensions of these materials minimize the impact of shear stress at the cellular interface. In fact the ability for nanotubes to penetrate cells has been well detailed (Kagan et al., 2006; Tian et al., 2006; Gilmour et al., 2013). Additionally, nanotube morphology has promising properties for neural tissue engineering, with most coatings having a fibrillar surface, as shown in **Figure 2**. This morphology presents the cells with a nanometric roughness that is thought to create a more intimate cell-electrode interface (Keefer et al., 2008; Seidlits et al., 2008) suitable for cellular attachment.

Despite the promising electrical and physical properties of CNTs their biocompatibility is a subject of considerable discussion. Being small and biologically inert provides CNTs with the ability to infiltrate tissues without being identified by the immune system (Seidlits et al., 2008). While these nanoscale structures are less likely to be identified by reactive astrocytes and consequently may minimize scar tissue formation, (Kagan et al., 2006), it has been suggested this may represent a hazard as internalized CNTs can damage the intracellular bodies including the nuclei of cells. Additionally, it has been shown that high concentrations of CNTs induce cytotoxicity, either as un-functionalised SWCNTs or as composites with other polymers. Cell death in a dose dependent manner has been reported for lymphocytes (Bottini et al., 2006) and fibroblasts (Tian et al., 2006). Likewise, Webster et al. (2004) created CNT composites with polycarbonate urethane and their results showed that the toxicity of the composite increased whenever the proportion of the CNTs in the composite was 10% or more. It is clear that the biocompatibility of CNTs will remain a controversial subject, but coatings which can constrain the CNTs while utilizing their impressive electrical conductivity have significant potential in the future of neural interfaces.

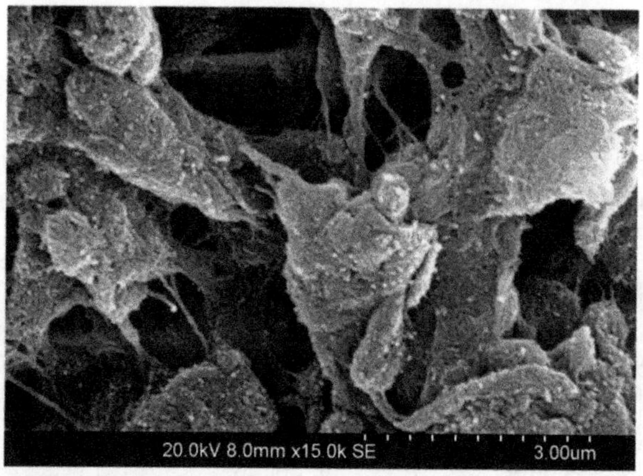

FIGURE 2 | Scanning electron microscope (SEM) image of multi-walled carbon nanotubes (MWNTs) coating a platinum disk electrode, demonstrate that CNTs produce fibrillar surface structures, imparting a high charge transfer area to the typically flat electrode. The platinum disk is not visible, as the entire substrate is covered with CNT bundles. Image produced at 15,000× magnification.

CONDUCTIVE POLYMERS

CPs are synthesized from chains of chemical compounds that present alternating double and single bonds in their structure (Guimard et al., 2007). This structure, known as a conjugated system, confers the conductive property to the polymer. When doped with an appropriately charged ion to stabilize the backbone, high conductivity can be obtained (Guimard et al., 2007). CPs can inject both electronic and ionic charge (Cogan, 2008) and have been used to both stimulate nerve tissue and record neuronal activity (Kim and Romero-Ortega, 2012). Among several conductive polymers, polypyrrole (PPy) (Cui et al., 2003; Kim et al., 2004; George et al., 2005; Stauffer and Cui, 2006; Green et al., 2008a) and poly(ethylene dioxythiophene) (PEDOT; Cui and Martin, 2003; Xiao et al., 2004; Yang et al., 2005; Ludwig et al., 2006, 2011; Green et al., 2008a), shown in **Figure 3** have been extensively used to coat neuroprosthetic electrode sites. Other CPs which have been investigated to a lesser extent include polyterthiophene (Stevenson et al., 2010), polyaniline (Huang et al., 2004; Bidez et al., 2006) and various modifications of PEDOT such as methoxy-PEDOT (PEDOT-MeOH), carboxylic acid modified PEDOT (PEDOT-COOH) and propylenedioxythiophene (Pro-DOT) (Martin and Feldman, 2012). PEDOT is considered one of the most promising CPs due its electrical and chemical stability in an oxygenated, hydrated environment (Cui and Martin, 2003; Guimard et al., 2007; Green et al., 2013b).

The fabrication method and the choice of CP components are critical to determining the resulting mechanical, chemical and electrical performance (Baek et al., 2013a). CPs can be fabricated by either chemical or electrochemical methods. While chemical synthesis enables the development of complex and highly ordered structures, the difficulties in applying these materials to metallic electrodes have largely hindered their investigation and application to neuroprosthetics. Additionally, chemically synthesized CPs require post-process doping to reach similar conductivities to electrochemically polymerized CPs. Electrodeposition is the most common method used to fabricate CP coatings on electrodes. This method enables direct formation of the polymer on the electrode site and by varying the time over which electrodeposition occurs, the thickness and roughness of the CP can be controlled (Fonner et al., 2008; Baek et al., 2013a). The dopant ion is included in the monomer electrolyte solution and is directly incorporated within the CP. Varying the dopant type and concentration also impacts on the CP electrical (Guimard et al., 2007) and morphological properties (Green et al., 2012a). While cations can be used to dope CPs, anions are almost exclusively used for electrodeposited CPs which are polymerized by oxidation producing a positively charge backbone, requiring a negatively charged dopant (Guimard et al., 2007). The most effective dopants for producing CPs with high charge transfer area and stable electrochemical properties are ions with sulfonate moieties, although phosphates and perchlorates have been successfully used to fabricate CP coatings with high charge transfer capacity. Common dopants which have been extensively investigated have included poly(styrene sulfonate) (PSS), para-toluene sulphonate (pTS), dexamethasone phosphate (Dex-P), and perchlorate (ClO_4).

CPs have been shown to improve on the electrical performance of Pt across various metrics important to electrode function, including the CSC (Cogan, 2008; Abidian et al., 2010; Green et al., 2013b), the electrochemical impedance (Kim et al., 2004, 2008; Abidian et al., 2010; Green et al., 2013b), and the charge injection limit (Kim et al., 2004, 2008; Green et al., 2012a,b). A summary of the various CPs and their electrical properties is shown in **Table 1**. In general CPs produced from PEDOT and doped with small sulfonate ions, namely pTS, have the highest charge storage capacity, lowest impedance and highest injection limit. Coating Pt electrodes with PEDOT/pTS can increase the CSC by one order of magnitude and the charge injection limit by up to two orders of magnitude (Cogan, 2008; Green et al., 2013b). Similarly, in the latter work the frequency dependant impedance is also reduced in the low frequency range, where it is proposed that capacitive double layers are the dominant mode of charge transfer (Green et al., 2013b). These improvements in electrical properties are primarily due to the increase in the charge transfer area of the electrode which occurs as a result of the intrinsic rough morphology of PEDOT. When large anions or polymers are used to dope PEDOT the surface is typically smoother which results in poorer electrical performance, such as that shown in **Table 1** for PEDOT/PSS. Small dopants enable more efficient polymerization than larger dopants, and structurally enable greater flexibility in the backbone during PEDOT formation. As a result these smaller

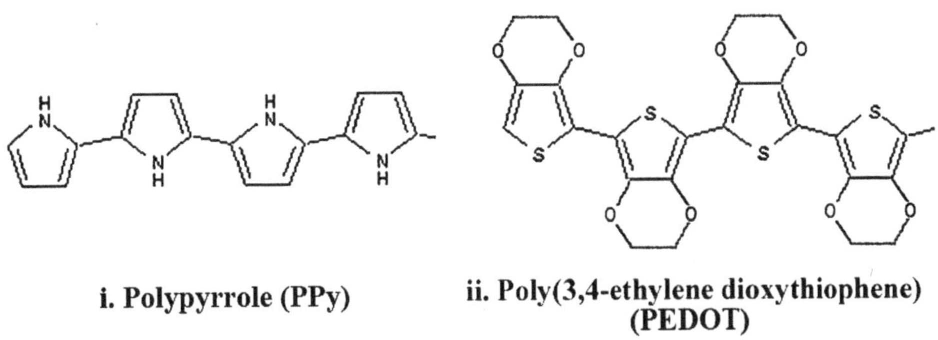

FIGURE 3 | Structure of PPy and PEDOT with alternating single and double bonds along the backbone which impart conductivity (Green et al., 2008a).

dopants create rougher, more nodular surfaces. The comparison of PEDOT/pTS and PEDOT/PSS surface morphology is shown in **Figure 4**. Since common analytical techniques such as stylus profilometry and indentation (including scanning AFM) can damage the CP surface, there are very few papers in the literature which quantify CP surface roughness. With the recent development of non-contact optical profilometry there is now an opportunity to provide measurements of roughness which can be related to the electrical performance of CPs. Using optical profilometry (Green et al., 2013b) have reported that PEDOT/pTS coatings can increase the surface area of a smooth electrode by a factor of 2, which closely correlated to the reduction in voltage drop across Pt electrodes coated with this CP (Green et al., 2013b). The electrical stability of CP electrode coatings is also related to the chemical constituents, with literature reporting minimal changes in PEDOT/pTS following more than 2 billion pulses (Boretius et al., 2011; Green et al., 2012a). However Yamato et al. (1995) reported loss of 95% of the electroactivity of PPy/PSS following 16 h of electrical polarization.

Mechanically CPs are largely claimed to reduce the stiffness of the electrode interface, however, few papers in the literature actually quantify the modulus of CPs. Several reports of dry CP films based on PEDOT demonstrate that the elastic modulus varies with dopant choice, but generally are in the range of 1–3 GPa (Yang and Martin, 2006; Baek et al., 2013a). More recent papers demonstrate that when hydrated the elastic modulus of CPs, in particular PEDOT/PSS can be as low as 40 MPa (Green et al., 2012b).This is substantially lower than the elastic modulus of Pt, but still more than two orders of magnitude higher than neural tissue. While CPs may have the capacity to dampen the mechanical mismatch at the neural interface, the mechanical stability is a greater concern. Several reports claim that delamination of these coatings can occur *in vivo* (Peixoto et al., 2009; Boretius et al., 2011) and moreover the surface, in particular of the highly rough PEDOT, is brittle and friable (Collier et al., 2000; Green et al., 2010b). While CPs have the benefit of being able to be functionalized to incorporate biological components, the addition of these large molecules further diminishes the mechanical stability of these coatings. Several approaches, including chemical tethering (Labaye et al., 2002) and mechanical interlocking (Green et al., 2012a) have been used to improve the adherence of CP coatings, but polymer cohesiveness requires improvement.

Various CPs have been shown *in vitro* to have cytocompatible properties, with several cell types including neuroblastomas (Bolin et al., 2009), spiral ganglion cells (Evans et al., 2009) and pheochromocytoma (PC12) neural model cells (Schmidt et al., 1997; Green et al., 2009). In spite of the promising results, little *in vivo* evidence has been presented to support the chronic stability and the benefit of applying CPs to neural interfacing electrodes. (Wilks et al., 2011) polymerized PEDOT *in vivo* within the rodent cerebral cortex, creating a direct CP interface with the neuronal tissue. In this work (Wilks et al., 2011) reported lowered impedance values, improved recording quality of local field potentials, and a tight cloud of PEDOT penetrating into the tissue surrounding the electrode. (Cui et al., 2003) were able to efficiently record neuronal activity for 2 weeks by implanting gold electrodes coated with PPy in guinea pigs cerebral cortex. After 2 weeks the polymer underwent structural changes and scar tissue encapsulation started to decrease electrode performance. Similarly, (Ludwig et al., 2006) demonstrated that CPs improve neural recordings using a PEDOT/PSS coated Michigan probe electrode array implanted in the rat motor cortex for 6 weeks. However impedance increased over time with a respective reduction in SNR correlating with a neural density decrease near the electrodes. It was suggested that neuronal loss was due to implant trauma. Recent evidence suggests that neurons not only may die following damage during the implantation process but can also migrate away from the electrode as the neuroglia isolates the device as a result of foreign body reactions (McConnell et al., 2009).

CPs address some of the limitations associated with reducing the size of Pt electrodes, providing electrical, mechanical and biological benefits. Despite the ability of CPs to enhance electrode performance, issues remain concerning mechanical stability and inflammatory reactions in the chronic implant environment. Approaches to improve the biological performance of CPs have included the development of composite CP-hydrogels and the use of biological inclusions intended to influence the cellular response.

Table 1 | Electrical properties of conductive polymers.

Conducting polymer	Charge storage capacity (CSC) (mC/cm^2)	Impedance @ 1000 kHz (Ω/cm^2)	Electrochemical charge injection limit (mC/cm^2)	Reference
PEDOT/pTS	245.59^S; 402.23^R	2.65×10^3	2.09 ± 0.2^S; 2.01 ± 0.4^R	Green et al. (2009, 2012a)
PEDOT/PSS	105.17^S; 243.48^R	2.03×10^3	1.36 ± 0.1^S; 1.52 ± 0.5^R	Green et al. (2012a), Baek et al. (2013a)
PEDOT/ClO_4	98.49^S; 389.88^R	2.03×10^3	2.39 ± 0.4^S; 2.09 ± 0.5^R	Baek et al. (2013a)
PPy/PSS	186.4	256.41×10^6	–	Cui et al. (2001a,b)
PTT/Dex-P	~35	–	–	Stevenson et al. (2010)
PProDOT	5.8	–	–	Rosario-Canales et al. (2011)
Poly(EDOT-COOH)	–	~10	–	Luo et al. (2012)
P(PRoDOT-OH)	–	~10	–	Luo et al. (2012)

S, coated on smooth platinum. R, coated on roughened platinum.

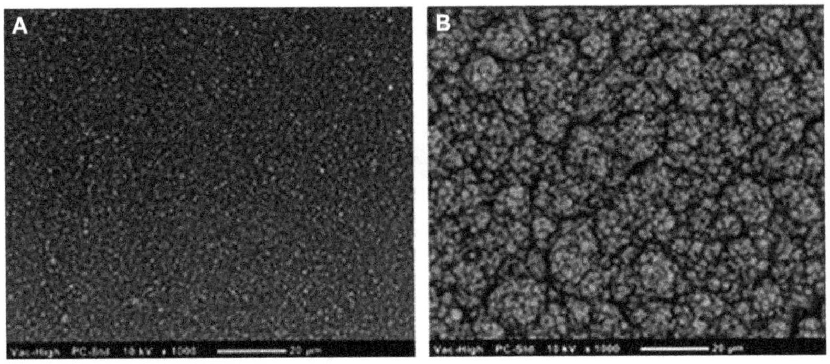

FIGURE 4 | Scanning electron microscope images show that (A) PEDOT doped with PSS produces a coating which is substantially smoother than that produced from (B) PEDOT doped with pTS.

HYDROGELS

The need to develop an electrode interfacing material with an elastic modulus similar to that of nerve tissue is a recurring concept (Kim et al., 2008). Hydrogels are polymer systems which have been extensively studied for tissue engineering (Lee and Mooney, 2001; Hoffman, 2002).The networks are held together by physical or chemical crosslinks and network design can incorporate a range of degradation profiles or may be non-degradable. Structure and mechanical properties of hydrogel networks can be controlled through selection of fabrication technique and chemical composition (Lacour et al., 2010). These crosslinked polymeric networks have high water contents making them an attractive platform for neural interfacing. Hydrogels are commonly fabricated from either natural materials such as collagen (Ma et al., 2004; Mao and Kisaalita, 2004; Suri and Schmidt, 2010), fibrin (Georges et al., 2006; Ahmed et al., 2008), and alginate (Novikova et al., 2006; Banerjee et al., 2009) or synthetic materials like polyvinyl alcohol (PVA) (Lu et al., 2009; Lim et al., 2012, 2013), polyethylene glycol (PEG; Drury and Mooney, 2003) and polyacrylamide (Georges et al., 2006). Synthetic polymers enable controlled hydrogel mechanical properties but lack cellular activity due to the absence of bioactive elements. On the other hand natural polymers support enhanced cellular interactions but form constructs that are less mechanically and dimensionally stable compared with synthetic hydrogels. Co-hydrogel or biosynthetic systems combine the benefits of natural and synthetic polymers and permit greater control over the polymer properties. While many hydrogel systems have been investigated for tissue engineering, only a few types have been applied to neuroprosthetic electrode arrays.

Although few hydrogels are considered conductive, most are poor insulators due to the open polymer mesh structure which swells in aqueous environments. Winter et al. applied poly(ethylene glycol)-poly(lactic acid) (PEGPLA) to multielectrode arrays and found that the electrochemical characteristics of the underlying IrOx coated electrode array were preserved (Winter et al., 2007) however, the thickness of the layer was not reported. Zhong and Bellamkonda coated electrode arrays with a nitrocellulose based hydrogel and found that impedance of the neural interface was reduced (Zhong and Bellamkonda, 2005). Hydrogel mesh structures provide minimal hindrance to the ions required for capacitive charge transfer. Furthermore, some hydrogels have a strongly charged backbone which encourages ion sequestering (Hoffman, 2002). These ions provide a ready source of charge for formation of a capacitive double layer at an underlying metallic electrode interface. However, it is also observed that when a hydrogel coating swells *in vivo*, it can push the target neural tissue further away from the electrode (Kim et al., 2010), necessitating higher charge delivery to activate the neurons.

By developing hydrogels with a mechanical modulus within the range of nerve tissue, less than 100 kPa (Lacour et al., 2010), it has been suggested that hydrogel coatings can reduce stress related to micromotion of stiff materials (Kim et al., 2010). The compression modulus of hydrogels is highly variable and strongly dependant on the type of polymer used for coating, a summary of hydrogel moduli is presented in **Table 2**. In a study by Baek, hydrophilic brushes fabricated from polyhydroxyethylmethacrylate (pHEMA) were applied to gold electrodes and found to reduce the modulus from 70 GPa to 143 MPa (Baek et al., 2013b). In a similar study by Green et al. (2012b), Pt was coated with the biosynthetic co-hydrogel polyvinyl alcohol-heparin (PVA-Hep) and the electrode modulus was reduced to near 100 kPa. Several studies on hydrogel chemistry and structure have shown that the mechanical properties of synthetic polymers can be controlled through varying the length of the polymer backbone, the number of crosslinks and the percentage polymer composition relative to the water content (LeRoux et al., 1999; Normand et al., 2000; Almany and Seliktar, 2005; Nilasaroya et al., 2008). However, a material that is as soft as the tissue presents difficulties during implantation (Kim et al., 2008; Richter et al., 2013). In an effort to address the latter issue, recent research has investigated novel hydrogel materials which have switchable properties when exposed to different environmental conditions. Capadona et al., developed a cellulose-whisker nanocomposite that softens when the temperature is increased from 25 to 37°C. It was shown that the initial stiffness of the arrays produced with this material were 4.2 GPa which was reduced to 1.6 MPa in 10 min following immersion in physiological fluid at 37°C (Capadona et al., 2008). It is conceivable that through choice of polymer and control of the hydrogel structural characteristics, the

Table 2 | Mechanical moduli of various hydrogels.

Hydrogel	Type (synthetic, natural, or biosynthetic)	Modulus range (kPa)	Reference
Polyvinyl alcohol (PVA)	Synthetic	2560–7360*	Baker et al. (2012)
Polyethylene glycol (PEG)	Synthetic		
Poly(2-hydroxyethyl methacrylate) (pHEMA)	Synthetic	440 ± 10	Jhaveri et al. (2008)
Poly(lactic-co-glycolic acid)	Synthetic	752 ± 54	Vaquette et al. (2010)
Collagen	Natural	0.5–12	Raub et al. (2010)
Agarose	Natural	1.5–2580**	Letherby and Young (1981), Normand et al. (2000), Aymard et al. (2001), Ahearne et al. (2005)
Alginate	Natural	1–8**	LeRoux et al. (1999)
PVA-heparin	Biosynthetic	60–68**	Nilasaroya et al. (2008)
PEG-Fibrinogen	Biosynthetic	0.01–2**	Almany and Seliktar (2005)

**Values change depending on confined compression **Values are proportional to the percent polymer composition.*

mechanical modulus of an electrode can be tailored for the neural interface.

Cell interactions with hydrogels, like the mechanical properties, depend on the polymer choice. Synthetic hydrogels generally have poor cell interactions which have made them useful as antifouling coatings for implants (Telford et al., 2010; Liu et al., 2012). This property may be of use in neural prosthetics where protein deposition, which increases the impedance of electrodes, can be prevented (Li et al., 2005; Green et al., 2010a). However, a significant benefit of synthetic hydrogel systems is that they can be modified to incorporate biological molecules. The ability to functionalize hydrogels has been extensively explored (Hoffman, 2002; Willerth and Sakiyama-Elbert, 2007) and they can be modified to include covalently bound bioactive molecules, to bind and release growth factors (Nilasaroya et al., 2008), or to degrade over time to allow controlled drug release (Anseth et al., 2002). (Zhong et al., 2001) demonstrated that natural hydrogels of collagen promoted cortical nerve cell attachment. Lim et al. have further shown that very small amounts of the collagen derivative gelatin, incorporated at 0.01–1 wt% within a synthetic PVA hydrogel can promote attachment of various cell types including neuronal cells (Lim et al., 2013). Further, Winter et al. used degradable PEGPLA to successfully deliver nerve growth factor (NGF) and promote the outgrowth of neuronal processes from PC12 cells (Winter et al., 2007). Several studies have examined release of drugs from hydrogel coatings (Zhong and Bellamkonda, 2005; Winter et al., 2007) and the issues related to drug delivery are discussed below in relation to bioactive coatings. Ultimately, further studies are required to develop a hydrogel which can soften device interfaces while limiting the gap between the electrode and tissue.

As hydrogels do not substantially improve the electrical properties of the underlying material, they can only go part of the way to addressing the limitations of metallic electrodes. However, there is a wealth of literature on the design, fabrication and characterisation of hydrogel systems for alternate biomedical applications (Lee and Mooney, 2001; Hoffman, 2002; Yu and Bellamkonda, 2003; Kurisawa et al., 2005; Lee et al., 2008; Nicodemus and Bryant, 2008; Winter et al., 2008; Zuidema et al., 2011; Abidian et al., 2012). It is expected that through consideration of this body of work a systematic assessment of various hydrogel chemistries and structures will allow selection of appropriate polymers for improving the mechanical softness and biological interaction of neural electrode arrays. It is proposed, however, that such a hydrogel will require additional modification to incorporate conductive components to ultimately improve charge transfer and facilitate the development of high density microelectrode arrays.

CONDUCTIVE HYDROGELS

Blending hydrogels with conductive components such as CNTs or CPs has provided an avenue for maintaining the desired electrical characteristics of a coated electrode while imparting reduced stiffness (Green et al., 2012b; Xiao et al., 2012). The hydrogel component also presents the opportunity to incorporate bioactive molecules at higher concentrations than in CNT or CP films alone. Since CNTs usually require a polymer matrix to constrain them within the electrode coating, composites based on CNTs have been discussed above. CP-hydrogel hybrids (known as conductive hydrogels) are a more recent development which address the limitations of homogenous CPs (Green et al., 2010a, 2012a). As the CP component is fabricated within the hydrogel matrix, the friable particulates are encapsulated, improving the mechanical stability of the coating. Few conductive hydrogel (CH) systems have been developed for neural interface purposes(Kim et al., 2004, 2010; Green et al., 2012a,b; Hassarati et al., 2014), but preliminary studies have demonstrated the potential of this coating technology.

The CSC, impedance and charge injection limit of CH coated electrodes are significantly better than bare metal electrodes, but are also often improved compared to homogenous CPs (Cheung, 2007; Green et al., 2012b; Hassarati et al., 2014). Kim et al. (2004) electrodeposited PPy through a 1% alginate hydrogel and found that the resulting construct had an impedance of 7 kΩ at 1 kHz (for a 1257 μm^2 electrode) which was approximately 14 times lower than the PPy films alone. In a similar study Chikar et al. (2012) deposited PEDOT through an alginate hydrogel and found that the CSC increased exponentially relative to the amount of PEDOT deposited within the hydrogel. This increase in CSC relative to the amount of PEDOT was more pronounced than that reported for PEDOT as a homogenous film, indicating that the same amount of material when deposited in a hydrogel had a greater impact on the electrical properties. It is generally thought that the hydrophilic mesh provided by the hydrogel promotes a large three-dimensional surface of conductive material which is available for charge transfer. This increase in surface area compared to the relatively dense and hydrophobic surface of a homogenous CP is expected to be the source of the enhanced electrochemical properties. The increase charge transfer area also leads to significant improvements in charge injection limit. In a study by Hassarati et al. (2014) a CH fabricated from PEDOT/PVA-Hep was applied to cochlear implants and increased the charge injection limit of the Pt electrodes by up to 24 times. This coating was also shown to be stable over 1 billion stimulations at clinically relevant levels.

Several CH systems have been shown to reduce the stiffness of electrodes, and as expected the modulus of these hybrids typically lies between that of the component CP and hydrogel (Aouada et al., 2006; Baek et al., 2013b; Green et al., 2012b). Double network polymers of chemically synthesized PEDOT:PSS and polyacrylamide (PAAm) were found to have elastic moduli which ranged between 27 and 350 kPa. The increased stiffness was a function of both the percentage content of the stiffer PEDOT:PSS and the cross-link density of the PAAm (Aouada et al., 2006). When chemically synthesized CPs are used as a component of a CH the amount of CP can be carefully controlled, and has an impact on both the electrical conductivity and stiffness of the hybrid. However, when electrodeposited CPs are grown through hydrogels the elastic moduli of the resulting hybrid appears to be minimally variable (Green et al., 2012b). In a recent study, the stiffness of two different CHs was found to be close to 1 MPa, despite the CHs being fabricated from hydrogels with different chemistries and percentage of polymer content (Green et al., 2012b). The morphology of these CH variants was also dissimilar, as depicted in **Figure 5**, but both the electrical and mechanical properties were not significantly different. While there are several studies which report combining hydrogels with electrodeposited CPs for application to electrodes, few have quantified the modulus of these hybrids.

Conductive hydrogels have shown negligible *in vitro* cytotoxicity and good compatibility with several cell types (Green et al., 2010a; Mario Cheong et al., 2013). The biological properties of these composites reflect the properties of the component polymers, which have been shown to be compatible with a range of cell types. Specifically, CH materials have been used to support the attachment and growth of PC12 cells, the interleukin-3 dependent pro-B cell line (BaF3) and Schwann cells (Runge et al., 2010; Mario Cheong et al., 2013). *In vivo* PEDOT-alginate CHs (Kim et al., 2010) have been implanted in the auditory cortex area of the guinea pig. Despite the impedance of the hydrogel electrodes being much lower *in vitro*, the CH had similar impedance *in vivo* to that of uncoated electrodes. However, a significant improvement in SNR was found in the initial period following implantation. The impact of the material on the surrounding tissue was not examined histologically, but it was proposed that swelling of the construct increased the distance between the electrodes and target tissue (Kim et al., 2010). In a related field Abidian et al. (2012) developed PEDOT-agarose nerve conduits which were found to support nerve regeneration, although control autografts supported regeneration of significantly greater nerve fiber numbers. It was proposed that the PEDOT within the agarose inhibited cellular access to essential nutrients, limiting the development of functional nerve fascicles. It is also important to note that these studies did not utilize any active stimulation of tissue. It is clear that more information is required to successfully develop CHs and it is critical to assess the performance of these constructs *in vivo* under active implant conditions.

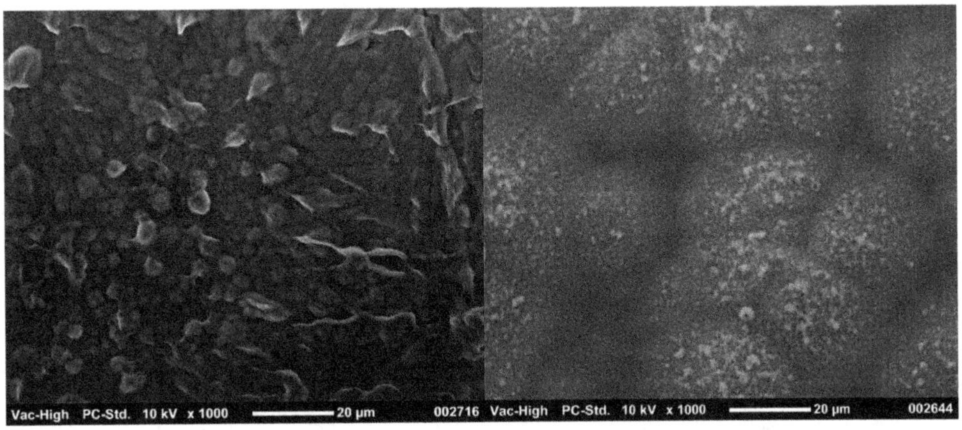

FIGURE 5 | Different morphologies of CHs can be produced through varying the hydrogel component. PEDOT grown through 30 wt% heparin has a more cobblestone appearance (left) compared to the nodular PEDOT grown through 20 wt% PVA-Hep (right).

In preliminary studies it has been shown that CHs have the properties which can address the limitations of both metallic and CP coated electrodes by reducing mechanical mismatch, while maintaining improved electrical properties. Initial *in vitro* studies demonstrate the benefit of these coatings, but there are no studies which systematically compare the different types of hydrogels and CPs used to fabricate these materials. Furthermore, the integration of the two polymer systems is poorly understood, which limits the ability to manipulate the CH structure and tailor the system to display specific characteristics for neural interfacing. Optimization of CHs will require studies which examine the long-term performance of coated electrodes in a stimulated biological environment.

BIOACTIVE COATINGS

All of the coating technologies discussed above can be modified to incorporate biological molecules. Cellular attachment molecules, anti-inflammatory agents and neurotrophins have been commonly investigated for improving the biological response of neural electrodes. Ideally, one of more of these molecules can be used to provide cues to bring neurons closer to electrodes and reduce the impact of the foreign body response. **Table 3** summarizes a range of biological molecules, which have been incorporated within or at electrode surfaces.

The provision of cell attachment molecules within coatings has been extensively explored. In studies which aim to restoring neuronal function, it has been proposed that extracellular matrix (ECM) molecules can provide structural and chemical cues to encourage regeneration at the neural interface (Chan and Mooney, 2008). ECM molecules such as collagen, laminin, and fibronectin among others, have been regarded as key elements in cellular attachment, cell growth, homeostasis, differentiation and cellular motility (Gumbiner, 1996; Banker and Goslin, 1998). Each molecule as well as related peptide sequences can provide mechanical, biological and chemical cues for neural tissue growth and development. Comprehensive reviews on the performance of specific proteins in the ECM have been previously published (Gumbiner, 1996; Banker and Goslin, 1998; Barros et al., 2011; Blau, 2013). **Table 3** lists some of the ECM molecules which have been included within synthetic polymers with an aim of imparting these cues at the device interface. The molecules are classified as proteins including laminin, fibronectin and collagen or related peptide sequences such as arginine–glycine-aspartic acid (RGD), polylysine and gelatin. Proteins and peptides can be incorporated within CNT, CP or CH coatings by simple adsorption, entrapment or covalent binding. It is known that adsorption does not produce a stable interface in the *in vivo* environment as competitive binding of the surrounding proteins can displace the adsorbed layer. Similarly, entrapped proteins can either diffuse through coatings, or if particularly large relative to the coating porosity, can be obstructed within the coating, such that they are not accessible to the cells. As a result cell attachment molecules are often covalently linked to either the coating surface or a component of the coating prior to fabrication. Such molecules have been bonded to CNTs or hydrogel macromer and alternatively used as a CP dopant ion (Cui et al., 2001b; Nguyen-Vu et al., 2007; Green et al., 2010b). Many studies have shown that these sequences encourage neural attachment, survival and differentiation *in vitro* (DeLong et al., 2005; Green et al., 2010b; Chikar et al., 2012). However, there is minimal evidence *in vivo* which supports the benefit of these components to the chronic neural interface. Cui et al. (2003) implanted PPy coated electrodes which were functionalized with laminin fragments in guinea pig cortex. It was shown that neuronal attachment was promoted on some of the electrodes but in spite of having good initial recordings, fibrotic tissues ultimately isolated the electrodes from the target tissue. While cell attachment proteins have clear benefit *in vitro*, there is a need to further explore their presentation and stability *in vivo*.

Anti-inflammatory molecules have been proposed for mitigating either the initial inflammatory reaction or the ongoing presence of fibrotic reactions at the neural interface. Unlike cell attachment proteins, anti-inflammatories must be delivered to the extracellular space to have an effect on the surrounding tissues. As a result these molecules are incorporated into coatings such that they can be delivered, either by passive diffusion or controlled delivery (Asplund et al., 2014). Dexamethasone is one of the most common drug molecules used to combat inflammation at the electrode interface, although hyaluronic acid (HA) and alpha-melanocyte-stimulating hormone (αMSH) have also been used. (Abidian et al., 2006) electrospun dexamethasone-loaded PLGA nanofibers, which were then encapsulated in PEDOT. In this highly conductive construct the dexamethasone could be delivered with a controlled dosage by electrical stimulation. However, due to the limited volume of the PEDOT coated nanofibres, the drug could only be delivered for 7 days at therapeutic levels. (Luo et al., 2011a) introduced dexamethasone to composite CNT-PPy coatings and also demonstrated release under electrical stimulation. The anti-inflammatory dose administered this way was enough to prevent microglia activation in a cell culture, but the ability to deliver therapeutic levels was restricted to a period of 24 h. In contrast (Zhong and Bellamkonda, 2005) entrapped α-MSH in nitrocellulose coatings which demonstrated slow, sustained release by diffusion over 21 days *in vitro*. The α-MSH was shown to retain bioactivity, and successfully inhibited microglial inflammatory responses. Nonetheless all of these approaches are limited as following depletion of the drug from the coating the desired low inflammation state was not maintained.

Inclusion of neurotrophins such as brain-derived neurotrophic factor (BDNF) (Richardson et al., 2007b) and nerve growth factor (NGF; Kim et al., 2007), within electrode coatings encourages the initial growth of neuronal processes towards implanted electrodes. This approach is designed to both initiate neural regeneration and also reduce the gap between the electrode and target tissue. However, several studies have shown that shrinkage of neurite growth occurs after the NGF supply is depleted (Fujita et al., 1989; Richardson et al., 2007a). While a substantial concentration of growth factor can be incorporated within hydrogels, there is only a very limited amount of any biological molecule which can be incorporated within CPs or CNTs (Richardson et al., 2007a). By removing the reliance on material loading and delivery rate (Gillespie et al., 2003) maintained spiral ganglion neurons for 28 days through BDNF administration via a mini-osmotic pump. It was expected that this method would provide a more controlled and

Table 3 | Summary of the combinations of coatings and biomolecules which have been investigated for improving the interaction of electrodes and neural cells.

Application	Coating	Biomolecule	Reference
Cell attachment	PEDOT	DCDPGYIGSR and DEDEDYFQRYLI	Green et al. (2010b)
	PEDOT	DCDPGYIGSR and DEDEDYFQRYLI	Green et al. (2009)
	PEDOT	Fibronectin fragments DCDPGYIGSR	Cui and Martin (2003)
	PPy	Fibronectin fragments Nonapeptide CDPGYIGSR	Cui et al. (2001b)
	CNT	Collagen type IV	Nguyen-Vu et al. (2006)
Anti-inflammatory	PPy	HA	Collier et al. (2000)
	PPy	Dexamethasone	Wadhwa et al. (2006)
	PEDOT electrodeposited on PLGA nanofibers	Dexamethasone	Abidian et al. (2006)
	Polyterthiophene	Dexamethasone phosphate	Stevenson et al. (2010)
	Alginate hydrogel loaded with Poly(lactic-co-glicolide)(PLGA) nanoparticles	Dexamethasone	Kim and Martin (2006)
	Nitrocellulose	αMSH	Zhong and Bellamkonda (2005, 2007)
	Silicon	αMSH	He et al. (2007)
	Multiwalled CNTs	Dexamethasone	Luo et al. (2011a)
Growth factors	Methylcellulose	PDGF-BB and IGF-1	Wells et al. (1997)
	Poly (ethylene-co-vinyl acetate) (EVA) (EVA rods)	NGF, NT-3, BDNF and GDNF,	Bloch et al. (2001), Barras et al. (2002), Fine et al. (2002)
	Agarose	NGF and Laminin	Yu and Bellamkonda (2003)
	Collagen	NT-3	Houweling et al. (1998)
	PEG and PEG-PLA	NT-3	Burdick et al. (2006), Piantino et al. (2006)
	Agarose	BNDF	Jain et al. (2006)
	Fibrin	Heparin binding delivery system (HBDS) and NT-3	Taylor and Sakiyama-Elbert (2006)
	PPy	Laminin fragments RNIAEIIKDI (p20)	Stauffer and Cui (2006)
	PEG-PLA	NGF,	Winter et al. (2007)
	pHEMA-lysine	NGF,	Jhaveri et al. (2008)
	Fibrin	NGF	Lee et al. (2003)
	Multiwalled CNT	NGF	Matsumoto et al. (2007)

HA, hyaluronic acid; αMSH, α-melanocyte stimulating hormone; NGF, nerve growth factor; PDGF-BB, platelet derived growth factor-BB; IGF-1, insulin-like growth factor-1; BDNF, brain derived neurotrophic factor; GDNF, glial cell-derived neurotrophic factor; NT-3 – neurotrophin 3; HBDS, heparin binding delivery system; PEG, poly(ethylene glycol); PEG-PLA, poly(ethylene glycol)-poly(lactic acid); and CNT, carbon nanotube.

longer treatment period than possible with coatings; however, an accelerated loss of neuronal survival occurred after cessation of the treatment. It is therefore expected that provision of neurotrophins at the neural interface will only be effective using a method which support chronic delivery. While current coating technologies do not meet this need, several tissue engineering constructs provide insight into approaches which may address this challenge.

While CNTs, CPs, and hydrogels can be functionalized with bioactive molecules to minimize inflammation and promote neuronal attachment, the main limitation is the ongoing administration of drugs at a therapeutic level. Additionally, at high concentrations it has been shown that these bulky molecules can severely impact on the coating physicochemical properties, in particular CP electrical and mechanical properties are diminished (Collier et al., 2000; Cui et al., 2001b; Green et al., 2009, 2010b). An advantage of CNTs is that their cylindrical morphology can been used as a reservoir for bioactive agents, however they require time intensive functionalization processes in order to be soluble and dispersed in common solvents and aqueous drug solutions (Georgakilas et al., 2002; Bianco et al., 2005).

Current coating technologies including CNTs, CPs, hydrogels, and CHs address several of the limitations of metallic electrodes used in neural interfacing. However, these materials by themselves do not provide a platform for chronic biochemical support which can prevent fibrotic tissue growth and encourage neural cell interactions. In the field of tissue engineering it has been shown that biochemical support (Bhatheja and Field, 2006; Allen and Barres, 2009). can be maintained through the provision of encapsulated cells (Johnson et al., 1989; Majumdar et al., 2011; Daud et al., 2012; Higashimori and Yang, 2012) which naturally produce a range of growth factors and extracellular matrix proteins (Bhatheja and Field, 2006; Allen and Barres, 2009).

A more complex, but highly functional interface will utilize coating technologies in combination with tissue engineered cellular constructs.

TISSUE ENGINEERING THE NEURAL INTERFACE

Ideally, materials used at the neural interface must both minimize the foreign body response as well as promote neuronal survival to maintain the target neurons in close proximity to the electrodes. A more recent idea which has evolved from the literature is the fabrication of electrodes which are intimately associated with neural tissue (Wilson and Dorman, 2008; Richter et al., 2011; Green et al., 2013a). This approach combines the principles of tissue engineering with neuroprosthetic electrode coatings and proposes the incorporation of neural cells within the device itself. Ultimately, polymer systems can be modified to not only improve the electrode properties, but also support the encapsulation and survival of neural cells.

The concept of integrating living cells with electrodes was first raised in 1980, when Ochiai et al. proposed using live blue-green algae embedded in an alginate gel to act as a solar to electric energy photoconverter (Ochiai et al., 1980). They coined the term, "living electrode." In a follow up study, (Ochiai et al., 1983) noted that although stability of these biological electrodes was good, the power conversion efficiency was very low at approximately 0.1%. The latter limitation in efficiency restricted further development of this concept. In 1999, non-nucleated cells were successfully embedded in the PPy electrodeposited onto metal electrodes (Campbell et al., 1999). Cell surface antigen integrity was maintained and because the biosensor application required only presentation of cell surface antigens, there was no requirement for long-term viability and cell function. More recently, Richardson-Burns et al. described electrodeposition of PEDOT on neuroblastoma-derived cell lines and primary mouse cortical cells grown on metal electrodes (Richardson-Burns et al., 2007). Cells survived initial short-term exposure to monomers, but apoptosis was observed at 72 h with up to a third of the cells dying by 120 h. Cytoskeletal disruption was noted soon after polymerization of PEDOT suggesting that focal adhesions may have been disrupted (Richardson-Burns et al., 2007). Despite subsequent research from the same group (Sarah et al., 2007; Ouyang et al., 2011), there has been little progress over the past 5 years on the concept of creating "living" electrodes that contain eukaryotic cells.

Pioneering studies by Richter et al. (2011) present polymeric devices seeded with stem cells. In this study, fibrin hydrogel was used to protect cells from shearing stress similar to that experienced upon neural electrode implantation. More recent reports have shown a proof of concept of the feasibility of building layered constructs of cell loaded hydrogels over CP coated Pt electrodes (Green et al., 2013a). This layered construct involves a hydrogel scaffold to hold neuronal cells while maintaining electrical characteristics of metallic electrodes coated with PEDOT. The concept behind this layered construct is that if neuroprogenitor cells can be supported and developed such that neurite processes are directed towards the target tissue, as depicted in **Figure 6**, then the electrode will be surrounded by a functional neural layer instead of fibrotic tissue. Several challenges arise in the fabrication of such a construct. Importantly, the hydrogel scaffold must be tailored to provide mechanical and biochemical properties that support the growth and differentiation of neural cells. Additionally, neurite outgrowth should be promoted in a vectorial fashion towards the target tissue. Finally, the encapsulated cells must form functional synaptic processes with the target neurons. These issues present great challenges, however, it is expected that recent

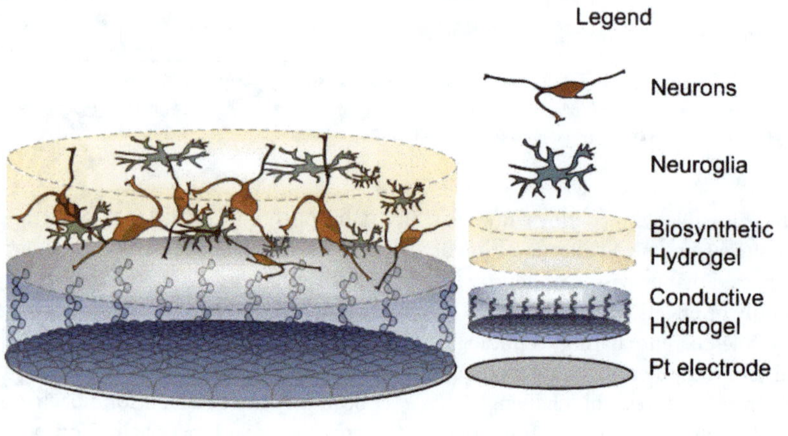

FIGURE 6 | Scheme of proposed construct, derived from Green et al. (2013a) bottom, Pt electrode site. Middle, conductive hydrogel coating and top, neural network encapsulated within degradable hydrogel.

research in tissue engineering will provide insights to guide development of such cellular constructs (Schmidt et al., 1997; Guimard et al., 2007; Sidhu et al., 2012). For example, it has been shown that cell survival and differentiation in three dimensional scaffolds is greatly improved by seeding cells with complementary accessory cells which would be normally present in the developing tissue (Sidhu et al., 2012). These cells generate a variety of biochemical cues producing ECM proteins and growth factors which support the attachment, survival, and differentiation of the functional cells within the scaffold. As such functional living electrodes are likely to require not only neural cells but also supporting neuroglia to achieve functional networks with target tissue.

Despite the substantial amount of research required to develop this technology, it has the potential to provide a pathway for maintaining neurons in close proximity with electrodes. Additionally, a fully realized tissue engineered electrode may prevent scar tissue encapsulation and provide a means of communicating with diseased or damaged cells using natural synaptic processes. Embedded neurons can provide single-cell electrodes which address individual target cells and this innovative method of communicating across the neural interface has the capacity to increase the spatial resolution of bionic devices.

CONCLUDING REMARKS

Carbon nanotubes, CPs, and hydrogels provide potential materials to enhance electrical performance of microelectrodes by increasing electrochemical area. However, to develop a long term neural interface it is critical to determine the interplay of the mechanical, electrical and biological properties. The true potential of these materials on neural interfaces is not completely understood as the many studies have been limited to characterization in the *in vitro* environment. An important component of future research is the assessment of organic coatings *in vivo* under chronic implant conditions. Systematic studies are required to assess the different coating technologies and provide direction on which material or combination of materials will provide the most beneficial characteristics for neural interfacing. Tissue engineered living electrodes may provide an alternate technology platform which will enable the development of a truly innovative way of communicating with the neural system through synaptic processes.

REFERENCES

Abidian, M. R., Corey, J. M., Kipke, D. R., and Martin, D. C. (2010). Conducting-polymer nanotubes improve electrical properties, mechanical adhesion, neural attachment, and neurite outgrowth of neural electrodes. *Small* 6, 421–429. doi: 10.1002/smll.200901868

Abidian, M. R., Daneshvar, E. D., Egeland, B. M., Kipke, D. R., Cederna, P. S., and Urbanchek, M. G. (2012b). Hybrid conducting polymer–hydrogel conduits for axonal growth and neural tissue engineering. *Adv. Healthc. Mater.* 1, 762–767. doi: 10.1002/adhm.201200182

Abidian, M. R., Kim, D. H., and Martin, D. C. (2006). Conducting-polymer nanotubes for controlled drug release. *Adv. Mater.* 18, 405–409. doi: 10.1002/adma.200501726

Abidian, M. R., and Martin, D. C. (2009). Multifunctional nanobiomaterials for neural interfaces. *Adv. Funct. Mater.* 19, 573–585. doi: 10.1002/adfm.200801473

Ahearne, M., Yang, Y., El Haj, A. J., Then, K. Y., and Liu, K. K. (2005). Characterizing the viscoelastic properties of thin hydrogel-based constructs for tissue engineering applications. *J. R. Soc. Interface* 2, 455–463. doi: 10.1098/rsif.2005.0065

Ahmed, T. A., Dare, E. V., and Hincke, M. (2008). Fibrin: a versatile scaffold for tissue engineering applications. *Tissue Eng. B Rev.* 14, 199–215. doi: 10.1089/ten.teb.2007.0435

Allen, N. J., and Barres, B. A. (2009). Neuroscience: glia – more than just brain glue. *Nature* 457, 675–677. doi: 10.1038/457675a

Almany, L., and Seliktar, D. (2005). Biosynthetic hydrogel scaffolds made from fibrinogen and polyethylene glycol for 3D cell cultures. *Biomaterials* 26, 2467–2477. doi: 10.1016/j.biomaterials.2004.06.047

Andrade, D. M., Zumsteg, D., Hamani, C., Hodaie, M., Sarkissian, S., Lozano, A. M., et al. (2006). Long-term follow-up of patients with thalamic deep brain stimulation for epilepsy. *Neurology* 66, 1571–1573. doi: 10.1212/01.wnl.0000206364.19772.39

Anseth, K. S., Metters, A. T., Bryant, S. J., Martens, P. J., Elisseeff, J. H., and Bowman, C. N. (2002). In situ forming degradable networks and their application in tissue engineering and drug delivery. *J. Control. Release* 78, 199–209. doi: 10.1016/S0168-3659(01)00500-4

Aouada, F. A., Guilherme, M. R., Campese, G. M., Girotto, E. M., Rubira, A. F., and Muniz, E. C. (2006). Electrochemical and mechanical properties of hydrogels based on conductive poly(3,4-ethylene dioxythiophene)/poly(styrenesulfonate) and PAAm. *Polym. Test.* 25, 158–165. doi: 10.1016/j.polymertesting.2005.11.005

Asplund, M., Boehler, C., and Stieglitz, T. (2014). Anti-inflammatory polymer electrodes for glial scar treatment. *Front. Neuroeng.* 7:9. doi: 10.3389/fneng.2014.00009

Aymard, P., Martin, D. R., Plucknett, K., Foster, T. J., Clark, A. H., and Norton, I. T. (2001). Influence of thermal history on the structural and mechanical properties of agarose gels. *Biopolymers* 59, 131–144. doi: 10.1002/1097-0282(200109)59:3<131::AID-BIP1013>3.0.CO;2-8

Babcock, A. A., Kuziel, W. A., Rivest, S., and Owens, T. (2003). Chemokine expression by glial cells directs leukocytes to sites of axonal injury in the CNS. *J. Neurosci.* 23, 7922–7930.

Baek, S., Green, R. A., and Poole-Warren, L. A. (2013a). Effects of dopants on the biomechanical properties of conducting polymer films on platinum electrodes. *J. Biomed. Mater. Res. A* doi: 10.1002/jbm.a.34945 [Epub ahead of print].

Baek, S., Green, R., Granville, A., Martens, P., and Poole-Warren, L. (2013b). Thin film hydrophilic electroactive polymer coatings for bioelectrodes. *J. Mat. Chem. B* 1, 3803–3810. doi: 10.1039/C3TB20152J

Baker, M. I., Walsh, S. P., Schwartz, Z., and Boyan, B. D. (2012). A review of polyvinyl alcohol and its uses in cartilage and orthopedic applications. *J. Biomed. Mater. Res. B Appl. Biomater.* 100, 1451–1457. doi: 10.1002/jbm.b.32694

Banati, R. B., Gehrmann, J., Schubert, P., and Kreutzberg, G. W. (1993). Cytotoxicity of microglia. *Glia* 7, 111–118. doi: 10.1002/glia.440070117

Banerjee, A., Arha, M., Choudhary, S., Ashton, R. S., Bhatia, S. R., Schaffer, D. V., et al. (2009). The influence of hydrogel modulus on the proliferation and differentiation of encapsulated neural stem cells. *Biomaterials* 30, 4695–4699. doi: 10.1016/j.biomaterials.2009.05.050

Banker, G., and Goslin, K. (1998). *Culturing Nerve Cells.* Cambridge, MA: MIT Press.

Barras, F. M., Pasche, P., Bouche, N., Aebischer, P., and Zurn, A. D. (2002). Glial cell line-derived neurotrophic factor released by synthetic guidance channels promotes facial nerve regeneration in the rat. *J. Neurosci. Res.* 70, 746–755. doi: 10.1002/jnr.10434

Barrese, J. C., Rao, N., Paroo, K., Triebwasser, C., Vargas-Irwin, C., Franquemont, L., et al. (2013). Failure mode analysis of silicon-based intracortical microelectrode arrays in non-human primates. *J. Neural Eng.* 10, 066014. doi: 10.1088/1741-2560/10/6/066014

Barros, C. S., Franco, S. J., and Müller, U. (2011). Extracellular matrix: functions in the nervous system. *Cold Spring Harb. Perspect. Biol.* 3, 1–24. doi: 10.1101/cshperspect.a005108

Bartlett, P., Baumberg, J., Birkin, P. R., Ghanem, M., and Netti, M. (2002). Highly ordered macroporous gold and platinum films formed by electrochemical deposition through templates assembled from submicron diameter monodisperse polystyrene spheres. *Chem. Mater.* 14, 2199–2208. doi: 10.1021/cm011272j

Bhatheja, K., and Field, J. (2006). Schwann cells: origins and role in axonal maintenance and regeneration. *Int. J. Biochem. Cell Biol.* 38, 1995–1999. doi: 10.1016/j.biocel.2006.05.007

Bianco, A., Kostarelos, K., Partidos, C. D., and Prato, M. (2005). Biomedical applications of functionalised carbon nanotubes. *Chem. Commun.* 571–577. doi: 10.1039/B410943K

Bidez, P. R., Li, S., Macdiarmid, A. G., Venancio, E. C., Wei, Y., and Lelkes, P. I. (2006). Polyaniline, an electroactive polymer, supports adhesion and proliferation of cardiac myoblasts. *J. Biomater. Sci. Polym. Ed.* 17, 199–212. doi: 10.1163/156856206774879180

Biran, R., Martin, D. C., and Tresco, P. A. (2005). Neuronal cell loss accompanies the brain tissue response to chronically implanted silicon microelectrode arrays. *Exp. Neurol.* 195, 115–126. doi: 10.1016/j.expneurol.2005.04.020

Blau, A. (2013). Cell adhesion promotion strategies for signal transduction enhancement in microelectrode array in vitro electrophysiology: an introductory overview and critical discussion. *Curr. Opin. Colloid Interface Sci.* 18, 481–492. doi: 10.1016/j.cocis.2013.07.005

Bloch, J., Fine, E. G., Bouche, N., Zurn, A. D., and Aebischer, P. (2001). Nerve Growth Factor- and Neurotrophin-3-releasing guidance channels promote regeneration of the transected rat dorsal root. *Exp. Neurol.* 172, 425–432. doi: 10.1006/exnr.2001.7778

Bolin, M. H., Svennersten, K., Wang, X., Chronakis, I. S., Richter-Dahlfors, A., Jager, E. W. H., et al. (2009). Nano-fiber scaffold electrodes based on PEDOT for cell stimulation. *Sens. Actuators B Chem.* 142, 451–456. doi: 10.1016/j.snb.2009.04.062

Boretius, T., Schuettler, M., and Stieglitz, T. (2011). On the stability of polyethylenedioxythiopene as coating material for active neural implants. *Artif. Organs* 35, 245–248. doi: 10.1111/j.1525-1594.2011.01210.x

Bottini, M., Bruckner, S., Nika, K., Bottini, N., Bellucci, S., Magrini, A., et al. (2006). Multi-walled carbon nanotubes induce T lymphocyte apoptosis. *Toxicol. Lett.* 160, 121–126. doi: 10.1016/j.toxlet.2005.06.020

Brummer, S. B., Robblee, L. S., and Hambrecht, F. T. (1983). Criteria for selecting electrodes for electrical stimulation: theoretical and practical considerations. *Ann. N. Y. Acad. Sci.* 405, 159–171. doi: 10.1111/j.1749-6632.1983.tb31628.x

Burdick, J. A., Ward, M., Liang, E., Young, M. J., and Langer, R. (2006). Stimulation of neurite outgrowth by neurotrophins delivered from degradable hydrogels. *Biomaterials* 27, 452–459. doi: 10.1016/j.biomaterials.2005.06.034

Campbell, T. E., Hodgson, A. J., and Wallace, G. G. (1999). Incorporation of erythrocytes into polypyrrole to form the basis of a biosensor to screen for rhesus (d) blood groups and rhesus (D) antibodies. *Electroanalysis* 11, 215–222. doi: 10.1002/(SICI)1521-4109(199904)11:4<215::AID-ELAN215>3.0.CO;2-#

Capadona, J. R., Shanmuganathan, K., Tyler, D. J., Rowan, S. J., and Weder, C. (2008). Stimuli-responsive polymer nanocomposites inspired by the sea cucumber dermis. *Science* 319, 1370-1374. doi: 10.1126/science.1153307

Chan, G., and Mooney, D. J. (2008). New materials for tissue engineering: towards greater control over the biological response. *Trends Biotechnol.* 26, 382–392. doi: 10.1016/j.tibtech.2008.03.011

Chen, Z., Ren, W., Gao, L., Liu, B., Pei, S., and Cheng, H.-M. (2011). Three-dimensional flexible and conductive interconnected graphene networks grown by chemical vapour deposition. *Nat. Mater.* 10, 424–428. doi: 10.1038/nmat3001

Cheung, K. C. (2007). Implantable microscale neural interfaces. *Biomed. Microdev.* 9, 923–938. doi: 10.1007/s10544-006-9045-z

Chikar, J. A., Hendricks, J. L., Richardson-Burns, S. M., Raphael, Y., Pfingst, B. E., and Martin, D. C. (2012). The use of a dual PEDOT and RGD-functionalized alginate hydrogel coating to provide sustained drug delivery and improved cochlear implant function. *Biomaterials* 33, 1982–1990. doi: 10.1016/j.biomaterials.2011.11.052

Cogan, S. F. (2008). Neural Stimulation and Recording Electrodes. *Annu. Rev. Biomed. Eng.* 10, 275–309. doi: 10.1146/annurev.bioeng.10.061807.160518

Cogan, S. F., Peramunage, D., Smirnov, A., Ehrlich, J., Mccreery, D. B., and Manoonkitiwongsa, P. S. (2007). *Polyethylenedioxythiophene (PEDOT) Coatings for Neural Stimulation and Recording Electrodes.* Norwood: EIC Laboratories, Inc.

Cogan, S. F., Troyk, P. R., Ehrlich, J., and Plante, T. D. (2005). In vitro comparison of the charge-injection limits of activated iridium oxide (AIROF) and platinum-iridium microelectrodes. *Biomed. Eng. IEEE Trans.* 52, 1612–1614. doi: 10.1109/TBME.2005.851503

Collier, J. H., Camp, J. P., Hudson, T. W., and Schmidt, C. E. (2000). Synthesis and characterization of polypyrrole–hyaluronic acid composite biomaterials for tissue engineering applications. *J. Biomed. Mater. Res.* 50, 574–584. doi: 10.1002/(SICI)1097-4636(20000615)50:4<574::AID-JBM13>3.0.CO;2-I

Collinger, J. L., Foldes, S., Bruns, T. M., Wodlinger, B., Gaunt, R., and Weber, D. J. (2013). Neuroprosthetic technology for individuals with spinal cord injury. *J. Spinal Cord Med.* 36, 258–272. doi: 10.1179/2045772313Y.0000000128

Cui, X., and Martin, D. C. (2003). Electrochemical deposition and characterization of poly(3,4-ethylenedioxythiophene) on neural microelectrode arrays. *Sens. Actuators B Chem.* 89, 92–102. doi: 10.1016/S0925-4005(02)00448-3

Cui, X., Wiler, J., Dzaman, M., Altschuler, R. A., and Martin, D. C. (2003). In vivo studies of polypyrrole/peptide coated neural probes. *Biomaterials* 24, 777–787. doi: 10.1016/S0142-9612(02)00415-5

Cui, X. T., Hetke, J. F., Wiler, J. A., Anderson, D. J., and Martin, D. C. (2001a). Electrochemical deposition and characterization of conducting polymer polypyrrole/PSS on multichannel neural probes. *Sens. Actuators A Phys.* 93, 8–18. doi: 10.1016/S0924-4247(01)00637-9

Cui, X. T., Lee, V. A., Raphael, Y., Wiler, J. A., Hetke, J. F., Anderson, D. J., et al. (2001b). Surface modification of neural recording electrodes with conducting polymer/biomolecule blends. *J. Biomed. Mater. Res.* 56, 261–272. doi: 10.1002/1097-4636(200108)56:2<261::AID-JBM1094>3.0.CO;2-I

Daud, M. F. B., Pawar, K. C., Claeyssens, F., Ryan, A. J., and Haycock, J. W. (2012). An aligned 3D neuronal-glial co-culture model for peripheral nerve studies. *Biomaterials* 33, 5901–5913. doi: 10.1016/j.biomaterials.2012.05.008

David-Pur, M., Bareket-Keren, L., Beit-Yaakov, G., Raz-Prag, D., and Hanein, Y. (2013). All-carbon-nanotube flexible multi-electrode array for neuronal recording and stimulation. *Biomed. Microdev.* 1–11. doi: 10.1007/s10544-013-9804-6

De Volder, M. F. L., Tawfick, S. H., Baughman, R. H., and Hart, A. J. (2013). Carbon nanotubes: present and future commercial applications. *Science* 339, 535–539. doi: 10.1126/science.1222453

DeLong, S. A., Gobin, A. S., and West, J. L. (2005). Covalent immobilization of RGDS on hydrogel surfaces to direct cell alignment and migration. *J. Control. Release* 109, 139–148. doi: 10.1016/j.jconrel.2005.09.020

Drury, J. L., and Mooney, D. J. (2003). Hydrogels for tissue engineering: scaffold design variables and applications. *Biomaterials* 24, 4337–4351. doi: 10.1016/S0142-9612(03)00340-5

Evans, A. J., Thompson, B. C., Wallace, G. G., Millard, R., O'Leary, S. J., Clark, G. M., et al. (2009). Promoting neurite outgrowth from spiral ganglion neuron explants using polypyrrole/BDNF-coated electrodes. *J. Biomed. Mater. Res. A* 91A, 241–250. doi: 10.1002/jbm.a.32228

Fan, Y. W., Cui, F. Z., Hou, S. P., Xu, Q. Y., Chen, L. N., and Lee, I. S. (2002). Culture of neural cells on silicon wafers with nano-scale surface topograph. *J. Neurosci. Methods* 120, 17–23. doi: 10.1016/S0165-0270(02)00181-4

Fieberg, A., and Reis, O. (2002). UV curable electrodeposition systems. *Prog. Org. Coat.* 45, 239–247. doi: 10.1016/S0300-9440(02)00065-6

Fine, E. G., Decosterd, I., Papaloïzos, M., Zurn, A. D., and Aebischer, P. (2002). GDNF and NGF released by synthetic guidance channels support sciatic nerve regeneration across a long gap. *Eur. J. Neurosci.* 15, 589–601. doi: 10.1046/j.1460-9568.2002.01892.x

Fitch, M. T., and Silver, J. (1997). Activated macrophages and the blood–brain barrier: inflammation after cns injury leads to increases in putative inhibitory molecules. *Exp. Neurol.* 148, 587–603. doi: 10.1006/exnr.1997.6701

Fitch, M. T., and Silver, J. (2008). CNS injury, glial scars, and inflammation: inhibitory extracellular matrices and regeneration failure. *Exp. Neurol.* 209, 294–301. doi: 10.1016/j.expneurol.2007.05.014

Fonner, J. M., Forciniti, L., Nguyen, H., Byrne, J. D., Kou, Y.-F., Syeda-Nawaz, J., et al. (2008). Biocompatibility implications of polypyrrole synthesis techniques. *Biomed. Mater.* 3:034124. doi: 10.1088/1748-6041/3/3/034124

Fujita, K., Lazarovici, P., and Guroff, G. (1989). Regulation of the differentiation of PC12 pheochromocytoma cells. *Environ. Health Perspect.* 80, 127–142. doi: 10.1289/ehp.8980127

Gabay, T., Ben-David, M., Kalifa, I., Sorkin, R., Abrams, Z. R., Ben-Jacob, E., et al. (2007). Electro-chemical and biological properties of carbon nanotube based multi-electrode arrays. *Nanotechnology* 18, 035201. doi: 10.1088/0957-4484/18/3/035201

Geddes, L. A., and Roeder, R. (2003). Criteria for the selection of materials for implanted electrodes. *Ann. Biomed. Eng.* 31, 879–890. doi: 10.1114/1.1581292

Georgakilas, V., Kordatos, K., Prato, M., Guldi, D. M., Holzinger, M., and Hirsch, A. (2002). Organic functionalization of carbon nanotubes. *J. Am. Chem. Soc.* 124, 760–761. doi: 10.1021/ja016954m

George, P. M., Lyckman, A. W., Lavan, D. A., Hegde, A., Leung, Y., Avasare, R., et al. (2005). Fabrication and biocompatibility of polypyrrole implants suitable for neural prosthetics. *Biomaterials* 26, 3511–3519. doi: 10.1016/j.biomaterials.2004.09.037

Georges, P. C., Miller, W. J., Meaney, D. F., Sawyer, E. S., and Janmey, P. A. (2006). Matrices with compliance comparable to that of brain tissue select neuronal over glial growth in mixed cortical cultures. *Biophys. J.* 90, 3012–3018. doi: 10.1529/biophysj.105.073114

Gillespie, L. N., Clark, G. M., Bartlett, P. F., and Marzella, P. L. (2003). BDNF-induced survival of auditory neurons in vivo: cessation of treatment leads to accelerated loss of survival effects. *J. Neurosci. Res.* 71, 785–790. doi: 10.1002/jnr.10542

Gilmour, A. D., Green, R. A., and Thomson, C. E. (2013). A low-maintenance, primary cell culture model for the assessment of carbon nanotube toxicity. *Toxicol. Environ. Chem.* 95, 1129–1144. doi: 10.1080/02772248.2013.844429

Green, R. A., Baek, S., Poole-Warren, L. A., and Martens, P. J. (2010a). Conducting polymer-hydrogels for medical electrode applications. *Sci. Technol. Adv. Mater.* 11, 014107. doi: 10.1088/1468-6996/11/1/014107

Green, R. A., Hassarati, R. T., Bouchinet, L., Lee, C. S., Cheong, G. L.M., Yu, J. F., et al. (2012a). Substrate dependent stability of conducting polymer coatings on medical electrodes. *Biomaterials* 33, 5875–5886. doi: 10.1016/j.biomaterials.2012.05.017

Green, R. A., Hassarati, R. T., Goding, J. A., Baek, S., Lovell, N. H., Martens, P. J., et al. (2012b). Conductive hydrogels: mechanically robust hybrids for use as biomaterials. *Macromol. Biosci.* 12, 494–501. doi: 10.1002/mabi.201100490

Green, R. A., Lim, K. S., Henderson, W. C., Hassarati, R. T., Martens, P. J., Lovell, N. H., et al. (2013a). "Living electrodes: tissue engineering the neural interface," in *Engineering in Medicine and Biology Society (EMBC), 2013 35th Annual International Conference of the IEEE)*, Osaka, 6957–6960.

Green, R. A., Lovell, N. H., and Poole-Warren, L. A. (2009). Cell attachment functionality of bioactive conducting polymers for neural interfaces. *Biomaterials* 30, 3637–3644. doi: 10.1016/j.biomaterials.2009.03.043

Green, R. A., Lovell, N. H., and Poole-Warren, L. A. (2010b). Impact of co-incorporating laminin peptide dopants and neurotrophic growth factors on conducting polymer properties. *Acta Biomater.* 6, 63–71. doi: 10.1016/j.actbio.2009.06.030

Green, R. A., Lovell, N. H., Wallace, G. G., and Poole-Warren, L. A. (2008a). Conducting polymers for neural interfaces: challenges in developing an effective long-term implant. *Biomaterials* 29, 3393–3399. doi: 10.1016/j.biomaterials.2008.04.047

Green, R. A., Matteucci, P. B., Hassarati, R. T., Giraud, B., Dodds, C. W., Chen, S., et al. (2013b). Performance of conducting polymer electrodes for stimulating neuroprosthetics. *J. Neural Eng.* 10, 016009. doi: 10.1088/1741-2560/10/1/016009

Green, R. A., Ordonez, J. S., Schuettler, M., Poole-Warren, L. A., Lovell, N. H., and Suaning, G. J. (2010c). Cytotoxicity of implantable microelectrode arrays produced by laser micromachining. *Biomaterials* 31, 886–893. doi: 10.1016/j.biomaterials.2009.09.099

Green, R. A., Toor, H., Dodds, C., and Lovell, N. H. (2012c). Variation in performance of platinum electrodes with size and surface roughness. *Sens. Mater.* 24, 15.

Green, R. A., Williams, C. M., Lovell, N. H., and Poole-Warren, L. A. (2008b). Novel neural interface for implant electrodes: improving electroactivity of polypyrrole through MWNT incorporation. *J. Mater. Sci. Mater. Med.* 19, 1625–1629. doi: 10.1007/s10856-008-3376-7

Guimard, N. K., Gomez, N., and Schmidt, C. E. (2007). Conducting polymers in biomedical engineering. *Prog. Polym. Sci.* 32, 876–921. doi: 10.1016/j.progpolymsci.2007.05.012

Gumbiner, B. M. (1996). Cell adhesion: the molecular basis of tissue architecture and morphogenesis. *Cell* 84, 345–357. doi: 10.1016/S0092-8674(00)81279-9

Haghighi, B., and Bozorgzadeh, S. (2011). Fabrication of a highly sensitive electrochemiluminescence lactate biosensor using ZnO nanoparticles decorated multiwalled carbon nanotubes. *Talanta* 85, 2189–2193. doi: 10.1016/j.talanta.2011.07.071

Hallab, N. J., Bundy, K. J., O'Connor, K., Moses, R. L., and Jacobs, J. J. (2001). Evaluation of metallic and polymeric biomaterial surface energy and surface roughness characteristics for directed cell adhesion. *Tissue Eng.* 7, 6. doi: 10.1089/107632700300003297

Hascup, E. R., Af Bjerkén, S., Hascup, K. N., Pomerleau, F., Huettl, P., Strömberg, I., et al. (2009). Histological studies of the effects of chronic implantation of ceramic-based microelectrode arrays and microdialysis probes in rat prefrontal cortex. *Brain Res.* 1291, 12–20. doi: 10.1016/j.brainres.2009.06.084

Hassarati, R., Dueck, W., Tasche, C., Carter, P., Poole-Warren, L., and Green, R. (2014). Improving Cochlear implant properties through conductive hydrogel coatings. *IEEE Trans. Neural Syst. Rehabil. Eng.* 22, 411–418. doi: 10.1109/TNSRE.2014.2304559

Hassler, C., Boretius, T., and Stieglitz, T. (2011). Polymers for neural implants. *J. Polym. Sci. B Polym. Phys.* 49, 18–33. doi: 10.1002/polb.22169

He, W., Mcconnell, G. C., Schneider, T. M., and Bellamkonda, R. V. (2007). A Novel Anti-inflammatory Surface for Neural Electrodes. *Adv. Mater.* 19, 3529–3533. doi: 10.1002/adma.200700943

Heim, M., Yvert, B., and Kuhn, A. (2012). Nanostructuration strategies to enhance microelectrode array (MEA) performance for neuronal recording and stimulation. *J. Physiol.* 106, 137–145. doi: 10.1016/j.jphysparis.2011.10.001

Higashimori, H., and Yang, Y. (2012). Imaging analysis of neuron to glia interaction in microfluidic culture platform (MCP)-based neuronal axon and glia co-culture system. *J. Vis. Exp.* 4448. doi: 10.3791/4448

Hoffman, A. S. (2002). Hydrogels for biomedical applications. *Adv. Drug Deliv. Rev.* 54, 3–12. doi: 10.1016/S0169-409X(01)00239-3

Houweling, D. A., Lankhorst, A. J., Gispen, W. H., Bär, P. R., and Joosten, E. A. J. (1998). Collagen containing neurotrophin-3 (NT-3) attracts regrowing injured corticospinal axons in the adult rat spinal cord and promotes partial functional recovery. *Exp. Neurol.* 153, 49–59. doi: 10.1006/exnr.1998.6867

Hsu, H.-L., Teng, I. J., Chen, Y.-C., Hsu, W.-L., Lee, Y.-T., Yen, S.-J., et al. (2010). Flexible UV-ozone-modified carbon nanotube electrodes for neuronal recording. *Adv. Mater.* 22, 2177–2181. doi: 10.1002/adma.200903413

Huang, J., Virji, S., Weiller, B. H., and Kaner, R. B. (2004). Nanostructured polyaniline sensors. *Chemistry* 10, 1314–1319. doi: 10.1002/chem.200305211

Humayun, M. S., Weiland, J. D., Fujii, G. Y., Greenberg, R., Williamson, R., Little, J., et al. (2003). Visual perception in a blind subject with a chronic microelectronic retinal prosthesis. *Vision Res.* 43, 2573–2581. doi: 10.1016/S0042-6989(03)00457-7

Jain, A., Kim, Y.-T., Mckeon, R. J., and Bellamkonda, R. V. (2006). In situ gelling hydrogels for conformal repair of spinal cord defects, and local delivery of BDNF after spinal cord injury. *Biomaterials* 27, 497–504. doi: 10.1016/j.biomaterials.2005.07.008

Jhaveri, S. J., Hynd, M. R., Dowell-Mesfin, N., Turner, J. N., Shain, W., and Ober, C. K. (2008). Release of nerve growth factor from HEMA hydrogel-coated substrates and its effect on the differentiation of neural cells. *Biomacromolecules* 10, 174–183. doi: 10.1021/bm801101e

Johnson, M. I., Higgins, D., and Ard, M. D. (1989). Astrocytes induce dendritic development in cultured sympathetic neurons. *Dev. Brain Res.* 47, 289–292. doi: 10.1016/0165-3806(89)90184-3

Kagan, V. E., Tyurina, Y. Y., Tyurin, V. A., Konduru, N. V., Potapovich, A. I., Osipov, A. N., et al. (2006). Direct and indirect effects of single walled carbon nanotubes on RAW 264.7 macrophages: role of iron. *Toxicol. Lett.* 165, 88–100. doi: 10.1016/j.toxlet.2006.02.001

Keefer, E. W., Botterman, B. R., Romero, M. I., Rossi, A. F., and Gross, G. W. (2008). Carbon nanotube coating improves neuronal recordings. *Nat. Nano* 3, 434–439. doi: 10.1038/nnano.2008.174

Kim, D. H., Abidian, M., and Martin, D. C. (2004). Conducting polymers grown in hydrogel scaffolds coated on neural prosthetic devices. *J. Biomed. Mater. Res. A* 71, 577–585. doi: 10.1002/jbm.a.30124

Kim, D.-H., and Martin, D. C. (2006). Sustained release of dexamethasone from hydrophilic matrices using PLGA nanoparticles for neural drug delivery. *Biomaterials* 27, 3031–3037. doi: 10.1016/j.biomaterials.2005.12.021

Kim, D.-H., Wiler, J. A., Anderson, D. J., Kipke, D. R., and Martin, D. C. (2010). Conducting polymers on hydrogel-coated neural electrode provide sensitive neural recordings in auditory cortex. *Acta Biomater.* 6, 57–62. doi: 10.1016/j.actbio.2009.07.034

Kim, D. H., Richardson-Burns, S., Povlich, L., Abidian, M. R., Spanninga, S., Hendricks, J. L., et al. (2008). "Soft, fuzzy, and bioactive conducting polymers for improving the chronic performance of neural prosthetic devices," in *Indwelling Neural Implants: Strategies for Contending with the In Vivo Environment*, ed. W. M. Reichert (Boca Raton, FL: CRC Press), 165–207.

Kim, D. H., Richardson-Burns, S. M., Hendricks, J. L., Sequera, C., and Martin, D. C. (2007). Effect of immobilized nerve growth factor on conductive polymers: electrical properties and cellular response. *Adv. Funct. Mater.* 17, 79–86. doi: 10.1002/adfm.200500594

Kim, Y.-T., and Romero-Ortega, M. I. (2012). Material considerations for peripheral nerve interfacing. *MRS Bull.* 37, 573–580. doi: 10.1557/mrs.2012.99

Krishnan, A., Dujardin, E., Ebbesen, T. W., Yianilos, P. N., and Treacy, M. M. J. (1998). Young's modulus of single-walled nanotubes. *Phys. Rev. B* 58, 14013–14019. doi: 10.1103/PhysRevB.58.14013

Kurisawa, M., Chung, J. E., Yang, Y. Y., Gao, S. J., and Uyama, H. (2005). Injectable biodegradable hydrogels composed of hyaluronic acid-tyramine conjugates for drug delivery and tissue engineering. *Chem. Commun.* 4312–4314. doi: 10.1039/B506989K

Labaye, D. E., Jérôme, C., Geskin, V. M., Louette, P., Lazzaroni, R., Martinot, L., et al. (2002). Full electrochemical synthesis of conducting polymer films chemically grafted to conducting surfaces. *Langmuir* 18, 5222–5230. doi: 10.1021/la011439n

Lacour, S. P., Benmerah, S., Tarte, E., Fitzgerald, J., Serra, J., Mcmahon, S., et al. (2010). Flexible and stretchable micro-electrodes for in vitro and in vivo neural interfaces. *Med. Biol. Eng. Comput.* 48, 945–954. doi: 10.1007/s11517-010-0644-8

LaVan, D. A., George, P. M., and Langer, R. (2003). Simple, three-dimensional microfabrication of electrodeposited structures. *Angew. Chem. Int. Ed. Engl.* 42, 1262–1265. doi: 10.1002/anie.200390323

Leach, J. B., Achyuta A. K. A., and Murthy, S. K. (2010). Bridging the Divide between Neuroprosthetic Design, Tissue Engineering and Neurobiology. *Front. Neuroeng.* 2:19. doi: 10.3389/neuro.16.018.2009

Lee, A. C., Yu, V. M., Lowe Iii, J. B., Brenner, M. J., Hunter, D. A., Mackinnon, S. E., et al. (2003). Controlled release of nerve growth factor enhances sciatic nerve regeneration. *Exp. Neurol.* 184, 295–303. doi: 10.1016/S0014-4886(03)00258-9

Lee, F., Chung, J. E., and Kurisawa, M. (2008). An injectable enzymatically crosslinked hyaluronic acid-tyramine hydrogel system with independent tuning of mechanical strength and gelation rate. *Soft Matter* 4, 880–887. doi: 10.1039/B719557E

Lee, K. Y., and Mooney, D. J. (2001). Hydrogels for tissue engineering. *Chem. Rev.* 101, 1869–1880. doi: 10.1021/cr000108x

LeRoux, M. A., Guilak, F., and Setton, L. A. (1999). Compressive and shear properties of alginate gel: effects of sodium ions and alginate concentration. *J. Biomed. Mater. Res.* 47, 46–53. doi: 10.1002/(SICI)1097-4636(199910)47:1<46::AID-JBM6>3.0.CO;2-N

Letherby, M. R., and Young, D. A. (1981). The gelation of agarose. *J. Chem. Soc.* 77, 1953–1966. doi: 10.1039/F19817701953

Li, Y.-T., Chang, C.-H., Chen, J.-J. J., Wang, C.-C., and Liang, C.-K. (2005). Dvelopment of implantable wireless biomicrosystem for measuring electrode-tissue impedance. *J. Med. Biol. Eng.* 25, 6.

Li, Y., and Mogul, D. J. (2007). Electrical control of epileptic seizures. *J. Clin. Neurophysiol.* 24, 197–204. doi: 10.1097/WNP.0b013e31803991c3

Lim, K. S., Alves, M. H., Poole-Warren, L. A., and Martens, P. J. (2013). Covalent incorporation of non-chemically modified gelatin into degradable PVA-tyramine hydrogels. *Biomaterials* 34, 7097–7105. doi: 10.1016/j.biomaterials.2013.06.005

Lim, K. S., Kundu, J., Reeves, A., Poole-Warren, L. A., Kundu, S. C., and Martens, P. J. (2012). The influence of silkworm species on cellular interactions with novel pva/silk sericin hydrogels. *Macromol. Biosci.* 12, 322–332. doi: 10.1002/mabi.201100292

Lin, C.-M., Lee, Y.-T., Yeh, S.-R., and Fang, W. (2009). Flexible carbon nanotubes electrode for neural recording. *Biosens. Bioelectron.* 24, 2791–2797. doi: 10.1016/j.bios.2009.02.005

Liu, S. Q., Yang, C., Huang, Y., Ding, X., Li, Y., Fan, W. M., et al. (2012). Antimicrobial and antifouling hydrogels formed in situ from polycarbonate and poly(ethylene glycol) via Michael addition. *Adv. Mater.* 24, 6484–6489. doi: 10.1002/adma.201202225

Lozano, A. M., and Lipsman, N. (2013). Probing and regulating dysfunctional circuits using deep brain stimulation. *Neuron* 77, 406–424. doi: 10.1016/j.neuron.2013.01.020

Lu, Y., Wang, D., Li, T., Zhao, X., Cao, Y., Yang, H., et al. (2009). Poly(vinyl alcohol)/poly(acrylic acid) hydrogel coatings for improving electrode–neural tissue interface. *Biomaterials* 30, 4143–4151. doi: 10.1016/j.biomaterials.2009.04.030

Ludwig, K. A., Langhals, N. B., Joseph, M. D., Richardson-Burns, S. M., Hendricks, J. L., and Kipke, D. R. (2011). Poly(3,4-ethylenedioxythiophene) (PEDOT) polymer coatings facilitate smaller neural recording electrodes. *J. Neural Eng.* 8, 014001. doi: 10.1088/17412560/8/1/014001

Ludwig, K. A., Uram, J. D., Yang, J., Martin, D. C., and Kipke, D. R. (2006). Chronic neural recordings using silicon microelectrode arrays electrochemically deposited with a poly(3,4-ethylenedioxythiophene) (PEDOT) film. *J. Neural Eng.* 3, 59–70. doi: 10.1088/1741-2560/3/1/007

Luo, S.-C., Sekine, J., Zhu, B., Zhao, H., Nakao, A., and Yu, H.-H. (2012). Polydioxythiophene nanodots, nonowires, nano-networks, and tubular structures: the effect of functional groups and temperature in template-free electropolymerization. *ACS Nano* 6, 3018–3026. doi: 10.1021/nn300737e

Luo, X., Matranga, C., Tan, S., Alba, N., and Cui, X. T. (2011a). Carbon nanotube nanoreservior for controlled release of anti-inflammatory dexamethasone. *Biomaterials* 32, 6316–6323. doi: 10.1016/j.biomaterials.2011.05.020

Luo, X., Weaver, C. L., Zhou, D. D., Greenberg, R., and Cui, X. T. (2011b). Highly stable carbon nanotube doped poly(3,4-ethylenedioxythiophene) for chronic neural stimulation. *Biomaterials* 32, 5551–5557. doi: 10.1016/j.biomaterials.2011.04.051

Ma, W., Fitzgerald, W., Liu, Q.-Y., O'Shaughnessy, T., Maric, D., Lin, H., et al. (2004). CNS stem and progenitor cell differentiation into functional neuronal circuits in three-dimensional collagen gels. *Exp. Neurol.* 190, 276–288. doi: 10.1016/j.expneurol.2003.10.016

Mahadevappa, M., Weiland, J. D., Yanai, D., Fine, I., Greenberg, R. J., and Humayun, M. S. (2005). Perceptual thresholds and electrode impedance in three retinal prosthesis subjects. *IEEE Trans. Neural Syst. Rehabil. Eng.* 13, 201–206. doi: 10.1109/TNSRE.2005.848687

Majumdar, D., Gao, Y., Li, D., and Webb, D. J. (2011). Co-culture of neurons and glia in a novel microfluidic platform. *J. Neurosci. Methods* 196, 38–44. doi: 10.1016/j.jneumeth.2010.12.024

Mao, C., and Kisaalita, W. S. (2004). Characterization of 3-D collagen hydrogels for functional cell-based biosensing. *Biosens. Bioelectron.* 19, 1075–1088. doi: 10.1016/j.bios.2003.10.008

Mario Cheong, G., Lim, K. S., Jakubowicz, A., Martens, P. J., Poole-Warren, L. A., and Green, R. A. (2013). Conductive hydrogels with tailored bioactivity for implantable electrode coatings. *Acta Biomater.* 10, 1216–1226. doi: 10.1016/j.actbio.2013.12.032

Martin, D. C., and Feldman, K. E. (2012). *Substituted 3,4-Propylenedioxythiophene Monomers and 3,4-Propylenedioxythiophene-Based Crosslinkers And Polymers Thereof.* Google Patents).

Matsumoto, K., Sato, C., Naka, Y., Kitazawa, A., Whitby, R. L.D., and Shimizu, N. (2007). Neurite outgrowths of neurons with neurotrophin-coated carbon nanotubes. *J. Biosci. Bioeng.* 103, 216–220. doi: 10.1263/jbb.103.216

McConnell, G. C., Rees, H. D., Levey, A. I., Gutekunst, C. A., Gross, R. E., and Bellamkonda, R. V. (2009). Implanted neural electrodes cause chronic, local inflammation that is correlated with local neurodegeneration. *J. Neural Eng.* 6, 056003. doi: 10.1088/1741-2560/6/5/056003

McCreery, D. B. (2008). Cochlear nucleus auditory prostheses. *Hear. Res.* 242, 64–73. doi: 10.1016/j.heares.2007.11.014

McCreery, D. B., Yuen, T. G. H., Agnew, W. F., and Bullara, L. A. (1997). A characterization of the effects on neuronal excitability due to prolonged microstimulation with chronically implanted microelectrodes. *IEEE Trans. Biomed. Eng.* 44, 931–939. doi: 10.1109/10.634645

Merker, J., Lupton, D., Töpfer, M., and Knake, H. (2001). High temperature mechanical properties of the platinum group metals. *Plat. Metals Rev.* 45, 74–82.

Merrill, D. R., Bikson, M., and Jefferys, J. G. R. (2005). Electrical stimulation of excitable tissue: design of efficacious and safe protocols. *J. Neurosci. Methods* 141, 171–198. doi: 10.1016/j.jneumeth.2004.10.020

Nakayama, Y., and Matsuda, T. (1995). Surface microarchitectural design in biomedical applications: preparation of microporous polymer surfaces by an excimer laser ablation technique. *J. Biomed. Mater. Res.* 29, 1295–1301. doi: 10.1002/jbm.820291017

Nguyen-Vu, T. D. B., Chen, H., Cassell, A. M., Andrews, R. J., Meyyappan, M., and Li, J. (2006). Vertically aligned carbon nanofiber arrays: an advance toward electrical–neural interfaces. *Small* 2, 89–94. doi: 10.1002/smll.200500175

Nguyen-Vu, T. D. B., Chen, H., Cassell, A. M., Andrews, R. J., Meyyappan, M., and Li, J. (2007). Vertically Aligned Carbon Nanofiber Architecture as a Multifunctional 3-D Neural Electrical Interface. *IEEE Trans. Biomed. Eng.* 54, 1121–1128. doi: 10.1109/TBME.2007.891169

Nicodemus, G. D., and Bryant, S. J. (2008). Cell encapsulation in biodegradable hydrogels for tissue engineering applications. *Tissue Eng. B Rev.* 14, 16 doi: 10.1089/ten.teb.2007.0332

Niina, O., Hirotaka, T., Yoshiuki, K., Toshiya, K., Risato, K., Tetsu, T., et al. (2011). Comparison of electrode materials for the use of retinal prosthesis. *Biomed. Mater. Eng.* 21, 83–97. doi: 10.3233/BME-2011-0658

Nilasaroya, A., Poole-Warren, L. A., Whitelock, J. M., and Jo Martens, P. (2008). Structural and functional characterisation of poly(vinyl alcohol) and heparin hydrogels. *Biomaterials* 29, 4658–4664. doi: 10.1016/j.biomaterials.2008.08.011

Normand, V., Lootens, D. L., Amici, E., Plucknett, K. P., and Aymard, P. (2000). New insight into agarose gel mechanical properties. *Biomacromolecules* 1, 730–738. doi: 10.1021/bm005583j

Normann, R. A. (2007). Technology insight: future neuroprosthetic therapies for disorders of the nervous system. *Nat. Clin. Pract. Neurol.* 3, 444–452. doi: 10.1038/ncpneuro0556

Novikova, L. N., Mosahebi, A., Wiberg, M., Terenghi, G., Kellerth, J.-O., and Novikov, L. N. (2006). Alginate hydrogel and matrigel as potential cell carriers for neurotransplantation. *J. Biomed. Mater. Res. A* 77A, 242–252. doi: 10.1002/jbm.a.30603

Ochiai, H., Shibata, H., Sawa, Y., and Katoh, T. (1980). "Living electrode" as a long-lived photoconverter for biophotolysis of water. *Proc. Natl. Acad. Sci. U.S.A.* 77, 2442–2444. doi: 10.1073/pnas.77.5.2442

Ochiai, H., Shibata, H., Sawa, Y., Shoga, M., and Ohta, S. (1983). Properties of semiconductor electrodes coated with living films of cyanobacteria. *Appl. Biochem. Biotechnol.* 8, 289–303. doi: 10.1007/BF02779496

Ouyang, L., Green, R., Feldman, K. E., and Martin, D. C. (2011). "Direct local polymerization of poly(3,4-ethylene dioxythiophene in rat cortex," in *Progress in Brain Research*, eds J. Schouenborg, M. Garwicz, and N. Danielsen (Oxford: Elsevier), 263–272.

Peixoto, N., Jackson, K., Samiyi, R., and Minnikanti, S. (2009). "Charge storage: stability measures in implantable electrodes," in *Engineering in Medicine and Biology Society, 2009. Annual International Conference of the IEEE*, Farifax.

Perlmutter, J. S., and Mink, J. W. (2006). DEEP BRAIN STIMULATION. *Annu. Rev. Neurosci.* 29, 229–257. doi: 10.1146/annurev.neuro.29.051605.112824

Piantino, J., Burdick, J. A., Goldberg, D., Langer, R., and Benowitz, L. I. (2006). An injectable, biodegradable hydrogel for trophic factor delivery enhances axonal rewiring and improves performance after spinal cord injury. *Exp. Neurol.* 201, 359–367. doi: 10.1016/j.expneurol.2006.04.020

Polikov, V. S., Tresco, P. A., and Reichert, W. M. (2005). Response of brain tissue to chronically implanted neural electrodes. *J. Neurosci. Methods* 148, 1–18. doi: 10.1016/j.jneumeth.2005.08.015

Poole-Warren, L., Lovell, N. H., Baek, S., and Green, R. (2010). Development of bioactive conducting polymers for neural interfaces. *Exp. Rev. Med. Dev.* 7, 35–49. doi: 10.1586/erd.09.58

Rao, L., Zhou, H., Li, T., Li, C., and Duan, Y. Y. (2012). Polyethylene glycol-containing polyurethane hydrogel coatings for improving the biocompatibility of neural electrodes. *Acta Biomater.* 8, 2233–2242. doi: 10.1016/j.actbio.2012.03.001

Raub, C. B., Putnam, A. J., Tromberg, B. J., and George, S. C. (2010). Predicting bulk mechanical properties of cellularized collagen gels using multiphoton microscopy. *Acta Biomater.* 6, 4657–4665. doi: 10.1016/j.actbio.2010.07.004

Richardson-Burns, S. M., Hendricks, J. L., Foster, B., Povlich, L. K., Kim, D.-H., and Martin, D. C. (2007). Polymerization of the conducting polymer poly(3,4-ethylenedioxythiophene) (PEDOT) around living neural cells. *Biomaterials* 28, 1539–1552. doi: 10.1016/j.biomaterials.2006.11.026

Richardson, R. T., Thompson, B., Moulton, S., Newbold, C., Lum, M. G., Cameron, A., et al. (2007a). The effect of polypyrrole with incorporated neurotrophin-3 on the promotion of neurite outgrowth from auditory neurons. *Biomaterials* 28, 513–523. doi: 10.1016/j.biomaterials.2006.09.008

Richardson, R. T., Thompson, B., Moulton, S., Newbold, C., Lum, M. G., Cameron, A., et al. (2007b). The effect of polypyrrole with incorporated neurotrophin-3 on the promotion of neurite outgrowth from auditory neurons. *Biomaterials* 28, 513–523. doi: 10.1016/j.biomaterials.2006.09.008

Richter, A., Kruse, C., Moser, A., Hofmann, U. G., and Danner, S. (2011). Cellular modulation of polymeric device surfaces: promise of adult stem cells for neuro-prosthetics. *Front. Neurosci.* 5:114. doi: 10.3389/fnins.2011.00114

Richter, A., Xie, Y., Schumacher, A., Loffler, S., Kirch, R. D., Al-Hasani, J., et al. (2013). A simple implantation method for flexible, multisite microelectrodes into rat brains. *Front. Neuroeng.* 6:6. doi: 10.3389/fneng.2013.00006

Rosario-Canales, M. R., Deria, P., Therien, M. J., and Santiago-Avilés, J. J. (2011). Composite Electronic Materials Based on Poly(3,4-propylenedioxythiophene) and Highly Charged Poly(aryleneethynylene)-Wrapped Carbon Nanotubes for Supercapacitors. *ACS Appl. Mater. Interf.* 4, 102–109. doi: 10.1021/am201041p

Rose, T. L., and Robblee, L. S. (1990). *Electrical stimulation with Pt electrodes. VIII. Electrochemically safe charge injection limits with 0.*2 ms pulses (neuronal application). *IEEE Trans. Biomed. Eng.* 37, 1118–1120. doi: 10.1109/10.61038

Rousche, P. J., Pellinen, D. S., Pivin, D. P. Jr., Williams, J. C., Vetter, R. J., et al. (2001). Flexible polyimide-based intracortical electrode arrays with bioactive capability. *IEEE Trans. Biomed. Eng.* 48, 361–371. doi: 10.1109/10.914800

Runge, M. B., Dadsetan, M., Baltrusaitis, J., Ruesink, T., Lu, L., Windebank, A. J., et al. (2010). Development of electrically conductive oligo(polyethylene glycol) fumarate-polypyrrole hydrogels for nerve regeneration. *Biomacromolecules* 11, 2845–2853. doi: 10.1021/bm100526a

Sarah, M. R.-B., Jeffrey, L. H., and David, C. M. (2007). Electrochemical polymerization of conducting polymers in living neural tissue. *J. Neural Eng.* 4, L6. doi: 10.1088/1741-2560/4/2/L02

Schmidt, C. E., Shastri, V. R., Vacanti, J. P., and Langer, R. (1997). Stimulation of neurite outgrowth using an electrically conducting polymer. *Proc. Natl. Acad. Sci. U.S.A.* 94, 8948–8953. doi: 10.1073/pnas.94.17.8948

Schuettler, M. (2007). "Electrochemical properties of platinum electrodes in vitro: comparison of six different surface qualities," in *Proceedings of the 29th Annual International Conference of the IEEE EMBS*, Freiburg.

Schuettler, M., Stiess, S., King, B. V., and Suaning, G. J. (2005). Fabrication of implantable microelectrode arrays by laser cutting of silicone rubber and platinum foil. *J. Neural Eng.* 2, S121–128. doi: 10.1088/1741-2560/2/1/013

Seidlits, S. K., Lee, J. Y., and Schmidt, C. E. (2008). Nanostructured scaffolds for neural applications. *Nanomedicine* 3, 183–199. doi: 10.2217/17435889.3.2.183

Shannon, R. V. (2012). Advances in auditory prostheses. *Curr. Opin. Neurol.* 25, 6. doi: 10.1097/WCO.0b013e32834ef878

Shepherd, R. K., Shivdasani, M. N., Nayagam, D. A. X., Williams, C. E., and Blamey, P. J. (2013). Visual prostheses for the blind. *Trends Biotechnol.* 31, 562–571. doi: 10.1016/j.tibtech.2013.07.001

Shoval, A., Adams, C., David-Pur, M., Shein, M., Hanein, Y., and Sernagor, E. (2009). Carbon nanotube electrodes for effective interfacing with retinal tissue. *Front. Neuroeng.* 2:4. doi: 10.3389/neuro.16.004.2009

Sidhu, K., Kim, J., Chayosumrit, M., Dean, S., and Sachdev, P. (2012). Alginate Microcapsule as a 3D platform for propagation and differentiation of human embryonic stem cells (hesc) to different lineages. *J. Vis. Exp.* 61, e3608. doi: 10.3791/3608

Stauffer, W. R., and Cui, X. T. (2006). Polypyrrole doped with 2 peptide sequences from laminin. *Biomaterials* 27, 2405–2413. doi: 10.1016/j.biomaterials.2005.10.024

Stevenson, G., Moulton, S. E., Innis, P. C., and Wallace, G. G. (2010). Polyterthiophene as an electrostimulated controlled drug release material of therapeutic levels of dexamethasone. *Synth. Metals* 160, 1107–1114. doi: 10.1016/j.synthmet.2010.02.035

Suri, S., and Schmidt, C. E. (2010). Cell-laden hydrogel constructs of hyaluronic acid, collagen, and laminin for neural tissue engineering. *Tissue Eng.* 16, 1703–1716. doi: 10.1089/ten.tea.2009.0381

Suzuki, I., Fukuda, M., Shirakawa, K., Jiko, H., and Gotoh, M. (2013). Carbon nanotube multi-electrode array chips for noninvasive real-time measurement of dopamine, action potentials, and postsynaptic potentials. *Biosens. Bioelectron.* 49, 1–6. doi: 10.1016/j.bios.2013.05.023

Taylor, S. J., and Sakiyama-Elbert, S. E. (2006). Effect of controlled delivery of neurotrophin-3 from fibrin on spinal cord injury in a long term model. *J. Control. Release* 116, 204–210. doi: 10.1016/j.jconrel.2006.07.005

Telford, A. M., James, M., Meagher, L., and Neto, C. (2010). Thermally cross-linked PNVP films as antifouling coatings for biomedical applications. *ACS Appl. Mater. Interfaces* 2, 2399–2408. doi: 10.1021/am100406j

Tian, F., Cui, D., Schwarz, H., Estrada, G. G., and Kobayashi, H. (2006). Cytotoxicity of single-wall carbon nanotubes on human fibroblasts. *Toxicology Vitro* 20, 1202–1212. doi: 10.1016/j.tiv.2006.03.008

Turner, J. N., Shain, W., Szarowski, D. H., Andersen, M., Martins, S., Isaacson, M., et al. (1999). Cerebral astrocyte response to micromachined silicon implants. *Exp. Neurol.* 156, 33–49. doi: 10.1006/exnr.1998.6983

Tyler, D. J., and Durand, D. M. (2002). Functionally selective peripheral nerve stimulation with a flat interface nerve electrode. *IEEE Trans. Neural Syst. Rehabil. Eng.* 10, 294–303. doi: 10.1109/TNSRE.2002.806840

Vaquette, C., Slimani, S., Kahn, C. J. F., Tran, N., Rahouadj, R., and Wang, X. (2010). A poly(lactic-co-glycolic acid) knitted scaffold for tendon tissue engineering: an in vitro and in vivo study. *J. Biomater. Sci. Polym. Ed.* 21, 1737–1760. doi: 10.1163/092050609X12560455246676

Wadhwa, R., Lagenaur, C. F., and Cui, X. T. (2006). Electrochemically controlled release of dexamethasone from conducting polymer polypyrrole coated electrode. *J. Control. Release* 110, 531–541. doi: 10.1016/j.jconrel.2005.10.027

Wang, K., Fishman, H. A., Dai, H., and Harris, J. S. (2006). Neural stimulation with a carbon nanotube microelectrode array. *Nano Lett.* 6, 2043–2048. doi: 10.1021/nl061241t

Ward, M. P., Rajdev, P., Ellison, C., and Irazoqui, P. P. (2009). Toward a comparison of microelectrodes for acute and chronic recordings. *Brain Res.* 1282, 183–200. doi: 10.1016/j.brainres.2009.05.052

Webster, T. J., Waid, M. C., Mckenzie, J. L., Price, R. L., and Ejiofor, J. U. (2004). Nano-biotechnology: carbon nanofibres as improved neural and orthopaedic implants. *Nanotechnology* 15, 48–54. doi: 10.1088/0957-4484/15/1/009

Weldon, D. T., Rogers, S. D., Ghilardi, J. R., Finke, M. P., Cleary, J. P., O'Hare, E., et al. (1998). Fibrillar β-amyloid induces microglial phagocytosis, expression of inducible nitric oxide synthase, and loss of a select population of neurons in the rat cns in vivo. *J. Neurosci.* 18, 2161–2173.

Wells, M. R., Kraus, K., Batter, D. K., Blunt, D. G., Weremowitz, J., Lynch, S. E., et al. (1997). Gel matrix vehicles for growth factor application in nerve gap injuries repaired with tubes: a comparison of biomatrix, collagen, and methylcellulose. *Exp. Neurol.* 146, 395–402. doi: 10.1006/exnr.1997.6543

Wester, B. A., Lee, R. H., and Laplaca, M. C. (2009). Development and characterization of in vivo flexible electrodes compatible with large tissue displacements. *J. Neural Eng.* 6, 024002. doi: 10.1088/1741-2560/6/2/024002

White, R. L., and Gross, T. J. (1974). An evaluation of the resistance to electrolysis of metals for use in biostimulation microprobes. *IEEE Trans. Biomed. Eng.* 21, 487–490. doi: 10.1109/TBME.1974.324339

Whitney, N. P., Eidem, T. M., Peng, H., Huang, Y., and Zheng, J. C. (2009). Inflammation mediates varying effects in neurogenesis: relevance to the pathogenesis of brain injury and neurodegenerative disorders. *J. Neurochem.* 108, 1343–1359. doi: 10.1111/j.1471-4159.2009.05886.x

World Health Organization. (2006). "Public health principles and neurological disorders," in *Neurological Disorders: Public Health Challenges.* Geneva, Switzerland: WHO Press.

Wilks, S. J., Woolley, A. J., Ouyang, L., Martin, D. C., and Otto, K. J. (2011). In vivo polymerization of poly (3, 4-ethylenedioxythiophene)(PEDOT) in rodent cerebral cortex. *Conf. Proc. IEEE Eng. Med. Biol. Soc.* 2011, 5412–5415. doi: 10.1109/IEMBS.2011.6091338

Willerth, S. M., and Sakiyama-Elbert, S. E. (2007). Approaches to neural tissue engineering using scaffolds for drug delivery. *Adv. Drug Deliv. Rev.* 59, 325–338. doi: 10.1016/j.addr.2007.03.014

Wilson, B. S., and Dorman, M. F. (2008). Cochlear implants: a remarkable past and a brilliant future. *Hear. Res.* 242, 3–21. doi: 10.1016/j.heares.2008.06.005

Winter, J. O., Cogan, S. F., and Rizzo, J. F. (2007). Neurotrophin-eluting hydrogel coatings for neural stimulating electrodes. *J. Biomed. Mater. Res.* 81B, 551–563. doi: 10.1002/jbm.b.30696

Winter, J. O., Gokhale, M., Jensen, R. J., Cogan, S. F., and Rizzo Iii, J. F. (2008). Tissue engineering applied to the retinal prosthesis: neurotrophin-eluting polymeric hydrogel coatings. *Mater. Sci. Eng. C* 28, 448–453. doi: 10.1016/j.msec.2007.04.011

Woolley, A. J., Desai, H. A., Steckbeck, M. A., Patel, N. K., and Otto, K. J. (2011). In situ characterization of the brain–microdevice interface using device capture histology. *J. Neurosci. Methods* 201, 67–77. doi: 10.1016/j.jneumeth.2011.07.012

Xiao, Y., Cui, X., Hancock, J. M., Bouguettaya, M., Reynolds, J. R., and Martin, D. C. (2004). Electrochemical polymerization of poly(hydroxymethylated-3,4-ethylenedioxythiophene) (PEDOT-MeOH) on multichannel neural probes. *Sens. Actuators B Chem.* 99, 437–443. doi: 10.1016/j.snb.2003.12.067

Xiao, Y., He, L., and Che, J. (2012). An effective approach for the fabrication of reinforced composite hydrogel engineered with SWNTs, polypyrrole and PEGDA hydrogel. *J. Mater. Chem.* 22, 8076–8082. doi: 10.1039/C2JM30601H

Yamato, H., Ohwa, M., and Wernet, W. (1995). Stability of polypyrrole and poly(3,4-ethylenedioxythiophene) for biosensor application. *J. Electroanal. Chem.* 397, 163–170. doi: 10.1016/0022-0728(95)04156-8

Yang, J., Kim, D. H., Hendricks, J. L., Leach, M., Northey, R., and Martin, D. C. (2005). Ordered surfactant-templated poly(3,4-ethylenedioxythiophene) (PEDOT) conducting polymer on microfabricated neural probes. *Acta Biomater.* 1, 125–136. doi: 10.1016/j.actbio.2004.09.006

Yang, J., and Martin, D. C. (2006). Impedance spectroscopy and nanoindentation of conducting poly(3,4-ethylenedioxythiophene) coatings on microfabricated neural prosthetic devices. *J. Mater. Res.* 21, 1124–1132. doi: 10.1557/jmr.2006.0145

Yang, S., Xia, B., Zeng, X., Luo, S., Wei, W., and Liu, X. (2010). Fabrication of DNA functionalized carbon nanotubes/Cu2+ complex by one-step electrodeposition and its sensitive determination of nitrite. *Anal. Chim. Acta* 667, 57–62. doi: 10.1016/j.aca.2010.03.063

Yu, X., and Bellamkonda, R. V. (2003). Tissue-engineered scaffolds are effective alternatives to autografts for bridging peripheral nerve gaps. *Tissue Eng.* 9, 421–430. doi: 10.1089/107632703322066606

Yu, Z., Mcknight, T. E., Ericson, M. N., Melechko, A. V., Simpson, M. L., and Morrison, B. (2007). Vertically aligned carbon nanofiber arrays record electrophysiological signals from hippocampal slices. *Nano Lett.* 7, 2188–2195. doi: 10.1021/nl070291a

Zhong, Y., and Bellamkonda, R. V. (2005). Controlled release of anti-inflammatory agent α-MSH from neural implants. *J. Control. Release* 106, 309–318. doi: 10.1016/j.jconrel.2005.05.012

Zhong, Y., and Bellamkonda, R. V. (2007). Dexamethasone-coated neural probes elicit attenuated inflammatory response and neuronal loss compared to uncoated neural probes. *Brain Res.* 1148, 15–27. doi: 10.1016/j.brainres.2007.02.024

Zhong, Y., and Bellamkonda, R. V. (2008). Biomaterials for the central nervous system. *J. R. Soc. Interface* 5, 957–975. doi: 10.1098/rsif.2008.0071

Zhong, Y., Yu, X., Gilbert, R., and Bellamkonda, R. V. (2001). Stabilizing electrode-host interfaces: a tissue engineering approach. *J. Rehabil. Res. Dev.* 38, 627–632.

Zuidema, J. M., Pap, M. M., Jaroch, D. B., Morrison, F. A., and Gilbert, R. J. (2011). Fabrication and characterization of tunable polysaccharide hydrogel blends for neural repair. *Acta Biomater.* 7, 1634–1643. doi: 10.1016/j.actbio.2010.11.039

17

Muscarinic cholinergic receptors modulate inhibitory synaptic rhythms in hippocampus and neocortex

Bradley E. Alger[1,2,3]*, Daniel A. Nagode[4] and Ai-Hui Tang[1]

[1] Department of Physiology, University of Maryland School of Medicine, Baltimore, MD, USA
[2] Department of Psychiatry, University of Maryland School of Medicine, Baltimore, MD, USA
[3] Program in Neuroscience, Graduate School, University of Maryland Baltimore, Baltimore, MD, USA
[4] Department of Biology, University of Maryland College Park, College Park, MD, USA

Edited by:
Sukumar Vijayaraghavan, University of Colorado Health Science Center, USA

Reviewed by:
Rodrigo Andrade, Wayne State University School of Medicine, USA
Rory McQuiston, Virginia Commonwealth University, USA
David A. Brown, University College London, UK

***Correspondence:**
Bradley E. Alger, Department of Physiology, University of Maryland School of Medicine, 655 West Baltimore Street, Rm 5-025, Baltimore, MD 21201, USA
e-mail: balgerlab@gmail.com

Activation of muscarinic acetylcholine (ACh) receptors (mAChRs) powerfully affects many neuronal properties as well as numerous cognitive behaviors. Small neuronal circuits constitute an intermediate level of organization between neurons and behaviors, and mAChRs affect interactions among cells that compose these circuits. Circuit activity is often assessed by extracellular recordings of the local field potentials (LFPs), which are analogous to *in vivo* EEGs, generated by coordinated neuronal interactions. Coherent forms of physiologically relevant circuit activity manifest themselves as rhythmic oscillations in the LFPs. Frequencies of rhythmic oscillations that are most closely associated with animal behavior are in the range of 4–80 Hz, which is subdivided into theta (4–14 Hz), beta (15–29 Hz) and gamma (30–80 Hz) bands. Activation of mAChRs triggers rhythmic oscillations in these bands in the hippocampus and neocortex. Inhibitory responses mediated by GABAergic interneurons constitute a prominent feature of these oscillations, and indeed, appear to be their major underlying factor in many cases. An important issue is which interneurons are involved in rhythm generation. Besides affecting cellular and network properties directly, mAChRs can cause the mobilization of endogenous cannabinoids (endocannabinoids, eCBs) that, by acting on the principal cannabinoid receptor of the brain, CB1R, regulate the release of certain neurotransmitters, including GABA. CB1Rs are heavily expressed on only a subset of interneurons and, at lower density, on glutamatergic neurons. *Exogenous* cannabinoids typically disrupt oscillations in the theta (θ) and gamma (γ) ranges, which probably contributes to the behavioral effects of these drugs. It is important to understand how neuronal circuit activity is affected by mAChR-driven eCBs, as this information will provide deeper insight into the actions of ACh itself, as well as into the effects of eCBs and exogenous cannabinoids in animal behavior. After covering some basic aspects of the mAChR system, this review will focus on recent findings concerning the mechanisms and circuitry that generate θ and γ rhythms in hippocampus and neocortex. The ability of optogenetic methods to probe the many roles of ACh in rhythm generation is highlighted.

Keywords: optogenetics, GABA, interneuron, endocannabinoid, opioid, theta, cholecystokinin, parvalbumin

INTRODUCTION

The numerous effects that acetylcholine (ACh) has in the nervous system are mediated by both muscarinic (mAChR) and nicotinic (nAChR) receptors. Initially, attention focused on the mAChRs, following the classical experiments of Otto Loewi that showed that chemical transmission at synapses in the heart was mediated by ACh acting at mAChRs. With the recognition that nAChRs are also present in the brain and are directly relevant to the understanding of, e.g., the addictive potency of nicotine and its importance in schizophrenia, an enormous effort has gone into investigating the nAChRs in the central nervous system, although work continued on the molecular structure and pharmacology of the mAChRs. In addition, electrophysiological studies have provided a wealth of data on their cellular actions, the ion channels that they control, and their downstream biochemical mechanisms. Yet, despite these efforts, there remain important gaps in our knowledge of how the mAChRs affect neuronal circuits. Neuronal oscillations are among the most prominent and readily detected signs of neuronal circuit behavior. Certain oscillations, particularly those in the theta (θ, 4–14 Hz) and gamma (γ, 30–80 Hz) frequency ranges, are widely believed to be essential for the performance of various behavioral and cognitive functions. A general cholinergic agonist, carbachol (CCh), is often used to induce these rhythms which are mediated by mAChRs in hippocampus and neocortex in model experimental systems. However, a full understanding of the cellular and molecular mechanisms of rhythm generation has not been achieved. GABAergic inhibitory interneurons are key elements in rhythm generation, and mAChRs affect their behavior in many ways.

This review will highlight some new results on the generation of oscillations in hippocampus and neocortex; useful reviews of earlier work (e.g., Lawrence, 2008) have appeared. We will discuss the types of mAChRs, their influence on the some of the main interneuron subtypes and to lesser extent on principal cells. An emerging but still under-investigated theme is the ability of certain mAChRs to stimulate the synthesis and release of endogenous cannabinoids (endocannabinoids, eCBs), the natural ligands for the cannabinoid receptors (CB1Rs) in the brain (see diagram in **Figure 1**). In many regions, certain interneurons are heavily invested with CB1Rs while other interneurons have none; glutamatergic neurons often have far lower densities (up to 30 times lower) of the CB1Rs than do the interneurons. The great majority of CB1Rs are located on or near synaptic nerve terminals where their activation by exogenous cannabinoids and eCBs inhibit transmitter release. There has been little concerted effort to understand the implications of the mAChR-eCB link on complex nervous system activity, however. In view of the potency of mAChRs to mobilize eCBs, and thereby indirectly alter neuronal activity, it will be of great interest to work out the details and functional implications of this association. A key issue that has been difficult to explore with conventional methods concerns endogenously released ACh. The bulk of all experimental work on mAChRs and their physiological effects has been carried out either with gross tissue stimulation delivered by extracellular electrodes or perfusion with pharmacological agents. These methods lack specificity and selectivity of action, and the conclusions they permit are accordingly limited. We will discuss recent experiments in which optogenetic techniques have been used to probe the workings of the ACh system in unprecedented detail.

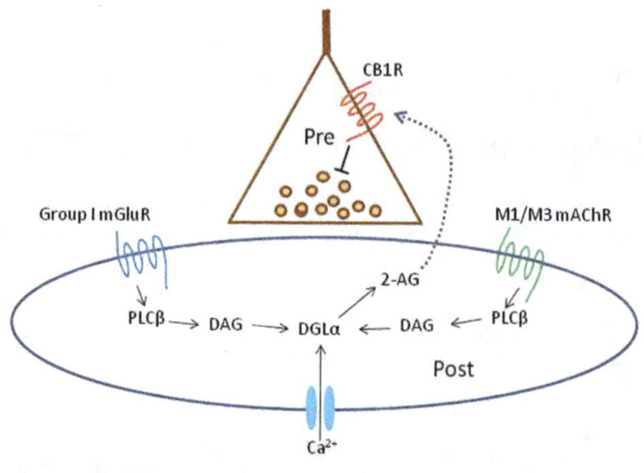

FIGURE 1 | Schematic summary diagram of the endocannabinoid system. A presynaptic nerve terminal is shown synapsing on a postsynaptic cell. Agonist binding of either group I mGluRs or M1 or M3 mAChRs activates phospholipase Cβ (PLCβ) in the postsynaptic cell. The product of the reaction catalyzed by PLCβ, diacylglycerol (DAG), is metabolized by the enzyme diacylglycerol lipase α (DGLα) to form the endocannabinoid, 2-arachidonyl glycerol (2-AG). DGLα can also be activated by Ca^{2+} influx via a PLC-independent mechanism. 2-AG is membrane permeant and gains access through an unknown mechanism to the cannabinoid receptor, CB1R, on the presynaptic nerve terminal. Binding of CB1R by 2-AG inhibits transmitter release, mainly by inhibiting Ca^{2+} influx into the terminal, although other mechanisms can be involved. This is the simplest conventional model of the system and various details are controversial or have been omitted for the sake of simplicity; see a comprehensive review, e.g., Kano et al. (2009), for more information.

CENTRAL CHOLINERGIC PROJECTION NEURONS ASSOCIATED WITH mAChR-INDUCED RHYTHM GENERATION

Almost all of the ACh in the hippocampus and neocortex comes from distal axons of cholinergic projection neurons that are highly concentrated in the basal forebrain (Lewis and Shute, 1967; see Woolf, 1991; van der Zee and Luiten, 1999; for review). This collection of nuclei includes the medial septum (MS) and lateral septum, the horizontal and vertical limb of the diagonal band of Broca (DBB), and the nucleus basalis magnocellularis (NBM). In rodents, cholinergic neurons in the MS/DBB project to olfactory-related structures, cingulate cortex, retrospenial cortex, medial prefrontal cortex, hippocampus and parahippocampus (Gaykema et al., 1989). The cholinergic projection from the MS/DBB to the hippocampus via the fornix/fimbria system is quite large, and selective ablation of the cholinergic cells in the MS/DBB or transection of the fimbria-fornix leads to a virtual loss of ACh fibers in the hippocampus (Lee et al., 1994; Naumann et al., 1994). Cholinergic neurons in the NBM project to the entire cortical mantle, with laminar projection patterns varying with cortical area. NBM also projects to the amygdala and olfactory bulb (see Woolf, 1991; van der Zee and Luiten, 1999 for reviews).

An important anatomical feature of the ACh system in the brain is that cholinergic fibers only rarely (e.g., 3% in hippocampus and neocortex, Yamasaki et al., 2010) make classical morphologically defined synapses onto their target neurons (one-to-one, or "wired transmission", Zoli et al., 1999). Rather, large vesicle-filled varicosities appear along the axons, and ACh is released into the local environment (Vizi and Kiss, 1998), where it diffuses in a paracrine-like way to receptors on target neurons and glia. This has been referred to as "volume conduction" (Zoli et al., 1999) and may be especially relevant for understanding mAChR-mediated effects, as they tend to have slow kinetics themselves and may involve the release of other modulators for which rapid kinetics is also not a key feature. A correlational EM study for the localization of M1 mAChRs and presynaptic synaptic specializations, including the presynaptic active-zone protein, bassoon, along cortical and hippocampal pyramidal cell (PC) dendrites, found that, unlike glutamate terminals and AMPA receptors, there was no close relationship between a cholinergic varicosity (identified by either the choline transporter, CHT1, or choline acetyl transferase, ChAT) near a dendrite and postsynaptic clusters of M1 receptors (Yamasaki et al., 2010). These findings appear to be consistent with the volume transmission mode. Sarter et al. (2009) question the relevance of the distinction between wired and volume transmission, since both can mediate responses with very slow kinetics, but admit that the difference may still be significant in the spatial domain—proximity of the release site to the receptors—which is the one most relevant to the present discussion.

DISTRIBUTION, ACTION, AND CELLULAR LOCALIZATION OF mAChR SUBTYPES IN HIPPOCAMPUS AND NEOCORTEX

Muscarinic acetylcholine receptors (mAChRs) are G-protein coupled receptors of the Class A, rhodopsin-like family, with ACh being the main endogenous agonist (the ACh precursor, choline, reportedly induces γ activity in an atropine-sensitive way at 2–5 mM, Fischer et al., 2014). mAChRs are widely distributed throughout the central nervous system. The five subtypes, designated M1-5 (Bonner, 1989; Caulfield and Birdsall, 1998) can be divided into two broad groups based on their primary coupling to G-proteins. M1, M3 and M5 receptors (M1-class) are preferentially coupled to $G_{q/11}$ proteins and activate phospholipase C, which initiates the IP3—diacylglycerol (DAG) cascade leading to intracellular Ca^{2+} mobilization, and activation of protein kinase C and mitogen-activated protein kinase (MAPK) pathways. M2 and M4 receptors (M2-class) couple to the pertussis-toxin sensitive $G_{i/o}$ proteins and inhibit adenylyl cyclase activity.

Although widespread in the brain, there is considerable regional variability in the distribution of mAChR subtypes. Throughout the brain, M1 is the most abundant subtype and M5 the least. In the hippocampus and neocortex, M1 is present at high levels; M3 is present at moderate levels (though generally low elsewhere). M4 is very high almost everywhere in the brain, while M2 is found at much lower densities. M5 mRNA is relatively sparse except in hippocampal CA1 PCs and some scattered subcortical nuclei. M1-class receptors are often located on somato-dendritic regions of neurons, and their activation leads to membrane depolarization and increases in cellular excitability by enhancing the mixed-cation Na^+/K^+ current (I_h), Ca^{2+} -dependent, non-selective cation current (e.g., Fisahn et al., 2002), and by inhibiting certain potassium channels, such as Kv7 (M-current), K_{sAHP}, and K ("leak" channels) (e.g., Brown and Adams, 1980; Cole and Nicoll, 1983; Halliwell, 1990; Cobb and Davies, 2005; Lawrence et al., 2006b; Broicher et al., 2008). M2-class receptors frequently reside on presynaptic axonal terminals (although there are exceptions), and agonist binding can activate Kir3 potassium channels and inhibit some voltage-gated Ca^{2+} channels (especially $Ca_{v2.2}$), which in turn hyperpolarizes the neuron or inhibits transmitter release (Hájos et al., 1998; Brown, 2010) (It should be noted that cholinergic axon terminals, including the axons of the MS/DBB fibers, generally express mAChRs, often M2-types, that probably act as presynaptic autoreceptors and regulate ACh outflow; this review will not cover this topic and interested readers can consult, e.g., Vizi and Kiss, 1998; Zoli et al., 1999 for reviews). While the exact cellular location and functional role of each subtype has not been fully elucidated, some correlations between different forms of cholinergic neuromodulation and the neurochemical identities of distinct neuron classes have been established in both hippocampus and neocortex.

mAChRs ON PYRAMIDAL CELLS AND INTERNEURONS IN HIPPOCAMPUS AND NEOCORTEX

In the hippocampal CA1 region, PCs provide excitatory output to other cortical and subcortical areas, and carry information about spatial location and episodic memories (e.g., Eichenbaum, 2013). The functions of PCs are supported by local inhibitory circuits comprising more than 20 types of GABAergic interneurons (Freund and Katona, 2007; Klausberger and Somogyi, 2008; Whittington et al., 2011). The majority of these interneurons are morphologically and neurochemically distinct (Klausberger and Somogyi, 2008), yet their detailed functions have not been worked out. One broad distinction is based on whether the interneurons participate in feedback or feedforward inhibition; another is whether they synapse on dendritic or somatic regions of their target cells. There is some overlap between these classifications, with feedforward inhibition often mediated by dendritic targeting interneurons, and feedback inhibition mediated by perisomatic (i.e., including the soma and proximal dendrites 50–100 μm away) regions. However, there are many exceptions to this generalization (Bartos et al., 2011) and we will focus on the dendritic vs. perisomatic targeting distinction, which seems to be quite general across many brain regions.

Perisomatic targeting interneurons include two non-overlapping classes of basket cells (BCs): the parvalbumin-expressing (PV+), fast-spiking interneurons, and cholecystokinin-expressing (CCK+) regular-spiking interneurons (Freund and Katona, 2007; Bartos and Elgueta, 2012). A third type, the PV+ axo-axonic interneurons (often referred to as "chandelier cells" especially in the neocortex, e.g., Povysheva et al., 2013), innervates only the initial segments of PC axons; we will not discuss axo-axonic cells in detail.

The CCK+ and PV+ BCs differ in a number of fundamental features (Freund and Katona, 2007; Bartos and Elgueta, 2012). In addition to differences in firing patterns—non-accommodating, γ-synchronized action potentials in PV+ BCs; accommodating, poorly γ-synchronized action potentials in CCK+ BCs—one other distinction is that CCK+ BCs express the main receptor for the cannabinoids, CB1R, while PV+ BCs express the mu-opioid (μOR) receptor (Drake and Milner, 2002), which responds to certain opioids. Traditional anatomical and physiological evidence suggests that these two receptor populations have virtually no overlap (recent evidence that suggests this conclusion should be modified will be discussed below). These distinctions between PV+ and CCK+ BCs hold for both hippocampus and cortex, but not everywhere. For example, in the striatum PV+ BCs express CB1Rs (Kano et al., 2009). Additional differences between PV+ and CCK+ BCs can be found in their complement of mAChRs, as discussed below.

A well-studied representative of the dendritic targeting class of interneurons is the somatostatin (SOM)- and mGluR1a-expressing interneuron. Hippocampal interneurons in this class have their somata in the stratum oriens and the great bulk of their axonal arbor in the stratum lacunosum-moleculare, and are referred to as oriens-lacunosum moleculare (O-LM) cells. O-LM cells target the dendrites rather than perisomatic regions of PCs and have different phase preferences for firing within θ rhythm oscillations than do the BCs (or axo-axonic cells). Therefore O-LM cells play distinctive functional roles in regulating both PC excitability and temporal patterning of PC activity (Buzsáki, 2002; Klausberger and Somogyi, 2008; Bartos et al., 2011).

These classes of interneurons are not unique to the CA1 region; most other regions of the hippocampus and the neocortex have similar inhibitory configurations (Lund and Lewis, 1993; Curley and Lewis, 2012). The BCs in the neocortex have essentially the same properties as in the hippocampus, as do the axo-axonic cells (Curley and Lewis, 2012), although it appears the cortical axo-axonic cells have not received as much attention as the hippocampal ones have. In the cortex, the Martinotti cells are also SOM+ /mGluR1α+, and target PC dendrites, and seem generally analogous to the O-LM cells of the hippocampus. Therefore, understanding how mAChR activation regulates these interneurons and consequently the dynamics of hippocampal network activity may be applicable to the neocortex.

mAChRs are widely distributed on the principal cells of the hippocampus and neocortex. PCs in CA1-CA3 and granule cells in dentate gyrus all have abundant postsynaptic expression of M1 receptors, and weaker expression of M3 receptors (Levey et al., 1995). Activation of M1 or M3 usually increases cellular excitability. Therefore, the most dramatic direct effect of either exogenously applied cholinergic agonists or endogenously released ACh on PCs is a pronounced membrane potential depolarization and decrease in membrane conductance (Dodd et al., 1981; Cole and Nicoll, 1983; Pitler and Alger, 1990). This response, together with a decrease of the afterhyperpolarization (AHP; Cole and Nicoll, 1983) and the activation of a persistent, voltage-dependent sodium current (Yamada-Hanff and Bean, 2013), often results in sustained action potential firing (Cobb and Davies, 2005), particularly in hippocampal CA3, where the PCs form a strong recurrent intercollateral network. Neocortical PCs are similarly affected by muscarinic agonists (McCormick and Prince, 1986; Haj-Dahmane and Andrade, 1999).

For the inhibitory interneurons, the major muscarinic response is also depolarization, but with a less prominent associated change in cell input resistance. Generalizations are somewhat difficult to make however, given the diversity of mAChR subtypes, interneurons, and the specific distributions of mAChRs along the cells. For example, M1 is predominantly expressed on PCs but found in very low abundance, if at all, on GAD67-expressing interneurons, including O-LM cells (Yamasaki et al., 2010). These factors make the muscarinic modulation of interneurons much more complicated than that of the PCs. Besides the depolarizing effects of mAChR activation, some interneurons exhibit pure hyperpolarizations or biphasic responses, in which an initial hyperpolarization is followed by a secondary depolarizing phase (McQuiston and Madison, 1999a; Widmer et al., 2006; Bell et al., 2013); the hyperpolarizing responses are attributable to activation of M4 receptors, which activate inwardly rectifying K^+ channels (Bell et al., 2013).

Both CCK+ and PV+ BCs are depolarized by mAChR activation, but some CCK+ Schaffer collateral-associated (SCA) cells also express M2 and M4 receptors to some extent and show biphasic responses when a cholinergic agonist is applied (Cea-del Rio et al., 2010, 2011). CCK+ BCs and SCA cells have strong expression of both M1 and M3 mAChRs, while PV+ BCs and axo-axonic cells express only M1 receptors in their somato-dendritic regions (Cea-del Rio et al., 2010, 2011). Therefore, CCK+ cells are more sensitive to ACh stimulation. More importantly, M3 receptor activation controls the mAChR-mediated increase in firing frequency, and both M1 and M3 mAChR activation is required for the full conversion of the spike AHP into a spike afterdepolarization. mAChR activation increases action potential duration and frequency and reduces spike adaptation in CCK+ cells, as in O-LM cells (Lawrence et al., 2006a), but not in PV+ cells (Cea-del Rio et al., 2010). On the other hand, the outputs of both types of interneurons are also modulated by mAChRs. PV+ cells express M2 receptors on their presynaptic axon terminals; activation of these receptors directly inhibits Ca^{2+} channels and suppresses GABA release (Hájos et al., 1998; Fukudome et al., 2004). ACh and muscarinic agonists also inhibit GABA release from CCK+ cells, but rather than directly activating presynaptic mAChRs, postsynaptic mAChRs on PCs reduce GABA release via an indirect retrograde signaling mechanism, as discussed in the section on eCBs and mAChRs, below.

The O-LM cells express both M1 and M3 receptors (Lawrence et al., 2006a) and generate large depolarizing responses upon mAChR activation (Kawaguchi, 1997; Widmer et al., 2006). Besides direct depolarization by inhibition of M-current, M1 or M3 activation also greatly accelerates action potential firing rate and generates a prominent suprathreshold afterdepolarization in these cells (Lawrence et al., 2006a,b).

ACh GENERATION AND MODULATION OF OSCILLATIONS

IN VIVO OSCILLATIONS IN HIPPOCAMPUS AND NEOCORTEX

Rhythmic fluctuations in cell membrane potentials produce field potential oscillations. Depending on how many cells are synchronously involved, the oscillations can coordinate neuronal activity both locally and across brain regions and are considered to be essential for various cognitive functions. The two most prominent oscillations in the hippocampus are in the θ and γ ranges, which are often concatenated such that γ activity is observed "riding" on a θ carrier wave. ACh can have either a causal or modulatory role in these oscillations, most notably in the θ band, and the mechanisms by which ACh influences them are controversial. It is generally agreed that mAChRs play a more prominent role than nAChRs in rhythm generation.

θ-frequency firing is a basic operational mode of the hippocampus, and is proposed to underlie the formation of episodic memories and spatial maps of the environment (Buzsáki, 2005). θ can be detected in all layers of the CA1 hippocampus, although its amplitude and phase change with depth, with a current source located in s. pyramidale and a current sink near the border of s. radiatum and s.l.m. θ rhythms can modulate plasticity, particularly at the CA3-CA1 Schaffer collateral pathway. For instance, LTP is optimally induced if a train of electrical stimuli coincides with the peak of the θ rhythm, and stimulation given at θ frequency ("theta burst") is optimal for the induction of LTP in CA1 neurons (Larson and Lynch, 1986).

Output from the MS/DBB is necessary for generating hippocampal θ-frequency rhythms *in vivo*, and lesioning the septum abolishes these rhythms and decreases the rate of learning by rats on a spatial maze task (Winson, 1978). However, the mechanisms of θ generation are not homogeneous, and differ depending on the behavior or state of an animal. "Type 1" θ occurs during active, exploratory behavior and is relatively insensitive to the mAChR antagonist atropine. This does not mean, however, that ACh has no role in Type I θ or associated behaviors. The mAChR antagonist, scopolamine, reduces the positive correlation between hippocampal θ and maze-running speed, and also diminishes the normally sharp spatial tuning of "grid" cells in the entorhinal cortex that provide a coordinate system for spatial navigation and memory formation (Newman et al., 2014). It is not known if scopalamine's effects can be attributed to disruptions of the network oscillations, although this seems likely. In contrast to Type I θ, "Type II" θ occurs under urethane anesthesia and during REM sleep, and is abolished by atropine or selective immunolesioning of the septal cholinergic neurons (Stewart and Fox, 1989). Type II is often referred to as "atropine sensitive" θ. Injection of CCh, physostigmine, or muscarine into the hippocampus of an awake cat elicits θ rhythms in the EEG that can also be blocked by atropine, but not by the broad spectrum nAChR antagonist, mecamylamine (Konopacki and Goebiewski, 1992), again suggesting that nicotinic signaling does not play a major role in ACh associated rhythms. The causal role of ACh in Type II θ is not without controversy; ACh release appears to lag behind Type II θ onset during urethane anesthesia (Zhang et al., 2010). MS/DBB cholinergic neurons fire in a manner that is phase-locked to the hippocampal θ rhythm *in vivo* (Brazhnik and Fox, 1997), although given the slow kinetics of mAChR activation and the bulk or volume transmission that probably characterizes most ACh release, the cholinergic cells are unlikely to be true pacemakers for θ rhythms.

Higher frequency γ oscillations in the hippocampus may act in concert with θ oscillations to encode and retrieve memory traces (Bragin et al., 1995; Csicsvari et al., 2003). γ and θ can occur concurrently, particularly in deeper hippocampal layers, and γ is strongest during periods of θ (Bragin et al., 1995; Buzsáki, 2005). A cross-frequency correlation (CFC) analysis showed that the degree of θ–γ coupling in CA3 *in vivo* increased during a context learning task in rats, and the strength of the coupling was directly correlated with the increase in performance accuracy (Tort et al., 2009). Their interaction provides a mechanism for the temporal ordering of individual episodic events (θ) and the reconstruction of different facets of a memory (γ). The latter, the so-called "binding phenomenon", occurs when disparate cortical areas encoding different facets of a memory, such as the shape, color, and texture of an object, must be activated simultaneously in order to form a coherent representation of the object (Singer and Gray, 1995). However, the hypothesis that neural synchrony through coherent γ oscillation solves the binding problem is controversial. γ rhythms have also been proposed to provide the exact temporal framework for spike-timing-dependent plasticity to occur, as θ oscillations would be too slow for the rapid and precise coordination required (Axmacher et al., 2006).

GABA inhibition is widely agreed to be a major factor in the generation of γ (Whittington and Traub, 2003; Whittington et al., 2011). Nevertheless, the details of the connection between endogenous ACh in hippocampus are less clear for γ than for θ rhythms. Atropine reduces hippocampal γ power in awake, behaving animals (Leung, 1985; Hentschke et al., 2007), and reduces θ–γ coupling (Hentschke et al., 2007). *In vivo*, however, hippocampal γ is abolished by lesioning the entorhinal cortex (Buzsáki, 2002, 2005), suggesting a requirement for glutamatergic, but not cholinergic, inputs in the generation of γ. After this ablation a somewhat slower γ appears in CA3 and CA1, suggesting that, under some conditions, the hippocampus can generate a form of γ without the extrinsic glutamatergic inputs from the entorhinal cortex. One hypothesis is that ACh could trigger the intrinsic γ oscillations: γ can be pharmacologically-induced by CCh in hippocampal slices (Fisahn et al., 1998; Traub et al., 2003). Muscarine-induced γ rhythm in the CA3 region *in vitro* depends on the activation of M1 mAChRs in PCs, and is absent in M1 mAChR$^{-/-}$ mice. This M1-dependent γ is produced by modulation of the mixed-cation Na^+/K^+ current and the Ca^{2+}-dependent non-selective cation current, but does not involve modulation of the M-current (Fisahn et al., 2002).

Although ACh-induced oscillations are prominent in the hippocampus, other brain regions can generate them locally as well, especially the neocortex. Stimulus-evoked γ activity in visual cortex is blocked by intracortical infusion of atropine (Rodriguez et al., 2004), for example. Unlike the MS/DBB cholinergic projection, which drives primarily the lower frequency θ oscillations in the hippocampus, the NBM is believed to underlie cortical "activation", or a decrease in lower frequency synchronized EEG activity accompanied by an increase in local γ frequency. Such a mechanism may underlie, among other things, selective attention (review by Wang, 2010). The discharge rate of NBM cholinergic neurons is much higher during cortical activation, ACh release in the cortex is higher, and lesions of NBM decrease both cortical ACh release and cortical activation (Dringenberg and Vanderwolf, 1998). Despite a lack of direct projections to the hippocampus, activity in the NBM does affect hippocampal activity, and lesions of the NBM can modulate event-related oscillations in the delta (δ, 0.1–3 Hz), θ, β (15–29 Hz), and γ frequency ranges in dorsal hippocampus, as well as in the amygdala and pre-frontal cortex (PFC). Cholinergic neurons in the MS/DBB and NBM could modulate oscillations between and within brain regions, respectively—excitotoxic lesions of MS/DBB decrease γ frequency event-related oscillations in frontal cortex, and reduce phase locking between frontal cortex and hippocampus in the θ band (Sanchez-Alavez et al., 2014). Similar lesions of NBM cause increases in frontal cortex δ and θ, decreases in γ, and reductions in phase-locking between frontal cortex and hippocampus in the γ band. The NBM mediates increases in cortical δ activity during stress in the PFC (a direct target) and retrosplenial cortex (an indirect target; Knox and Berntson, 2008).

IN VITRO MODELS OF ACh-GENERATED OSCILLATIONS IN HIPPOCAMPUS AND NEOCORTEX

Whether ACh plays a causal or modulatory role in rhythm generation *in vivo* is controversial. *In vitro*, cholinergic agonists or released ACh generate rhythmic cell firing, synaptic currents, and local field potentials (LFPs). These effects have been reported most frequently in hippocampal slices, but also occur in neocortical slices. Thus, the brain slice preparation has been an invaluable tool for studying the mechanisms by which ACh can generate oscillations at multiple levels, especially when considering the "inverse problem" of the LFP (Buzsáki et al.,

2012), i.e., the task of inferring microscopic variables (e.g., synaptic or cellular components) from macroscopic data (e.g., a current source density analysis). Solving the "forward problem" i.e., identifying the synaptic or non-synaptic events generating the LFP by correlating them with the LFP, may be a prerequisite for solving the inverse problem.

Application of CCh to hippocampal slices induces θ frequency membrane potential oscillations and firing in a majority of cells in CA1, CA3, and DG (Bland et al., 1988). The mixed ACh agonist CCh induces oscillations in the LFP (Hájos et al., 2004), membrane potentials or firing patterns (Williams and Kauer, 1997), and rhythmic inhibitory post-synaptic responses in CA1 PCs (Reich et al., 2005). It has been proposed that ACh-generated rhythms are initiated in CA3 and transmitted into CA1 via the Schaffer collaterals (Williams and Kauer, 1997; Fisahn et al., 1998; Buzsáki, 2002), although using a novel slicing procedure, Pietersen et al. (2014) report evidence for intrinsic γ generation in CA1. *In vivo* Type II (atropine sensitive) θ might additionally require rhythmic inhibition onto interneurons from septal GABAergic afferents (Stewart and Fox, 1990; Tóth et al., 1997; Buzsáki, 2002). These models cannot explain all of the data however, since θ-frequency rhythmic sIPSP/Cs in CA1 PCs can be induced by CCh application to slices in the presence of iGluR antagonists (**Figure 2C**; Reich et al., 2005; Karson et al., 2008) or in small isolated sections of CA1 (Reich et al., 2005).

Rhythmic inhibition is thought to be essential for the generation of hippocampal oscillations, including ACh-mediated oscillations (Stewart and Fox, 1990; Buzsáki, 2002; Mann and Paulsen, 2007; Klausberger and Somogyi, 2008). Electrical stimulation of cholinergic afferents in hippocampal slices increases the frequency of spontaneous IPSPs in CA1 PCs (Pitler and Alger, 1992b). Stimulation of single hippocampal BCs at θ frequency produces unitary IPSPs in synaptically connected PCs that are sufficient to entrain the PC firing (Cobb et al., 1995). As noted earlier, most interneuron types in CA1 are modulated by ACh (McQuiston and Madison, 1999a,b; Widmer et al., 2006). Hippocampal interneurons are very heterogeneous, and different interneuron classes will fire in a distinct pattern (or not at all) within a given type of oscillation (Klausberger et al., 2003).

The two populations of perisomatic-targeting interneurons, PV+ and CCK+ BCs, are activated by ACh (Karson et al., 2009; Cea-del Rio et al., 2010), and have been functionally implicated in fast and slow oscillations, respectively, generated by cholinergic agonists (Reich et al., 2005; Gulyás et al., 2010). Fast, iGluR-mediated excitatory stimulation of PV+ cells produces IPSPs that contribute to atropine-insensitive, but not atropine-sensitive θ rhythms (Korotkova et al., 2010). Exogenous muscarinic agonists or endogenous ACh activate PV+ cells (Cea-del Rio et al., 2010). At the same time, M2 mAChR activation suppresses GABA release from PV+ terminals, but does not entirely eliminate it (Hájos et al., 1998; Gulyás et al., 2010). Application of CCh, or release of endogenous ACh, generates θ frequency IPSP/Cs in CA1 PCs which can be disrupted by exogenous or endogenous cannabinoids, suggesting that ACh generates θ in CA1 by activating CCK+ BCs (discussed below, and cf Cea-del Rio et al., 2012). In addition to the perisomatic-targeting interneurons, the dendritic targeting O-LM cells exhibit rhythmic membrane potential oscillations in response to CCh application, even in the absence of fast glutamatergic signaling (Chapman and Lacaille, 1999; Lawrence, 2008).

In CA3, CCh application generates γ-frequency oscillations (Hájos et al., 2004; Oren et al., 2006, 2010). The γ LFPs are greatly suppressed by a μOR agonist (μORs are predominantly located on PV+ terminals, where their activation suppresses GABA release), and PV+ BCs show the highest degree of phase modulation by the LFP (Gulyás et al., 2010). *In vitro*, morphine also suppresses CA3 γ rhythms that arise from tetanic stimulation of the s. oriens, and this effect is blocked by the μOR antagonist cyprodime (Whittington et al., 1998). Thus, it would appear that in CA3, unlike in CA1, ACh generates oscillations by selectively activating the PV+ network.

Whereas θ and γ are the two prominent ACh-generated oscillations in hippocampus, several different frequency ranges have been observed in neocortical slices. Unlike hippocampal slices, where atropine-sensitive θ or γ oscillations can be reliably elicited by CCh alone, oscillations in neocortical slices are frequently generated by applying kainate, or GABA-A receptor antagonists along with CCh. For example, CCh application generates β oscillations in rat PFC (van Aerde et al., 2009). The combination of CCh plus kainate also elicits β oscillations in primary motor cortical slices that are unaffected by AMPA blockers but prevented by GABA-A or a gap junction blocker (carbenoxolone) (Yamawaki et al., 2008). CCh generates β activity in an intact preparation of newborn rat neocortex that is dependent on mAChRs and AMPA/kainate receptors, but not GABA-A receptors (Kilb and Luhmann, 2003). CCh plus kainate elicits γ in somatosensory and visual cortex slices (Oke et al., 2010). Both CCh and bicuculline application are required to generate oscillations in neonatal rat cortical slices (Lukatch and MacIver, 1997). CCh and bicuculline also generate 3–22 Hz LFP activity in slices of occipital lobe, including "spiral" waves (Huang and Hsu, 2010). Thus, the differences in frequency ranges and pharmacology of ACh generated oscillations in neocortical slices might reflect the different circuitry activated by ACh in various cortical regions.

eCBs AND mAChRs

Depolarization-induced suppression of inhibition (DSI) is profound, reversible disinhibition of principal cells that was initially described in the hippocampus as a transient suppression of sIPSPs or sIPSCs that followed a brief, 1 or 2 s, depolarizing current injection into a CA1 PC (Pitler and Alger, 1992a). A great deal of evidence showed that DSI was mediated by a retrograde signal process, i.e., as a result of Ca^{2+} entry into a PC, a chemical messenger was released and traveled backwards across the synaptic cleft, and by activating an initially unidentified G-protein coupled receptor on certain GABAergic nerve terminals, temporarily prevented GABA release (Alger, 2002, for review). CCh markedly increased IPSP frequency by activating mAChRs on hippocampal interneurons (Pitler and Alger, 1992b) and in addition enhanced and prolonged DSI (Pitler and Alger, 1992a). nAChRs were found to have no role in enhancing DSI (Martin and Alger, 1999): nicotine did not mimic the effects of CCh and a broad spectrum nAChR-antagonist, mecamylamine, did not antagonize them. In contrast, the CCh-effects on DSI were abolished by

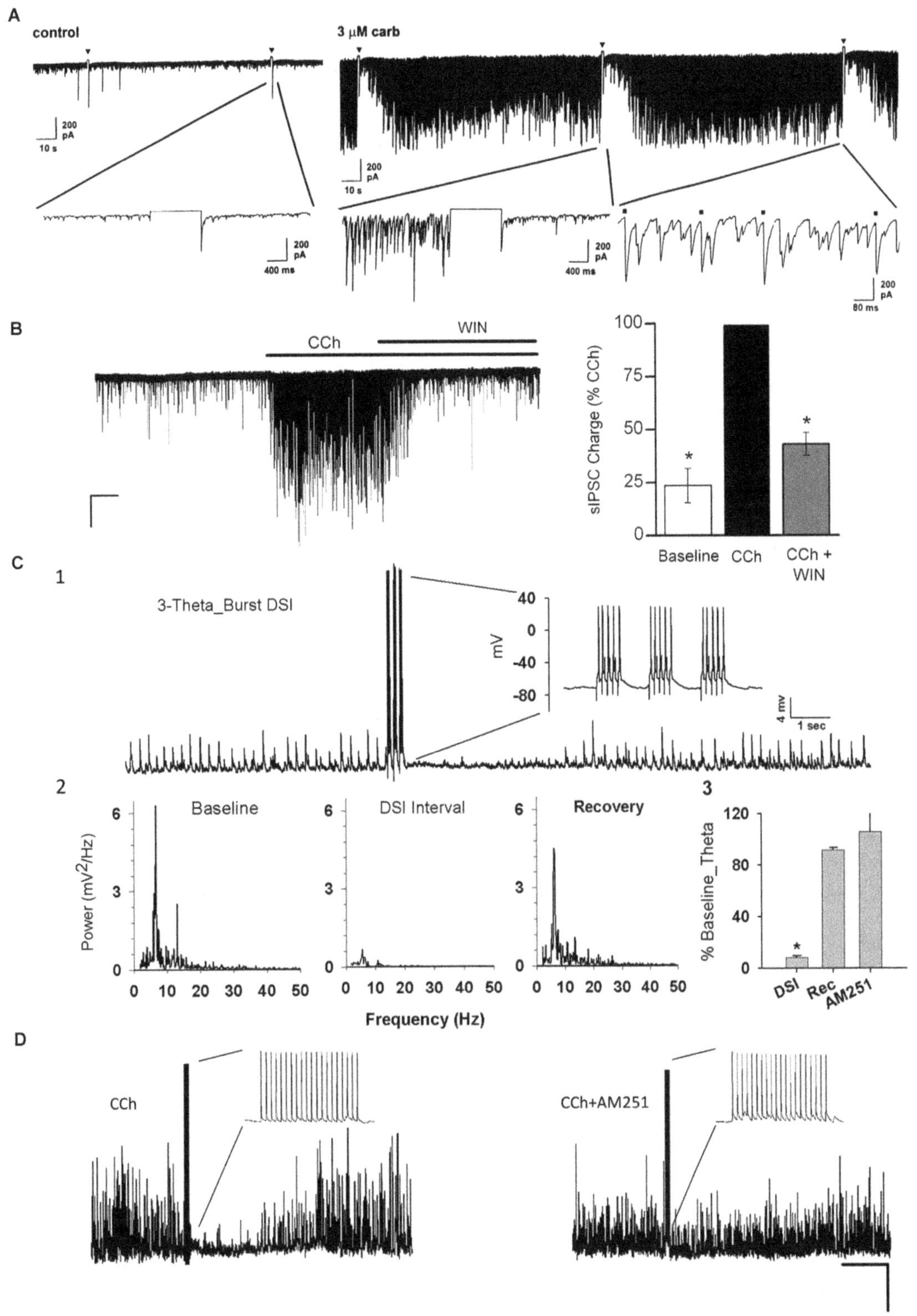

FIGURE 2 | Carbachol (CCh) elicits persistent occurrence of large, rhythmic inhibitory synaptic responses in hippocampus and neocortex. **(A)** Representative whole-cell recording from a Sprague/Dawley rat CA1 pyramidal cell (PC) in control saline (iGluR antagonists present in experiments shown in all panels) *in vitro* and a 1-s depolarizing voltage-step (downward triangles) has no effect on the small spontaneous IPSCs visible on the baseline. Bath application of 3 μM CCh induces a persistent barrage of large IPSCs that are transiently interrupted by the periods of DSI that occur after the voltage steps (From Martin and Alger, 1999; with permission). **(B)** Representative trace from a layer II/III neocortical PC from a Swiss CD-1 mouse slice. A large barrage of IPSCs occurs after CCh (5 μM) is added to the bath, and the IPSCs are suppressed by further addition of the CB1R agonist WIN55212-2 (5 μM). From Trettel et al. (2004) with permission.

(*Continued*)

FIGURE 2 | Continued
(C1) Representative sharp electrode recording of large, rhythmic IPSPs induced by 5 μM CCh in a rat CA1 PC in a hippocampal slice. Brief bursts of action potentials induced by depolarizing current injections induced a period of DSI. **(C2)** Power spectral analyses of the IPSPs before, during and after DSI. Note peak power in the theta frequency range. **(C3)** Group data showing "relative theta power" (integral of power from 4–14 Hz/total power from 2–50 Hz) from experiments as in **C1**, **C2**. DSI strongly suppressed the theta power (which recovered fully following DSI). DSI was abolished by the CB1R antagonist, AM251 (3 μM). From Reich et al. (2005) with permission. **(D)** DSI of 5 μM, CCh-induced IPSPs produced by an action potential train in a layer II/III PC in a mouse neocortical slice. DSI was abolished by 5 μM AM251. From Trettel et al. (2004) with permission.

atropine and other mAChR antagonists, and were mimicked by selective mAChR agonists, such as Oxo-M. A battery of mAChR antagonists, including pirenzepine, 4-DAMP, and AFDX-116, led to the conclusion that either the M1 or M3, but not the M2 receptor, were responsible for inducing persistent action potential firing of the interneurons that were most highly sensitive to DSI (Martin and Alger, 1999; cf Trettel et al., 2004), i.e., the firing of these interneurons produced GABAergic IPSCs that were readily suppressed by DSI (**Figure 2**). The results explained the great sensitivity of CCh-induced sIPSCs to DSI, but provided no insight into the actual mechanism of DSI itself.

In 2001 the retrograde messenger for DSI was reported to be an eCB, and the GPCR-coupled receptor on the interneuron terminals was the cannabinoid receptor, CB1R (Ohno-Shosaku et al., 2001; Wilson and Nicoll, 2001). There are two major eCBs, anandamide and 2-arachidonyl glycerol (2-AG), and 2-AG was demonstrated to be the main signaling eCB (see Kano et al., 2009 for review and **Figure 1** DSI). It was soon found that a mGluR agonist, (±)-1-aminocyclopentane-trans-1,3-dicarboxylic acid (ACPD) or the selective group I mGluR agonist, (S)-3,5-dihydroxyphenylglycine (DHPG), markedly increased DSI (Varma et al., 2001). At low concentrations, DHPG enhanced DSI without affecting the IPSCs directly, while at higher concentrations DHPG directly suppressed the IPSCs as well. Most significantly, the three phenomena, DSI, the enhancement of DSI by mGluRs, and the direct suppression of IPSCs by high concentrations of an mGluR agonist were all abolished by a CB1R antagonist, and absent in the $CB1R^{-/-}$ mouse. The explanation was that mGluRs on PCs either enhanced the mobilization of eCBs by DSI, or directly caused eCB mobilization from these cells, and the eCBs crossed the synaptic cleft and inhibited the IPSCs by activating the CB1Rs on the interneuron terminals (**Figure 1**; "mobilized" is the preferred term because the processes of eCB synthesis and release cannot be distinguished electrophysiologically and are not inextricably linked, see Alger and Kim, 2011, for review). eCBs are also retrograde signals at excitatory synapses (Kreitzer and Regher, 2001) and mGluRs mobilize eCBs there as well (Maejima et al., 2001). Thus eCBs are not only produced by high levels of Ca^{2+} in principal cells, but are intermediaries in modulating synaptic transmitter release by glutamate, and hence were likely to have a broad range of actions.

Both group I mGluRs and M1-class mAChRs are GPCRs that are coupled to $G_{q/11}$ type G-proteins. Kim et al. (2002) found that activating mAChRs with low μM concentrations of CCh markedly enhanced DSI without affecting the IPSCs directly, but at higher concentrations directly suppressed them. For concentrations up to ~5 μM CCh, the suppressive effects on the IPSCs were entirely reversed by a CB1R antagonist, demonstrating that, like the type I mGluRs, mAChRs could mobilize eCBs. Above 5 μM, a portion of the CCh-induced IPSC suppression could not be prevented by CB1R antagonists, suggesting that a distinct, eCB-independent form of synaptic depression also occurred. Significantly, bath-application of the AChE inhibitor, physostigmine, in the absence of other treatments, induced an atropine- and CB1R-dependent suppression of IPSCs, indicating that the low, tonic levels of ACh present in hippocampal slices were sufficient to induce persistent mobilization of eCBs (Kim et al., 2002). In accordance with this suggestion, Colgin et al. (2003) found that an AChE inhibitor depressed fEPSPs in the dentate gyrus and CA1 of hippocampal slices. This effect was absent when, prior to the *in vitro* experiments, the fimbria/fornix was lesioned and allowed to deteriorate. Most importantly, the effect was abolished by atropine and a CB1R antagonist, but unaffected by an M2 mAChR inhibitor, clearly arguing that ACh from cholinergic afferents could suppress glutamate transmission heterosynaptically via mAChR-induced, eCB release. Presumably *in vivo* release of ACh can have the same ability to regulate synaptic transmission indirectly by stimulating the release of eCBs. It is important to note that, in addition to glutamate and GABA, eCBs may also directly regulate the release of ACh itself (Gifford and Ashby, 1996; Kathmann et al., 2001; Tzavara et al., 2003; Degroot et al., 2006), although detailed physiological mechanisms of these effects have yet to be worked out.

Neither the mAChR-dependent increase of DSI, nor the direct mobilization of eCBs by mAChR activation was associated with any change in $[Ca^{2+}]_i$ (Kim et al., 2002), suggesting that the GPCR-dependent pathway of eCB mobilization and the Ca^{2+}-dependent pathways were independent. Indeed, the ability of mAChRs to mobilize eCBs was occluded when $GTP_{\gamma}S$, a generalized activator of G-proteins, was infused into the cells, but unaffected when intracellular Ca^{2+} was chelated by high concentrations of intracellular BAPTA (Kim et al., 2002). Hence, mAChR-dependent eCB mobilization is independent of changes in $[Ca^{2+}]_i$ but entirely dependent on G-protein activation, whereas, conversely, DSI is totally dependent on a rise in $[Ca^{2+}]_i$ and unaffected by $GTP_{\gamma}S$. Thus the two pathways for eCB mobilization are independent, but, importantly, can interact, as shown by the enhancement of DSI (Ca^{2+}-dependent pathway) by co-activation of a GPCR pathway (Varma et al., 2001; Kim et al., 2002).

The findings on mAChRs and eCBs were confirmed and extended in paired recordings from principal cells and interneurons in tissue-cultured primary hippocampal neurons (Ohno-Shosaku et al., 2003). Ohno-Shosaku et al. (2003) observed no real change in the ability of CCh (or Oxo-M) to mobilize eCBs in tissue cultured cells from knock out mice with either $M1^{-/-}$ or $M3^{-/-}$ mAChRs eliminated, but a virtual elimination of the eCB-related effects in the combined $M1^{-/-}/M3^{-/-}$ line. This demonstrated involvement of both M1 and M3 mAChRs, and suggested that activation of either receptor alone could produce enough eCBs for maximal suppression of IPSCs. In the dorsal striatum, tonic activity of the cholinergic interneurons leads to a persistent enhancement of DSI in the medium spiny neurons, which is blocked by the M1 antagonist, pirenzepine, and is absent in the $M1^{-/-}$ mouse, and hence is also mediated via M1 mAChRs (Narushima et al., 2007).

Although these issues have not been dissected as thoroughly in the neocortex as in the hippocampus, the apparently identical observations of IPSC frequency enhancement by CCh and eCB-dependent DSI in neocortical slices (**Figure 2**; cf. Fortin et al., 2004; Trettel et al., 2004; Yoshino et al., 2011) makes it likely that the association between M1/M3 receptors and eCBs holds there as well. Fukudome et al. (2004) showed, also in paired principal cell-interneuron recordings in hippocampal tissue-culture, that the *eCB-independent*, CCh-induced suppression of GABA release was mediated by M2 receptors, as it was mimicked by the M2 preferring agonist, gallamine, and absent in tissue from the $M2^{-/-}$ mouse. Importantly, the M2-mediated suppression occurred in those interneurons that were not sensitive to suppression by eCBs, and vice versa, interneurons from which GABA release was suppressed by eCBs were insensitive to suppression by gallamine. It is therefore likely that the interneurons from which GABA release is inhibited indirectly by M1/M3 (i.e., eCB-sensitive) actions and those inhibited by M2 mAChRs are of different classes. Undoubtedly, the former represented the CCK+/CB1R+ interneurons and the latter the CCK−/CB1R− interneurons, probably the PV+ cells, although the cells were not immunologically identified. The results from slices (Martin and Alger, 1999; Kim et al., 2002) and tissue-culture (Ohno-Shosaku et al., 2003; Fukudome et al., 2004) are in substantial agreement in identifying the M1/M3 receptors as the likely stimulants of the eCB mobilization, while M2 receptors mediate an eCB-independent form of presynaptic inhibition.

Studies with tissue from phospholipase C beta (PLC_β) isoform-specific, knock-out mice, $PLC_{\beta 1}^{-/-}$ and $PLC_{\beta 4}^{-/-}$ showed that PLC_β is an essential element in the G-protein signaling pathway between mAChRs, or mGluRs, and eCBs in hippocampus and cerebellum, with the different isoforms being predominant in different brain structures (Hashimotodani et al., 2005; Maejima et al., 2005); in the absence of PLC_β neither of these GPCRs can mobilize eCBs. Another key observation was that DSI is independent of PLC_β (Hashimotodani et al., 2005), which confirms that the Ca^{2+} -dependent and GPCR-dependent forms of eCB mobilization utilize distinct biochemical pathways, although 2-AG is the eCB produced by both of them. PLC_β is activated by M1/M3 mAChRs and requires Ca^{2+} for its enzymatic activity, hence it is proposed that PLC_β acts as a coincidence-detector (Hashimotodani et al., 2005) that can integrate the actions of Ca^{2+} and G-proteins and thereby explain the ability of mAChRs to enhance DSI. Some challenges to this straightforward story exist (Edwards et al., 2006, 2008) and future work should provide more mechanistic detail. Nevertheless, PLC is a part of the molecular cascade that produces 2-AG, though not anandamide, and so the involvement of PLC also confirmed that 2-AG was the major eCB produced by mAChRs. 2-AG is produced by the enzyme diacylglycerol lipase alpha (DGL_α) and the absence of this enzyme in $DGL_\alpha^{-/-}$ mice prevents the mAChRs from mobilizing eCBs (Tanimura et al., 2010; Yoshino et al., 2011). DSI is also absent in $DGL\alpha^{-/-}$ mice (Gao et al., 2010; Tanimura et al., 2010; Yoshino et al., 2011), unlike the case with $PLC_\beta{}^{-/-}$ mice in which DSI is unaffected. Evidently, if diacylglycerol is the common precursor for the production of 2-AG, two independent pathways supply diacylglycerol to DGL_α for the production of 2-AG.

The summary picture is that M1 and M3 mAChRs mobilize the eCB 2-AG via a molecular pathway involving PLC_β and DGL_α.

OPTOGENETIC STUDIES

Release of endogenous ACh via bulk tissue electrical stimulation activates interneurons in hippocampus (Pitler and Alger, 1992b; Widmer et al., 2006), and drives inhibitory oscillations in CA1 PCs (Martin and Alger, 1999). However, bulk stimulation of tissue can also affect non-cholinergic fibers and glia, and complete pharmacological isolation of ACh responses is often not possible. The advent of optogenetics has allowed for stimulation or silencing of specific neuron populations in slice preparations as well as *in vivo*, and the cholinergic system was one of the first targeted for optogenetic manipulation (see Fenno et al., 2011, for review). Expression of the light-activated non-selective cation channel, Channelrhodopsin2 (ChR2, Boyden et al., 2005), in cholinergic neurons allows for specific stimulation of cholinergic cells or fibers and release of endogenous ACh in slice preparations. ChR2 is commonly delivered *in vivo* to target nuclei via an adeno-associated virus (AAV) vector, which has a high tropism for neural tissue and can result in expression levels exceeding 90% in target cells (**Figure 3**). To ensure specificity of ChR2 expression in cholinergic cells, the cre-loxP system has been utilized: the vector constructs carry a double-floxed inverted (FLEXED) ChR2 sequence (Atasoy et al., 2008), and the vectors are injected into the brains of ChAT-Cre mice, which express cre recombinase only in cholinergic cells. Injection of AAV-ChR2 into cholinergic nuclei results in expression of ChR2 in distal axon terminals of projection neurons in ~2–5 weeks (**Figure 3A**; cf Gu and Yakel, 2011; Nagode et al., 2011, 2014; Tang et al., 2011; Kalmbach et al., 2012; Kalmbach and Waters, 2014), allowing for stimulation of ACh release in slice preparations which do not retain the cholinergic cell bodies (e.g., the hippocampus). The variability in expression time may have to do with differences in viral serotype used (AAV2/1—2/9 have all been used), viral titer (typically higher than 10^{12} genome copies/ml), or ChR2 variant. In general the AAVs appear to have equal tropism for all cells, although selective transformation of inhibitory cells in the cortex was reported with low titer levels (e.g., Nathanson et al., 2009) and specific tropism for cholinergic neurons has apparently not been reported. AAV2/1, 2/5, and 2/9 have all been used successfully with the cre/lox strategy in the Chat-Cre mice. The ChR2-variant, ChIEF, which has faster kinetics, hence greater suitability for high frequency stimulation, and increased steady-state photocurrent, than does the more commonly used H134R ChR2, has also been targeted to septal cholinergic cells and used to stimulate ACh release in hippocampal slices (Bell et al., 2011, 2013). ChIEF appears to show superior expression and transport to plasma membranes when compared to H134R ChR2 (Mattis et al., 2011),

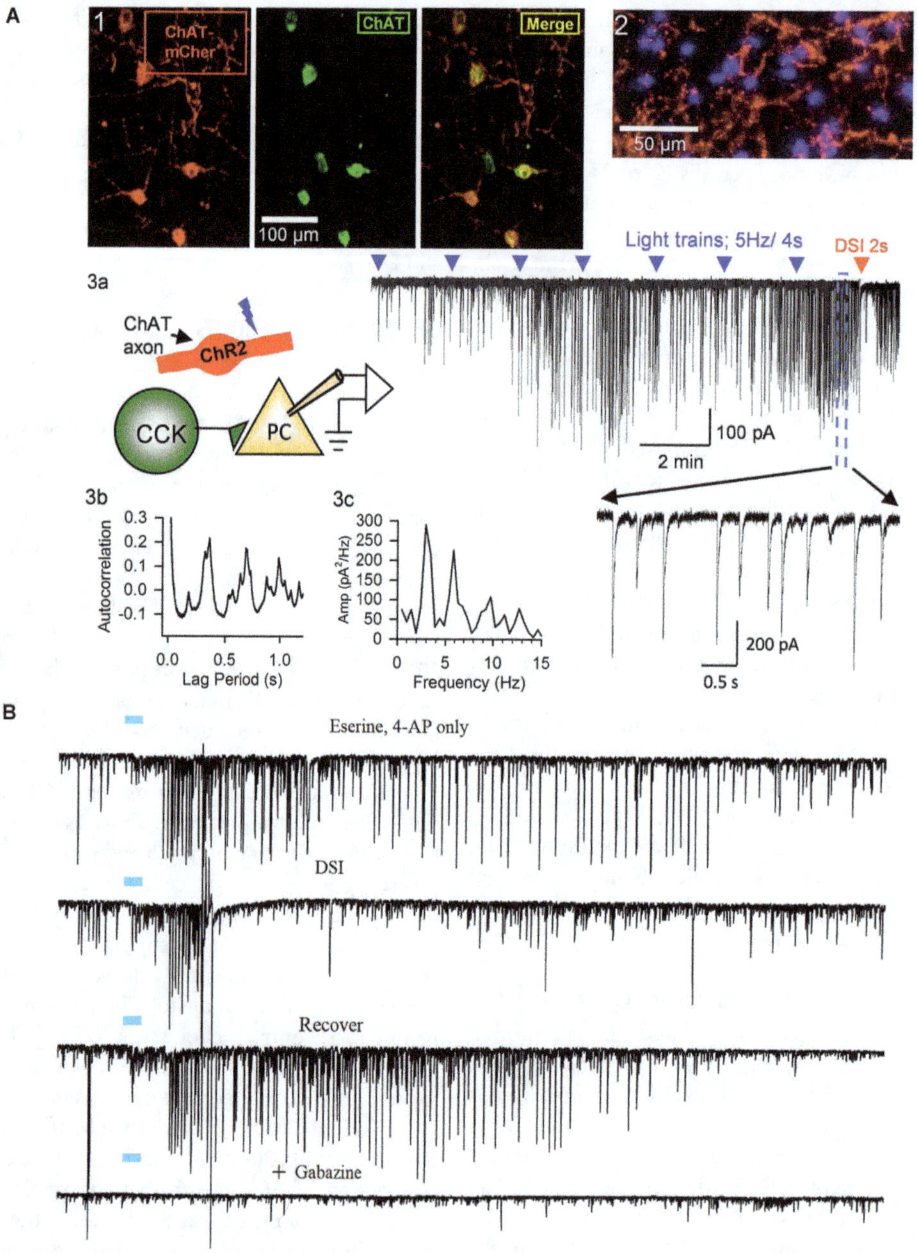

FIGURE 3 | Release of ACh by light-stimulation of ChR2 in ChAT-expressing axons induces bursts of rhythmic IPSCs in the CA1 region of hippocampal slices. (A1) Examples of ChAT-positive cells in MS/DBB expressing ChR2+mCherry following viral injection of AAV (see text) into a ChAT-Cre mouse (from Nagode et al., 2011, with permission), and **(A2)** ChR2+mCherry axons plus DAPi staining showing cholinergic axons in proximity to cells in CA1. Details of procedures are found in Nagode et al. (2011). **(A3)** Diagram of experimental setup; light-stimulation of ChR2-expressing axons in CA1 release ACh onto CCK+ interneurons that fire trains of action potentials and thereby induce IPSPs in CA1 PCs. Sample trace to the right shows trains of blue-light pulses (blue triangles) given at 2 min intervals gradually come to induce prolonged bursts of GABAergic IPSCs (downward deflections in the presence of iGluR blockers to prevent EPSC occurrence in experiments shown in this panel; cf. expanded portion, below) in a PC. A 2-s voltage step was given to the PC near the end of the trace (red arrow) to induce DSI, the transient interruption of the IPSCs. **(A3b,c)** Autocorrelation function and power spectrum of data from this cell illustrate the rhythmic nature of the ACh-induced IPSCs. Neither physostigmine nor 4-AP were used in this experiment. **(B)** Top trace, light pulse (blue bar) delivered to ChR2-expressing axons in a slice from a ChAT-Cre, AAV-injected mouse induced a burst of large IPSCs in a CA1 PC; second trace, the burst of IPSCs was interrupted during the period of DSI produced by a brief depolarization of the PC; third trace, recovery of the IPSC burst after the DSI trial; fourth trace, application of the GABA-A receptor antagonist, gabazine, blocks all light-induced activity, confirming their identity as IPSCs. Physostigmine, 1 μM, and 4-AP, 20 μM, were present in the bathing solution. Results are typical of numerous experiments. **(A2, B)** from D.A. Nagode Ph.D. thesis at http://archive.hshsl.umaryland.edu/handle/10713/2315. **(A3a–c)** is a typical result (c.f. Nagode et al., 2011).

although whether this translates into advantages of ChIEF over H134R ChR2 for release of ACh from terminals is not yet known.

In addition to the viral strategy, transgenic mouse lines constitutively expressing ChR2 have been developed. The most widely-used strain is the ChAT-ChR2-EYFP mouse (Strain 014546; Jackson Laboratories; e.g., Ren et al., 2011; Pinto et al., 2013). *In vivo* stimulation of basal forebrain ACh neurons, or their axon terminals in visual cortex, has also been achieved using this mouse. Pinto et al. (2013) found that ChR2 activation of basal forebrain cell bodies or axon terminals desynchronized cortical activity and enhanced visual discrimination. On the other hand, crossing Chat-Cre mice with the inhibitory halorhodopsin or archerhodopsin-expressing mice to silence basal forebrain cholinergic neurons synchronized cortical activity and decreased visual discrimination. However, the ChAT-ChR2-EYFP strain exhibits some deficits in attention and working and spatial memory, due to increased copy number and expression of VAChT (Kolisnyk et al., 2013), which should be considered before using them, especially for behavioral studies. Indeed, because efficiency of optogenetic activators or silencers is low, the high protein expression required to affect neuronal activity, especially during brain development, might permanently alter brain circuitry and therefore behavior. The expression of opsins in ChAT-Cre mice also varies across brain regions. The viral transduction method in adults, though more invasive, may be more advantageous than constitutively expressing mouse models in some cases.

It must be noted that in some parts of the nervous system ACh is reportedly co-localized with other neurotransmitters, including glutamate (e.g., Allen et al., 2006; Lamotte d'Incamps and Ascher, 2008) and GABA (Bayraktar et al., 1997, but see Chédotal et al., 1994), and furthermore that they may be co-released with ACh (e.g., Allen et al., 2006; Lamotte d'Incamps and Ascher, 2008; Ren et al., 2011). In principle co-release of glutamate by ChR2-induced depolarization could confound studies of optogenetic ACh release. Although we have seen no evidence for this in our experiments (Nagode et al., 2011, 2014), the possibility should be explored. Therefore, even precise cellular targeting of light-activated molecules to ChAT-expressing cells may not absolutely guarantee that light stimulation will cause the release of only ACh, or conversely, that any light-induced biological effects can unambiguously be attributed to ACh *a priori*. This will probably be true whether the opsins are expressed in the target cells virally or transgenically. Additional pharmacological or perhaps molecular biological controls would have to be taken to identify the active agent. For the use of pharmacological tools, *in vitro* slice preparations will undoubtedly be most effective. Of course, from the point of view of behavioral relevance, *in vivo* preparations will be most desirable. Thus, it seems that combinations of *in vivo* and *in vitro* approaches will be required to achieve definitive conclusions regarding axonally released transmitter actions, even using optogenetic techniques, for the forseeable future.

For the study of ACh effects in slice preparations, particularly oscillations or other network phenomena, generating sufficient ACh release is a significant concern. ChR2 expression in axon terminals is usually weaker than in somata, and axons from the basal nuclei are unavoidably severed by the slicing. If the "bulk transmission" hypothesis is correct (Vizi and Kiss, 1998), large amounts of ACh release might be required to activate receptors on target cells, especially since acetylcholinesterase (AChE) hydrolyzes ACh very efficiently. It is nevertheless possible to stimulate long bursts of DSI-sensitive IPSCs that closely mimic those induced by mAChR agonists (e.g., **Figures 3**, **4**). While these IPSCs can be elicited by light-induced ACh release in slices in normal recording saline (**Figure 3A**), we (Tang et al., 2011; Nagode et al., 2011, 2014) often use physostigmine to inhibit AChE, and a low concentration of the K-channel blocker, 4-AP, to enhance ChR2-induced ACh release (as has been done by others, e.g., Petreanu et al., 2007; Hull et al., 2009). This greatly increases the occurrence of ChR2-induced rhythmic activity without otherwise altering the IPSCs (**Figures 2B** and **3**; cf Nagode et al., 2011). Such pharmacological enhancement is not necessary for evoking post-synaptic ACh currents (Bell et al., 2011, 2013) or nAChR-dependent plasticity of EPSCs in CA1 PCs (Gu and Yakel, 2011), suggesting that less ACh is required to generate single cell firing than sustained network activity.

An important new finding (Nagode et al., 2014) was that light-induced ACh release triggers IPSCs that are sensitive to DSI, and that most of them are also sensitive to μOR agonists even when the output of PV+ cells (which express the great majority of hippocampal μORs) has been abolished (**Figure 4B**). Dual CB1R/μOR sensitivity has been reported (e.g., Neu et al., 2007; Glickfeld et al., 2008) but it was surprising to encounter it so frequently in the optogenetic experiments. The explanation for this observation is not understood, but may imply that axonally released ACh has an unexpectedly strong tendency to activate dually sensitive interneurons, which could be important for understanding cannabinoid/opioid interactions *in vivo*. It will be of great interest to explore the effects of silencing septal cholinergic neurons with halorhodopsin or archerhodopsin *in vivo* during ongoing hippocampal θ oscillations. The unique ability to release ACh from cholinergic axons optogenetically probably made this discovery possible.

While dramatic effects of optogentically released ACh are on the induction of θ rhythm frequency oscillations of IPSPs via activation of mAChRs, a pulse of released ACh also elicits a burst of IPSCs by activating nAChRs and a highly novel mechanism involving T-type Ca^{2+} channel activation and Ca^{2+} stores (Tang et al., 2011). These events occur even in the presence of TTX, strongly suggesting that the nAChRs are on the GABAergic nerve terminals. Moreover, since there are no morphologically defined synapses along these axons, this appears to be a direct example of a non-synaptic effect of axonally released ACh. Non-synaptic stimulation of GABA release can also be produced by optogenetic stimulation of striatal cholinergic interneurons. Interestingly, the same ionic mechanism as proposed in hippocampus (Tang et al., 2011) appears to operate in striatum (Nelson et al., 2014).

mAChRs, eCBs, AND NEURONAL NETWORK OSCILLATIONS IN HIPPOCAMPUS

mAChR-activation induces the firing of CCK+/CB1R+ cells and IPSCs from these cells are a major factor in inhibitory θ rhythms. However, there is extremely good evidence that the M1 and M3 mAChRs are also very effective in stimulating the mobilization

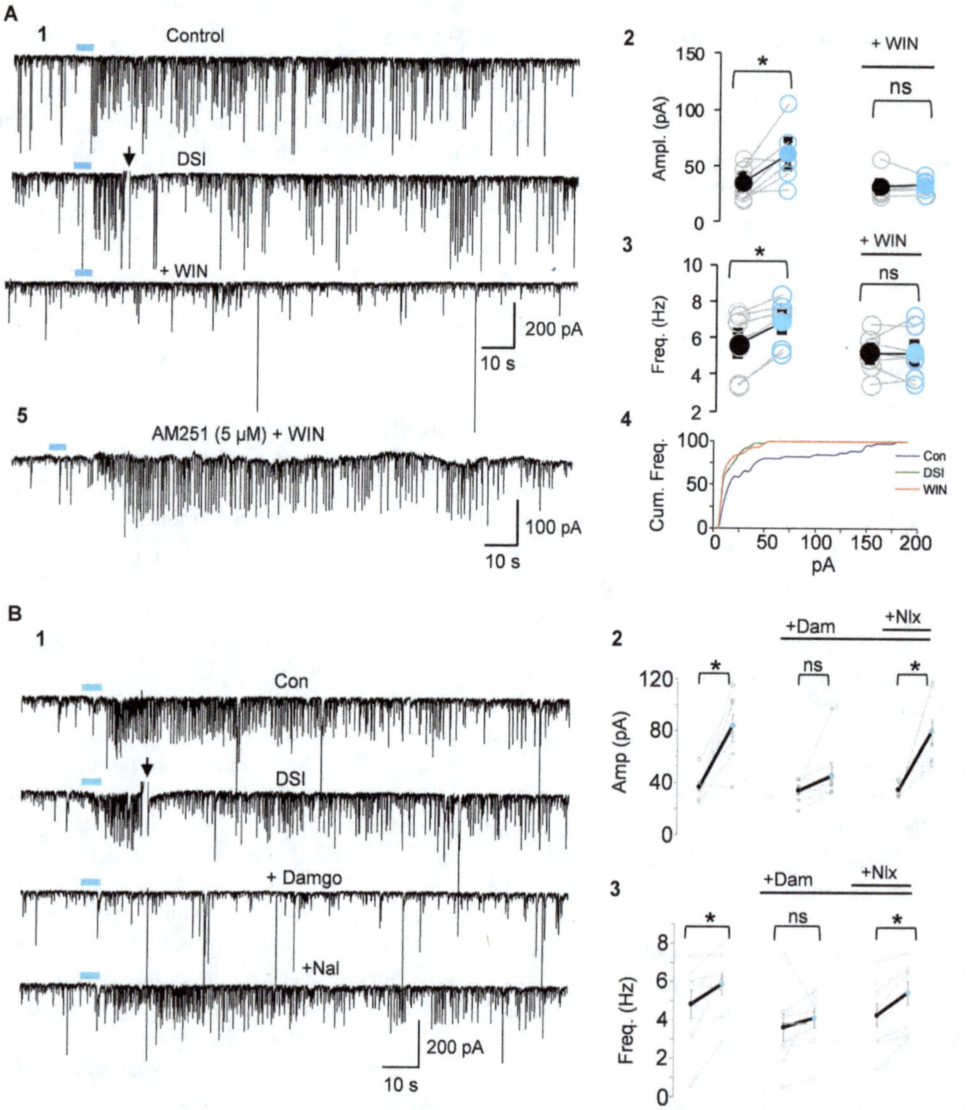

FIGURE 4 | IPSCs triggered by light-induced ACh release arise from CB1R+ interneurons. (A1) Top two traces as in **Panel 3B**, the CB1R agonist, WIN55212-2 (WIN) was then applied to the bathing solution of the same cell, and prevented the ability of ACh to induce repetitive IPSCs. **(A2–A4)** Group data showing that the increases in IPSC amplitudes **(A2)** or frequency **(A3)** or cumulative frequency **(A4)** induced by light in control solution (left graphs in **A2,A3**), were occluded in WIN-treated slices; i.e., that they arose from CB1R+ interneurons. **(A5)** Shows that pretreatment with the CB1R antagonist, AM251, prevented the ability of WIN to suppress the ACh-induced IPSCs. **(B1)** DSI-sensitive IPSCs induced by ACh release can also be reversibly suppressed by the μOR agonist, DAMGO, and recover when the μOR antagonist, naloxone, is applied. **(B2,3)** Show group data for experiments such as in **(A)**. Physostigmine, 1 μM, and 4-AP, 5–20 μM, were present in the bathing solution. Figures taken from D. Nagode Ph.D. Thesis, at http://archive.hshsl.umaryland.edu/handle/10713/2315.

of eCBs. One might expect that the GABAergic output from CCK+/CB1R+ cells would be rapidly eliminated by the eCBs, and indeed it has been proposed that CCh-generated eCBs silence the CB1R+ cells during rhythm generation in CA3 (Gulyás et al., 2010; Holderith et al., 2011). Nevertheless, on the contrary, the CCh-induced IPSCs are highly susceptible to inhibition by DSI (e.g., Pitler and Alger, 1992b; Alger et al., 1996; Martin and Alger, 1999; Wilson and Nicoll, 2001; Kim et al., 2002; Hampson et al., 2003; Fortin et al., 2004; Trettel et al., 2004; Yoshino et al., 2011). Thus the CB1R+ interneurons are not entirely silenced by the mAChR-induced eCBs. As noted, studies from DGL$\alpha^{-/-}$ mice, which are incapable of generating the major eCB, 2-AG, confirm that both mAChR-dependent eCB effects and DSI are mediated by 2-AG (Tanimura et al., 2010; Yoshino et al., 2011), so differences in eCB identity cannot account for the continued sensitivity of CCh-induced θ IPSCs to DSI.

An entirely different mechanism was described by Makara et al. (2007) who reported that, in the presence of CCh, the eCB-system becomes dependent on nitric oxide (NO) production. When mAChRs were activated DSI could be prevented by inhibitors of NO synthesis or NO scavengers. NO scavengers injected into the postsynaptic PCs prevented the action of NO and soluble cGMP, a proposed intracellular target of NO, was selectively located in presynaptic CB1R+ nerve terminals. Hence the picture was that NO was released as a retrograde signal from the PCs, affected cGMP in the presynaptic CB1R+ terminals and acted in concert with eCBs to inhibit GABA release. It was proposed that NO acted at a step downstream of CB1R, although activation of CB1R via the synthetic CB1R agonist, WIN55212-2, was not affected. It was unclear why eCB-mediated actions were immune to NO in the absence of CCh. To our knowledge, these provocative observations have not been replicated, hence although mAChRs do generate NO at neuromuscular synapses (Malomouzh et al., 2007; Newman et al., 2007), even interacting with eCBs at other synapses (e.g., via M3 activation at vertebrate neuromuscular synapses, Newman et al., 2007), a role for NO in mAChR actions in hippocampus remains conceivable but undefined.

Resolution of the puzzle that mAChRs both mobilize eCBs and stimulate the activity of eCB-sensitive interneurons could well involve a mechanism that modulates presynaptic CB1R actions and partially offsets their depressive effects on GABA release. Several candidates exist (**Figure 5**), including: (1) K^+ channel antagonists—blocking K^+ channels pharmacologically can completely abolish DSI (Alger et al., 1996; Morishita et al., 1998; Diana and Marty, 2003), probably because voltage-gated Ca^{2+} channel opening and intra-terminal $[Ca^{2+}]_i$ increase when K^+ channels are blocked (Varma et al., 2002). ACh-induced blockade of presynaptic K^+ channels (or other factors, e.g., retrograde release of arachidonic acid; Carta et al., 2014) might thus overcome CB1R-induced depression during ACh action. (2) Direct effects on the transmitter release machinery via application of N-ethylmaleimide (NEM), which blocks pertussis toxin-sensitive G-proteins, increases GABA release and reverses DSI through an unknown mechanism (Morishita et al., 1997). (3) The firing frequency of the interneuron—the degree of eCB-mediated suppression of GABA release decreases as the firing of the interneuron increases (Losonczy et al., 2004; Földy et al., 2007). Since CCh stimulates interneuron firing (Pitler and Alger, 1992a; Martin and Alger, 1999; Cea-del Rio et al., 2010; Gulyás et al., 2010), the net effect of eCBs on persistently occurring IPSCs will represent a balance between inhibition and excitation of interneuronal output.

If indeed mAChR-released eCBs suppress, but do not abolish, CCK+/CB1R+ interneuron output, then a CB1R antagonist should increase the IPSCs coming from these cells. That is, we predict that action of mAChRs on the interneurons will cause them to fire and release GABA, while the CB1R antagonist will prevent the eCBs generated by the PCs from simultaneously retarding the occurrence of the IPSCs. Thus a given ACh stimulus should give rise to more IPSCs in the presence of CB1R antagonism than it normally would. While concerted effort will be required to test this hypothesis in detail, we have observed (Nagode et al., 2011) that indeed the CB1R antagonist AM251 increases the number of IPSCs triggered by optogenetically released ACh (**Figure 6**). This example shows that the number and mean amplitude of the IPSCs triggered by ChR2-induced ACh release are increased after AM251 was applied. This suggests that eCBs generated by mAChRs can influence the IPSC rhythms. It will also be important to determine whether similar influences can be detected on atropine-sensitive, inhibitory rhythms *in vivo*, as this would suggest that mAChR-induced eCBs could be involved in regulation of persistent, behaviorally significant rhythms.

Finally, CB1R+ interneurons are electrically interconnected (Galarreta et al., 2004) and eCBs can indirectly strengthen electrical synapses (Pereda, 2014). Additionally, weakening of inhibition between electrically connected interneurons (as might occur during enhanced eCB release), also strengthens electrical coupling (Iball and Ali, 2011). Strengthening of electrical coupling will enhance the synchrony of firing within such networks. Thus complex interactions among chemical and electrical synapses and eCBs could help to rationalize the role of mAChRs in θ inhibitory oscillations. Unraveling the details of the modulation of eCB actions initiated by the cholinergic system will be an important task for the future.

mAChR DRIVEN eCB RELEASE AND ELECTRICAL SYNAPTIC CONNECTIONS SHARPEN DISTINCTIONS AMONG INTERNEURON CIRCUITS AND TUNE INTERNEURONAL OSCILLATIONS

The two major BC interneuron subtypes, the CCK+ (regular-spiking, RS) and the PV+ (fast-spiking, FS) cells are sharply segregated by their divergent properties (Freund and Katona, 2007), including their complements of mAChRs. These cellular and molecular differences imply that the two cell types are activated under different circumstances, by different neurotransmitters and modulators, and cause different effects on their target cells. Another factor is critical to ensuring that the cells within each group do not act in isolation, but participate in coordinated circuit based activity. As noted, electrical synaptic coupling often exists among like cells in hippocampus and neocortex (Galarreta and Hestrin, 1999; Gibson et al., 1999), although some interneurons are electrically coupled to cells of different classes (e.g., Krook-Magnuson et al., 2011). Generally, PV+ cells are electrically coupled to other PV+ cells, but not to PCs or other types of interneurons, including the CCK+ cells. CCK+ cells are electrically coupled to other CCK+ cells (Galarreta et al., 2004), but not to PCs or other types of interneurons, including the PV+ cells. The steady-state electrotonic coupling (coupling coefficient) among the cells averages from 4–7%, meaning that, e.g., a 10 mV change in membrane potential in one cell changes the potential in the coupled cell from 0.4–0.7 mV. This is enough to induce a cell to fire if it is near threshold. Injection of two random noise signals (Galarreta and Hestrin, 1999) or small sinusoidal voltages (Gibson et al., 1999) into two electrically coupled interneurons can cause both of the cells to fire synchronously when either of them reaches threshold. Thus the PV+ cells would tend to fire together as a circuit and the CCK+ cells would also tend to fire as an independent circuit. Interneuron circuit-wide activity will powerfully influence PC population activity.

The existence of electrical gap junctions between the cells is also noteworthy because it confers susceptibility to modulation by various regulatory factors. The strength of gap junctional

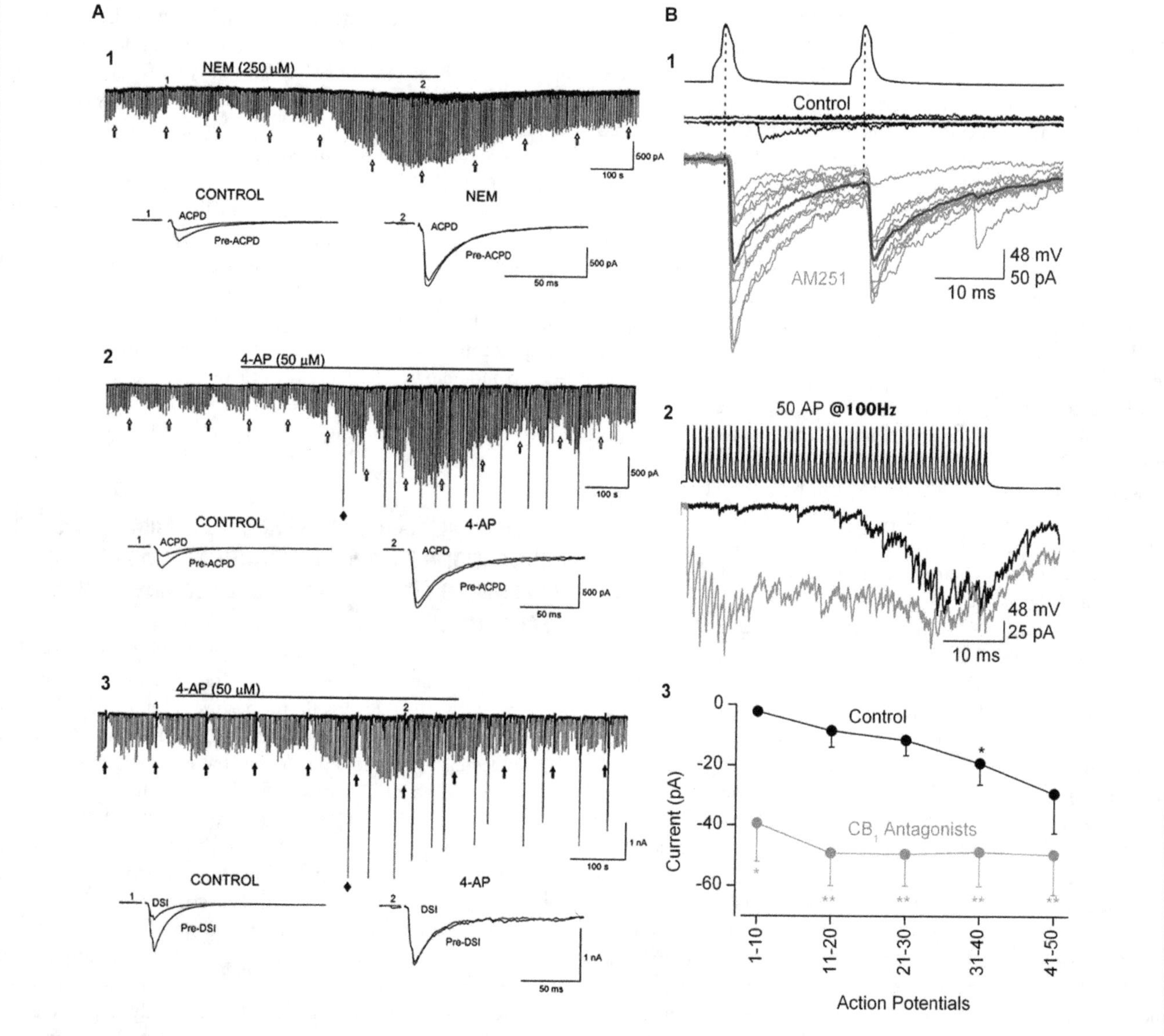

FIGURE 5 | The ability of eCBs to inhibit GABA release can be modulated by manipulations that increase transmitter release. (A1) Bath-application N-ethylmaleimide, an organic compound that affects G-proteins, ion channels and other biochemical processes, increases GABA release and abolishes the GPCR-dependent, eCB-mediated depression of IPSCs, as well as DSI (not shown; cf. Morishita et al., 1997). **(A2,A3)** The K^+ channel blocker, 4-AP, increases IPSCs and abolishes mGluR-dependent, eCB-mediated IPSC suppression and DSI. From Morishita et al. (1998) with permission. **(B)** Paired recording from mossy-fiber associated (MFA), CCK+ interneurons and CA3 PCs. **(B1)** Top two sets of traces show two presynaptic action potentials in the interneuron and the absence of a response in the PC in control saline. After addition of the CB1R antagonist, AM251, the interneuron action potentials reliably elicit large unitary IPSCs. **(B2)** A train of 50 interneuron action potentials initially produces only a few sparse IPSCs in the PC towards the end of the train in control solution (black trace). In the presence of AM251 (gray trace) the IPSCs are detected from the first action potential and occur throughout the train. **(B3)** Group data showing the difference in the IPSC currents, integrated within 100-ms time windows, in control and CB1R antagonist conditions. The conclusion is that a tonic, eCB mediated suppression of GABA release can be overcome by vigorous stimulation of interneuron activity. From Losonczy et al. (2004) with permission.

transmission is dependent on the input (leak) resistance of the target cells, and is frequency dependent, decreasing as the frequency of the voltage deflections through the junctional channels increases. When the leak resistance is low the coupling among cells is also low, because the currents, instead of passing via the gap junction into the coupled cells and depolarizing them, are shunted through the leak resistance to the extracellular space. When the leak resistance is high, the strength of electrical coupling increases. Interestingly the PV+ and CCK+ interneurons that are electrically coupled to each other are frequently also chemically coupled; that is, the target postsynaptic cells receive both electrical and chemical synaptic transmission from their upstream presynaptic partners (Galarreta and Hestrin, 1999; Gibson et al., 1999; Ali, 2007; Iball and Ali, 2011). The release

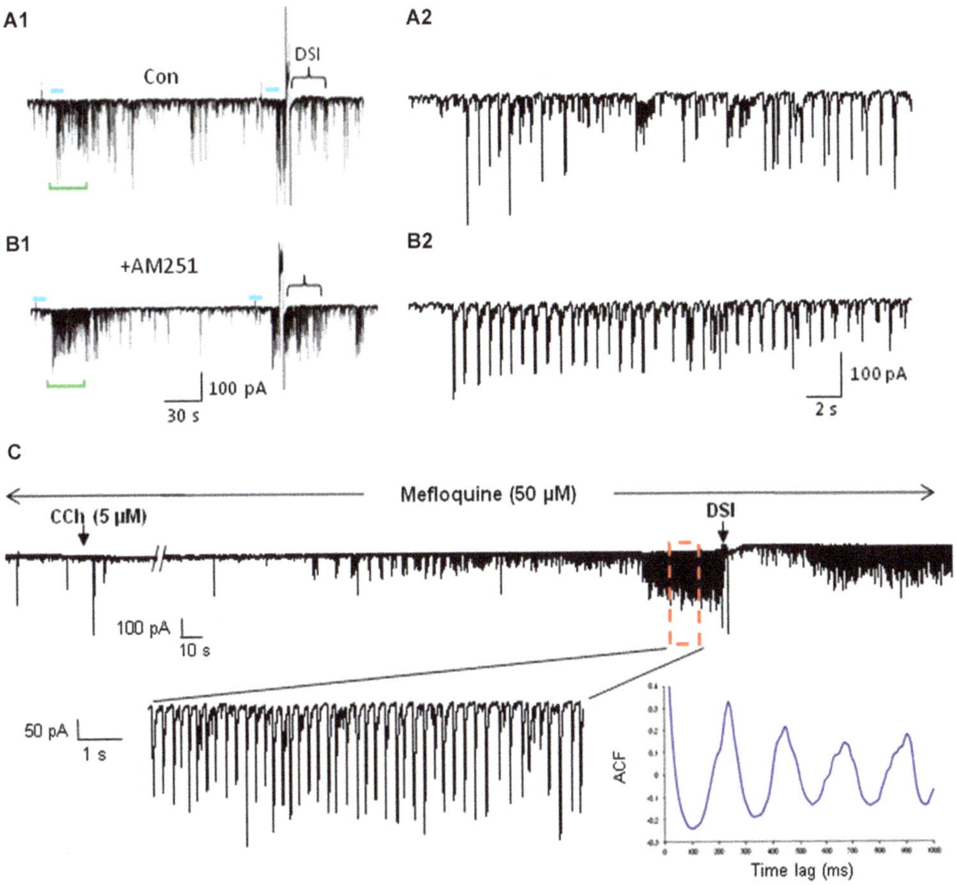

FIGURE 6 | mAChR-induced IPSCs are regulated by eCBs but do not depend on electrical coupling for their occurrence. **(A)** Bath application of the CB1R antagonist AM251 increases the occurrence of IPSCs evoked by optogenetic release of ACh (CA1 PC recording). Blue bars indicate the period of light stimulation (5 Hz). Traces in **(A2)** and **(B2)** depict an expansion of ~29 s of the traces (green brackets) in **(A1)** and **(B1)** beginning just before the onset of L-IPSC activity. The increase in number and average amplitude of the L-IPSCs caused by AM251 indicates that they had been partially suppressed by the eCBs mobilized by ACh. Bracket at the end of **(A1)** indicates approximate period of DSI after a voltage step given to the pyramidal cell. Comparable period in **(B1)** shows that AM251 prevents DSI, thus confirming that the L-IPSC activity (e.g., expanded trace in **A2**), despite being partially suppressed by the long-lasting ACh-induced mobilization of eCBs, could be further depressed by a sudden release of eCBs (i.e., DSI). Physostigmine and 4-AP are present. **(A)** and **(B)** modified with permission from Nagode et al. (2011). **(C)** Representative trace from a rat hippocampal slice pretreated and continuously perfused with the gap junction blocker, mefloquine (50 μM). Inset shows an expanded time scale of the indicated region in the top trace. The autocorrelogram of the expanded region demonstrates rhythmic, CCh-induced IPSCs despite the presence of mefloquine. Typical results ($n = 5$). From D.A. Nagode Ph.D. thesis at http://archive.hshsl.umaryland.edu/handle/10713/2315.

of GABA from CCK+ cells can be suppressed by eCBs (Ohno-Shosaku et al., 2001; Wilson and Nicoll, 2001), and when eCBs are released from other CCK+ cells the eCBs reduce the strength of chemical inhibition (Iball and Ali, 2011). By decreasing the chemical synaptic inhibition among CCK+ cells this simultaneously strengthens the electrical coupling between them. The release of eCBs depresses the strengths of individual GABAergic synapses onto other CCKs cells *and* increases their tendency to fire together. Importantly, the two kinds of synaptic junctions are independently regulated in the hippocampus; eCBs only suppress the release of GABA, they do not affect the electrical coupling. Thus inhibition can do more than simply veto or permit cell firing, it can directly shift the mode of firing within interneuronal circuits. The functional aspects of this concept has not been explored in the context of mAChR control of oscillations. However, given the ability of mAChRs to mobilize eCBs, mAChR-dependent stimulation of CCK+ cell mediated oscillations could in part reflect dual regulation of chemical and electrical signaling, although the gap junction blocker, mefloquine (Cruikshank et al., 2004), did not alter the ACh-induced θ IPSCs (**Figure 6C**).

PV+ cells are also electrically as well as chemically coupled and their tendency to fire together is facilitated by electrical synapses (Galarreta and Hestrin, 1999). Activation of mAChRs induces the occurrence of γ rhythms driven by PV+ cells in hippocampal CA3, but PV+ cells but do not express CB1Rs and are therefore not directly affected by eCBs. The PV+ cell-mediated inhibitory γ rhythms are suppressed by *exogenous* cannabinoids because activation of the CB1Rs on the glutamate terminals that excite the PV+ cells is suppressed and the resulting loss of excitatory drive keeps the cells from firing (Holderith et al., 2011). Surprisingly, the eCBs released by activation of M1/M3 mAChRs on PC apparently do not affect the CB1Rs on the glutamate terminals. This conclusion follows from the observation that the CB1R antagonist that prevents the inhibition of γ by exogenous eCBs, when applied by itself does not alter mAChR-driven oscillations (Gulyás et al., 2010). Given that a mAChR agonist very efficiently suppressed GABA release via eCB action in these experiments, it is clear that the eCBs were mobilized. Probably the eCBs simply did not reach the CB1Rs on glutamatergic terminals. The powerful eCB uptake and degradation systems, together with the fact that eCBs cannot travel far from their site of production/release (Kano et al., 2009) could have limited their movements. The restricted actions of the eCB system help sharpen the targeting of ACh actions, even if ACh is released in the volume conduction mode.

Release of GABA from PV+ cells is regulated by opioids, because these cells strongly express μORs on their nerve terminals (Drake and Milner, 2002). Thus μOR agonists, such as enkephalins, may have the analogous effects on the development of PV+ driven inhibitory rhythms as eCBs do on the CCK+ cell rhythms. Mobilization of endogenous opioids in the hippocampus by ACh has not yet been explored in this context to the best of our knowledge.

It is established that the CCK+ cells and the PV+ cells predominate in different kinds of neuronal oscillations. The preferred frequencies of the oscillations, γ for the PV/FS cells and the slower θ rhythms for the CCK/RS, cells will largely be set by intrinsic membrane properties, including the kinetics of their AHPs, that enable the PV/FS cells to fire at higher frequency than the CCK/RS cells, as well as by the kinetics of the chemical transmission that they each mediate—IPSPs mediated by PV/FS cells are faster than those of the CCK/RS cells. Most importantly, the circuitry underlying the rhythms, at least in the hippocampus, is likely to be quite different. The inhibitory θ in CA1 is probably generated by an interconnected inhibitory network of CCK+ cells that express CB1Rs, and perhaps also μORs. This rhythm is independent of fast excitatory glutamatergic synaptic input. Rather, the rhythmic output of this circuit is produced when the cells receive a slow cholinergic input that activates their mAChRs for at least several seconds. Inhibitory synaptic interactions among the interneurons then gives rise to synchronous rhythmic firing within the network, and IPSCs are projected onto groups of PCs. In contrast, the faster inhibitory γ rhythms in CA3 are generated mainly by excitatory synaptic interactions among CA3 PCs, which activate PV+ interneurons that then feed back inhibitory inputs to the PCs. These rhythms are abolished by iGluR blockers, or CB1R agonists, which prevent stimulation of the PV+ cells; they are also abolished by activation of μORs on the PV+ cell terminals. The schematic diagram in **Figure 7** summarizes these conclusions. Note that this schematic is intended only to illustrate the circuitry for the inhibitory rhythms, it does not include other circuitry such as that described by Pietersen et al. (2014) that produces an intrinsic γ rhythm that is entrained by cholinergic inputs and is dependent on excitatory synaptic inputs (hence a PING model) in CA1.

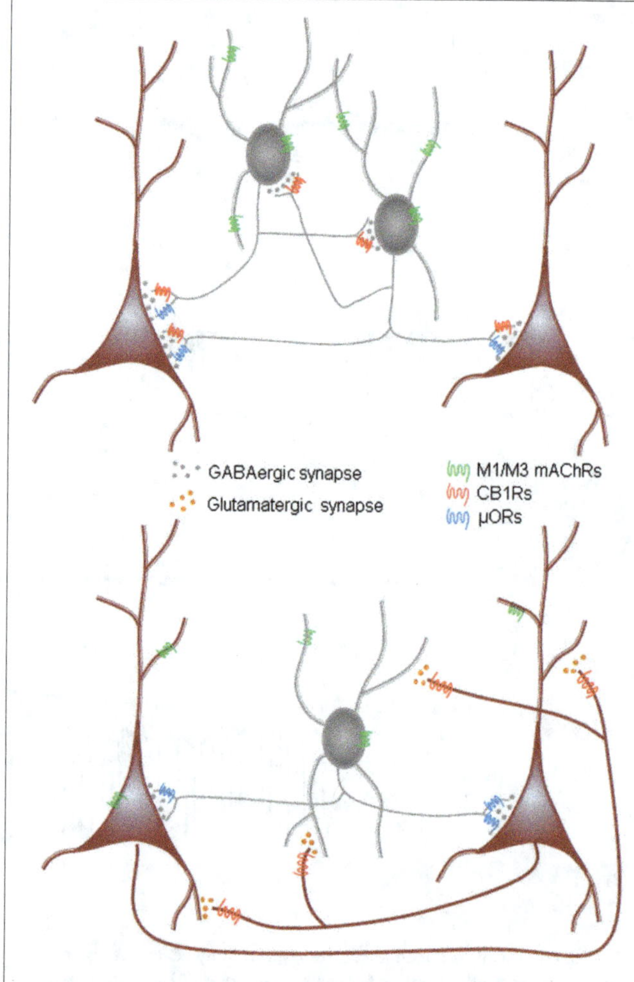

FIGURE 7 | Diagrams of two models for mACh-induced inhibitory rhythmic IPSCs in hippocampus. Top, synaptically connected interneuron network is tonically activated by activation of M1/M3 mAChRs on interneurons in CA1. Interneuron firing is induced by mAChR-induced depolarization that, when integrated with intrinsic interneuron firing properties and incoming GABAergic IPSPs from other interneurons of the group, generates rhythmic synchronous interneuron firing. The target PCs receive a rhythmic barrage of IPSPs. This is analogous to the ING ("interneuron gamma") model of gamma rhythms. Cannabinoids interrupt rhythms generated by this network by inhibiting the release of GABA from the CB1R-expressing (mainly CCK+) interneurons; opioids probably inhibit the network by acting on μORs present on a subset of the CB1R+ cells. Note evidence of Pietersen et al. (2014) for an intrinsic γ generator in CA1 that would involve a PING mechanism. **Bottom**, ACh drives action potential firing in an interconnected excitatory network (such as the CA3, but not the CA1, PCs) as well as in the interneurons. The glutamatergic output of the PCs excites interneurons that feed GABAergic IPSPs back onto the PCs. Interactions between the excitatory and inhibitory cells generates the rhythms. This is analogous to the PING ("pyramidal-interneuron gamma") model. Cannabinoids inhibit rhythms generated by this network by inhibiting the release of glutamate from the PCs; opioids inhibit the rhythms by acting on the μORs on the (mainly PV+) interneurons.

FUTURE AREAS FOR EXPLORATION OF mAChR FUNCTION IN THE BRAIN

Despite the enormous amount of investigation into muscarinic cholinergic systems in the brain there are still many areas about which little is known. We highlight a few opportunities related to their roles of in hippocampal and cortical oscillations or behaviors related to them.

mAChRs, PAMs, and endocannabinoids

Deficiencies in mAChR actions are implicated in various kinds of cognitive dysfunction. Attempts to develop effective therapeutic agents that act directly on specific brain mAChRs have not been successful, largely because of difficulties in restricting the agents to particular mAChR subtypes (Bubser et al., 2012). These agents are generally agonists that bind to the active site of the molecule, or generally enhance the availability of ACh (by preventing its uptake, for example). In either case, side effects occur when unintended receptors are also activated. It has been difficult to devise agonists that only activate one mAChR subtype because the agonist binding site is highly conserved across subtypes. An alternative approach targets sites that are away from this highly conserved region. Ligands at these sites, allosteric modulators, are more specific because they bind to relatively less well-conserved parts of the receptor molecule, i.e., sites that vary widely between subtypes and hence offer more opportunities for specific binding. Allosteric modulators do not directly activate the receptor but enhance the effects of ACh or other ligands that activate it directly. For example, positive allosteric modulators (PAMs) that are specific for M1, M4 or M5 mAChRs have been developed (Bubser et al., 2012). In the presence of a PAM for M1, a low concentration of ACh that produces predominantly M1 mAChR dependent effects would increase the ability of naturally released ACh to activate M1 selectively on its normal postsynaptic target cells. This approach should improve the specificity of action over the usual systemic therapeutic drug application method. Similar strategies have been used in the case of nAChRs; e.g., the weak AChE inhibitor and PAM of nAChRs, galantamine, attenuates nicotine self-administration and seeking rats (Hopkins et al., 2012).

Because activation of M1 (or M3) mAChRs potently stimulates the release of eCBs, an M1-specific PAM should enhance the ability of cholinergic agonists to mobilize eCBs. This hypothesis has not been tested, but could easily be investigated in *in vitro* brain slice preparations. If PAMs do facilitate eCB mobilization by mAChRs, it might have clinical applications, particularly in view of the preliminary results suggesting efficacy of CB1R agonists in alleviating certain consequences of Alzheimer's dementia (agitation, lack of nutritional intact, sleep disturbances; Aso and Ferrer, 2014). Perhaps a mAChR PAM given in conjunction with low concentrations of a CB1R agonist would be beneficial and further reduce the possibility of untoward side effects of either drug alone. Alternatively, an eCB uptake inhibitor, by increasing the concentration of eCBs near their normal site of action, might be beneficial in boosting the eCB mobilizing ability of M1 mAChR activation.

mAChRs, glia, and eCBs

No longer thought to be passive supporting partners of neurons, glia are now understood to have active roles in the regulation of synaptic transmission. Glial cells, mainly astrocytes, express a diversity of mAChRs including M1 and M3 (Pap et al., 2009). In several brain regions activation of mAChRs on glia cause elevations in intracellular glial $[Ca^{2+}]_i$ (Araque et al., 2002; Pap et al., 2009; Takata et al., 2011; Navarrete et al., 2012). Glia participate in the induction of synaptic plasticity in the hippocampus, including a form of LTP at the CA3-CA1 synapses that is dependent on activation of mAChRs (Navarrete et al., 2012). Stimulation of glial mAChRs by application of cholinergic agonists, or stimulation of ACh release from septal cholinergic fibers causes an increase in hippocampal Ca^{2+} in glia (Araque et al., 2002). *In vivo* sensory stimulation or electrical stimulation of the MS increases Ca^{2+} in hippocampal astrocytes and induces LTP of CA3-CA1 synapses (Navarrete et al., 2012). This cholinergic LTP induction depends on activation of mAChRs and mGluRs. Rises in glial cell Ca^{2+} result from activation of IP_3Rs (Takata et al., 2011; Navarrete et al., 2012), and are associated with the release of various factors (Sul et al., 2004) including glutamate (Halassa and Haydon, 2010, for review). Astrocytes are also activated by endocannabinoids (Navarrete and Araque, 2008; Min and Nevian, 2012). The glial induction of LTP in the hippocampus is caused by Ca^{2+}-dependent glutamate release from the astrocytes and subsequent activation of hippocampal PC mGluRs. A similar cholinergically-driven, astrocyte-Ca^{2+} mediated synaptic plasticity in the mouse barrel cortex is dependent on mAChRs and NMDARs (Takata et al., 2011), indicating that mAChR activation stimulates glutamate release there as well. Given that glutamate activation of mGluRs is a potent stimulus for eCB mobilization from PCs (Maejima et al., 2001; Varma et al., 2001) elevation of glial cell $[Ca^{2+}]_i$ should also mobilize eCBs indirectly from the PCs following mGluR stimulation. Given the eCB-mediated influences on cortical and hippocampal rhythms, glia could also participate in regulation of rhythms via eCBs. This hypothesis has evidently not been tested, but if true, would add another potent element to the array of effects mediated by mAChR.

mAChR regulation of rhythms by controlling ectopic axonal activity

It is generally assumed that axons simply transmit signals from neuronal somata to synaptic terminals, and therefore that they automatically follow somatic activity. Two corollaries follow from this assumption: (1) somatic action potential activity is an accurate guide to the activity reaching the terminals; and (2) axons do not act independently of somata.

However, under some circumstances axonal action potentials can be initiated independently of somatic depolarizations. These were initially described in the context of disease or other aberrant conditions, but new challenges to the simple picture have arisen in physiological contexts. In hippocampal slices, Dugladze et al. (2012) report that kainic acid-induced γ oscillations in the field potentials around the PCs of the CA3 region are accompanied by much higher frequency firing in the distal axonal branches of the PCs. Remarkably, this high frequency of axonal firing was not reflected in the somatic action potential firing of the PC somato-dendritic regions. It appeared that the two cellular compartments—axon and soma-dendrite—were in essence operating independently. When GABA-A receptors were pharmacologically blocked, however, the axonal action potentials did invade the somato-dendritic region, implying that normally they were actively prevented from doing so by a persistent GABAergic inhibition. The investigators discovered that a continual high frequency firing of the axo-axonic interneurons, which specifically target the axon hillock region of the PCs, were responsible. In fact, a single axo-axonic cell was capable of fully controlling the antidromic invasion of the somato-dendritic region of a PC. As noted earlier, the axo-axonic cells in CA3 are strongly activated by mAChR activation, but the IPSPs produced by these cells do not directly contribute to oscillations. Rather, Dugladze et al. (2012) suggest that the main function of the axo-axonic cells is to preserve the independence of axonal and somato-dendritic signaling. It will be important to determine if mAChR-induced oscillations share the ability to modulate PC function in this novel and powerful way.

mAChRs, eCBs, and Fragile X Syndrome

Endocannabinoid modulation of CCK+ cells may underlie some of the deficits in oscillations in Fragile X Syndrome (FXS). In the hippocampus of a mouse model of FXS, *Fmr1*$^{-/-}$ mice, there is enhanced coupling of mGluRs to eCB release at inhibitory synapses in both hippocampus (Zhang and Alger, 2010) and striatum (Maccarrone et al., 2010). Surprisingly, the eCB actions at excitatory synapses are actually decreased, not increased, in this model (Jung et al., 2012). While the molecular basis for this striking difference is not fully understood, the distinctive molecular architecture of excitatory and inhibitory synapses will undoubtedly constitute a major factor. DGL_{α} is normally precisely localized in the spine heads of excitatory synapses (Katona et al., 2006), and it has been found that the disease is associated with an enhanced distance between mGluRs and DGL_{α} (Jung et al., 2012) which could explain the decreased efficiency of eCB production. DGL_{α} has not yet been found at inhibitory synapses (e.g., Lafourcade et al., 2007), and the explanation for enhanced eCB actions at those synapses is unknown, although biochemical targets are being identified (Busquets-Garcia et al., 2013). It should be emphasized that the functional consequences of both decreased eCB action at excitatory synapses and increased eCB action at inhibitory synapses will be the same: an overall increase in network excitability. The same could be true of mAChR-induced eCB release, as overactive signaling through M1 mAChRs has been hypothesized to contribute to the FXS phenotype (D'Antuono et al., 2003). There is enhanced CCh-induced LTD in CA1 hippocampal slices from FRX mice (Volk et al., 2007), and M1 and M4 antagonists reduce the induction of audiogenic seizures (Veeraragavan et al., 2011a,b). The relationship between mAChRs and eCBs deserves further study in the context of FXS, in part because the availability of clinically tested CB1R ligands that could be candidates for inclusion in the therapeutic arsenal for treatment of symptoms of this serious disorder.

CONCLUSION

Studies of the mAChR system in the brain continue to yield exciting new insights and information on a wide variety of neurophysiological problems. Undoubtedly the future holds enormous promise for novel and valuable advances both in the basic understanding of this powerful and ubiquitous regulatory system, and in eventual clinical applications.

CONTRIBUTIONS OF AUTHORS

This review was written jointly by all of the authors. The recent research referred to from the Alger laboratory was supervised by Bradley E. Alger and conducted by Daniel A. Nagode and Ai-Hui Tang, who also had major roles in the experimental design, data analysis, and interpretation of results.

ACKNOWLEDGMENTS

This work was supported by the NIH RO1 MH077277 and RO1 DA014625 grants to Bradley E. Alger and F31 NS-074880 to Daniel A. Nagode, as well as a grant from the FRAXA Research Foundation, Newburyport, MA, USA to Bradley E. Alger.

REFERENCES

Alger, B. E. (2002). Retrograde signaling in the regulation of synaptic transmission: focus on endocannabinoids. *Prog. Neurobiol.* 68, 247–286. doi: 10.1016/s0301-0082(02)00080-1

Alger, B. E., and Kim, J. (2011). Supply and demand for endocannabinoids. *Trends Neurosci.* 34, 304–315. doi: 10.1016/j.tins.2011.03.003

Alger, B. E., Pitler, T. A., Wagner, J. J., Martin, L. A., Morishita, W., Kirov, S. A., et al. (1996). Retrograde signaling in depolarization-induced suppression of inhibition in rat hippocampal CA1 cells. *J. Physiol.* 496, 197–209.

Ali, A. B. (2007). Presynaptic inhibition of GABAA receptor-mediated unitary IPSPs by cannabinoid receptors at synapses between CCK-positive interneurons in rat hippocampus. *J. Neurophysiol.* 98, 861–869. doi: 10.1152/jn.00156.2007

Allen, T. G., Abogadie, F. C., and Brown, D. A. (2006). Simultaneous release of glutamate and acetylcholine from single magnocellular "cholinergic" basal forebrain neurons. *J. Neurosci.* 26, 1588–1595. doi: 10.1523/jneurosci.3979-05.2006

Araque, A., Martín, E. D., Perea, G., Arellano, J. I., and Buño, W. (2002). Synaptically released acetylcholine evokes Ca2+ elevations in astrocytes in hippocampal slices. *J. Neurosci.* 22, 2443–2450.

Aso, E., and Ferrer, I. (2014). Cannabinoids for treatment of Alzheimer's disease: moving toward the clinic. *Front. Pharmacol.* 5:37. eCollection 2014. doi: 10.3389/fphar.2014.00037

Atasoy, D., Aponte, Y., Su, H. H., and Sternson, S. M. (2008). A FLEX switch targets channelrhodopsin-2 to multiple cell types for imaging and long-range circuit mapping. *J. Neurosci.* 28, 7025–7030. doi: 10.1523/JNEUROSCI.1954-08.2008

Axmacher, N., Mormann, F., Fernandez, G., Elger, C. E., and Fell, J. (2006). Memory formation by neuronal synchronization. *Brain Res. Rev.* 52, 170–182. doi: 10.1016/j.brainresrev.2006.01.007

Bartos, M., Alle, H., and Vida, I. (2011). Role of microcircuit structure and input integration in hippocampal interneuron recruitment and plasticity. *Neuropharmacology* 60, 730–739. doi: 10.1016/j.neuropharm.2010.12.017

Bartos, M., and Elgueta, C. (2012). Functional characteristics of parvalbumin- and cholecystokinin- expressing basket cells. *J. Physiol.* 590, 669–681. doi: 10.1113/jphysiol.2011.226175

Bayraktar, T., Staiger, J. F., Acsady, L., Cozzari, C., Freund, T. F., and Zilles, K. (1997). Co-localization of vasoactive intestinal polypeptide, gamma-aminobutyric acid and choline acetyltransferase in neocortical interneurons of the adult rat. *Brain Res.* 757, 209–217. doi: 10.1016/s0006-8993(97)00218-7

Bell, L. A., Bell, K. A., and McQuiston, A. R. (2013). Synaptic muscarinic response types in hippocampal CA1 interneurons depend on different levels of presynaptic activity and different muscarinic receptor subtypes. *Neuropharmacology* 73, 160–173. doi: 10.1016/j.neuropharm.2013.05.026

Bell, K. A., Shim, H., Chen, C. K., and McQuiston, A. R. (2011). Nicotinic excitatory postsynaptic potentials in hippocampal ca1 interneurons are predominantly mediated by nicotinic receptors that contain $\alpha4$ and $\beta2$ subunits. *Neuropharmacology* 61, 1379–1388. doi: 10.1016/j.neuropharm.2011.08.024

Bland, B. H., Colom, L. V., Konopacki, J., and Roth, S. H. (1988). Intracellular records of carbachol-induced theta rhythm in hippocampal slices. *Brain Res.* 447, 364–368. doi: 10.1016/0006-8993(88)91141-9

Bonner, T. I. (1989). New subtypes of muscarinic acetylcholine receptors. *Trends Pharmacol. Sci.* Suppl.15.

Boyden, E. S., Zhang, F., Bamberg, E., Nagel, G., and Deisseroth, K. (2005). Millisecond-timescale, genetically targeted optical control of neural activity. *Nat. Neurosci.* 8, 1263–1268. doi: 10.1038/nn1525

Bragin, A., Jando, G., Nadasdy, Z., Hetke, J., Wise, K., and Buzsaki, G. (1995). Gamma (40–100 hz) oscillation in the hippocampus of the behaving rat. *J. Neurosci.* 15, 47–60.

Brazhnik, E. S., and Fox, S. E. (1997). Intracellular recordings from medial septal neurons during hippocampal theta rhythm. *Exp. Brain Res.* 114, 442–453. doi: 10.1007/pl00005653

Broicher, T., Wettschureck, N., Munsch, T., Coulon, P., Meuth, S. G., Kanyshkova, T., et al. (2008). Muscarinic ACh receptor-mediated control of thalamic activity via G(q)/G (11)-family G-proteins. *Pflugers Arch.* 456, 1049–1060. doi: 10.1007/s00424-008-0473-x

Brown, D. A. (2010). Muscarinic acetylcholine receptors (mAChRs) in the nervous system: some functions and mechanisms. *J. Mol. Neurosci.* 41, 340–346. doi: 10.1007/s12031-010-9377-2

Brown, D. A., and Adams, P. R. (1980). Muscarinic suppression of a novel voltage-sensitive K+ current in a vertebrate neurone. *Nature* 283, 673–676. doi: 10.1038/283673a0

Bubser, M., Byun, N., Wood, M. R., and Jones, C. K. (2012). Muscarinic receptor pharmacology and circuitry for the modulation of cognition. *Handb. Exp. Pharmacol.* 208, 121–166. doi: 10.1007/978-3-642-23274-9_7

Busquets-Garcia, A., Gomis-González, M., Guegan, T., Agustín-Pavón, C., Pastor, A., Mato, S., et al. (2013). Targeting the endocannabinoid system in the treatment of fragile X syndrome. *Nat. Med.* 19, 603–607. doi: 10.1038/nm.3127

Buzsáki, G. (2002). Theta oscillations in the hippocampus. *Neuron* 33, 325–340. doi: 10.1016/s0896-6273(02)00586-x

Buzsáki, G. (2005). Theta rhythm of navigation: link between path integration and landmark navigation, episodic and semantic memory. *Hippocampus* 15, 827–840. doi: 10.1002/hipo.20113

Buzsáki, G., Anastassiou, C. A., and Koch, C. (2012). The origin of extracellular fields and currents—EEG, ECoG, LFP and spikes. *Nat. Rev. Neurosci.* 13, 407–420. doi: 10.1038/nrn3241

Carta, M., Lanore, F., Rebola, N., Szabo, Z., Da Silva, S. V., Lourenço, J., et al. (2014). Membrane lipids tune synaptic transmission by direct modulation of presynaptic potassium channels. *Neuron* 81, 787–799. doi: 10.1016/j.neuron.2013.12.028

Caulfield, M. P., and Birdsall, N. J. (1998). International union of pharmacology. XVII. Classification of muscarinic acetylcholine receptors. *Pharmacol. Rev.* 50, 279–290.

Cea-del Rio, C. A., Lawrence, J. J., Erdelyi, F., Szabo, G., and McBain, C. J. (2011). Cholinergic modulation amplifies the intrinsic oscillatory properties of CA1 hippocampal cholecystokinin-positive interneurons. *J. Physiol.* 589, 609–627. doi: 10.1113/jphysiol.2010.199422

Cea-del Rio, C. A., Lawrence, J. J., Tricoire, L., Erdelyi, F., Szabo, G., and McBain, C. J. (2010). M3 muscarinic acetylcholine receptor expression confers differential cholinergic modulation to neurochemically distinct hippocampal basket cell subtypes. *J. Neurosci.* 30, 6011–6024. doi: 10.1523/JNEUROSCI.5040-09.2010

Cea-del Rio, C. A., McBain, C. J., and Pelkey, K. A. (2012). An update on cholinergic regulation of cholecystokinin-expressing basket cells. *J. Physiol.* 590, 695–702. doi: 10.1113/jphysiol.2011.225342

Chapman, C. A., and Lacaille, J. C. (1999). Cholinergic induction of theta-frequency oscillations in hippocampal inhibitory interneurons and pacing of pyramidal cell firing. *J. Neurosci.* 19, 8637–8645.

Chédotal, A., Cozzari, C., Faure, M. P., Hartman, B. K., and Hamel, E. (1994). Distinct choline acetyltransferase (ChAT) and vasoactive intestinal polypeptide (VIP) bipolar neurons project to local blood vessels in the rat cerebral cortex. *Brain Res.* 646, 181–193. doi: 10.1016/0006-8993(94)90076-0

Cobb, S. R., Buhl, E. H., Halasy, K., Paulsen, O., and Somogyi, P. (1995). Synchronization of neuronal activity in hippocampus by individual GABAergic interneurons. *Nature* 378, 75–78. doi: 10.1038/378075a0

Cobb, S. R., and Davies, C. H. (2005). Cholinergic modulation of hippocampal cells and circuits. *J. Physiol.* 562, 81–88. doi: 10.1113/jphysiol.2004.076539

Cole, A. E., and Nicoll, R. A. (1983). Acetylcholine mediates a slow synaptic potential in hippocampal pyramidal cells. *Science* 221, 1299–1301. doi: 10.1126/science.6612345

Colgin, L. L., Kramár, E. A., Gall, C. M., and Lynch, G. (2003). Septal modulation of excitatory transmission in hippocampus. *J. Neurophysiol.* 90, 2358–2366. doi: 10.1152/jn.00262.2003

Cruikshank, S. J., Hopperstad, M., Younger, M., Connors, B. W., Spray, D. C., and Srinivas, M. (2004). Potent block of Cx36 and Cx50 gap junction channels by mefloquine. *Proc. Natl. Acad. Sci. U S A* 101, 12364–12369. doi: 10.1073/pnas.0402044101

Csicsvari, J., Jamieson, B., Wise, K. D., and Buzsaki, G. (2003). Mechanisms of gamma oscillations in the hippocampus of the behaving rat. *Neuron* 37, 311–322. doi: 10.1016/S0896-6273(02)01169-8

Curley, A. A., and Lewis, D. A. (2012). Cortical basket cell dysfunction in schizophrenia. *J. Physiol.* 590, 715–724. doi: 10.1113/jphysiol.2011.224659

D'Antuono, M., Merlo, D., and Avoli, M. (2003). Involvement of cholinergic and gabaergic systems in the fragile x knockout mice. *Neuroscience* 119, 9–13. doi: 10.1016/s0306-4522(03)00103-9

Degroot, A., Kofalvi, A., Wade, M. R., Davis, R. J., Rodrigues, R. J., Rebola, N., et al. (2006). CB1 receptor antagonism increases hippocampal acetylcholine release: site and mechanism of action. *Mol. Pharmacol.* 70, 1236–1245. doi: 10.1124/mol.106.024661

Diana, M. A., and Marty, A. (2003). Characterization of depolarization-induced suppression of inhibition using paired interneuron—Purkinje cell recordings. *J. Neurosci.* 23, 5906–5918.

Dodd, J., Dingledine, R., and Kelly, J. S. (1981). The excitatory action of acetylcholine on hippocampal neurones of the guinea pig and rat maintained in vitro. *Brain Res.* 207, 109–127. doi: 10.1016/0006-8993(81)90682-x

Drake, C. T., and Milner, T. A. (2002). Mu opioid receptors are in discrete hippocampal interneuron subpopulations. *Hippocampus* 12, 119–136. doi: 10.1002/hipo.1107

Dringenberg, H. C., and Vanderwolf, C. H. (1998). Involvement of direct and indirect pathways in electrocorticographic activation. *Neurosci. Biobehav. Rev.* 22, 243–257. doi: 10.1016/s0149-7634(97)00012-2

Dugladze, T., Schmitz, D., Whittington, M. A., Vida, I., and Gloveli, T. (2012). Segregation of axonal and somatic activity during fast network oscillations. *Science* 336, 1458–1461. doi: 10.1126/science.1222017

Edwards, D. A., Kim, J., and Alger, B. E. (2006). Multiple mechanisms of endocannabinoid response initiation in hippocampus. *J. Neurophysiol.* 95, 67–75. doi: 10.1152/jn.00813.2005

Edwards, D. A., Zhang, L., and Alger, B. E. (2008). Metaplastic control of the endocannabinoid system at inhibitory synapses in hippocampus. *Proc. Natl. Acad. Sci. U S A* 105, 8142–8147. doi: 10.1073/pnas.0803558105

Eichenbaum, H. (2013). Memory on time. *Trends Cogn. Sci.* 17, 81–88. doi: 10.1016/j.tics.2012.12.007

Fenno, L., Yizhar, O., and Deisseroth, K. (2011). The development and application of optogenetics. *Annu. Rev. Neurosci.* 34, 389–412. doi: 10.1146/annurev-neuro-061010-113817

Fisahn, A., Pike, F. G., Buhl, E. H., and Paulsen, O. (1998). Cholinergic induction of network oscillations at 40 Hz in the hippocampus in vitro. *Nature* 394, 186–189. doi: 10.1038/28179

Fisahn, A., Yamada, M., Duttaroy, A., Gan, J. W., Deng, C. X., McBain, C. J., et al. (2002). Muscarinic induction of hippocampal gamma oscillations requires coupling of the M1 receptor to two mixed cation currents. *Neuron* 33, 615–624. doi: 10.1016/s0896-6273(02)00587-1

Fischer, V., Both, M., Draguhn, A., and Egorov, A. V. (2014). Choline-mediated modulation of hippocampal sharp wave-ripple complexes in vitro. *J. Neurochem.* 129, 792–805. doi: 10.1111/jnc.12693

Földy, C., Lee, S. Y., Szabadics, J., Neu, A., and Soltesz, I. (2007). Cell type-specific gating of perisomatic inhibition by cholecystokinin. *Nat. Neurosci.* 10, 1128–1130. doi: 10.1038/nn1952

Fortin, D. A., Trettel, J., and Levine, E. S. (2004). Brief trains of action potentials enhance pyramidal neuron excitability via endocannabinoid-mediated suppression of inhibition. *J. Neurophysiol.* 92, 2105–2112. doi: 10.1152/jn.00351.2004

Freund, T. F., and Katona, I. (2007). Perisomatic inhibition. *Neuron* 56, 33–42. doi: 10.1016/j.neuron.2007.09.012

Fukudome, Y., Ohno-Shosaku, T., Matsui, M., Omori, Y., Fukaya, M., Tsubokawa, H., et al. (2004). Two distinct classes of muscarinic action on hippocampal inhibitory synapses: M2-mediated direct suppression and M1/M3-mediated indirect suppression through endocannabinoid signalling. *Eur. J. Neurosci.* 19, 2682–2692. doi: 10.1111/j.0953-816x.2004.03384.x

Galarreta, M., Erdélyi, F., Szabó, G., and Hestrin, S. (2004). Electrical coupling among irregular-spiking GABAergic interneurons expressing cannabinoid receptors. *J. Neurosci.* 24, 9770–9778. doi: 10.1523/jneurosci.3027-04.2004

Galarreta, M., and Hestrin, S. (1999). A network of fast-spiking cells in the neocortex connected by electrical synapses. *Nature* 402, 72–75. doi: 10.1038/47029

Gao, Y., Vasilyev, D. V., Goncalves, M. B., Howell, F. V., Hobbs, C., Reisenberg, M., et al. (2010). Loss of retrograde endocannabinoid signaling and reduced adult neurogenesis in diacylglycerol lipase knock-out mice. *J. Neurosci.* 30, 2017–2024. doi: 10.1523/JNEUROSCI.5693-09.2010

Gaykema, R. P., Luiten, P. G., Nyakas, C., and Traber, J. (1989). Cortical projection patterns of the medial septum-diagonal band complex. *J. Comp. Neurol.* 293, 103–124. doi: 10.1002/cne.902930109

Gibson, J. R., Beierlein, M., and Connors, B. W. (1999). Two networks of electrically coupled inhibitory neurons in neocortex. *Nature* 402, 75–79. doi: 10.1038/47035

Gifford, A. N., Ashby, C. R. Jr. (1996). Electrically evoked acetylcholine release from hippocampal slices is inhibited by the cannabinoid receptor agonist, WIN 552122 and is potentiated by the cannabinoid antagonist, SR 141716A. *J. Pharmacol. Exp. Ther.* 277, 1431–1436.

Glickfeld, L. L., Atallah, B. V., and Scanziani, M. (2008). Complementary modulation of somatic inhibition by opioids and cannabinoids. *J. Neurosci.* 28, 1824–1832. doi: 10.1523/JNEUROSCI.4700-07.2008

Gu, Z., and Yakel, J. L. (2011). Timing-dependent septal cholinergic induction of dynamic hippocampal synaptic plasticity. *Neuron* 14, 155–165. doi: 10.1016/j.neuron.2011.04.026

Gulyás, A. I., Szabó, G. G., Ulbert, I., Holderith, N., Monyer, H., Erdélyi, F., et al. (2010). Parvalbumin-containing fast-spiking basket cells generate the field potential oscillations induced by cholinergic receptor activation in the hippocampus. *J. Neurosci.* 30, 15134–15145. doi: 10.1523/JNEUROSCI.4104-10.2010

Haj-Dahmane, S., and Andrade, R. (1999). Muscarinic receptors regulate two different calcium-dependent non-selective cation currents in rat prefrontal cortex. *Eur. J. Neurosci.* 11, 1973–1980. doi: 10.1046/j.1460-9568.1999.00612.x

Hájos, N., Pálhalmi, J., Mann, E. O., Németh, B., Paulsen, O., and Freund, T. F. (2004). Spike timing of distinct types of GABAergic interneuron during hippocampal gamma oscillations in vitro. *J. Neurosci.* 24, 9127–9137. doi: 10.1523/jneurosci.2113-04.2004

Hájos, N., Papp, E. C., Acsády, L., Levey, A. I., and Freund, T. F. (1998). Distinct interneuron types express m2 muscarinic receptor immunoreactivity on their dendrites or axon terminals in the hippocampus. *Neurosci.* 82, 355–376. doi: 10.1016/s0306-4522(97)00300-x

Hájos, N., and Paulsen, O. (2009). Network mechanisms of gamma oscillations in the CA3 region of the hippocampus. *Neural Netw.* 22, 1113–1119. doi: 10.1016/j.neunet.2009.07.024

Halassa, M. M., and Haydon, P. G. (2010). Integrated brain circuits: astrocytic networks modulate neuronal activity and behavior. *Annu. Rev. Physiol.* 72, 335–355. doi: 10.1146/annurev-physiol-021909-135843

Halliwell, J. V. (1990). Physiological mechanisms of cholinergic action in the hippocampus. *Prog. Brain Res.* 84, 255–272. doi: 10.1016/s0079-6123(08)60910-3

Hampson, R. E., Zhuang, S. Y., Weiner, J. L., and Deadwyler, S. A. (2003). Functional significance of cannabinoid-mediated, depolarization-induced suppression of inhibition (DSI) in the hippocampus. *J. Neurophysiol.* 90, 55–64. doi: 10.1152/jn.01161.2002

Han, J., Kesner, P., Metna-Laurent, M., Duan, T., Xu, L., Georges, F., et al. (2012). Acute cannabinoids impair working memory through astroglial CB1 receptor modulation of hippocampal LTD. *Cell* 148, 1039–1050. doi: 10.1016/j.cell.2012.01.037

Hashimotodani, Y., Ohno-Shosaku, T., Tsubokawa, H., Ogata, H., Emoto, K., Maejima, T., et al. (2005). Phospholipase Cbeta serves as a coincidence detector through its Ca2+ dependency for triggering retrograde endocannabinoid signal. *Neuron* 45, 257–268. doi: 10.1016/j.neuron.2005.01.004

Hentschke, H., Perkins, M. G., Pearce, R. A., and Banks, M. I. (2007). Muscarinic blockade weakens interaction of gamma with theta rhythms in mouse hippocampus. *Eur. J. Neurosci.* 26, 1642–1656. doi: 10.1111/j.1460-9568.2007.05779.x

Holderith, N., Nemeth, B., Papp, O. I., Veres, J. M., Nagy, G. A., and Hajos, N. (2011). Cannabinoids attenuate hippocampal gamma oscillations by suppressing excitatory synaptic input onto ca3 pyramidal neurons and fast spiking basket cells. *J. Physiol.* 589, 4921–4934. doi: 10.1113/jphysiol.2011.216259

Hopkins, T. J., Rupprecht, L. E., Hayes, M. R., Blendy, J. A., and Schmidt, H. D. (2012). Galantamine, an acetylcholinesterase inhibitor and positive allosteric modulator of nicotinic acetylcholine receptors, attenuates nicotine taking and seeking in rats. *Neuropsychopharmacology* 37, 2310–2321. doi: 10.1038/npp.2012.83

Huang, C. C., and Hsu, K. S. (2010). Activation of muscarinic acetylcholine receptors induces a nitric oxide-dependent long-term depression in rat medial prefrontal cortex. *Cereb. Cortex* 20, 982–996. doi: 10.1093/cercor/bhp161

Hull, C., Adesnik, H., and Scanziani, M. (2009). Neocortical disynatpic inhibition requires somatodendritic integration in interneurons. *J. Neurosci.* 29, 8991–8995. doi: 10.1523/JNEUROSCI.5717-08.2009

Iball, J., and Ali, A. B. (2011). Endocannabinoid release modulates electrical coupling between cck cells connected via chemical and electrical synapses in CA1. *Front. Neural Circuits* 5:17. doi: 10.3389/fncir.2011.00017

Jung, K. M., Sepers, M., Henstridge, C. M., Lassalle, O., Neuhofer, D., Martin, H., et al. (2012). Uncoupling of the endocannabinoid signalling complex in a mouse model of fragile X syndrome. *Nat. Commun.* 3:1080. doi: 10.1038/ncomms2045

Kalmbach, A., Hedrick, T., and Waters, J. (2012). Selective optogenetic stimulation of cholinergic axons in neocortex. *J. Neurophysiol.* 107, 2008–2019. doi: 10.1152/jn.00870.2011

Kalmbach, A., and Waters, J. (2014). Modulation of high- and low-frequency components of the cortical local field potential via nicotinic and muscarinic acetylcholine receptors in anesthetized mice. *J. Neurophysiol.* 111, 258–272. doi: 10.1152/jn.00244.2013

Kano, M., Ohno-Shosaku, T., Hashimotodani, Y., Uchigashima, M., and Watanabe, M. (2009). Endocannabinoid-mediated control of synaptic transmission. *Physiol. Rev.* 89, 309–380. doi: 10.1152/physrev.00019.2008

Karson, M. A., Tang, A.-H., Milner, T. A., and Alger, B. E. (2009). Synaptic cross talk between perisomatic-targeting interneuron classes expressing cholecystokinin and parvalbumin in hippocampus. *J. Neurosci.* 29, 4140–4154. doi: 10.1523/JNEUROSCI.5264-08.2009

Karson, M. A., Whittington, K. C., and Alger, B. E. (2008). Cholecystokinin inhibits endocannabinoid-sensitive hippocampal IPSPs and stimulates others. *Neuropharmacology* 54, 117–128. doi: 10.1016/j.neuropharm.2007.06.023

Kathmann, M., Weber, B., Zimmer, A., and Schlicker, E. (2001). Enhanced acetylcholine release in the hippocampus of cannabinoid CB(1) receptor-deficient mice. *Br. J. Pharmacol.* 132, 1169–1173. doi: 10.1038/sj.bjp.0703987

Katona, I., Urbán, G. M., Wallace, M., Ledent, C., Jung, K. M., Piomelli, D., et al. (2006). Molecular composition of the endocannabinoid system at glutamatergic synapses. *J. Neurosci.* 26, 5628–5637. doi: 10.1523/jneurosci.0309-06.2006

Kawaguchi, Y. (1997). Selective cholinergic modulation of cortical GABAergic cell subtypes. *J. Neurophysiol.* 78, 1743–1747.

Kilb, W., and Luhmann, H. J. (2003). Carbachol-induced network oscillations in the intact cerebral cortex of the newborn rat. *Cereb. Cortex* 13, 409–421. doi: 10.1093/cercor/13.4.409

Kim, J., Isokawa, M., Ledent, C., and Alger, B. E. (2002). Activation of muscarinic acetylcholine receptors enhances the release of endogenous cannabinoids in the hippocampus. *J. Neurosci.* 22, 10182–10191.

Klausberger, T., Magill, P. J., Márton, L. F., Roberts, J. D., Cobden, P. M., Buzsáki, G., et al. (2003). Brain-state- and cell-type-specific firing of hippocampal interneurons in vivo. *Nature* 421, 844–848. doi: 10.1038/nature01374

Klausberger, T., and Somogyi, P. (2008). Neuronal diversity and temporal dynamics: the unity of hippocampal circuit operations. *Science* 321, 53–57. doi: 10.1126/science.1149381

Knox, D., and Berntson, G. G. (2008). Cortical modulation by nucleus basalis magnocellularis corticopetal cholinergic neurons during anxiety-like states is reflected by decreases in delta. *Brain Res.* 1227, 142–152. doi: 10.1016/j.brainres.2008.06.060

Kolisnyk, B., Guzman, M. S., Raulic, S., Fan, J., Magalhães, A. C., Feng, G., et al. (2013). ChAT-ChR2-EYFP mice have enhanced motor endurance but show deficits in attention and several additional cognitive domains. *J. Neurosci.* 33, 10427–10438. doi: 10.1523/JNEUROSCI.0395-13.2013

Konopacki, J., and Goebiewski, H. (1992). Theta rhythms in the rat medial entorhinal cortex in vitro: evidence for involvement of muscarinic receptors. *Neurosci. Lett.* 141, 93–96. doi: 10.1016/0304-3940(92)90342-5

Korotkova, T., Fuchs, E. C., Ponomarenko, A., von Engelhardt, J., and Monyer, H. (2010). NMDA receptor ablation on parvalbumin-positive interneurons impairs hippocampal synchrony, spatial representations and working memory. *Neuron* 68, 557–569. doi: 10.1016/j.neuron.2010.09.017

Kreitzer, A. C., and Regher, W. G. (2001). Retrograde inhibition of presynaptic calcium influx by endogenous cannabinoids at excitatory synapses onto Purkinje cells. *Neuron* 29, 717–727. doi: 10.1016/s0896-6273(01)00246-x

Krook-Magnuson, E., Luu, L., Lee, S. H., Varga, C., and Soltesz, I. (2011). Ivy and neurogliaform interneurons are a major target of μ-opioid receptor modulation. *J. Neurosci.* 31, 14861–14870. doi: 10.1523/JNEUROSCI.2269-11.2011

Lafourcade, M., Elezgarai, I., Mato, S., Bakiri, Y., Grandes, P., and Manzoni, O. J. (2007). Molecular components and functions of the endocannabinoid system in mouse prefrontal cortex. *PLoS One* 2:e709. doi: 10.1371/journal.pone.0000709

Lamotte d'Incamps, B., and Ascher, P. (2008). Four excitatory postsynaptic ionotropic receptors coactivated at the motoneuron-Renshaw cell synapse. *J. Neurosci.* 28, 14121–14131. doi: 10.1523/JNEUROSCI.3311-08.2008

Larson, J., and Lynch, G. (1986). Induction of synaptic potentiation in hippocampus by patterned stimulation involves two events. *Science* 232, 985–988. doi: 10.1126/science.3704635

Lawrence, J. J. (2008). Cholinergic control of GABA release: emerging parallels between neocortex and hippocampus. *Trends Neurosci.* 31, 317–327. doi: 10.1016/j.tins.2008.03.008

Lawrence, J. J., Grinspan, Z. M., Statland, J. M., and McBain, C. J. (2006a). Muscarinic receptor activation tunes mouse stratum oriens interneurones to amplify spike reliability. *J. Physiol.* 571, 555–562. doi: 10.1113/jphysiol.2005.103218

Lawrence, J. J., Statland, J. M., Grinspan, Z. M., and McBain, C. J. (2006b). Cell type-specific dependence of muscarinic signalling in mouse hippocampal stratum oriens interneurones. *J. Physiol.* 570, 595–610. doi: 10.1113/jphysiol.2005.100875

Lee, M. G., Chrobak, J. J., Sik, A., Wiley, R. G., and Buzsaki, G. (1994). Hippocampal theta activity following selective lesion of the septal cholinergic system. *Neuroscience* 62, 1033–1047. doi: 10.1016/0306-4522(94)90341-7

Leung, L. W. (1985). Spectral analysis of hippocampal EEG in the freely moving rat: effects of centrally active drugs and relations to evoked potentials. *Electroencephalogr. Clin. Neurophysiol.* 60, 65–77. doi: 10.1016/0013-4694(85)90952-6

Levey, A. I., Edmunds, S. M., Koliatsos, V., Wiley, R. G., and Heilman, C. J. (1995). Expression of m1–m4 muscarinic acetylcholine receptor proteins in rat hippocampus and regulation by cholinergic innervation. *J. Neurosci.* 15, 4077–4092.

Lewis, P. R., and Shute, C. C. (1967). The cholinergic limbic system: projections to hippocampal formation, medial cortex, nuclei of the ascending cholinergic reticular system and the subfornical organ and supra-optic crest. *Brain* 90, 521–540. doi: 10.1093/brain/90.3.521

Losonczy, A., Biró, A. A., and Nusser, Z. (2004). Persistently active cannabinoid receptors mute a subpopulation of hippocampal interneurons. *Proc. Natl. Acad. Sci. U S A* 101, 1362–1367. doi: 10.1073/pnas.0304752101

Lukatch, H. S., and MacIver, M. B. (1997). Physiology, pharmacology and topography of cholinergic neocortical oscillations in vitro. *J. Neurophysiol.* 77, 2427–2445.

Lund, J. S., and Lewis, D. A. (1993). Local circuit neurons of developing and mature macaque prefrontal cortex: golgi and immunocytochemical characteristics. *J. Comp. Neurol.* 328, 282–312. doi: 10.1002/cne.903280209

Maccarrone, M., Rossi, S., Bari, M., De Chiara, V., Rapino, C., Musella, A., et al. (2010). Abnormal mGlu 5 receptor/endocannabinoid coupling in mice lacking FMRP and BC1 RNA. *Neuropsychopharmacology* 35, 1500–1509. doi: 10.1038/npp.2010.19

Maejima, T., Hashimoto, K., Yoshida, T., Aiba, A., and Kano, M. (2001). Presynaptic inhibition caused by retrograde signal from metabotropic glutamate to cannabinoid receptors. *Neuron* 31, 463–475. doi: 10.1016/s0896-6273(01)00375-0

Maejima, T., Oka, S., Hashimotodani, Y., Ohno-Shosaku, T., Aiba, A., Wu, D., et al. (2005). Synaptically driven endocannabinoid release requires Ca2+-assisted metabotropic glutamate receptor subtype 1 to phospholipase Cbeta4 signaling cascade in the cerebellum. *J. Neurosci.* 25, 6826–6835. doi: 10.1523/jneurosci.0945-05.2005

Makara, J. K., Katona, I., Nyíri, G., Németh, B., Ledent, C., Watanabe, M., et al. (2007). Involvement of nitric oxide in depolarization-induced suppression of inhibition in hippocampal pyramidal cells during activation of cholinergic receptors. *J. Neurosci.* 27, 10211–10222. doi: 10.1523/jneurosci.2104-07.2007

Malomouzh, A. I., Mukhtarov, M. R., Nikolsky, E. E., and Vyskocil, F. (2007). Muscarinic M1 acetylcholine receptors regulate the non-quantal release of acetylcholine in the rat neuromuscular junction via NO-dependent mechanism. *J. Neurochem.* 102, 2110–2117. doi: 10.1111/j.1471-4159.2007.04696.x

Mann, E. O., and Paulsen, O. (2007). Role of GABAergic inhibition in hippocampal network oscillations. *Trends Neurosci.* 30, 343–349. doi: 10.1016/j.tins.2007.05.003

Manzanares, J., Corchero, J., Romero, J., Fernandez-Ruiz, J. J., Ramos, J. A., and Fuentes, J. A. (1999). Pharmacological and biochemical interactions between opioids and cannabinoids. *Trends Pharmacol. Sci.* 20, 287–294. doi: 10.1016/s0165-6147(99)01339-5

Martin, L. A., and Alger, B. E. (1999). Muscarinic facilitation of the occurrence of depolarizationinduced suppression of inhibition in rat hippocampus. *Neuroscience* 1999, 61–71. doi: 10.1016/s0306-4522(98)00745-3

Mattis, J., Tye, K. M., Ferenczi, E. A., Ramakrishnan, C., O'Shea, D. J., Prakash, R., et al. (2011). Principles for applying optogenetic tools derived from direct comparative analysis of microbial opsins. *Nat. Methods* 9, 159–172. doi: 10.1038/nmeth.1808

McCormick, D. A., and Prince, D. A. (1986). Mechanisms of action of acetylcholine in the guinea-pig cerebral cortex in vitro. *J. Physiol.* 375, 169–194.

McQuiston, A. R., and Madison, D. V. (1999a). Muscarinic receptor activity has multiple effects on the resting membrane potentials of CA1 hippocampal interneurons. *J. Neurosci.* 19, 5693–5702.

McQuiston, A. R., and Madison, D. V. (1999b). Muscarinic receptor activity induces an afterdepolarization in a subpopulation of hippocampal CA1 interneurons. *J. Neurosci.* 19, 5703–5710.

Min, R., and Nevian, T. (2012). Astrocyte signaling controls spike timing-dependent depression at neocortical synapses. *Nat. Neurosci.* 15, 746–753. doi: 10.1038/nn.3075

Morishita, W., Kirov, S. A., and Alger, B. E. (1998). Evidence for metabotropic glutamate receptor activation in the induction of depolarization-induced suppression of inhibition in hippocampal CA1. *J. Neurosci.* 18, 4870–4882.

Morishita, W., Kirov, S. A., Pitler, T. A., Martin, L. A., Lenz, R. A., and Alger, B. E. (1997). N-ethylmaleimide blocks depolarization-induced suppression of inhibition and enhances GABA release in the rat hippocampal slice in vitro. *J. Neurosci.* 17, 941–950.

Nagode, D. A., Tang, A.-H., Karson, M. A., Klugmann, M., and Alger, B. E. (2011). Optogenetic release of ACh induces rhythmic bursts of perisomatic ipscs in hippocampus. *PLoS One* 6:e27691. doi: 10.1371/journal.pone.0027691

Nagode, D. A., Tang, A. H., Yang, K., and Alger, B. E. (2014). Optogenetic identification of an intrinsic cholinergically driven inhibitory oscillator sensitive to cannabinoids and opioids in hippocampal CA1. *J. Physiol.* 592, 103–123. doi: 10.1113/jphysiol.2013.257428

Narushima, M., Uchigashima, M., Fukaya, M., Matsui, M., Manabe, T., Hashimoto, K., et al. (2007). Tonic enhancement of endocannabinoid-mediated retrograde suppression of inhibition by cholinergic interneuron activity in the striatum. *J. Neurosci.* 27, 496–506. doi: 10.1523/jneurosci.4644-06.2007

Nathanson, J. L., Yanagawa, Y., Obata, K., and Callaway, E. M. (2009). Preferential labeling of inhibitory and excitatory cortical neurons by endogenous tropism of adeno-associated virus and lentivirus vectors. *Neuroscience* 161, 441–450. doi: 10.1016/j.neuroscience.2009.03.032

Naumann, T., Kermer, P., and Frotscher, M. (1994). Fine structure of rat septohippocampal neurons. III. Recovery of choline acetyltransferase immunoreactivity after fimbria-fornix transection. *J. Comp. Neurol.* 350, 161–170. doi: 10.1002/cne.903500202

Navarrete, M., and Araque, A. (2008). Endocannabinoids mediate neuron-astrocyte communication. *Neuron* 57, 883–893. doi: 10.1016/j.neuron.2008.01.029

Navarrete, M., Perea, G., Fernandez de Sevilla, D., Gómez-Gonzalo, M., Núñez, A., Martín, E. D., et al. (2012). Astrocytes mediate in vivo cholinergic-induced synaptic plasticity. *PLoS Biol.* 10:e1001259. doi: 10.1371/journal.pbio.1001259

Nelson, A. B., Hammack, N., Yang, C. F., Shah, N. M., Seal, R. P., and Kreitzer, A. C. (2014). Striatal cholinergic interneurons drive GABA release from dopamine terminals. *Neuron* 82, 63–70. doi: 10.1016/j.neuron.2014.01.023

Neu, A., Foldy, C., and Soltesz, I. (2007). Postsynaptic origin of CB1-dependent tonic inhibition of GABA release at cholecystokinin-positive basket cell to pyramidal cell synapses in the ca1 region of the rat hippocampus. *J. Physiol.* 578, 233–247. doi: 10.1113/jphysiol.2006.115691

Newman, E. L., Climer, J. R., and Hasselmo, M. E. (2014). Grid cell spatial tuning reduced following systemic muscarinic receptor blockade. *Hippocampus* 24, 643–655. doi: 10.1002/hipo.22253

Newman, Z., Malik, P., Wu, T. Y., Ochoa, C., Watsa, N., and Lindgren, C. (2007). Endocannabinoids mediate muscarine-induced synaptic depression at the vertebrate neuromuscular junction. *Eur. J. Neurosci.* 25, 1619–1630. doi: 10.1111/j.1460-9568.2007.05422.x

Ohno-Shosaku, T., Maejima, T., and Kano, M. (2001). Endogenous cannabinoids mediate retrograde signals from depolarized postsynaptic neurons to presynaptic terminals. *Neuron* 29, 729–738. doi: 10.1016/s0896-6273(01)00247-1

Ohno-Shosaku, T., Matsui, M., Fukudome, Y., Shosaku, J., Tsubokawa, H., Taketo, M. M., et al. (2003). Postsynaptic M1 and M3 receptors are responsible for the muscarinic enhancement of retrograde endocannabinoid signalling in the hippocampus. *Eur. J. Neurosci.* 18, 109–116. doi: 10.1046/j.1460-9568.2003.02732.x

Oke, O. O., Magony, A., Anver, H., Ward, P. D., Jiruska, P., Jefferys, J. G., et al. (2010). High-frequency gamma oscillations coexist with low-frequency gamma oscillations in the rat visual cortex in vitro. *Eur. J. Neurosci.* 31, 1435–1445. doi: 10.1111/j.1460-9568.2010.07171.x

Oren, I., Hajos, N., and Paulsen, O. (2010). Identification of the current generator underlying cholinergically induced gamma frequency field potential oscillations in the hippocampal CA3 region. *J. Physiol.* 588, 785–797. doi: 10.1113/jphysiol.2009.180851

Oren, I., Mann, E. O., Paulsen, O., and Hajos, N. (2006). Synaptic currents in anatomically identified CA3 neurons during hippocampal gamma oscillations in vitro. *J. Neurosci.* 26, 9923–9934. doi: 10.1523/jneurosci.1580-06.2006

Pap, P., Koszeghy, A., Szucs, G., and Rusznák, Z. (2009). Cytoplasmic Ca(2+) concentration changes evoked by cholinergic stimulation in primary astrocyte cultures prepared from the rat cochlear nucleus. *Hear. Res.* 255, 73–83. doi: 10.1016/j.heares.2009.05.006

Pereda, A. E. (2014). Electrical synapses and their functional interactions with chemical synapses. *Nat. Rev. Neurosci.* 15, 250–263. doi: 10.1038/nrn3708

Petreanu, L., Huber, D., Sobczyk, A., and Svoboda, K. (2007). Channelrhodopsin-2-assisted circuit mapping of long-range callosal projections. *Nat. Neurosci.* 10, 663–668. doi: 10.1038/nn1891

Pietersen, A. N., Ward, P. D., Hagger-Vaughan, N., Wiggins, J., Jefferys, J. G., and Vreugdenhil, M. (2014). Transition between fast and slow gamma modes in rat hippocampus area CA1 in vitro is modulated by slow CA3 gamma oscillations. *J. Physiol.* 592, 605–620. doi: 10.1113/jphysiol.2013.263889

Pinto, L., Goard, M. J., Estandian, D., Xu, M., Kwan, A. C., Lee, S. H., et al. (2013). Fast modulation of visual perception by basal forebrain cholinergic neurons. *Nat. Neurosci.* 16, 1857–1863. doi: 10.1038/nn.3552

Pitler, T. A., and Alger, B. E. (1990). Activation of the pharmacologically defined M3 muscarinic receptor depolarizes hippocampal pyramidal cells. *Brain Res.* 534, 257–262. doi: 10.1016/0006-8993(90)90137-z

Pitler, T. A., and Alger, B. E. (1992a). Postsynaptic spike firing reduces synaptic GABAA responses in hippocampal pyramidal cells. *J. Neurosci.* 12, 4122–4132.

Pitler, T. A., and Alger, B. E. (1992b). Cholinergic excitation of GABAergic interneurons in the rat hippocampal slice. *J. Physiol.* 450, 127–142.

Povysheva, N. V., Zaitsev, A. V., Gonzalez-Burgos, G., and Lewis, D. A. (2013). Electrophysiological heterogeneity of fast-spiking interneurons: chandelier versus basket cells. *PLoS One* 12:e70553. doi: 10.1371/journal.pone.0070553

Ramírez, B. G., Blazquez, C., Gomez del Pulgar, T., Guzman, M., and de Ceballos, M. L. (2005). Prevention of Alzheimer's disease pathology by cannabinoids: neuroprotection mediated by blockade of microglial activation. *J. Neurosci.* 25, 1904–1913. doi: 10.1523/jneurosci.4540-04.2005

Reich, C. G., Karson, M. A., Karnup, S. V., Jones, L., and Alger, B. E. (2005). Regulation of IPSP theta rhythms by muscarinic receptors and endocannabinoids in hippocampus. *J. Neurophysiol.* 94, 4290–4299. doi: 10.1152/jn.00480.2005

Ren, J., Qin, C., Hu, F., Tan, J., Qiu, L., Zhao, S., et al. (2011). Habenula "cholinergic" neurons co-release glutamate and acetylcholine and activate postsynaptic neurons via distinct transmission modes. *Neuron* 69, 445–452. doi: 10.1016/j.neuron.2010.12.038

Rodriguez, R., Kallenbach, U., Singer, W., and Munk, M. H. (2004). Short- and long-term effects of cholinergic modulation on gamma oscillations and response synchronization in the visual cortex. *J. Neurosci.* 24, 10369–10378. doi: 10.1523/jneurosci.1839-04.2004

Sanchez-Alavez, M., Robledo, P., Wills, D. N., Havstad, J., and Ehlers, C. L. (2014). Cholinergic modulation of event-related oscillations (ERO). *Brain Res.* 1559, 11–25. doi: 10.1016/j.brainres.2014.02.043

Sarter, M., Parikh, V., and Howe, W. M. (2009). Phasic acetylcholine release and the volume transmission hypothesis: time to move on. *Nat. Rev. Neurosci.* 10, 383–390. doi: 10.1038/nrn2635

Singer, W., and Gray, C. M. (1995). Visual feature integration and the temporal correlation hypothesis. *Annu. Rev. Neurosci.* 18, 555–586. doi: 10.1146/annurev.neuro.18.1.555

Stewart, M., and Fox, S. E. (1989). Detection of an atropine-resistant component of the hippocampal theta rhythm in urethane-anesthetized rats. *Brain Res.* 500, 55–60. doi: 10.1016/0006-8993(89)90299-0

Stewart, M., and Fox, S. E. (1990). Do septal neurons pace the hippocampal theta rhythm? *Trends Neurosci.* 13, 163–168. doi: 10.1016/0166-2236(90)90040-h

Sul, J. Y., Orosz, G., Givens, R. S., and Haydon, P. G. (2004). Astrocytic connectivity in the hippocampus. *Neuron Glia Biol.* 1, 3–11. doi: 10.1017/s1740925x04000031

Takata, N., Mishima, T., Hisatsune, C., Nagai, T., Ebisui, E., Mikoshiba, K., et al. (2011). Astrocyte calcium signaling transforms cholinergic modulation to cortical plasticity in vivo. *J. Neurosci.* 31, 18155–18165. doi: 10.1523/JNEUROSCI.5289-11.2011

Tang, A. H., Karson, M. A., Nagode, D. A., McIntosh, J. M., Uebele, V. N., Renger, J. J., et al. (2011). Nerve terminal nicotinic acetylcholine receptors initiate quantal GABA release from perisomatic interneurons by activating axonal T-type (Cav3) Ca^{2+} channels and Ca^{2+} release from stores. *J. Neurosci.* 31, 13546–13561. doi: 10.1523/JNEUROSCI.2781-11.2011

Tanimura, A., Yamazaki, M., Hashimotodani, Y., Uchigashima, M., Kawata, S., Abe, M., et al. (2010). The endocannabinoid 2-arachidonoylglycerol produced by diacylglycerol lipase alpha mediates retrograde suppression of synaptic transmission. *Neuron* 65, 320–327. doi: 10.1016/j.neuron.2010.01.021

Tóth, K., Freund, T. F., and Miles, R. (1997). Disinhibition of rat hippocampal pyramidal cells by GABAergic afferents from the septum. *J. Physiol.* 500, 463–474.

Tort, A. B., Komorowski, R. W., Manns, J. R., Kopell, N. J., and Eichenbaum, H. (2009). Theta-gamma coupling increases during the learning of item-context associations. *Proc. Natl. Acad. Sci. U S A* 106, 20942–20947. doi: 10.1073/pnas.0911331106

Traub, R. D., Cunningham, M. O., Gloveli, T., LeBeau, F. E., Bibbig, A., Buhl, E. H., et al. (2003). GABA-enhanced collective behavior in neuronal axons underlies persistent gamma-frequency oscillations. *Proc. Natl. Acad. Sci. U S A* 100, 11047–11052. doi: 10.1073/pnas.1934854100

Trettel, J., Fortin, D. A., and Levine, E. S. (2004). Endocannabinoid signalling selectively targets perisomatic inhibitory inputs to pyramidal neurones in juvenile mouse neocortex. *J. Physiol.* 556, 95–107. doi: 10.1113/jphysiol.2003.058198

Tzavara, E. T., Wade, M., and Nomikos, G. G. (2003). Biphasic effects of cannabinoids on acetylcholine release in the hippocampus: site and mechanism of action. *J. Neurosci.* 23, 9374–9384.

van Aerde, K. I., Mann, E. O., Canto, C. B., Heistek, T. S., Linkenkaer-Hansen, K., Mulder, A. B., et al. (2009). Flexible spike timing of layer 5 neurons during dynamic beta oscillation shifts in rat prefrontal cortex. *J. Physiol.* 587, 5177–5196. doi: 10.1113/jphysiol.2009.178384

van der Zee, E. A., and Luiten, P. G. M. (1999). Muscarinic acetylcholine receptors in the hippocampus, neocortex and amygdala: a review of immunocytochemical localization in relation to learning and memory. *Prog. Neurobiol.* 58, 409–471. doi: 10.1016/s0301-0082(98)00092-6

Varma, N., Brager, D., Morishita, W., Lenz, R. A., London, B., and Alger, B. E. (2002). Presynaptic factors in the regulation of DSI expression in hippocampus. *Neuropharmacology* 43, 550–562. doi: 10.1016/s0028-3908(02)00168-5

Varma, N., Carlson, G. C., Ledent, C., and Alger, B. E. (2001). Metabotropic glutamate receptors drive the endocannabinoid system in hippocampus. *J. Neurosci.* 21, RC188.

Veeraragavan, S., Bui, N., Perkins, J. R., Yuva-Paylor, L. A., and Paylor, R. (2011a). The modulation of fragile X behaviors by the muscarinic M4 antagonist, tropicamide. *Behav. Neurosci.* 125, 783–790. doi: 10.1037/a0025202

Veeraragavan, S., Bui, N., Perkins, J. R., Yuva-Paylor, L. A., Carpenter, R. L., and Paylor, R. (2011b). Modulation of behavioral phenotypes by a muscarinic M1 antagonist in a mouse model of fragile X syndrome. *Psychopharmacology (Berl)* 217, 143–151. doi: 10.1007/s00213-011-2276-6

Vizi, E. S., and Kiss, J. P. (1998). Neurochemistry and pharmacology of the major hippocampal transmitter systems: synaptic and nonsynaptic interactions. *Hippocampus* 8, 566–607. doi: 10.1002/(sici)1098-1063(1998)8:6<566::aid-hipo2>3.0.co;2-w

Volk, L. J., Pfeiffer, B. E., Gibson, J. R., and Huber, K. M. (2007). Multiple Gq-coupled receptors converge on a common protein synthesis-dependent long-term depression that is affected in fragile x syndrome mental retardation. *J. Neurosci.* 27, 11624–11634. doi: 10.1523/jneurosci.2266-07.2007

Wang, X. J. (2010). Neurophysiological and computational principles of cortical rhythms in cognition. *Physiol. Rev.* 90, 1195–1268. doi: 10.1152/physrev.00035.2008

Whittington, M. A., Cunningham, M. O., LeBeau, F. E., Racca, C., and Traub, R. D. (2011). Multiple origins of the cortical γ rhythm. *Dev. Neurobiol.* 71, 92–106. doi: 10.1002/dneu.20814

Whittington, M. A., and Traub, R. D. (2003). Interneuron diversity series: inhibitory interneurons and network oscillations in vitro. *Trends Neurosci.* 26, 676–682. doi: 10.1016/j.tins.2003.09.016

Whittington, M. A., Traub, R. D., Faulkner, H. J., Jefferys, J. G., and Chettiar, K. (1998). Morphine disrupts long-range synchrony of gamma oscillations in hippocampal slices. *Proc. Natl. Acad. Sci. U S A* 95, 5807–5811. doi: 10.1073/pnas.95.10.5807

Widmer, H., Ferrigan, L., Davies, C. H., and Cobb, S. R. (2006). Evoked slow muscarinic acetylcholinergic synaptic potentials in rat hippocampal interneurons. *Hippocampus* 16, 617–628. doi: 10.1002/hipo.20191

Williams, J. H., and Kauer, J. A. (1997). Properties of carbachol-induced oscillatory activity in rat hippocampus. *J. Neurophysiol.* 78, 2631–2640.

Wilson, R. I., and Nicoll, R. A. (2001). Endogenous cannabinoids mediate retrograde signaling at hippocampal synapses. *Nature* 410, 588–592. doi: 10.1038/35069076

Winson, J. (1978). Loss of hippocampal theta rhythm results in spatial memory deficit in the rat. *Science* 201, 160–163. doi: 10.1126/science.663646

Woolf, N. J. (1991). Cholinergic systems in mammalian brain and spinal cord. *Prog. Neurobiol.* 37, 475–524. doi: 10.1016/0301-0082(91)90006-m

Yamada-Hanff, J., and Bean, B. P. (2013). Persistent sodium current drives conditional pacemaking in CA1 pyramidal neurons under muscarinic stimulation. *J. Neurosci.* 33, 15011–15021. doi: 10.1523/JNEUROSCI.0577-13.2013

Yamasaki, M., Matsui, M., and Watanabe, M. (2010). Preferential localization of muscarinic M1 receptor on dendritic shaft and spine of cortical pyramidal cells and its anatomical evidence for volume transmission. *J. Neurosci.* 30, 4408–4418. doi: 10.1523/JNEUROSCI.5719-09.2010

Yamawaki, N., Stanford, I. M., Hall, S. D., and Woodhall, G. L. (2008). Pharmacologically induced and stimulus evoked rhythmic neuronal oscillatory activity in the primary motor cortex in vitro. *Neuroscience* 151, 386–395. doi: 10.1016/j.neuroscience.2007.10.021

Yoshino, H., Miyamae, T., Hansen, G., Zambrowicz, B., Flynn, M., Pedicord, D., et al. (2011). Postsynaptic diacylglycerol lipase mediates retrograde endocannabinoid suppression of inhibition in mouse prefrontal cortex. *J. Physiol.* 589, 4857–4884. doi: 10.1113/jphysiol.2011.212225

Zhang, L., and Alger, B. E. (2010). Enhanced endocannabinoid signaling elevates neuronal excitability in fragile X syndrome. *J. Neurosci.* 30, 5724–5729. doi: 10.1523/JNEUROSCI.0795-10.2010

Zhang, H., Lin, S. C., and Nicolelis, M. A. (2010). Spatiotemporal coupling between hippocampal acetylcholine release and theta oscillations in vivo. *J. Neurosci.* 30, 13431–13440. doi: 10.1523/JNEUROSCI.1144-10.2010

Zoli, M., Jansson, A., Syková, E., Agnati, L. F., and Fuxe, K. (1999). Volume transmission in the CNS and its relevance for neuropsychopharmacology. *Trends Pharmacol. Sci.* 20, 142–150. doi: 10.1016/s0165-6147(99)01343-7

18

A simple implantation method for flexible, multisite microelectrodes into rat brains

Anja Richter[1†], Yijing Xie[2,3†], Anett Schumacher[4], Susanne Löffler[1], Robert D. Kirch[3], Jaafar Al-Hasani[5], Daniel H. Rapoport[5], Charli Kruse[5], Andreas Moser[1], Volker Tronnier[1], Sandra Danner[5] and Ulrich G. Hofmann[3]*

[1] Neurochemistry Group, Department of Neurology, University of Luebeck, Luebeck, Germany
[2] Graduate School for Computing in Medicine and Life Sciences, University of Luebeck, Luebeck, Germany
[3] Neuroelectronic Systems, Department of General Neurosurgery, University Hospital Freiburg, Freiburg, Germany
[4] Department of Psychology, University of Toronto Scarborough, Toronto, ON, Canada
[5] Fraunhofer Institution for Marine Biotechnology, Fraunhofer Society, Lübeck, Germany

Edited by:
Jürgen Krüger, University of Freiburg, Switzerland

Reviewed by:
Anja Kunze, University of California, Los Angeles, USA
Victor Pikov, Huntington Medical Research Institutes, USA

***Correspondence:**
Ulrich G. Hofmann, Neuroelectronic Systems, Department of General Neurosurgery, University Hospital Freiburg, c/o Engesserstr. 4, 5th floor, 79108 Freiburg, Germany
e-mail: ulrich.hofmann@uniklinik-freiburg.de

† These authors have contributed equally to this work.

A long term functional and reliable coupling between neural tissue and implanted microelectrodes is the key issue in acquiring neural electrophysiological signals or therapeutically excite neural tissue. The currently often used rigid micro-electrodes are thought to cause a severe foreign body reaction resulting in a thick glial scar and consequently a poor tissue-electrode coupling in the chronic phase. We hypothesize, that this adverse effect might be remedied by probes compliant to the soft brain tissue, i.e., replacing rigid electrodes by flexible ones. Unfortunately, this flexibility comes at the price of a low stiffness, which makes targeted low trauma implantation very challenging. In this study, we demonstrate an adaptable and simple method to implant extremely flexible microprobes even to deep areas of rat's brain. Implantation of flexible probes is achieved by rod supported stereotactic insertion fostered by a hydrogel (2% agarose in PBS) cushion on the exposed skull. We were thus able to implant very flexible micro-probes in 70 rats as deep as the rodent's subthalamic nucleus. This work describes in detail the procedures and steps needed for minimal invasive, but reliable implantation of flexible probes.

Keywords: neuroelectrophysiology, brain, implantation, flexible device, rat, deep brain, microprobes

INTRODUCTION

Electrical stimulation of discrete brain areas is a clinically increasingly used symptomatic treatment for neurological movement and affective disorders (Schlapfer and Bewernick, 2009; Pizzolato and Mandat, 2012). To further improve this treatment, the necessity arises to optimize the brain-device-interface on the cellular scale (Martens et al., 2010). With respect to this goal, pre-clinically often used microprobes for brain stimulation and recording are tethered to the skull (Hiller et al., 2007) and by nature of their rigidity present strong mechanical provocation to the surrounding tissue (Szarowski et al., 2003; Biran et al., 2007; McConnell et al., 2009). Traditionally implantable electrodes are rigid, thus showing no probe deformation during insertion (Campbell et al., 1991; Rousche and Normann, 1992). Furthermore, clinical implantation equipment provides precise location control to access brain areas specifically (Schjetnan and Luczak, 2011). After implantation, however, electrophysiological connection is impaired e.g., due to chronic gliosis, mechanical trauma or long-term inflammation (Turner et al., 1999; Polikov et al., 2005; Leach et al., 2010).

Recently, flexible microprobes have been developed from different polymers to offset this tissue scar formation by better adapting the probe's mechanical properties to the target tissue (Takeuchi et al., 2005; Kozai and Kipke, 2009; Rubehn and Stieglitz, 2010; Lee et al., 2012; Kim et al., 2013). In contrast to rigid ones, flexible implants are supposed to follow intrinsic movements of the brain resulting from breathing, blood circulation, or body movements (Rousche et al., 2001; Mercanzini et al., 2009; Rubehn and Stieglitz, 2010; Andrei et al., 2012). To test the assumption, we needed to stereotactically implant flexible microprobes in brain structures (Williams, 2008; Hassler et al., 2011). However, thin (~20 μm), film-like Polyimide microprobes are impossible to implant like the well-known rigid shank electrodes, since their inherent flexibility results in a buckling force leading to uncontrolled bending still outside the brain tissue. Instead we developed and present here a supported insertion method with the support removed after reaching the target requiring no change in Polyimide probe design. This method enables the insertion of Polyimide-based, ~20 μm thick, 350 μm wide and 1.5 cm long electrodes down to the subthalamic nucleus (~8.5 mm) of rat's brain using commercially available stereotactic equipment (David Kopf Instruments, Model 900).

MATERIALS AND METHODS

See the accompanying video for a visualized version of the protocol. A list of materials required for this procedure can be found in **Table 1**. We strongly recommend to practice this procedure with already euthanized animals from other experiments prior to *in vivo* application. A competent handling of all instruments is strongly recommended to achieve reproducible results.

Table 1 | Specific reagents and equipment required for this approach.

Name of the reagent	Company	Catalog number
Surgical disposable scalpel #21	Braun Aesculap AG	5518075
Surgical disposable scalpel #23	Braun Aesculap AG	5518016
Cotton swabs, walnut sized	Henry Schein Medical GmbH	9003187
5/0 Premilene-DS16 surgical sutures	Braun Aesculap AG	2090212
Leukofix fixing tape	Henry Schein Medical GmbH	220-544
Tungsten rod ø 140 μm	A-M Systems, Inc.	7166
Loctite 4061 rapid glue	Henkel Loctite GmbH	26085
0.9 mm drill bit	FineScienceTools, USA	19007-09
Rechargeable Cordless Micro Drill	Stoelting Co., USA	58610
Small Animal Stereotaxic Instrument	David Kopf Instruments, USA	Model 900
7.5% betaisodona solution	B. Braun Melsungen AG	3864154
Softasept (74.1% Ethanol and 10% 2-Propanol)	B. Braun Melsungen AG	3887138
Agarose, low gelling temperature (<65°C)	Sigma-Aldrich Co.	A9414
Anaesthetics and other medicine according to approved procedures.		

PRESURGICAL PREPARATION PROCEDURE

Aseptic technique should be used for all survival surgical procedures. Disinfect the surgical work surface with commercial disinfectant and prepare sterile surgical packs of instruments, drapes, gauze, swabs, sutures, and scalpel blades. A surgical mask, hair bonnet and sterile gloves should be worn. A Germinator dry bead sterilizer is also used to re-sterilize surgical instruments between procedures if multiple rat surgeries will be done during one session. Preparation of the rats including disinfection, anesthesia and positioning in the stereotactic frame was performed according to standardized stereotactic procedures, which were reviewed and approved by committees of the University of Lübeck and the responsible Ministry for Agriculture, Environment and Rural Areas, Schleswig-Holstein, Germany.

Adult, male Wistar rats (250–300 g) were anesthetized using an i.p. injection of a Ketamine/Xylazine cocktail [100 mg/kg Ketamine (100 mg/ml), 8 mg/kg Xylazine (2%)]. This amount is generally sufficient for a typical 60 min surgery. If needed, rats can be redosed using a fraction of the original dose. Disinfectant (Softasept) was applied to the scalp starting from the center of the surgical region, spiraling outward and then rinsed with Ringer's solution. The surgical field was prepared by shaving the area using small animal shears. Protective ointment (Bepanthene® nose and eye cream) was applied to the eyes to prevent drying and to provide a physical barrier during surgery. Anesthetized and shaved rats were placed in a stereotactic frame with atraumatic ear bars (tooth bar = 0.0)[1].

As an insertion tool we clamped a tungsten rod (ø140–175 μm) to the head of a stereotactic arm. The length of the tungsten rod below the clamp head should be ~2 cm to provide sufficient space for manipulations. The rod must be perfectly straight, as can be tested by rolling it on a flat ground.

SKIN INCISION AND PREPARATION OF SUBCUTANEOUS TISSUE TO EXPOSE SKULL

A midline incision of ~1.5 cm length starting between the ears (bregma) and extending toward the nose was made with a scalpel. The subcutaneous tissue was prepared bluntly with two cotton swabs by vigorous but slow rubbing from the center to the periphery of the wound. This stretches the cutaneous and subcutaneous tissues and opens the operation area above the skull. It has to be performed until the necessary operation area is free of all tissues above the skull bone and bleeding has stopped. A well prepared skull is indicated by a typical squeaking sound when rubbing the swab on the bone.

WIDENING OF THE SURGICAL FIELD

A wide, flat operation area is essential for successful implantation. Wound rims were fixed using surgical suture loops (5/0 Premilene-DS16). Loop ends are fixed at the frame with a non-residue tape (Leukofix) while carefully pulling the wound boundaries apart and thus widening the surgical area. That way the desired anatomical orientation points become visible, in our case lambda and the interaural line. We strongly recommend folding the skin on the rostral end by a double stitch which lessens traumatization. If necessary such a loop can be used to fix the caudal end of the wound rim as well.

ADJUSTMENT OF THE STEREOTACTIC FRAME AND TARGETING

The wound area was washed with Ringer's solution and cleaned with walnut sized cotton swabs prior to targeting. The stereotactic arm is positioned such that the securely mounted insertion tool was moved to the anatomical reference point of choice (lambda in our case). The target coordinates were determined according to the medial:lateral and anterior:posterior axes found in a stereotactic atlas. The insertion arm of the stereotactic frame was positioned over the target point and the tungsten rod was carefully lowered until it touched the skull. The z-position was noted and the target depth was calculated[1].

TREPANNING THE SKULL

First, the target point was marked on the skull by careful circular nicking the bone with a 20 G needle below the tungsten rod. The produced cavity is used as starting point for drilling—otherwise the skull may be too slippery for precise drilling. When

[1]One of the reviewers recommends for improved animal welfare the following steps in addition to the demonstrated ones:

(a) Before securing ears in earbars, apply Antipyrine-Benzocaine otic solution to ears.

(b) For monitoring depth of anesthesia and overall animal health, it is helpful to insert rectal thermometer probe.

(c) Removal of subcutaneous tissue can be done more effectively by cutting the muscle with the scalpel and scraping periosteum with a Freer chisel while controlling the skull bleeding with bone wax.

(d) After drilling the skull and before puncturing the meninges, it is suggested to apply Sensorcaine (bupivacaine with epinephrine) to the cortex to produce local anesthesia and vasospasms (to reduce cortical bleeding).

not needed *in situ*, the stereotactic arm was moved out of harms way to carefully maintain insertion rod registration.

A handheld microdrill with a small drill bit (here 0.9 mm ø) was then used to make the burr hole. Drilling was done in short intervals (depending upon the power output of the drill) and drill progress was controlled visually in between. The complete penetration of the skull bone is clearly noticeable by a sudden loss in resistance to the drill bit. Carefully remove it from the drill site and flush all bone fragments with Ringer's solution. Lesser experienced surgeons may want to use a stop above the drill tip by slipping a cylinder, cut from a medical tubing, over the drill. For the price of a slightly diminished view, the drill won't penetrate deeper than the catch allows and thus minimizes uncontrolled brain penetration (Pohl et al., 2011).

PENETRATION OF THE MENINGES

A successful drilling procedure will leave meninges intact, shimmering opaque at the base of the burr hole. Removing them in a controlled way was done with a slightly nicked 23 G cannula tip. Twisting the cannula's now ridgy tip on the base of the hole and pulling it produces a noticeable rupture of the elastic dura mater. Severing the pia mater results in bleeding, which has to be flushed away until it stops. The repetition of this step along the boundary of the hole may be necessary until no more elastic resistance exists. If successfully performed, this step leaves no opaque meninges remaining in the burr hole. This part of the procedure may impair recordings from superficial layers of the cortex.

INTRODUCING AN AGAROSE BLOCK INTO THE OPERATION AREA

All of the steps up until this point are standard for any type of stereotactic intervention in a rat's brain. Next, we introduced a novel tool to facilitate implantation of flexible microprobes. A block of 2 mm height from 2% (w/v) agarose gel was placed over the burr hole on the skull with a sterile spatula. One edge of the block was lodged under the anterior wound fold with close contact to the anterior borders. The posterior part of the gel block extended over the caudal wound boundaries thus increasing the working area. This afforded a slight slope down to the anterior edge of the wound, which facilitated the subsequent microprobe insertion. The airspace between the agar block and the skull was filled by injecting Ringer's solution, which released trapped air bubbles from beneath the surface of the gel block. Ringer's solution was also used to maintain a moist and slippery working surface.

Using this agarose gel block improves the positioning of the flexible probes, keeps the exposed brain surface moist, and avoids scratching the probe's surface on skull bone. In addition, the 2% agarose gel block facilitates close wrapping of the probe around the insertion rod. To estimate the effects of using 2% agarose gel in probe insertion, we performed a dummy insertion experiment in a brain-tissue-like phantom (**Figures 1A,B**). **Figures 1C,D.** demonstrate the difference of implantation channel width without and with 2% agarose block in a brain phantom (Chen et al., 2004).

POSITIONING OF THE IMPLANT AND INSERTION START

The flexible microprobe was transferred with a pair of tweezers from its sterile storage onto the gel block, as precise and flat as possible, with the tip positioned 5–6 mm past the insertion site. The stereotactically mounted insertion rod was again positioned above the target point (**Figure 2A1**). As soon as the tungsten rod is inserted, it pushes the probe into the burr hole (**Figures 2A2–A4**). The flexible microprobe aligns itself along the rod, thus minimizing cross-section and trauma upon insertion into brain tissue (**Figures 2A5,A6**). To visualize and evaluate the insertion procedure, we showed here in **Figure 2B** a sequence of side-view images of probe insertion with a tungsten rod into a translucent brain-tissue-like phantom.

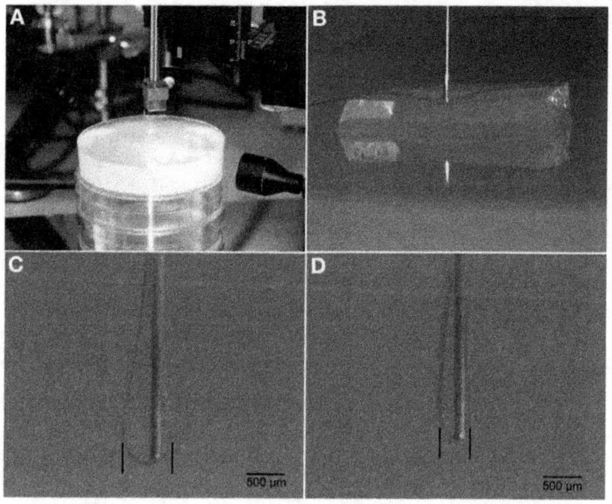

FIGURE 1 | Illustrations of test insertions of flexible probes into a brain phantom. (A). Experimental setup including 2% agarose gel. **(B).** Micrograph of insertion rod on top of flex probe and agarose cushion. **(C).** Insertion result in brain phantom without agarose cushion. **(D).** Insertion result with agarose cushion. Note the difference of spread of flex probe around the implantation rod.

The transparent agarose block allowed for visual control of the relative alignment of the microprobe and the insertion rod. The diffraction at the gel/air boundary may give the appearance of missing the burr hole, which is a known optical illusion. Additional Ringer's solution applied to the gel block minimizes friction, which is essential for maintaining mobility of the microprobe during the insertion procedure. Additional bleedings upon insertion is usually a result of an incomplete disruption of the pia mater and thus must be avoided with proper preparation of the entry hole. Finally, the microprobe was partially inserted by advancing the insertion rod until a desired length of the microprobe remained outside of the skull.

REMOVAL OF THE AGAROSE BLOCK AND INSERTION FINISHING

The part of the agarose gel anterior to the insertion rod was cut parallel to the interaural line using a scalpel. The anterior gel block can now be removed by shoving it away from the insertion rod. The microprobe's connector pad, meanwhile, was very gently flipped toward the tungsten rod and thus moved out of harm's way. Subsequently, the posterior triangle of the gel is shoved out of the wound area. Manipulation of agarose gel was accomplished with a sharp scalpel tip, as it is too slippery for forceps, but easily pinned down by the blade. After the agarose block had been

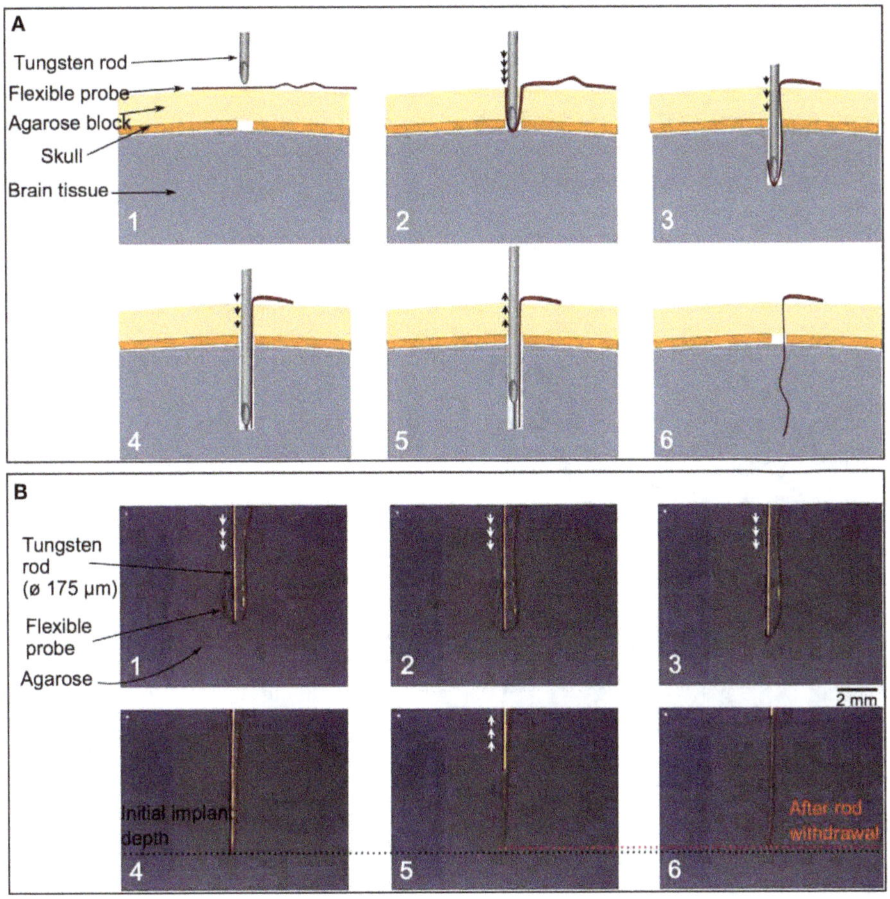

FIGURE 2 | A schematic cross-section of the insertion field (A). The arrows indicate the tungsten rod movement direction. Above the brain tissue (gray) the skull and meningeal layer (dark orange) display a burr hole (white space). The tailored agarose cushion (light orange) is used as an insertion matrix for the flexible probe (red) (A: 1). Advancing the insertion tungsten rod (upper grey structure) along the planned trajectory the probe wraps around the rod's tip and is thus arranged by the gel for optimal control (A: 2–4). After the flexible probe is completely straightened, the insertion rod is withdrawn slowly from the remaining probe (A: 5, 6). Image sequence of inserting a flexible probe with a tungsten rod (with flat tip, ø 175 μm) to a 0.5 % agarose gel **(B)**. The arrows indicate the tungsten rod movement direction. During the insertion, the flexible probe first folds and wraps around the rod (B: 1–3). Until it reaches the planned depth position (the black dotted line) and cis ompletely straightened, the insertion rod is withdrawn (B: 4, 6). The red dotted line in panels B5 and B6 indicates the depth position of the flexible probe tip after the rod is removed. It illustrates a misplacement of around 100 μm from the initial depth position.

removed completely, the microprobe insertion was finalized until the desired target depth was reached.

MOUNTING OF THE IMPLANT

Remaining Ringer's solution was removed and the skull thoroughly dried using cotton swabs. The microprobe was fixed to the skull using a small spot of medical super glue (Loctite) deposited at least 5 mm posterior to the burr hole. The connector pad was pushed down into the glue using a scalpel tip. Forceps are not recommended here, since the glue may rapidly fix their arms shut, which will destroy the entire implantation upon the ensuing struggle to free them. A scalpel, however, easily cuts itself free through gentle twisting.

The connector pad was covered with another drop of glue and upon solidifying, the tungsten rod was removed from the brain by smooth and continuous upward movements. The entire area is flushed clean with Ringer's solution, which polymerizes all leftover super glue. A pair of forceps were used to carefully scrape all inadvertently fixed connective tissue free.

The wound closure may be performed according to the experimental needs. In our histological study we sutured the skin over the implantation site, cleaned the suture with Ringer's solution and applied iodide disinfectant and local anesthetic. The animal was monitored and kept warm on a temperature controlled plate until it was fully awake.

RESULTS

The most significant result of this method is the successful implantation of very flexible, film-like microprobes into deep brain regions with minimal tissue disruption. Cross-sectional histology demonstrated that we reliably reached our target point deep in the brain of rats.

One week after surgery we observed in the implanted rats the inevitable lesion caused by the insertion needle next to the implant (**Figure 3**). The tissue reaction was evident from a thin glial layer homogeneously surrounding the implantation lesion. A clear, but thin brain-probe-interface without cysts is indicative for a good connectivity to the target area adjacent to the implant. After four weeks a cyst-free tissue next to the implantation-site was visible (the central free space is the original position of the implant, moved upon slicing), indicating a good mechanical connectivity of the implant to the target area (**Figure 4**).

High precision and successful implantation was corroborated by recording electrophysiological signals from neuronal tissue adjacent to the target area (subthalamic nucleus) immediately following implantation (**Figure 5**) and four weeks post-surgery with flex probes of slightly different design. Detailed histological data will be published elsewhere. Seventy animals have undergone this procedure to date and all of them survived without incident until the planned euthanasia six months following surgery.

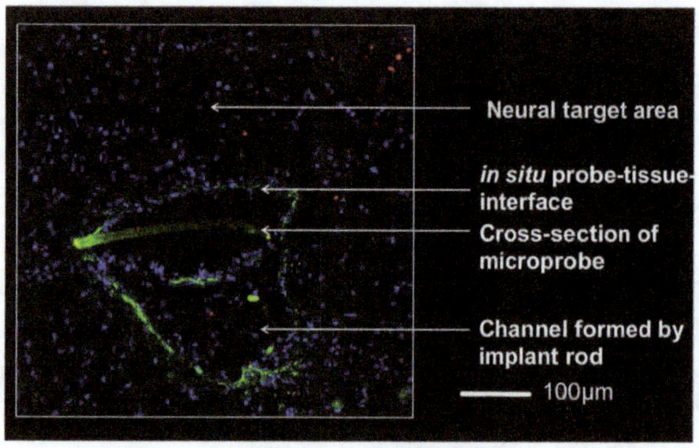

FIGURE 3 | Micrograph of the implantation area one week after implantation 4,5 mm below the brain surface. The rod supported insertion of the microprobe yields an implantation channel on one side of the slightly crescent-shaped probe (350 μm wide). Invading cells to this region are indicated by stained nuclei (DAPI, blue). A thin glial layer (glial fibrillary acidic protein, green) surrounds the lesion and reflects a mild tissue reaction. The lack of a pronounced extracellular matrix layer (chondroitinsulfate proteoglycan, red) supports this observation. The brain-probe-interface showed no cysts. Magnification 20x with an PlanApochromat-Objective at AxioObserver Z.1 (Carl Zeiss MicroImaging GmbH, Germany).

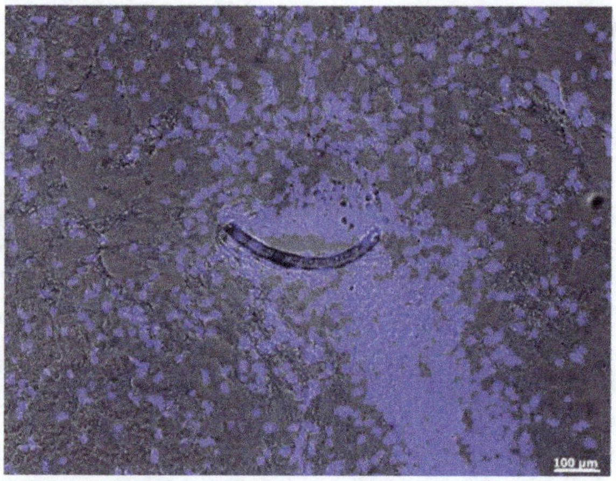

FIGURE 4 | Microprobe cross-section (crescent-shaped strip) in an horizontal slice of the subthalamic nucleus of an implanted rat 4 weeks after surgery. This micrograph combines fluorescence and bright-field illumination, where nuclei (blue) are stained with DAPI. Magnification 10x with an PlanApochromat-Objective using an AxioObserver Z.1 (Carl Zeiss MicroImaging GmbH, Germany).

DISCUSSION

Although the hypothesis on the beneficial effect of the probe's elasticity matching the brain's was mentioned more than a decade ago (Stieglitz and Meyer, 1999), all efforts to use flexible probes on a large scale were less efficient due to the difficulty to implant them in a reliable way in deeper brain regions (Rousche et al., 2001; Kozai and Kipke, 2009). We thus started with an established procedure for implantation of rigid electrodes and modified it to our needs. The animals implanted with our technique all survived the implantation without exception. No abnormalities of movements and/or behavior were developed post operatively. Histological examination confirmed the positioning of the implant in the target area with minimal tissue disruption. To ensure reproducibility and best possible use of limited time under anesthesia, we strongly recommend to exercise this procedure with agarose dummies or dead animals before starting on living ones. There are several finely tuned handling steps, which require sensitive use of instruments, microprobe and surgical technique. A well experienced experimenter will need less than one hour for the entire procedure, for which the initial dose of Ketamine/Xylazine-cocktail may not quite suffice. Deep anesthesia has to be maintained at all times by re-injecting fractions of the initial dose.

The extremely cautious use of the miniature power drill and the subsequent removal of the meninges is essential for exerting minimal tissue damage. An automatized drill system may reduce the risk of severe brain trauma (Pohl et al., 2012).

However, in our view the highest optimization potential remaining is the design of the insertion tool/microprobe connection. This study was based on temporarily fixating both by dynamic forces, a removable anchoring of the probe to the insertion tool might improve positioning even further as was

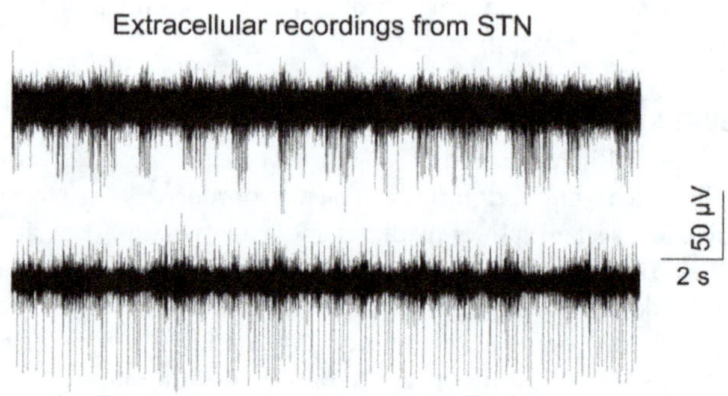

FIGURE 5 | Typical signal trace recorded from the subthalamic nucleus right after insertion of a flexible microprobe; bandpass filtered (400–4000 kHz) and sampled with 24414 kHz. Recording was done with an electrical connected flexible microprobe as described in Löffler et al. (2012).

19

Major unsolved points in adult neurogenesis: doors open on a translational future?

Paolo Peretto*[1,2]* *and Luca Bonfanti*[1,3]

[1] *Neuroscience Institute Cavalieri Ottolenghi, Orbassano, Italy*
[2] *Department of Life Sciences and System Biology, University of Turin, Torino, Italy*
[3] *Department of Veterinary Sciences, University of Turin, Torino, Italy*

Edited by:
Verdon Taylor, University of Sheffield, UK

Reviewed by:
Hans Georg Kuhn, University of Gothenburg, Sweden
Nicolas Toni, University of Lausanne, Switzerland

****Correspondence:***
Paolo Peretto, Department of Life Sciences and Systems Biology, University of Turin, Via Accademia Albertina 13, 10123 Torino, Italy
e-mail: paolo.peretto@unito.it;
Luca Bonfanti, Department of Veterinary Sciences, University of Turin, Via Leonardo da Vinci, 44, 10095 Grugliasco, Italy
e-mail: luca.bonfanti@unito.it

In spite of many data gathered during the last two decades on adult neurogenesis (AN) it is evident that such knowledge is not sufficient for granting translational outcomes in brain repair, especially if the ultimate goal is to promote cell replacement. Alternative strategies aimed at fostering AN physiological functions (restorative approaches) are still undefined. By asking the question whether AN research field has to be considered as a dead end in the context of brain repair, here we review some unresolved issues: multifaceted evolutionary constraints in mammals, stem/progenitor cell type/availability and tissue permissivity, impact on other brain functions, interplay with other forms of plasticity, and relevance in humans. We suggest that full understanding of AN biology is an essential step for its possible exploitation in brain repair, and that further fundamental, multidisciplinary research is required to reach translational outcomes. Scientist's attitude and their communication skills are also important. To avoid overestimation of AN reparative potential in a translational perspective, more distant goals of cell replacement should be kept clearly distinct from restorative approaches involving AN functional plasticity.

Keywords: brain repair, neurodegenerative diseases, regenerative medicine, therapeutic approaches, neural stem cells, parenchymal progenitors, cell therapy, brain evolution

Two decades of investigation on adult neurogenesis (AN) yielded an utterly new vision of brain plasticity and opened new perspectives for brain repair/regeneration strategies. Nevertheless, the ultimate goal of exploiting neurogenic processes for obtaining cell replacement is still far from being achieved. Starting from this antinomy, the big question is: should be the AN research field considered as a dead end in the perspective of brain repair, or, alternatively, is it worthwhile to put in place further efforts in order to solve the problem? By reading the scientific literature, it is clear that all neurobiologists, even believing in an AN translational future, do not share the same answer. Non-univocal visions are normal in a field that has developed by progressively ramifying in many directions accordingly to the different goals pursued by each research group. Some scientists primarily deal with AN physiological roles/mechanisms, apparently being less interested in direct translation of results. Others are mainly focused on aspects that implement AN, or directly address the issue of injury-induced, reactive neurogenesis, paying less attention to the peculiar limits of the mammalian CNS in repairing damage. New translational perspectives in "restorative" rather than "structural reparative" neurology have been recently raised, what could be useful in slowing down the impact of various neurologic impairments (e.g., those occurring in neurodegenerative, vascular, traumatic diseases, age-related cognitive decline), even in the absence of cell replacement. Nevertheless, it is evident that knowledge gathered during the last two decades is not yet sufficient for granting translation of basic neurobiological research. Such inability is linked to several unresolved issues in both physiological and lesion-induced neurogenesis, and to scarcely integrated views between different approaches used to address AN studies. In other words, even in the absence of current, effective therapeutic outcomes, we may not be at a dead end, rather we are in the middle of a route with many new "perfectly reasonable deviations from the beaten track" (Feynman, 2005).

THE PRESENT KNOWLEDGE IN MAMMALS: SOME LIGHTS IN THE DARK

Our knowledge of AN in mammals might be grouped in two domains: first, some facts and concepts which are definitively accepted and substantially understood by the scientific community ("acquired knowledge"), and second, a number of issues which remain largely obscure and/or underestimated ("gaps of knowledge"). The main blocks of acquired knowledge can be summarized as follows: (i) two canonical neurogenic zones (subventricular zone, SVZ, and subgranular zone, SGZ) harboring stem cell niches provide neural cell addition into the olfactory bulb and hippocampus (Ming and Song, 2011); we know a lot about their anatomical organization and functional regulation as well as the integration of the newly born neurons (Fuentealba et al., 2012; Tong and Alvarez-Buylla, 2014; Vadodaria and Gage, 2014); (ii) wide areas of the central nervous system (CNS) out of the canonical neurogenic sites host cycling and/or quiescent progenitors which give rise to different processes of non-canonical cell genesis: parenchymal gliogenesis (Boda and Buffo, 2010; Trotter et al., 2010), parenchymal neurogenesis (Bonfanti and Peretto, 2011) and periventricular neurogenesis (Migaud et al.,

2010); little is known about non-canonical cell genesis, which seems to lack integration within the parenchyma; (iii) progenitors in both canonical and non-canonical neurogenic sites are activated in different pathological conditions (Arvidsson et al., 2002; Luzzati et al., 2011); in spite of such activation, the response to injury is substantially non-coordinated and/or abortive, not leading to effective brain repair (Kernie and Parent, 2010; Bonfanti, 2011; Bonfanti and Peretto, 2011).

Behind these blocks of acquired knowledge large amounts of unknown facts and concepts are still hidden. First of all, AN remarkable plasticity has introduced a new kind of complexity: that of dynamic, developmental-like processes related to neuronal addition occurring within a substantially static tissue. Moreover, in mammals, the CNS is structurally, functionally, and evolutionarily refractory to repair, healing, and regeneration. These facts make it extremely challenging to exploit AN as a therapeutic tool, also because the variables involved are dependent among each other and linked by different hierarchies (**Figure 1**). Here, we will analyze the key points still remaining open in the AN field, considering them as potential hurdles to a full understanding of the biological process itself, and, in turn, to its possible exploitation for brain repair.

AN PHYSIOLOGICAL FUNCTION(S) vs. BRAIN REPAIR: EVOLUTIONARY ASPECTS

Unlike most vertebrates, in adult mammals spontaneous neurogenesis is primarily linked to homeostatic/physiological roles and hardly directed to repair (Bonfanti, 2011). This view is supported by many studies which addressed the issue of reactive (lesion-induced) neurogenesis, indicating "activation" of neural progenitors which substantially do not provide cell replacement, most of the newly born/mobilized cells being fated to die (Kernie and Parent, 2010; Luzzati et al., 2011).

The fact that many non-mammalian vertebrates can perform brain repair/regeneration (Endo et al., 2007; Grandel and Brand, 2013) underlines the involvement of evolutionary aspects at the developmental, anatomical, stem cell types/availability and tissue-specific environment levels (Bonfanti, 2011). The occurrence of AN in the CNS of all vertebrates suggests the naive (and wrong) view of a direct relationship between neurogenic activity and regenerative capability (Ferretti, 2011): AN is not sufficient for regeneration to occur, and other aspects should be considered. Beside lower intrinsic regenerative properties (and lower availability of stem/progenitor cells), the mammalian CNS is characterized by more detrimental tissue reactions, in fact hampering regeneration. Immune cell activation leading to inflammation is an early response after injury that is common to most animal groups. Yet, whereas in many non-mammalian vertebrates initial acute inflammation stimulates regeneration without subsequent detrimental tissue responses, in mammals neuroinflammation leads to the formation of the glial scar with consequent impairment of regeneration (Mescher and Neff, 2006; Sofroniew, 2009; Kyritsis et al., 2014). In other words, stem/progenitor cell availability alone cannot grant regenerative capacity if glial cell activation and inflammatory reactions also occur. A theory explains the failure in mammalian brain repair as a result of evolutionary constraints in which the injured CNS would not favor a strategy of regeneration, but rather one of minimizing further damage (Weil et al., 2008). Hence, important gaps of knowledge still exist, both in mammals and other vertebrates, concerning homeostatic/metabolic functions and tissue reaction aspects linked to AN, and the role of the immune system, which still remain largely unexplored (Schwartz et al., 2013). All these variables are involved in determining the differences between neurogenic and non-neurogenic tissue local environments, and, in turn, their permissivity to reparative processes.

PROGENITOR CELLS, TISSUE ENVIRONMENT, AND AN OUTCOME(S)

Although cell proliferation exists throughout the intact CNS and is enhanced by several physiological/pathological conditions, it does not produce substantial neurogenic outcomes in the parenchyma out of the canonical sites (olfactory bulb, dentate gyrus). The main aspects that seem essential in granting CNS neurogenic/reparative capacity are: occurrence of specialized progenitor types and tissue permissivity. The SVZ and SGZ neurogenic niches harbor stem cells that appear very specified in their commitment (Obernier et al., 2014) and thus hard to divert toward other fates. As to parenchymal neural progenitors in non-canonical sites it is not yet clear what is their origin, nature, fate, and function(s). Yet, these cells do represent promising substrates for future research for several reasons (abundance, widespread distribution, region-specific differentiative commitment). Wherever stem/progenitor cells are located, both in canonical and non-canonical sites, unraveling the mechanisms underlying their quiescence or activation is also essential for their possible manipulation (Basak et al., 2012). Nevertheless, the functional availability of proper stem/progenitor cells is not sufficient to grant AN and repair in the absence of a receptive tissue environment: olfactory bulb and hippocampus circuits are permissive to neuronal integration, whereas the mature parenchyma allows less or no integration (Bonfanti and Peretto, 2011).

Taken together, these facts add hurdles to the ultimate goal of making mammalian AN processes useful for cell replacement. In spite of a large amount of data concerning the regulation of canonical AN (in terms of modulation; see Kempermann, 2011), very little is known about the cellular/molecular factors which allow the interaction between progenitors and the mature CNS tissue (permissivity) both in neurogenic and non-neurogenic sites. Such tissue permissivity is strictly linked to intrinsic features (adhesion molecules, extracellular matrix, availability of growth factors, etc.) which are maintained and/or delayed from development, thus allowing the AN process to persist during adulthood. In this context, a few studies have thoroughly investigated the steps that drive and regulate the shift between embryonic and AN.

ANIMAL MODELS vs. HUMANS

Most knowledge on AN has been gathered on laboratory rodents, what is a clear limit for translational approaches. Indeed, neurogenic processes differ quite among mammals as to their location, rate, niche organization, and the postnatal temporal windows in which they occur (Bonfanti and Peretto, 2011). For instance,

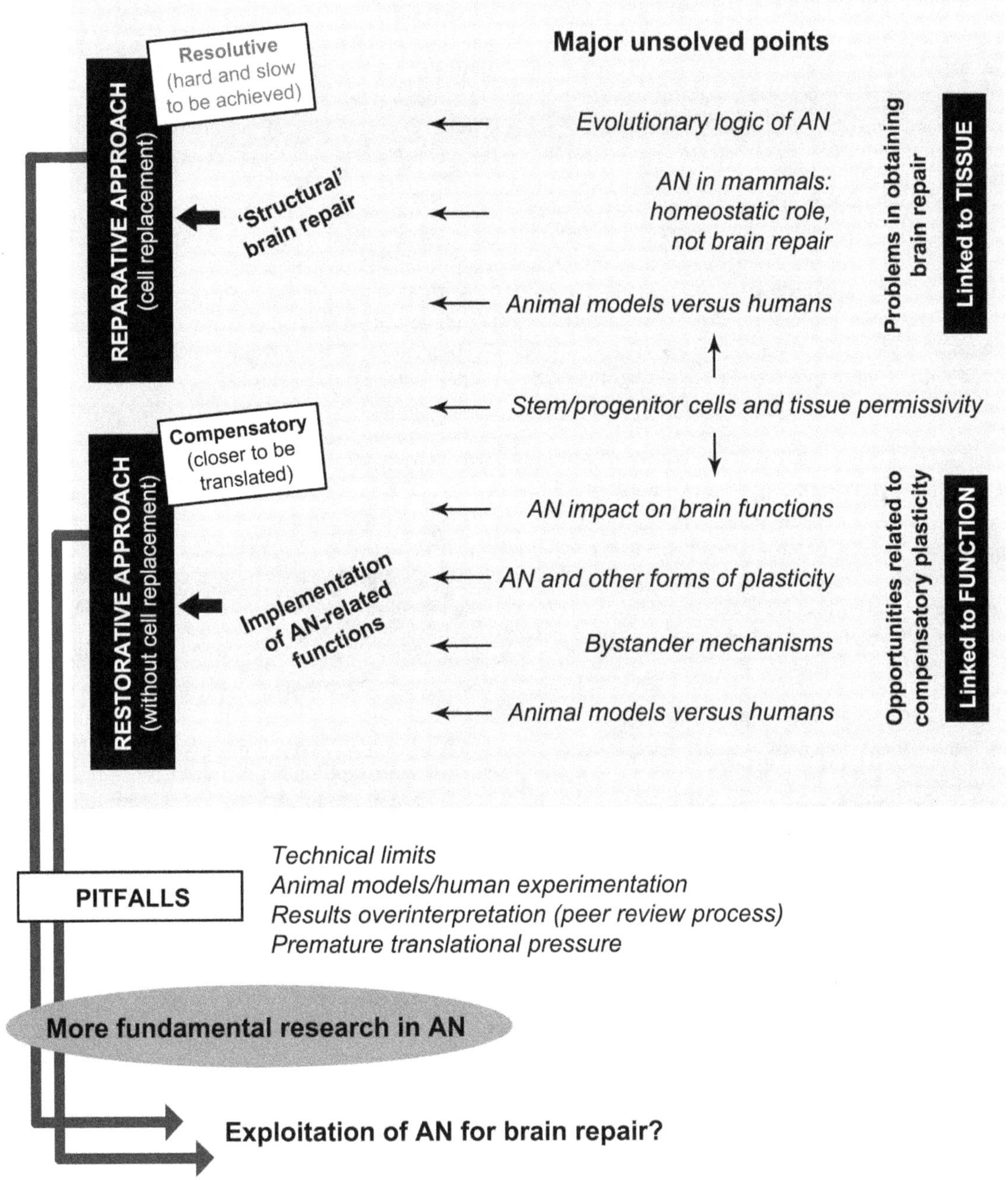

FIGURE 1 | Interplay between adult neurogenesis (AN), some of its major unsolved points, and possible perspectives for brain repair. Gray box: among many open issues still existing in the potential role of AN in neural plasticity (gaps of knowledge), a general distinction should be made between: (i) tissue-related problems depending on evolutionary issues and hampering brain repair/regeneration (top), and (ii) function-related opportunities depending on possible homeostatic roles of AN which could be exploited/implemented for restorative approaches (bottom). Stem/progenitor cell availability and tissue permissivity (middle) are essential aspects for allowing translational perspectives to be figured out in both directions. Reparative approaches, which imply cell replacement as the ultimate goal of regenerative medicine, are not available at present. Restorative approaches include different therapeutic perspectives linked to the implementation of physiological functions of AN aimed at obtaining compensatory plasticity in the absence of cell replacement, both in the damaged and undamaged (age-related decline) brain. Successful achievement of these goals is linked to further investments in fundamental research by overcoming of current pitfalls in the AN field.

while cell migration from SVZ to olfactory bulb persists throughout life in mice, it is exhausted very early in human infants (Sanai et al., 2011). In the human hippocampus, measures of ^{14}C concentration in genomic DNA show a substantially constant rate of AN through ages, in contrast with an evident decrease in young rodents (Spalding et al., 2013). Also parenchymal neurogenesis remarkably varies among mammals, showing species-specific regional localizations (Luzzati et al., 2006; Ponti et al., 2008).

Other inter-mammalian differences concern specific functions related to the ecological needs and behavioral activity of the animals (Barker et al., 2011).

Besides AN heterogeneity, mammals also differ in their brain anatomy and physiology (Carlson, 2012), and this can affect the impact AN might exert on the whole brain function (see below). Also the average lifespan varies among mammals, thus implying that differences in postnatal development of CNS areas, brain maturation, puberty, make it difficult to compare AN in different species (Lindsey and Tropepe, 2006; Kuhn and Blomgren, 2011). Hence, restraining AN research to laboratory rodents may introduce several bias in the search for translational outcomes. If comparative/evolutionary studies through phylogeny are essential to unravel the common logic of AN, the study of differences among mammals are also important for correctly interpreting/modeling the possible contribution of AN to homeostasis and brain repair in humans.

TO WHICH EXTENT AN IMPACTS THE BRAIN FUNCTION?

Addition of newborn neurons in the olfactory bulb and hippocampus optimizes neurological functions/behaviors such as social interaction/reproduction, memory, learning, and pattern separation (Sahay et al., 2011; Feierstein, 2012). These two brain regions are essential for behavioral outputs critical for survival of the individuals and species (Mucignat-Caretta et al., 2012; Snyder and Cameron, 2012). Accordingly, AN is assumed as a mechanism which promotes life-long adaptability of individuals to environmental complexity and novelty (Freund et al., 2013). Regulation of AN is achieved through integration of multiple external and internal stimuli, which implies activity of multiple brain regions/circuits and complex feedback loops (Kempermann, 2011). Thus, though restricted to the olfactory bulb and hippocampus, AN potentially impacts diverse brain functions (Snyder and Cameron, 2012; Lepousez et al., 2013), which might explain that in mammals it occurs only in two regions. Although little is known on this hypothesis, since the anatomical, functional, molecular bases underlying the above mentioned interactions are far from being clarified, the possible impact of AN on other brain functions/circuits can have important translational implications (Leuner and Gould, 2010; Kheirbek et al., 2012; Snyder and Cameron, 2012; Quadrato et al., 2014). Several data are already available on the link between hippocampus, pattern separation/overgeneralization of sensory stimuli and anxiety disorders (Leuner and Gould, 2010; Kheirbek et al., 2012). The recent finding that human hippocampal AN appears substantially maintained during adulthood (Spalding et al., 2013) adds new interest to this issue, also in the perspective of implementing cognitive functions during aging (Bordey, 2014). Yet, proper translational outcomes imply definitive clarification of the real rate/impact of AN in humans during postnatal development and adulthood, in physiological, and pathological condition.

Finally, if AN does extensively affect the brain function(s), it should be emphasized that it is only one among other forms of CNS plasticity and that very little is known about the mechanisms which underlie their mutual relationships.

AN AND OTHER FORMS OF PLASTICITY AND/OR REPAIR STRATEGIES

The CNS of mammals, in spite of having lost most of its regenerative/repair capacity with respect to other phyla, is endowed with different forms of structural plasticity involving pre-existing cellular elements (Bonfanti and Nacher, 2012). Among them, the most known and widespread is the experience-dependent synaptic plasticity that can occur in response to environmental enrichment and after a lesion in the form of compensatory events, i.e., synaptic formation/elimination and axonal sprouting/pruning (Brown et al., 2009; Chen and Nedivi, 2010; Fu and Zuo, 2011). Further levels of structural plasticity are found in a population of "immature," non-newly generated neurons of the cerebral cortex (Gomez-Climent et al., 2008). These cells, in spite of their differentiated neuronal morphology (Luzzati et al., 2009), express immature neuronal markers and show very few synapses on their membrane, thus not being integrated in the adult cortical circuits, like "stand by" elements (Bonfanti and Nacher, 2012). All these forms of structural plasticity could be useful in rehabilitation approaches that mostly exploit compensatory plasticity of undamaged, preexisting structures (Dobkin, 2004). If and how all these forms of plasticity are integrated with AN is a fully open question, also taking into account that mammalian AN itself consists of heterogeneous processes involving the canonical neurogenic niches and progenitors located throughout the CNS tissue (non-canonical cell genesis; Boda and Buffo, 2010; Bonfanti and Peretto, 2011).

A better knowledge of the mutual relationships existing within the vast landscape of neural plasticity is fundamental to correctly figure out restorative therapeutic approaches in neurology (**Figure 1**). In recent years, several studies have started to unravel new modes of communication between stem/progenitor cells (endogenous or transplanted) and resident cells of the CNS, also involving a cross-talk with the immune system. This communication is at the basis of the so called "bystander effects," namely a series of paracrine mechanisms which can exert beneficial effects even in the absence of cell replacement (Martino et al., 2011). An hypothesis supported by several works is that transplanted stem/progenitor cells can exert a bystander immune modulation by modifying the inhospitable microenvironment at the injury site through the release of soluble molecules such as chemokines and cytokines (Pluchino and Cossetti, 2013). More recently, it has been proposed that the same effects might be also exerted by cell mobilization/activation of endogenous stem/progenitor cells toward adjacent injured sites (Kokaia et al., 2012). In perspective, these studies have the added value of considering neural plasticity, AN, and brain repair in the context of a cross-talk between the CNS and the immune system, the latter being far more important than previously thought. Hence, the study of cell-cell interaction/paracrine communication does represent a fully open, promising field of research, aimed at developing "restorative" rather than "cell replacement" strategies.

SOME PITFALLS IN AN FIELD: INTERPRETATION OF RESULTS AND PEER REVIEW PROCESS

Since the beginning, following the emphasis of a new form of CNS plasticity, the reparative potential of AN has been overestimated by the scientific community, at least under its possible regenerative outcome. This fact is reflected by statements contained in many papers dealing with both spontaneous and lesion-induced AN in which the results obtained are more or less directly linked with potential therapeutic outcomes, in the absence of direct evidence for such a link. These statements, although originally intended as "possibilities" by the authors, are frequently amplified by the media, thus generating unjustified hopes in patients affected by neurological diseases (this aspect is analyzed in Cattaneo and Bonfanti, 2014). The source of this problem is well addressed by Kerner (2006): "Many individual research reports, while suggesting exciting new innovations that may lie ahead in the future, have little or no immediate application in public health and/or clinical practice. Thus, it may be difficult for the practice community to distinguish the signal about what is currently important to practice from the noise of what may or may not become important in the future."

In the neurological context, restorative approaches in the absence of cell replacement, including modulation of physiological/paracrine functions (Martino et al., 2011; Bordey, 2014; Quadrato et al., 2014) should always be kept clearly distinct from the true reparative/regenerative processes involving cell replacement. In the history of AN scientific publications, from the initial "naïve" belief that AN could easily represent the biological substrate for cell replacement in the CNS, to a more recent overestimation of the bystander effect therapeutic potential, it appears that too many unjustified claims actually bypass the filter of peer review. We feel that this habit is not rewarding for the public representation of science and even not for the future of AN field.

FUTURE PERSPECTIVES: AN AND FUNDAMENTAL RESEARCH

It appears evident that having introduced excessive and premature translational issues toward brain repair did not solve the problem of neurological diseases. Moreover, a simplistic view of AN as a ready-made therapeutic tool could even be counterproductive, since it might put down the interest in AN studies. In spite of some oversights along the route, the increasing knowledge gathered during the last 20 years is enormous, considering the changes that AN research has produced in our vision of brain plasticity. Non-invasive technologies are essential to study AN in humans (e.g., Spalding et al., 2013 for ^{14}C detection), although further technical advancements are needed (e.g., cell imaging enhanced resolution; Sierra et al., 2011). Yet, because the AN field has become widely diversified both in its goals and lines of research (**Figure 1**), obtaining of future breakthroughs will require a multidisciplinary integration of high specific expertise in order to gain a whole transversal view of the variables involved (for the several meanings of translation/implementation concepts see Kerner, 2006). The current gaps of knowledge should be filled with new basic research prior to put them into a translational view. We can be confident that applied (beneficial and profitable) products of fundamental research will be eventually achieved in the future, although not visible/predictable at the time of the experimental phases (Press, 2013). Confidence in the eventual usefulness of basic research should be sufficient to bring back AN in the normal context of science.

ACKNOWLEDGMENT

We thank Carlos Lois for reading the manuscript and for his precious advices.

REFERENCES

Arvidsson, A., Collin, T., Kirik, D., Kokaia, Z., and Lindvall, O. (2002). Neuronal replacement from endogenous precursors in the adult brain after stroke. *Nat. Med.* 8, 963–970. doi: 10.1038/nm747

Barker, J. M., Boonstra, R., and Wojtowicz, J. M. (2011). From pattern to pourpose: how comparative studies contribute to understanding the function of adult neurogenesis. *Eur. J. Neurosci.* 34, 963–977. doi: 10.1111/j.1460-9568.2011.07823.x

Basak, O., Giachino, C., Fiorini, E., Macdonald, H. R., and Taylor, V. (2012). Neurogenic subventricular zone stem/progenitor cells are Notch1-dependent in their active but not quiescent state. *J. Neurosci.* 32, 5654–5666. doi: 10.1523/JNEUROSCI.0455-12.2012

Boda, E., and Buffo, A. (2010). Glial cells in non-germinal territories: insights into their stem/progenitor properties in the intact and injured nervous tissue. *Arch. Ital. Biol.* 148, 119–136.

Bonfanti, L. (2011). From hydra regeneration to human brain structuralplasticity: a long trip through narrowing roads. *Sci.World J.* 11, 1270–1299. doi: 10.1100/tsw.2011.113

Bonfanti, L., and Nacher, J. (2012). New scenarios for neuronal structural plasticity in non-neurogenic brain parenchyma: the case of cortical layer II immature neurons. *Prog. Neurobiol.* 98, 1–15. doi: 10.1016/j.pneurobio.2012.05.002

Bonfanti, L., and Peretto, P. (2011). Adult neurogenesis in mammals–a theme with many variations. *Eur. J. Neurosci.* 34, 930–950. doi: 10.1111/j.1460-9568.2011.07832.x

Bordey, A. (2014). Endogenous stem cells for enhancing cognition in the diseased brain. *Front. Neurosci.* 8:98. doi: 10.3389/fnins.2014.00098

Brown, C. E., Aminoltejari, K., Erb, H., Winship, I. R., and Murphy, T. H. (2009). *In vivo* voltage-sensitive dye imaging in adult mice reveals that somatosensory maps lost to stroke are replaced over weeks by new structural and functional circuits with prolonged modes of activation within both the peri-infarct zone and distant sites. *J. Neurosci.* 29, 1719–1734. doi: 10.1523/JNEUROSCI.4249-08.2009

Carlson, B. A. (2012). Diversity matters: the importance of comparative studies and the potential for synergy between neuroscience and evolutionary biology. *Arch. Neurol.* 69, 987–993. doi: 10.1001/archneurol.2012.77

Cattaneo, E., and Bonfanti, L. (2014). Stem cell therapeutic potential is higher in society than in the brain. *Front. Neurosci.* 8:79. doi: 10.3389/fnins.2014.00079

Chen, J. L., and Nedivi, E. (2010). Neuronal structural remodeling: is it all about access? *Curr. Opin. Neurobiol.* 20, 557–562. doi: 10.1016/j.conb.2010.06.002

Dobkin, B. H. (2004). Neurobiology of rehabilitation. *Ann. N.Y. Acad. Sci.* 1038, 148–170. doi: 10.1196/annals.1315.024

Endo, T., Yoshino, J., Kado, K., and Tochinai, S. (2007). Brain regeneration in anuran amphibians. *Dev. Growth Differ.* 49, 121–129. doi: 10.1111/j.1440-169X.2007.00914.x

Feierstein, C. E. (2012). Linking adult olfactory neurogenesis to social behavior. *Front. Neurosci.* 6:173. doi: 10.3389/fnins.2012.00173

Ferretti, P. (2011). Is there a relationship between adult neurogenesis and neuron generation following injury across evolution? *Eur. J. Neurosci.* 34, 951–962. doi: 10.1111/j.1460-9568.2011.07833.x

Feynman, R. P. (2005). *Perfectly Reasonable Deviations (from the Beaten Track)*. New York, NY: Basic Books.

Freund, J., Brandmaier, A. M., Lewejohann, L., Kirste, I., Kritzler, M., Krüger, A., et al. (2013). Emergence of individuality in genetically identical mice. *Science* 340, 756–759. doi: 10.1126/science.1235294

Fu, M., and Zuo, Y. (2011). Experience-dependent structural plasticity in the cortex. *Trends Neurosci.* 34, 177–187. doi: 10.1016/j.tins.2011.02.001

Fuentealba, L. C., Obernier, K., and Alvarez-Buylla, A. (2012). Adult neural stem cells bridge their niche. *Cell Stem Cell* 10, 698–708. doi: 10.1016/j.stem.2012.05.012

Gomez-Climent, M. A., Castillo-Gomez, E., Varea, E., Guirado, R., Blasco-Ibanez, J. M., Crespo, C., et al. (2008). A population of prenatally generated cells in the rat paleocortex maintains an immature neuronal phenotype into adulthood. *Cereb. Cortex* 18, 2229–2240. doi: 10.1093/cercor/bhm255

Grandel, H., and Brand, M. (2013). Comparative aspects of adult neural stem cell activity in vertebrates. *Dev. Genes Evol.* 223, 131–147. doi: 10.1007/s00427-012-0425-5

Kempermann, G. (2011). Seven principles in the regulation of adult neurogenesis. *Eur. J. Neurosci.* 33, 1018–1024. doi: 10.1111/j.1460-9568.2011.07599.x

Kerner, J. F. (2006). Knowledge translation versus knowledge integration: a "funder's" perspective. *J. Contin. Educ. Health Prof.* 26, 72–80. doi: 10.1002/chp.53

Kernie, S. G., and Parent, J. M. (2010). Forebrain neurogenesis after focal ischemia and traumatic brain injury. *Neurobiol. Dis.* 37, 267–274. doi: 10.1016/j.nbd.2009.11.002

Kheirbek, M. A., Klemenhagen, K. C., Sahay, A., and Hen, R. (2012). Neurogenesis and generalization: a new approach to stratify and treat anxiety disorders. *Nat. Neurosci.* 15, 1613–1620. doi: 10.1038/nn.3262

Kokaia, Z., Martino, G., Schwartz, M., and Lindvall, O. (2012). Cross-talk between neural stem cells and immune cells: the key to better brain repair? *Nat. Neurosci.* 15, 1078–1087. doi: 10.1038/nn.3163

Kuhn, G. H., and Blomgren, K. (2011). Developmental dysregulation of adult neurogenesis. *Eur. J. Neurosci.* 33, 1115–1122. doi: 10.1111/j.1460-9568.2011.07610.x

Kyritsis, N., Kizil, C., and Brand, M. (2014). Neuroinflammation and central nervous system regeneration in vertebrates. *Trends Cell Biol.* 24, 128–135. doi: 10.1016/j.tcb.2013.08.004

Lepousez, G., Valley, M. T., and Lledo, P. M. (2013). The impact of adult neurogenesis on olfactory bulb circuits and computations. *Annu. Rev. Physiol.* 75, 339–363. doi: 10.1146/annurev-physiol-030212-183731

Leuner, B., and Gould, E. (2010). Structural plasticity and hippocampal function. *Annu. Rev. Psychol.* 61, 111–140. doi: 10.1146/annurev.psych.093008.100359

Lindsey, B. W., and Tropepe, V. (2006). A comparative framework for understanding the biological principles of adult neurogenesis. *Prog. Neurobiol.* 80, 281–307. doi: 10.1016/j.pneurobio.2006.11.007

Luzzati, F., Bonfanti, L., Fasolo, A., and Peretto, P. (2009). DCX and PSA-NCAM expression identifies a population of neurons preferentially distributed in associative areas of different pallial derivatives and vertebrate species. *Cereb. Cortex* 19, 1028–1041. doi: 10.1093/cercor/bhn145

Luzzati, F., De Marchis, S., Fasolo, A., and Peretto, P. (2006). Neurogenesis in the caudate nucleus of the adult rabbit. *J. Neurosci.* 26, 609–621. doi: 10.1523/JNEUROSCI.4371-05.2006

Luzzati, F., De Marchis, S., Parlato, R., Gribaudo, S., Schütz, G., Fasolo, A., et al. (2011). New striatal neurons in a mouse model of progressive striatal degeneration are generated in both the subventricular zone and the striatal parenchyma. *PLoS ONE* 6:e25088. doi: 10.1371/journal.pone.0025088

Martino, G. V., Pluchino, S., Bonfanti, L., and Schwartz, M. (2011). Brain regeneration in physiology and pathology: the immune signature driving therapeutic plasticity of neural stem cells. *Phys. Rev.* 91, 1281–1304. doi: 10.1152/physrev.00032.2010

Mescher, A. L., and Neff, A. W. (2006). Limb regeneration in amphibians: immunological considerations. *ScientificWorldJournal* 6, 1–11. doi: 10.1100/tsw.2006.323

Migaud, M., Batailler, M., Segura, S., Duittoz, A., Franceschini, I., and Pillon, D. (2010). Emerging new sites for adult neurogenesis in the mammalian brain: a comparative study between the hypothalamus and the classical neurogenic zones. *Eur. J. Neurosci.* 32, 2042–2052. doi: 10.1111/j.1460-9568.2010.07521.x

Ming, G. L., and Song, H. (2011). Adult neurogenesis in the mammalian brain: significant answers and significant questions. *Neuron* 70, 687–702. doi: 10.1016/j.neuron.2011.05.001

Mucignat-Caretta, C., Redaelli, M., and Caretta, A. (2012). One nose, one brain: contribution of the main and accessory olfactory system to chemosensation. *Front. Neuroanat.* 6:46. doi: 10.3389/fnana.2012.00046

Obernier, K., Tong, K. K., and Alvarez-Buylla, A. (2014). Restricted nature of adult neural stem cells: re-evaluation of their potential for brain repair. *Front. Neurosci.* 8:162. doi: 10.3389/fnins.2014.00162

Pluchino, S., and Cossetti, C. (2013). How stem cells speak with host immune cells in inflammatory brain diseases. *Glia* 61, 1379–1401. doi: 10.1002/glia.22500

Ponti, G., Peretto, P., and Bonfanti, L. (2008). Genesis of neuronal and glial progenitors in the cerebellar cortex of peripuberal and adult rabbits. *PLoS ONE* 3:e2366. doi: 10.1371/journal.pone.0002366

Press, W. H. (2013). What's so special about science (and how much should we spend on it?). *Science* 342, 817–822. doi: 10.1126/science.342.6160.817

Quadrato, G., Elnaggar, M. Y., and Di Giovanni, S. (2014). Adult neurogenesis in brain repair: cellular plasticity vs. cellular replacement. *Front. Neurosci.* 8:17. doi: 10.3389/fnins.2014.00017

Sahay, A., Wilson, D. A., and Hen, R. (2011). Pattern separation: a common function for new neurons in hippocampus and olfactory bulb. *Neuron* 70, 582–588. doi: 10.1016/j.neuron.2011.05.012

Sanai, N., Nguyen, T., Ihrie, R. A., Mirzadeh, Z., Tsai, H. H., Wong, M., et al. (2011). Corridors of migrating neurons in the human brain and their decline during infancy. *Nature* 478, 382–386. doi: 10.1038/nature10487

Schwartz, M., Kipnis, J., Rivest, S., and Prat, A. (2013). How do immune cells support and shape the brain in health, disease, and aging? *J. Neurosci.* 33, 17587–17596. doi: 10.1523/JNEUROSCI.3241-13.2013

Sierra, A., Encinas, J. M., and Maletic-Savatic, M. (2011). Adult human neurogenesis: from microscopy to magnetic resonance imaging. *Front. Neurosci.* 5:47. doi: 10.3389/fnins.2011.00047

Snyder, J. S., and Cameron, H. A. (2012). Could,adult,hippocampal,neurogenesis be relevant for human behavior? *Behav. Brain Res.* 14, 384–390. doi: 10.1016/j.bbr.2011.06.024

Sofroniew, M. V. (2009). Molecular dissection of reactive astrogliosis and glial scar formation. *Trends Neurosci.* 32, 638–647. doi: 10.1016/j.tins.2009.08.002

Spalding, K. L., Bergmann, O., Alkass, K., Bernard, S., Salehpour, M., Huttner, H. B., et al. (2013). Dynamics of hippocampal neurogenesis in adult humans. *Cell* 153, 1219–1227. doi: 10.1016/j.cell.2013.05.002

Tong, C. K., and Alvarez-Buylla, A. (2014). SnapShot: adult neurogenesis in the V-SVZ. *Neuron* 81:220-220.e1. doi: 10.1016/j.neuron.2013.12.004

Trotter, J., Karram, K., and Nishiyama, A. (2010). NG2 cells: Properties, progeny and origin. *Brain Res. Rev.* 63, 72–82. doi: 10.1016/j.brainresrev.2009.12.006

Vadodaria, K. C., and Gage, F. H. (2014). SnapShot: adult hippocampal neurogenesis. *Cell* 156:1114-1114.e1. doi: 10.1016/j.cell.2014.02.029

Weil, Z. M., Norman, G. J., DeVries, A. C., and Nelson, R. J. (2008). The injured nervous system: a Darwinian perspective. *Prog. Neurobiol.* 86, 48–59. doi: 10.1016/j.pneurobio.2008.06.001

The sinusoidal probe: a new approach to improve electrode longevity

Harbaljit S. Sohal[1,2], Andrew Jackson[1], Richard Jackson[2], Gavin J. Clowry[1], Konstantin Vassilevski[2], Anthony O'Neill[2] and Stuart N. Baker[1]*

[1] Newcastle Movement Lab, Institute of Neuroscience, Newcastle University, Newcastle Upon Tyne, UK
[2] School of Electrical and Electronic Engineering, Newcastle University, Newcastle Upon Tyne, UK

Edited by:
Ulrich G. Hofmann, Albert-Ludwigs-University Freiburg, Germany

Reviewed by:
Liang Guo, The Ohio State University, USA
Maria Asplund, Albert-Ludwigs Universität, Freiburg, Germany

***Correspondence:**
Stuart N. Baker, Newcastle Movement Lab, Institute of Neuroscience, Newcastle University, Framlington Place, Newcastle Upon Tyne NE2 4HH, UK
e-mail: stuart.baker@newcastle.ac.uk

Micromotion between the brain and implanted electrodes is a major contributor to the failure of invasive brain–machine interfaces. Movements of the electrode tip cause recording instabilities while spike amplitudes decline over the weeks/months post-implantation due to glial cell activation caused by sustained mechanical trauma. We have designed a sinusoidal probe in order to reduce movement of the recording tip relative to the surrounding neural tissue. The probe was microfabricated from flexible materials and incorporated a sinusoidal shaft to minimize tethering forces and a 3D spheroid tip to anchor the recording site within the brain. Compared to standard microwire electrodes, the signal-to-noise ratio and local field potential power of sinusoidal probe recordings from rabbits was more stable across recording periods up to 678 days. Histological quantification of microglia and astrocytes showed reduced neuronal tissue damage especially for the tip region between 6 and 24 months post-implantation. We suggest that the micromotion-reducing measures incorporated into our design, at least partially, decreased the magnitude of gliosis, resulting in enhanced longevity of recording.

Keywords: flexible, microelectrode, chronic, electrophysiology, gliosis, long term, electrode

INTRODUCTION

Brain–machine-interface (BMIs) decode motor information from cortical activity, providing control of computers, assistive devices or functional electrical stimulation to restore function after paralysis (Nicolelis, 2001; Taylor et al., 2002; Schwartz, 2004; Hochberg et al., 2006, 2012; Bartels et al., 2008; Zimmermann et al., 2011; Collinger et al., 2012). Invasive BMIs use intracortical microelectrodes to record from neurons in close proximity (~100–150 μm) to the recording tip (Biran et al., 2005, 2007; Polikov et al., 2005; Perge et al., 2013). Unfortunately, sustained immune activation caused by the foreign body response with time leads to neuronal loss around microelectrodes (Polikov et al., 2005). Furthermore, immune mediators such as astrocytes and microglia ensheath electrode recording sites, isolating the electrode from surrounding brain tissue and releasing detrimental immune factors that compromise neuronal function (Biran et al., 2005; Polikov et al., 2005; Winslow et al., 2010; Winslow and Tresco, 2010; Collinger et al., 2012). These mechanisms cause instabilities in the recordings obtained from both microwire and silicon probes (Jackson and Fetz, 2007; Dickey et al., 2009) and can lead to device failure within weeks or months after chronic implantation (Polikov et al., 2005; Ward et al., 2009; Collinger et al., 2012).

An important contributor to the sustained tissue response is the modulus mismatch between the brain and implanted microelectrodes (Kozai and Kipke, 2009). Typical electrode materials include silicon (e.g., the "Utah" array, Rousche and Normann, 1998 and "Michigan" probe, Kipke et al., 2003) and metal microwires (Nicolelis et al., 2003; Jackson and Fetz, 2007) which have a higher Young's modulus (YM, ~150 GPa) than brain tissue (5–30 KPa; Miller et al., 2000; Potter et al., 2012). This mismatch means microelectrodes anchored to the skull cannot accommodate movement of the brain within the cranial cavity (Biran et al., 2007; Thelin et al., 2011). Even if electrodes are designed to float with the brain, deformation of the tissue will change the position of deep neurons relative to an anchoring point at the brain surface (Biran et al., 2005; LaPlaca et al., 2005; Subbaroyan et al., 2005; Gilletti and Muthuswamy, 2006; Kozai and Kipke, 2009; Yoshida Kozai et al., 2012; Hwang and Andersen, 2013; Kim et al., 2013). Damage caused by electrode movement relative to surrounding tissue will be exacerbated by the sharp tip profiles typically used to aid insertion. The amount of damage around the tips can be estimated through cell loss over time for current electrode arrays. For the Utah array, 61% of cells that were recorded on the first recording session were lost after 2 weeks (Dickey et al., 2009). Similar neuronal loss has been shown for microwire electrodes (Nicolelis et al., 2003; Jackson and Fetz, 2007). Microelectrodes can record between 100 and 150 μm away from their recording sites (Polikov et al., 2005; Seymour et al., 2011). For a single electrode shank, this equates to a 6750 mm^3 (150 × 150 × 300 μm) volume around the electrode. For the human brain there are an estimated 6.66×10^4 neurons per mm^3 (Allen et al., 2005; Azevedo et al., 2009; Marblestone et al., 2013). Through extrapolation, if an estimated 61% of cells are lost for every two weeks of recording, then just a solitary cell will remain after ~40 weeks post-implant around a single shank, assuming the electrode can record from every cell in that given brain volume and neurons are lost linearly over time.

Micromotion can be reduced using flexible materials (Polikov et al., 2005; Kozai and Kipke, 2009; Harris et al., 2011) or by decreasing the overall footprint of the microelectrode (Yoshida Kozai et al., 2012; Suyatin et al., 2013). Flexible arrays require specialized insertion techniques to penetrate the dura or pia. Proposed methods include temporary stiffening with biodegradable solutions (Chorover and DeLuca, 1972; Kohler et al., 2009; Witteveen et al., 2010; Hassler et al., 2011) or soluble polymers such as polyethylene glycol (PEG; Takeuchi et al., 2004) prior to insertion. Some flexible arrays have sharp anchoring structures to restrict further the movement of the recording site relative to the surrounding neuronal tissue (Kohler et al., 2009; Wu et al., 2011). Nevertheless, while flexible materials can bend to shorten the distance between the anchoring point and the tip, a straight electrode, no matter how flexible, cannot accommodate deformations of the brain that increase this distance.

All current chronic electrode designs, which have evolved from the straight shafts traditionally used for acute recording share this fundamental limitation. We propose a simple yet radical solution: a novel flexible electrode which is not straight and can therefore lengthen and shorten to accommodate brain deformations. Specifically, we designed an electrode shaft with a sinusoidal profile mechanically to decouple the recording site from the fixed end of the electrode. Moreover, we incorporated a spherical tip to anchor the recording sites relative to the surrounding tissue and minimize damage. The novel electrode was microfabricated and tested *in vivo* over a 6–24 month period in rabbits. The electrode was compared to conventional rigid microwires of the same recording tip diameter. Microwires were chosen as a comparison as they have been well characterized in many species in chronic studies (Nicolelis et al., 2003; Jackson and Fetz, 2007; Winslow et al., 2010) and have reduced gliosis responses compared to standard silicon probes (Winslow et al., 2010; Yoshida Kozai et al., 2012).

The electrophysiological recordings and post-mortem characterization of the tissue response compared to conventional microwires suggest that the novel design features incorporated in our sinusoidal electrode may improve the long-term stability of recordings for BMI applications.

MATERIALS AND METHODS

SINUSOIDAL PROBE: DESIGN AND MICROFABRICATION

The probe consisted of three W/Ti (80/20 wt %) recording sites encased in parylene-C. Tungsten is a good recording metal (Hubel, 1959). However, with a YM of 400 GPa, it is not flexible compared to other metals (Geddes and Roeder, 2003). Therefore, tungsten was sintered with titanium to increase flexibility, resulting in a YM of ~200 GPa. Parylene-C was chosen as it is biocompatible, flexible, and a FDA-approved dielectric for biomedical applications (Seymour and Kipke, 2006; Kozai et al., 2010; Winslow et al., 2010; Yoshida Kozai et al., 2012).

The recording end of the electrode was a parylene disk of 100 μm diameter, with three protruding, exposed recording sites to aid single-unit isolation (Gray et al., 1995). Three metal tracks ran within an electrode shaft that was 20 μm deep, 35 μm wide and had a sinusoidal profile with cycles of 100 μm amplitude and 500 μm period. We report data from two design iterations, which differed in length and how connection to the electrode was made. The first generation electrode was 5.5 mm in length and had a bondpad (approximately 400 μm^2) at the end of the sinusoidal shaft, to which individual wires were attached. The second generation electrode was 3 mm in length (**Figure 1G**) and incorporated an integrated ribbon cable (3 cm long and 3 mm wide) leading to a standard connector (micro ps1/ps2 series, Omnetics Connector Corporation, USA).

Fabrication began with a three-inch silicon wafer (Compart, UK) onto which a 1 μm aluminum sacrificial layer was e-beam deposited (BOC-Edwards auto ebeam evaporator, UK) to increase adhesion between the first polymeric layer during the fabrication process and aid device release (**Figure 1A**). The first layer of parylene-C was deposited with a thickness up to 10 μm, through a chemical vapor deposition process (CVD; **Figure 1B**). Next, a 1 μm WTi layer (80/20 wt%) was magnetron sputter deposited (Kurt J. Lesker PVD 75 vacuum deposition, USA) with a power setting of 100 W (**Figure 1C**). After masking with AZ-5214e photoresist (HD microchemical, Germany), the metal layer was patterned with SF_6 reactive ion etch (RIE; Plasma-Therm 790, USA) using parameters of 200 W, 150 mTorr, and 10 sccm flow rate to define the overall electrode tracks, bondpad and recording site regions (**Figure 1C**). A slight over-etch was employed to surface roughen the first parylene-C layer to aid adhesion of the second layer, again deposited through CVD (**Figure 1D**). Subsequently both parylene-C layers were patterned using oxygen RIE (Plasma-Therm 790, USA) with parameters of 200 W, 50 mTorr, and 18 sccm flow rate to form the overall electrode shape and to re-open recording site/bond pad regions (**Figure 1E**). A 40 nm thick titanium mask was e-beamed deposited and patterned (Kurt J. Lesker PVD 75 vacuum deposition) for this process. Exposed WTi was unaffected by parylene-C oxygen RIE. Finally, the electrodes were released from the silicon substrate by etching the aluminum sacrificial layer using 3% tetramethylammonia hydroxide (TMAH) as found in AZ-326 MIF photoresist developer (HD MicroChemicals, Germany; **Figures 1E,H**). Post-release (**Figure 1F**), the recording end had three clearly isolated electrode recording sites (**Figure 1I**).

Connectors were attached to the bondpad region using conductive paint (RS Components, UK) and insulated with two-part epoxy (Araldite: Farnell, UK). A polyimide ball was added by dipping the recording end first in VM 652 adhesion promoter (HD Microchemicals, Germany) and then in PI-5878G (HD Microchemicals, Germany) forming a small sphere around the electrode tip. The added sphere had a diameter of less than 100 μm as confirmed through optical microscopy during fabrication and further confirmed through post-hoc histology via the implantation site size. The polyimide was soft-baked at 120°C for 30 min in a convection oven. To re-open the covered recording sites, the electrode tip was dipped into TMAH for a few seconds. Electrode tip exposure was confirmed by tip impedances (at 1 kHz in saline) comparable to pre-polyimide application.

To aid insertion in to the brain, we used carriers made from 0.229 mm diameter sharpened stainless steel electrodes (Microprobe INC., USA) emerging from 25 g hypodermic needles

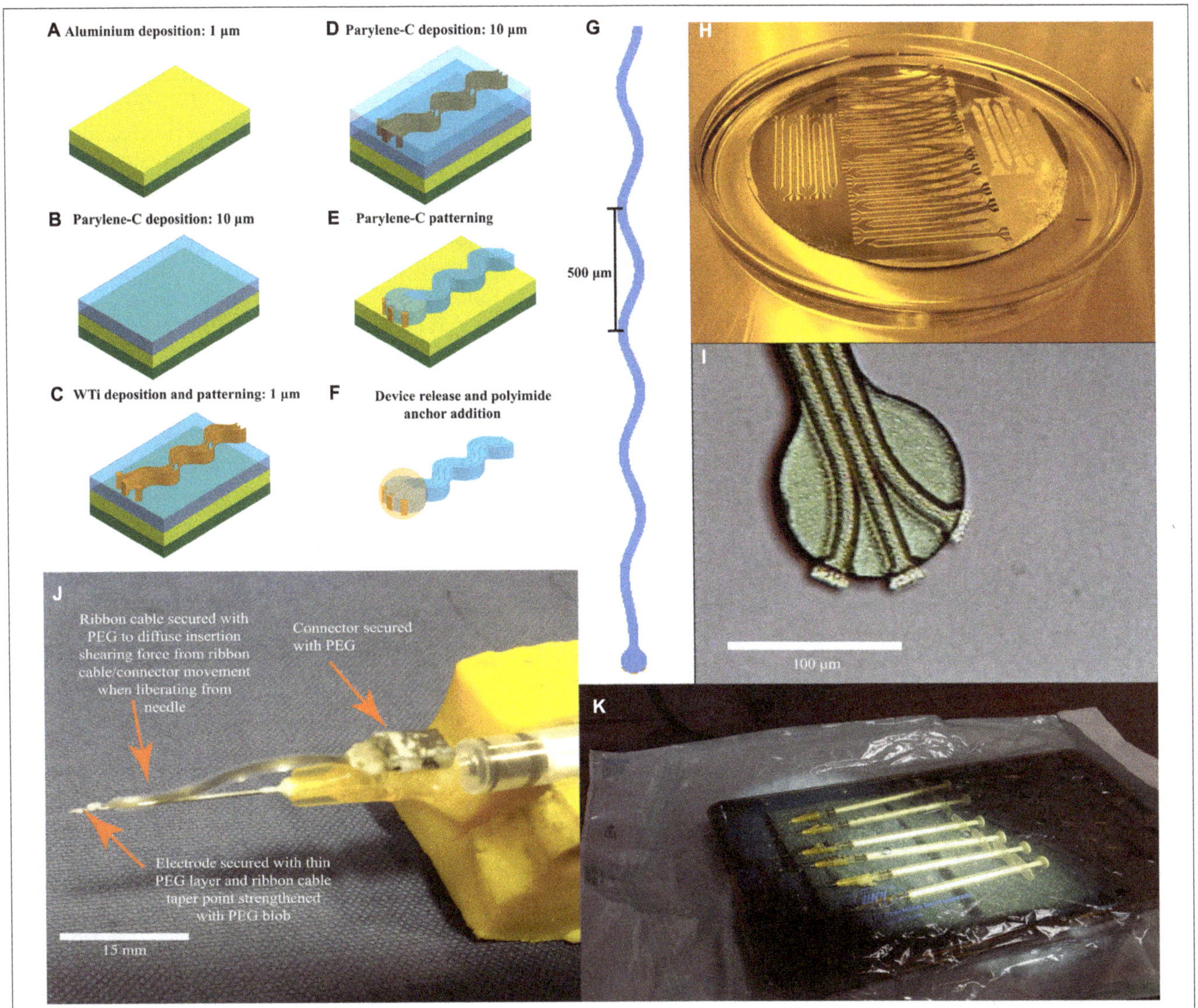

FIGURE 1 | Sinusoidal probe microfabrication and surgery preparation. (A–F) Sequential microfabrication steps for the sinusoidal probe concentrating on the recording end (illustrative and not to scale): **(A)** 1 µm aluminum ebeam deposition as a sacrificial layer on a silicon substrate. **(B)** Parylene-C deposition through a CVD process. **(C)** WTi sputter deposition and patterning to define electrode tracks, bondpad and recording site regions. **(D)** Second layer parylene-C deposition through CVD. **(E)** Patterning of both parylene-C layers using oxygen plasma. **(F)** Device release using a TMAH based photoresist developer and addition of 3D polyimide ball anchor. **(G)** Mask layout for the 3 mm version of the probe. Three metal tracks ran within an electrode shaft that was 20 µm deep, 35 µm wide and had a sinusoidal profile with cycles of 100 µm amplitude and 500 µm period. **(H)** Successful device release in TMAH. **(I)** Optical microscopy image of the recording end showing three separate and isolated electrode recording sites, pre-polyimide anchor addition. The protruding electrode recording sites may appear thicker due to the underlying first parylene-C layer, which is not removed during WTi etching. **(J)** Attached sinusoidal probe to improvised insertion carrier to allow for successful brain penetration and electrode insertion. **(K)** Electrodes under sterile conditions, placed in an autoclaved container and then into surgical bag primed for UV light sterilization.

(**Figure 1J**). Electrodes and carriers were cleaned with ethanol before being attached with PEG and sterilized with ultra-violet irradiation (**Figure 1K**).

ANIMALS AND SURGICAL PROCEDURES

All experiments were approved by the local ethics committee at Newcastle University and were performed under appropriate Home Office licenses in accordance with the UK Animals (Scientific Procedures) Act 1986. Electrodes were implanted into the sensorimotor representation of five New Zealand white rabbits (*Oryctolagus cuniculus*; Subjects R, J, N, L, Lo). After a midline skin incision and burr-hole craniotomies, electrodes were inserted stereotaxically at coordinates relative to bregma of 4 mm anterior to 4 mm posterior and 0.5 to 7 mm lateral (Gould, 1986; Swadlow, 1989, 1990, 1994; Swadlow and Hicks, 1996). Electrodes were inserted quickly (Bjornsson et al., 2006) using the stereotaxic manipulator. The PEG was dissolved with warm saline to release the electrode from the carrier, which was subsequently removed. Microwire electrodes (50 µm diameter Teflon-insulated tungsten) were inserted manually with surgical forceps. Connectors were attached to the skull with skull screws and dental cement. A wire wrapped around one skull screw served as ground and reference for the recordings. In this study, 4–5 sinusoidal electrodes were inserted per animal for both the first generation (Rabbit N, L) and second generation (Rabbit- R, J, Lo). Between 2 and 4 microwire electrodes were also inserted for comparison in each animal.

ELECTROPHYSIOLOGY DATA ACQUISITION

Tri-weekly recording sessions began one week post-surgery. Animals were individually placed in a custom-made restraining box while neuronal activity was amplified (10× MPA8I headstage followed by 1000× PGA1632 amplifier; Multichannel systems, Germany) and recorded (Power 1401, Cambridge Electronic Design, UK). Spike channels were filtered between 0.3 and 8 kHz and sampled at 25 kHz while local field potentials (LFP) were filtered between 1 and 300 Hz and sampled at 1 kHz.

CHRONIC RECORDING PERFORMANCE EVALUATION

In this study, statistical comparisons combined data across all electrodes of the same type implanted in each animal.

We analyzed LFP, spike activity and high voltage spindle responses (HVS) from both sinusoidal and microwire electrodes. The HVS activity is characterized by highly synchronous spike and wave patterns, typically only seen when the animal remains motionless with eyes open (Buzsáki et al., 1988).

All analysis was performed within the Matlab environment (version 2009a, MathWorks, USA). LFP power spectra for each electrode were constructed using a fast-Fourier transform and the spectrum was divided into distinct bands. The mean power in each band was calculated for each session across the chronic recording period.

For HVS responses and spiking, principle component analysis spike sorting was performed with custom written software GetSpike. This enabled spikes to be sorted by initial thresholding and cluster cutting with times recorded. Accepted waveforms consisted of sections five sampling points before and 15 after the threshold crossing. The mean peak-to-peak amplitude, noise and signal-to-noise ratio (SNR) were evaluated daily across the chronic period. The SNR was calculated in accordance to Suner et al. (2005). For the signal, the peak-to-peak amplitude (A) of the mean waveform was calculated. For the noise, the mean waveform was subtracted from all waveforms, with the standard deviation calculated from the resulting values. Noise was then calculated as 2× the average standard deviation (ε). SNR was then calculated as A/ε. For statistical analysis to compare recorded responses, percentile-bootstrapping was used because of unequal sample sizes: each sinusoidal probe had three recording sites compared to one microwire recording site. Spike events from the full dataset were drawn randomly (with replacement) to create surrogate datasets with the same number of events as the real data, but distributed evenly between sinusoidal and microwire electrodes. This procedure was repeated 10000 times to estimate the expected difference in each measure under the null hypothesis of no difference between electrode types. The null hypothesis was rejected if the observed difference fell outside the 2.5–97.5% percentile range of the bootstrapped distribution.

HISTOLOGY ANALYSIS

Post-mortem histology was used to assess tissue response to implanted electrodes. After anesthesia was induced with hypnorm (0.3 ml/kg i.m.) and midazolam (2 mg/kg i.v.), animals were perfused transcardially with phosphate buffered saline (PBS) and then formal saline (10%). The relevant brain regions were removed and transferred to incrementally increasing sucrose solutions (10–30%) for cryoprotection before cutting into 50 μm sections perpendicular to the electrode tracks.

The tissue was stained for microglia, astrocytes, and neurofilament. Slices were incubated with 3% normal horse serum (Vector Labs, UK: S-2000) to prevent non-specific binding, and incubated overnight with relevant concentrations of the primary antibodies GFAP (1:500, Sigma-Aldrich, UK), isolectin-b4 [1:200, Vector Labs, UK: Biotinylated Griffonia (Bandeiraea) Simplicifolia Lectin 1] and where appropriate, SMI-32 (1:1000, Cambridge Biosciences, UK: R-500) diluted in PBS at 4°C. GFAP and Neurofilament slices underwent incubation with biotinylated antimouse for 2 h. All slices were then incubated with horseradish peroxide streptavidin (Vector Labs, UK: SA-5004) for 1 h.

Finally, the diaminobenzidine (DAB) reaction was performed (Sigma–Aldrich, UK). Slices were incubated with DAB and placed in PBS after the reaction. Slices were dehydrated in an ascending alcohol series (5 min of 70, 95, 100, and 100% ethanol) and 2, 10 min histoclear washes (Sigma-Aldrich, UK), before cover slips were mounted with histomount (Sigma-Aldrich, UK).

Images were taken at 10× magnification at a pre-saturation exposure time dependent on the staining using axiovision software (Carl Zeiss Microimaging, Germany) before normalization using custom Matlab software. Background levels were assessed from tissue at least 1 mm away from the electrode implantation site, and subtracted from electrode tract images to leave the glial response around electrodes which was inverted (using the "imcomplement" function on Matlab) and normalized by the background level. Images were imported into ImageJ64 software (NIH, USA) to determine the radial distribution of staining intensity around electrode tracks. This analysis was carried out on all sections stained for microglia, astrocytes and where appropriate neurofilament. To compare the overall differences between sinusoidal and microwire electrodes, the mean of at least 15 tracks were compared between each electrode type.

Graphs were plotted of mean intensity as a function of radial distance from each electrodes type. Paired t-tests were performed for distances between 50 and 500 μm away, with a significance level of $P < 0.05$, in accordance with previous literature (Biran et al., 2005; Winslow et al., 2010; Winslow and Tresco, 2010; Potter et al., 2012). In addition, we assessed the Bonferroni-corrected significance of the smallest P value for each depth.

RESULTS

ELECTRODE IMPEDANCE

All sinusoidal probes had pre-implantation impedances less than the 4–5 MΩ considered the limit for single unit recordings (Ludwig et al., 2006, 2011). The mean (±SEM) impedance at 1 kHz was 559 ± 88 kΩ ($n = 99$), compared with 200–400 kΩ for microwires.

ELECTROPHYSIOLOGY: LFP RECORDINGS

Figures 2A–C shows example LFP power spectra for sinusoidal and microwire electrodes (Rabbit-J, second generation probe). Two clear oscillatory bands can be seen: theta (4–8 Hz) and beta (13–30 Hz) which were separated by band-pass filtering (**Figures 2D,E**). In this animal, LFP recordings were obtained from one sinusoidal and two microwire electrodes over a 163 day period (**Figures 2A–C**). The LFP signal obtained from each of the three recording sites of the sinusoidal electrode were very similar ($R^2 = 0.98$, **Figures 2D,E**). Although the microwire electrode had higher LFP power values for both theta and beta frequency bands, the sinusoidal electrode recording was more stable over time (**Figures 2F,G**). Across the duration of the implant period, the standard deviation of the recorded power was 3.5, 7.8, and 9.9 μV^2 (theta frequency) and 5.5, 11.2, and 11.6 μV^2 (beta frequency) for the one sinusoidal and two microwire electrodes, respectively. Lower standard deviation values, measured across the recording sessions on different days, indicated that the LFP signal obtained for the sinusoidal probe appeared more stable across the chronic recording period in this animal than the comparator microwires. This result was also replicated for electrodes implanted in rabbit-R.

ELECTROPHYSIOLOGY: HIGH VOLTAGE SPINDLE RESPONSES

Figure 3A shows example HVS activity observed in rabbit-R ($n = 15$ sinusoidal and $n = 2$ microwire recording sites, second generation probe). This activity comprised high frequency

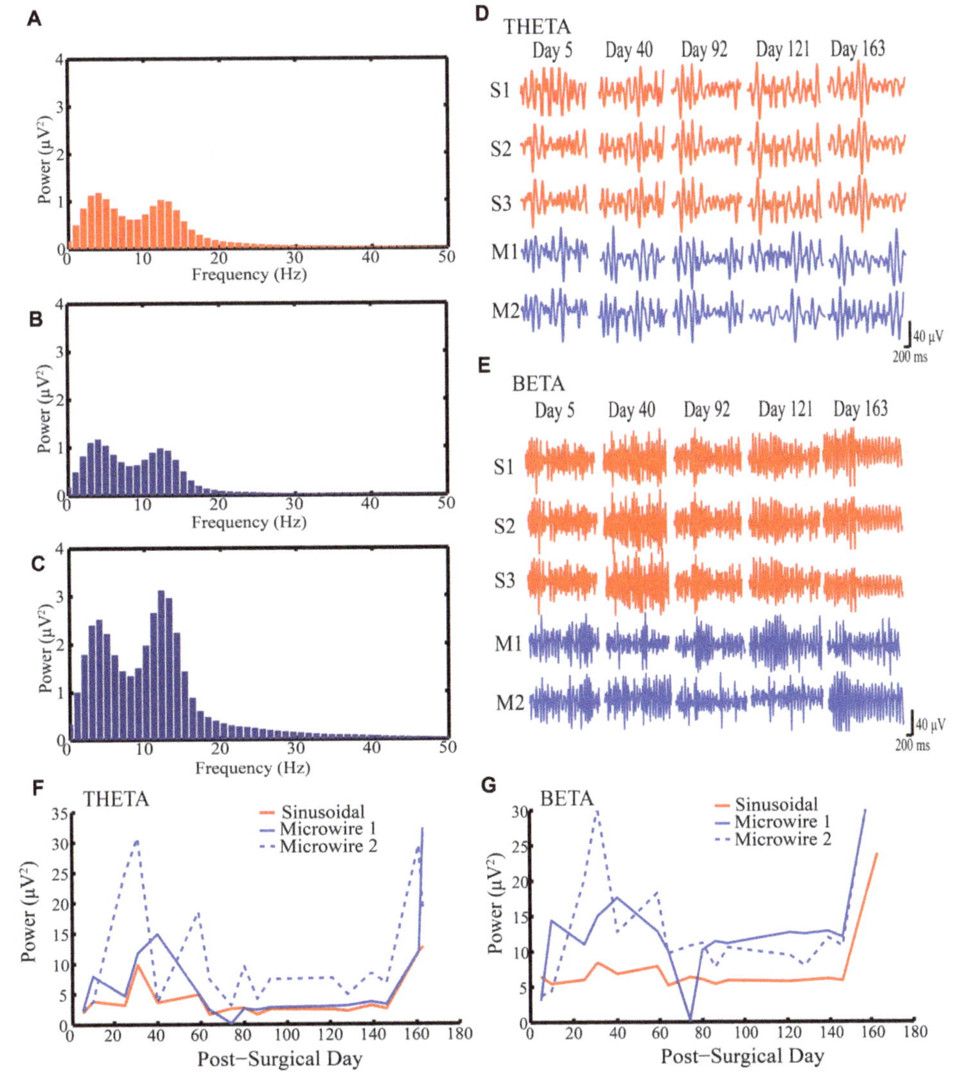

FIGURE 2 | Local field potential (LFP) recordings obtained from Rabbit-J over a 163 day indwelling period. (A–C) Example power spectra for one sinusoidal and two microwire electrodes respectively showing peaks at both theta and beta bands **(D)** Example of filtered recordings from selected days for theta band from all electrodes, S1–3 are the three individual electrode recording sites on the sinusoidal probe, M1–2 are two separate microwire electrodes. **(E)** Example of filtered recordings from selected days for beta band from all electrodes. **(F,G)** Daily recorded power over the indwelling period for both theta and beta activity, respectively. The same LFP signal was captured by all three electrode recording sites for the sinusoidal probe over the indwelling period. Note the stability in LFP power for the sinusoidal compared to the microwire electrode.

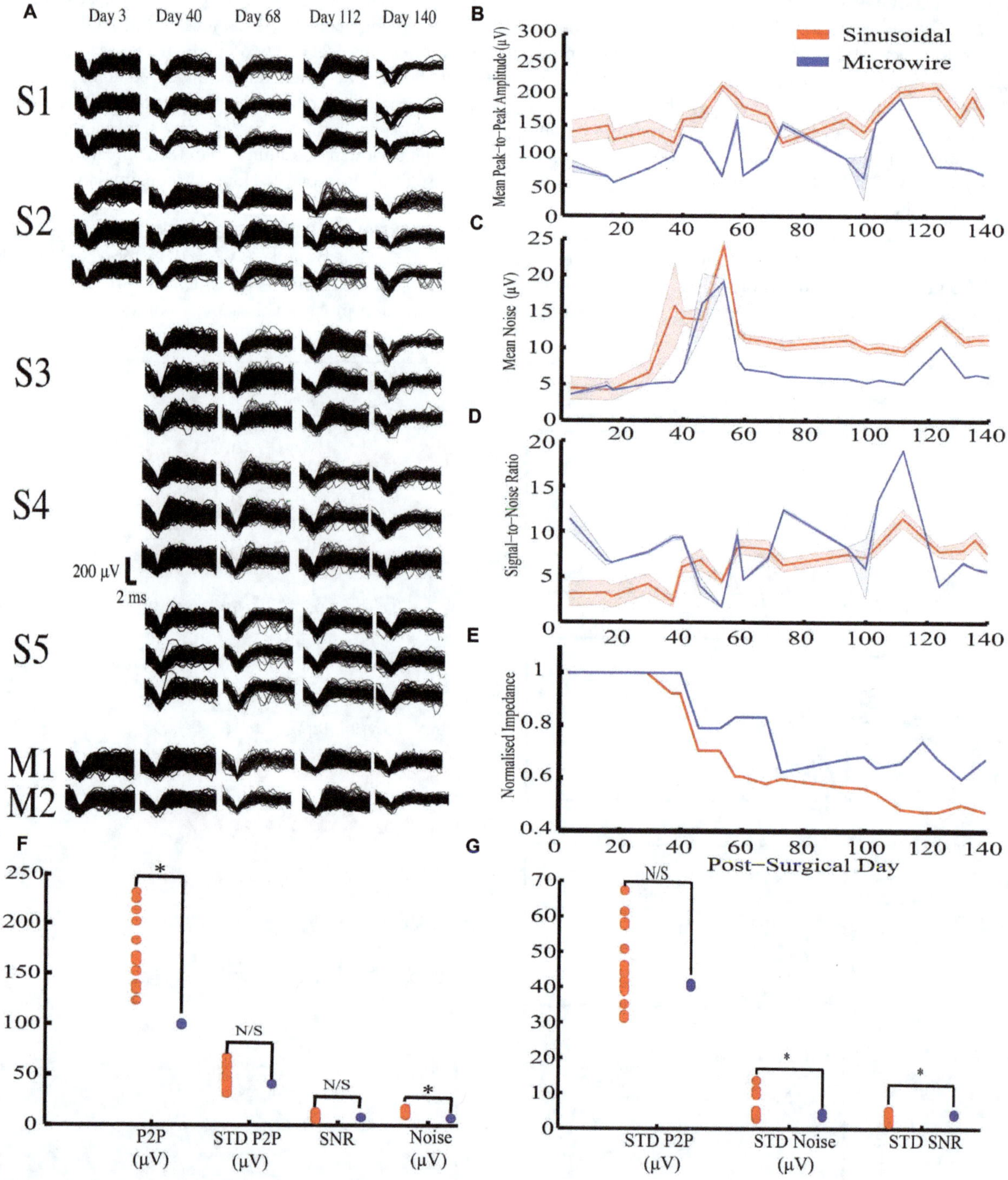

FIGURE 3 | Chronic high voltage spindle (HVS) responses from both sinusoidal and microwire electrode over a 140 day indwelling period from rabbit-R. (A) Selected overlain waveforms over the recording period, S1–5 are five different sinusoidal probes and M1–2 are two different microwire electrodes. **(B–E)** Overall sinusoidal (n = 15 recording sites) and microwire (n = 2 recording sites) chronic performance over a 140 day indwelling period (mean ± SEM): **(B)** Mean peak to peak amplitude recorded per recording session. **(C)** Average noise amplitude recorded per recording session. **(D)** Signal-to-noise ratio over the entire recording period. **(E)** Impedance normalized to the first recording session. There was an overall decrease in impedance for the sinusoidal (R^2 = 0.84) and microwire (R^2 = 0.78) electrode over the indwelling period. **(F)** Statistical comparison of daily obtained recording parameters using bootstrapping methods between the two electrode types. **(G)** Comparisons of standard deviation values obtained across the entire recording period to analyze overall recording parameter stability using bootstrapping methods between the two electrode types. P2P = peak-to-peak amplitude. STD = standard deviation. * indicates comparisons that fell outside the 2.5 to 97.5% percentile range of the bootstrapped distribution.

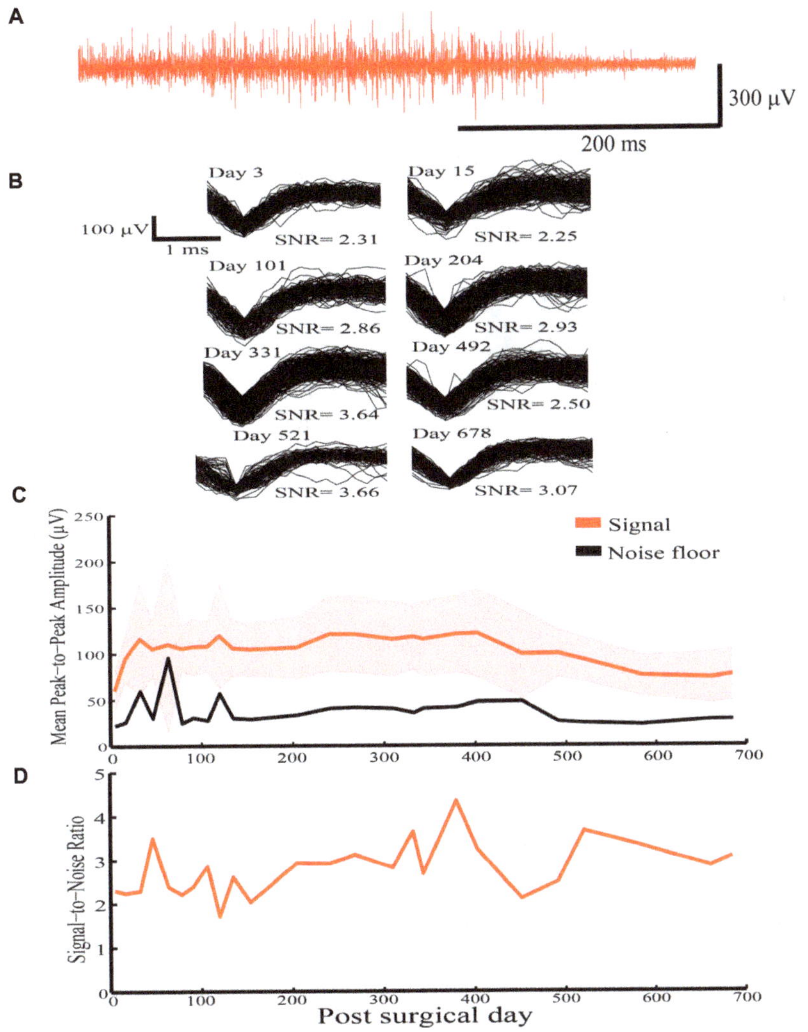

FIGURE 4 | High voltage spindle responses response recorded over a 678-indwelling period in Rabbit-N. (A) Example recording trace for the HVS activity. **(B)** Overlain waveforms for selected days for the HVS response. **(C)** Daily mean peak-to-peak amplitude (±SEM) with corresponding noise floor recorded across the recording period for HVS activity. **(D)** Daily signal-to-noise ratio (SNR) values recorded as a function of indwelling period for HVS activity.

spike-wave discharge, which was synchronous across all electrodes implanted on the same side of the brain, allowing accurate comparison of SNR across electrode types.

For this activity, the sinusoidal probes had higher mean peak-to-peak values compared to the microwire electrodes (**Figures 3B,F**) but also higher noise levels (**Figures 3C,F**). As a result there was no difference in the SNR between the two electrode types (**Figure 3D**). However, the SNR for the sinusoidal probe was more stable across the recording period, as revealed by a lower standard deviation across recording sessions (**Figure 3G**).

Overall impedance values were not significantly correlated with either mean peak-to-peak A ($R^2 = 0.037$) or noise ($R^2 = 0.015$) across all electrodes. However, impedance declined for both electrode types over the course of the implant period (**Figure 3E**). For the sinusoidal probe this resulted in improved SNR across the recording period ($R^2 = 0.76$), an effect not seen for microwire electrodes ($R^2 = 0.01$).

In summary, the sinusoidal electrode recorded higher mean peak-to-peak amplitude values with comparable stability to the microwire electrodes. Similar SNR values were obtained, however, the sinusoidal electrode had more stable SNR values across the recording period.

In Rabbit-N (first generation probe), HVS activity was recorded for a 678-day period on a solitary sinusoidal probe (**Figure 4A**). Similar waveforms were extracted over the 678-day indwelling period (**Figure 4B**). Further, stable mean peak-to-peak amplitude (**Figure 4C**) and SNR (**Figure 4D**) were recorded over the indwelling period. This initial result shows the potential for the sinusoidal electrode to record stable neuronal activity over chronic indwelling periods for >2 years.

ELECTROPHYSIOLOGY: SINGLE-UNIT RECORDING EXAMPLE

Figure 5 shows an example of a putative single unit obtained across all three electrode-recording sites of a sinusoidal electrode

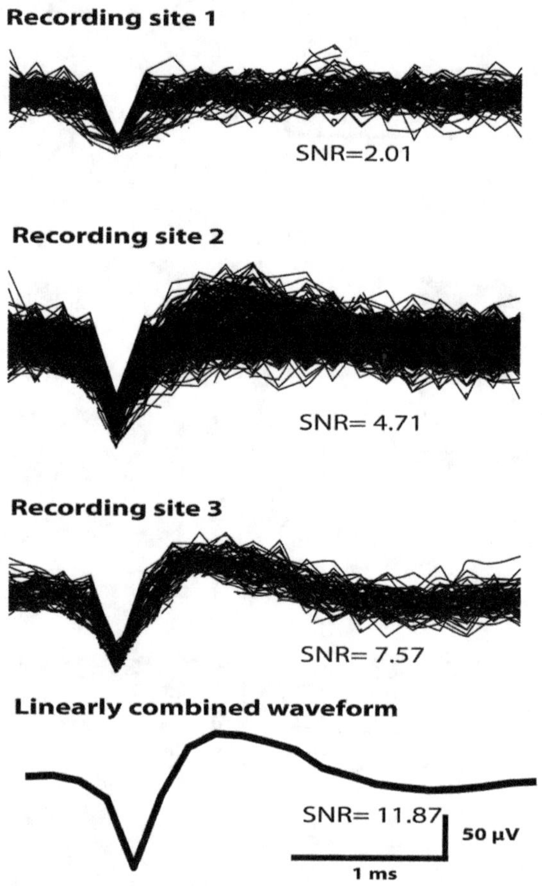

FIGURE 5 | A single unit recorded across all three sinusoidal recording sites in Rabbit-Lo. An algorithm was used that optimized the SNR by forming a linear combination of the three available channels; the SNR of the combined waveform was 11.87. The SNR values from the individual recording sites were lower than this value.

in Rabbit-Lo (second generation probe). The unit had different SNR and mean peak-to-peak amplitude on each contact, which allowed for effective unit isolation. Since the same action potential is observed on all three recordings, it is possible to improve SNR by linear combination. The three individual recording sites had SNR values of 2.01, 4.71, and 7.57. We used an algorithm, which chose the optimal linear combination to maximize the SNR; this achieved an SNR of 11.87. This example shows the utility of recording the same single unit across three electrode recording sites. An additional advantage of recording the same waveform on different electrodes is that differences in A may provide information additional to waveform shape that can be used for spike sorting (Gray et al., 1995; Harris et al., 2000).

THE GLIAL RESPONSE TO IMPLANTED ELECTRODES

The glial response to both electrode types was assessed over a 6–24 month chronic indwelling period by staining for astrocytes (**Figure 6**), microglia (**Figure 7**) and neurofilament (**Figure 8**). Overall there was a decrease in the astrocytic response at both 6 (**Figures 6A,D**) and 24 months (**Figures 6C,F**) close to the sinusoidal probe implantation site and where the classical astrocytic response is usually found (Polikov et al., 2005). No difference was found between the two electrode types at 12 months (**Figures 6B,E**). We found a decrease in overall microgliosis over a region of 0–500 μm at both 12 (**Figures 7A,C**) and 24 months (**Figures 7B,D**). Interestingly, for the same time points we also found an increase in neurofilament staining around the sinusoidal probe (**Figure 8**). Therefore it appears that the sinusoidal electrodes were better integrated into the neural tissue with decreased gliosis compared to microwires.

DISCUSSION

MICROFABRICATION

Microfabrication was successful with high functional yields generated from a single wafer. As dilute TMAH was used to release devices, a clean room wet bench was not needed for device release. This is an advantage over other polymeric probes requiring strong acids or bases (Kohler et al., 2009; Kozai and Kipke, 2009; Wu et al., 2011) for a similar release process. In some previous work, polymeric probes have been successfully peeled off the silicon wafer substrate without the inclusion of a sacrificial layer (e.g., Takeuchi et al., 2004). We found a similar approach to be problematic during initial testing as some probes remained attached, decreasing the yield of finished probe. Inclusion of the sacrificial aluminum layer in our process aided device adhesion during fabrication, but allowed reliable and straightforward release. This led to high functional yields.

Adhesion between two parylene-C layers can be problematic. Multiple groups bake parylene-C post device fabrication to promote this adhesion, however, this is time consuming and risks damaging devices as temperatures (200°C) above the parylene-C glass transition are used (Pang et al., 2005; Metzen and Stieglitz, 2012; Kim et al., 2013; Kuo et al., 2013). Here we show that a slight RIE over-etch when etching the WTi metal layer has the benefit of surface roughening the first parylene-C layer, improving parylene adhesion and preventing subsequent device delamination.

Other groups have attempted to increase neuronal recordings longevity by decreasing the footprint of the probe (Lind et al., 2010; Yoshida Kozai et al., 2012). Using the equation for the deflection of a rectangular cantilever beam, which takes into account the material dimensions and YM, a decrease in dimensions will lead to a decrease in overall stiffness values (Lempka et al., 2006; Yoshida Kozai et al., 2012). Decreasing the material's YM will have a similar effect. A limitation to decreasing probe dimensionality is the reduction in recording site area, which leads to higher obtained impedances (Ludwig et al., 2006). Electrodeposition of materials (e.g. PEDOT) onto the small recording site is required to achieve suitable impedance values for single-unit recording (Ludwig et al., 2011; Yoshida Kozai et al., 2012). However, these materials often have delamination issues >1 month post-implant (Yoshida Kozai et al., 2012).

The primary focus of this study was to compare the sinusoidal electrode to more conventional probes currently used for recording in non-human primates or humans. The improved performance over the rigid microwire electrode was largely due to reduced implant stiffness and reduced movement of the recording tip relative to the surrounding tissue. The contribution of the

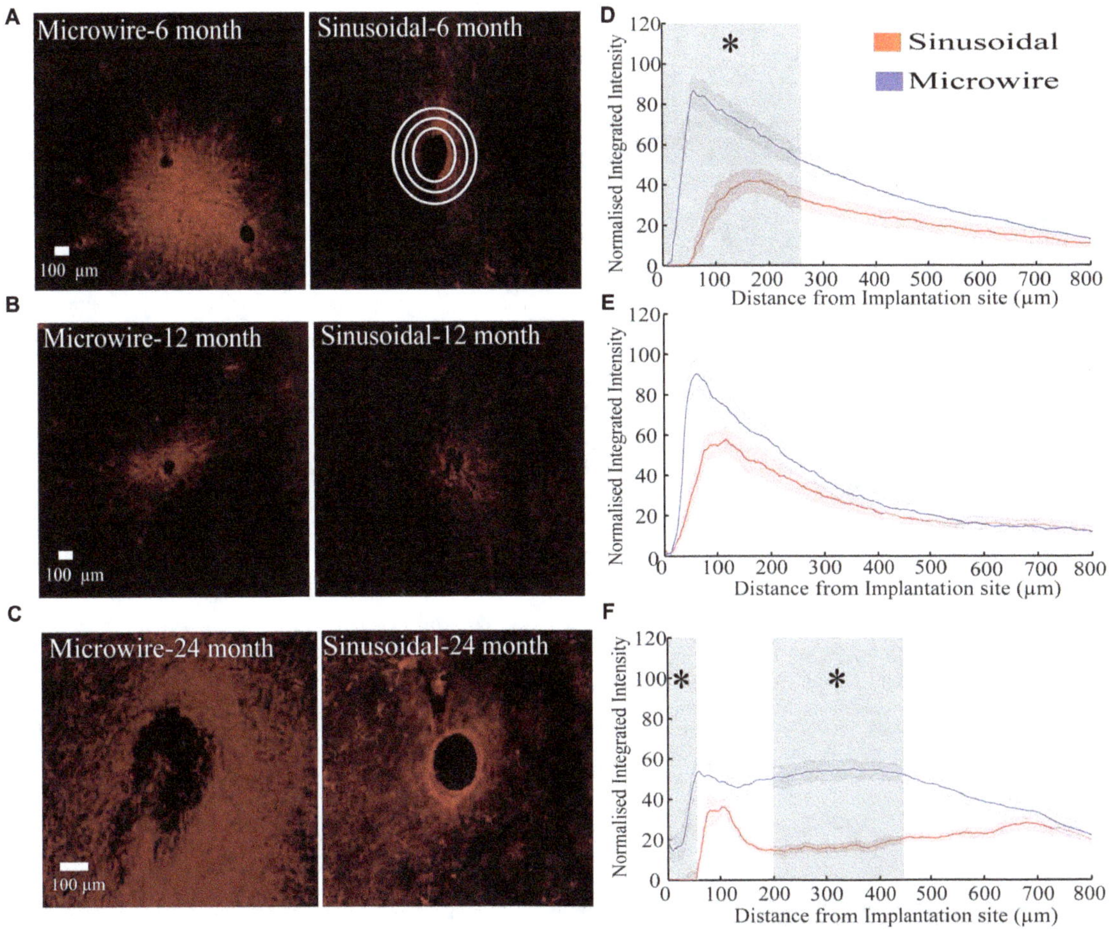

FIGURE 6 | The astrocytic response over a 6 (rabbit J, L), 12(rabbit P), and 24 (rabbit-N) month chronic indwelling period. (A) Representative images for the astrocytic response for both electrode types at the 6 month time point. Note the interaction between the two microwire recording sites. White concentric rings show an illustrative example of measurements taken for the radial distribution intensity as a function of distance from the electrode implantation site. **(B)** Representative images for the astrocytic response for both electrode types at the 12 month time point. **(C)** Representative images for the astrocytic response for both electrode types at the 24 month time point. **(D)** Overall normalized integrated intensity response (±SEM) for both electrode types for the 6 month time point ($n = 30$ electrode tracts). Significant differences (gray shading) were found at 50–250 μm away from the electrode implantation site ($P < 0.05$). **(E)** Overall normalized integrated intensity response (±SEM) for both electrode types for the 12 month time point ($n = 15$ electrode tracts). No significant differences were found. **(F)** Overall normalized integrated intensity response (±SEM) for both electrode types for the 24 month time point ($n = 15$ electrode tracts). Significant differences were found at 50 and 150–450 μm away from the electrode implantation site ($P < 0.05$).

sinusoidal shaft to the success of the design is difficult to quantify from this study, as a straight-shafted control was not used. This comparison can be addressed in future studies both with a modeling approach and through *in vivo* implantation of a straight-shaft version of the probe.

CHRONIC NEURONAL RECORDING

A striking result was the ability to record neuronal activity for >2 year period with stable recording parameters with the sinusoidal probe. Chronic recordings have also been obtained from other probes, such as the Utah array (>1–2 years; Rousche and Normann, 1998; Suner et al., 2005; Hochberg et al., 2006, 2012; Simeral et al., 2011; Collinger et al., 2012), Michigan probe (>6 weeks; Kipke et al., 2003; Vetter et al., 2004) and microwire probes (>1.5 years; Nicolelis et al., 2003; Jackson and Fetz, 2007). However, a distinct problem for all these probes is the lack of recording parameter stability. For microwires, Nicolelis et al. (2003) recorded activity from primate cortex. Based on the similarity of unsorted waveform clusters in principle component space, that study found 80% of the original units were still present after 2 days and 55% after 8 days (Nicolelis et al., 2003). Jackson and Fetz (2007) used the correlation coefficient between unsorted waveform averages and reported that 50% of original units were stable for a week, and 10% were stable through to 2 weeks. Dickey et al. (2009) used both average spike waveforms and interspike interval histograms to show that for a Utah array implanted in rhesus macaque monkeys 57, 43, and 39% of original units were stable for 7, 10, and 15 days respectively. In our hands, the sinusoidal probe provided more stable recordings judged from LFP and HVS activity than microwire electrodes.

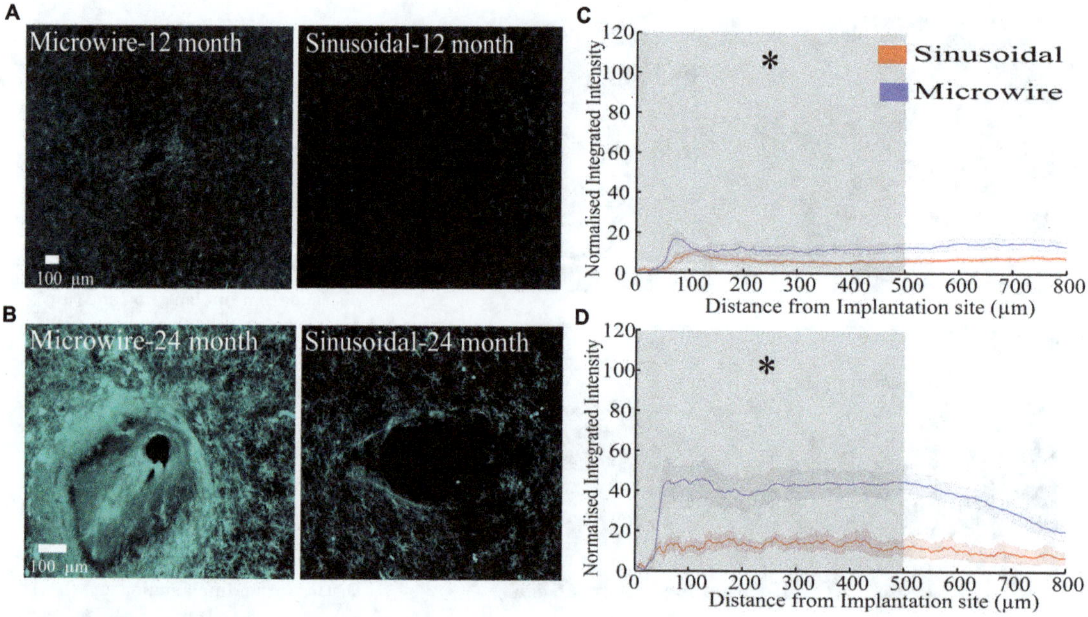

FIGURE 7 | The microglial response over a 12 (rabbit-P) and 24 (rabbit-N) month chronic indwelling period. (A) Representative images for the microglial response for both electrode types at the 6 month time point. **(B)** Representative images for the microglial response for both electrode types at the 12 month time point. **(C)** Overall normalized integrated intensity response (±SEM) for both electrode types for the 12 month time point ($n = 15$ electrode tracts per electrode comparison). Significant differences were found at 50–500 μm away from the electrode implantation site ($P < 0.05$). **(D)** Overall normalized integrated intensity response (±SEM) for both electrode types for the 24 month time point ($n = 15$ electrode tracts per electrode comparison). For the bottom profile representation, significant differences were found at 50–500 μm away from the electrode implantation site ($P < 0.05$).

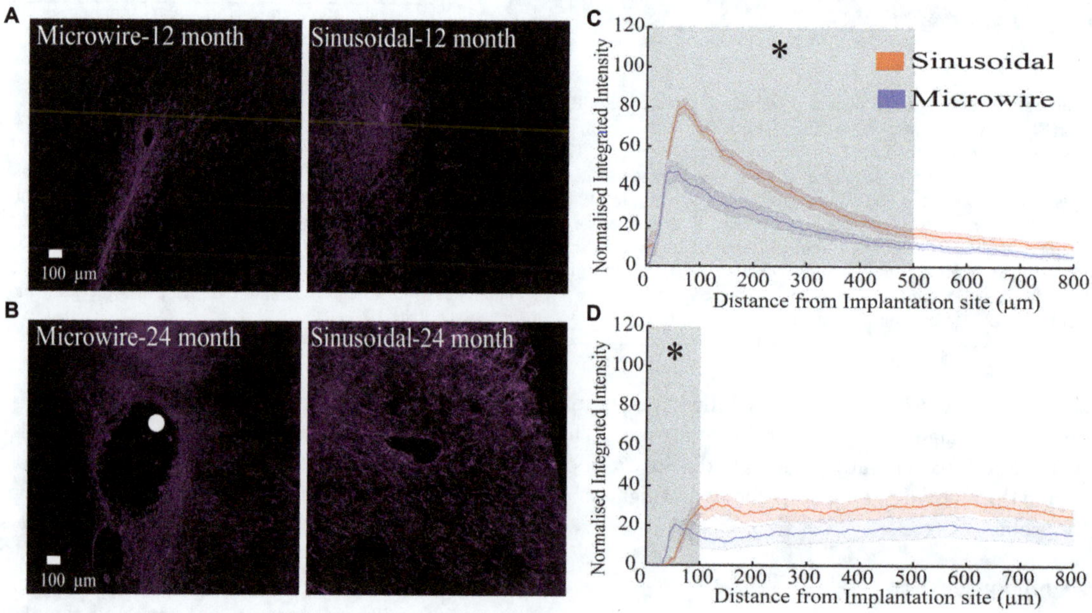

FIGURE 8 | The neurofilament response over a 12 (rabbit p) and 24 (rabbit-N) month chronic indwelling period. (A) Representative images for the neurofilament response for both electrode types at the 6 month time point. **(B)** Representative images for the neurofilament response for both electrode types at the 12 month time point. The white dot represents the microwire electrode implantation site. **(C)** Overall normalized integrated intensity response (±SEM) for both electrode types for the 12 month time point ($n = 15$ electrode tracts per electrode comparison). Significant differences were found at 50–500 μm away from the electrode implantation site ($P < 0.05$). **(D)** Overall normalized integrated intensity response (±SEM) for both electrode types for the 24 month time point ($n = 15$ electrode tracts per electrode comparison). Significant differences were found at 50 and 100 μm away from the electrode implantation site ($P < 0.05$).

However, further testing is needed to corroborate this recording stability.

To compare our electrode performance with other commercially available electrodes a commonly used SNR measure was used. For our electrode, peak SNR values for HVS were between 3 and 6. An appropriate comparison is the SNR measured from other electrode designs using multi-unit activity. Jackson and Fetz (2007) obtained values around 7 for their microwire electrode. Ward et al. (2009) obtained values between 6 and 7 for multiple electrode types including the Utah array, microwire, and Michigan probe electrodes over a 30 day recording period. For novel carbon fiber electrodes, SNR values of 3–8 were obtained over a 5 week indwelling period (Yoshida Kozai et al., 2012). Our electrode had comparable or slightly lower SNR values, although variability in recording stability was less than the microwire electrode.

Signal amplitudes of 60–400 μV (Ward et al., 2009), 120–250 μV (Suner et al., 2005), 60–100 μV (Vetter et al., 2004), and 60–200 μV (Yoshida Kozai et al., 2012) have been obtained for microwire, Utah array, Michigan probe and carbon fiber electrodes for chronic recording. We show recording amplitude of 100–230 μV for HVS responses, which is comparable to these electrode types.

Noise values are rarely reported in chronic electrode studies, however, from the Michigan probe, a value of 6–13 μV has been described (Vetter et al., 2004). We here report noise values of 7–13 μV during HVS responses. This is comparable to the Michigan probe electrode.

Overall, the SNR for a recorded unit can be increased by capturing that single unit across all three sinusoidal probe-recording sites. In addition, being able to record the same neuron on different sites on the probe may help sorting spikes in multi-unit recordings, as is commonly done with tetrode recording (Tseng et al., 2011).

Measurements of electrode impedance were not correlated with noise or signal values. For saline impedance testing, thermal noise is the main component of noise as there is no neuronal activity present. *In vivo*, SNR should follow impedance trends as thermal noise is directly related to the electrode impedance (Ludwig et al., 2006). As there was no correlation, it is possible that other sources of noise (e.g., biological or instrumentation noise) may have dominated the overall noise floor, as sources of noise summate in quadrature. Other groups have reported this phenomenon: SNR measurements are not related to 1 kHz *in vivo* impedance in both rodents and non-human primates for a variety of microelectrodes (Suner et al., 2005; Ward et al., 2009; Kim et al., 2013). Therefore, long-term impedance measurements may not be the best indicator for understanding chronic electrode performance.

Overall, our electrode had stable or initially declining impedances that stabilized over the indwelling period, similar to the microwire electrode. In contrast, silicon based probes have increasing impedances over both a 30 (Ward et al., 2009) and 81(Vetter et al., 2004) day indwelling period. For the Utah array there is a drop in impedance >1 year post-implant, which is related to electrode degradation (Suner et al., 2005). The drop in microwire impedance is related to the gradual insulation delamination surrounding the recording site, which increases the geometric surface area (GSA) available for recording (Patrick et al., 2011; Prasad et al., 2012).

For HVS responses, a few sinusoidal electrodes had drops in impedance after >20 days post-surgery, leading to improved recording characteristics. This may be related to the polyimide ball anchor. Gradual polyimide ball dissolution may have resulted in an increase in available GSA for recording. An alternative anchor which is more stable may need to be considered for future studies.

GLIAL RESPONSE

In this study, the sinusoidal probe was compared to microwire electrodes. Although the electrode was not compared to standard silicon probes, an emergent hierarchy is evident from the literature. In general silicon probes give a heightened immune response in relation to microwire style probes (Winslow et al., 2010; Yoshida Kozai et al., 2012). As we show decreased overall gliosis at multiple time points, it is reasonable to assume that we should also have a decreased response when comparing to standard silicon probes.

The sinusoidal probe had decreased overall gliosis measured by astrocytosis for the 6 month time point and by both astrocytosis and microgliosis for the 12 and 24 month time point. There was an increase in neurofilament staining around the sinusoidal probe at the 12 and 24 month time point. It appears that electrode designs incorporating micromotion-reducing measures can reduce gliosis and promote neuronal integration. Interestingly, we show an increase in neurofilament staining without the use of neurotropic factors, such as that used in the cone electrode (Kennedy, 1989; Kennedy et al., 1992; Bartels et al., 2008). The addition of a three dimension ball anchor seemed to attract neurites similar to the effect observed by Winslow and Tresco (2010) with cylindrical microwire electrodes over a 12-week indwelling period. The decreased microglial response is most likely the cause for the better neuronal integration seen with neurofilament staining for the sinusoidal probe. A heightened microglial response is associated with the loss of neurons in the immediate vicinity of the probe (~100 μm away), designated the "kill zone" (Biran et al., 2007); this is also the maximum theorized distance over which an implanted neuronal probe can record neuronal activity (Polikov et al., 2005). Therefore, an advantage of the sinusoidal probe is a decreased microgliosis response over a chronic indwelling period that limits the "kill zone" region.

Intriguingly individual microwire electrode tracts can interact with one another, producing interacting tracks of glial scarring over chronic indwelling period of >6 months. This is not ideal, as interaction between two electrode tracts may induce biological noise and alter overall network effects for the specific recording cells of interest as astrocytes can interact with neurons (Giaume et al., 2010; Gourine et al., 2010; Sasaki et al., 2012).

There are reports that at long times post-implant, gliosis extends beyond a reported distance of 500 μm (Biran et al., 2005; Polikov et al., 2005). This raises the possibility that on-going gliosis could continue to spread far beyond the original implantation site, affecting considerable volumes of brain tissue. Such chronic spreading gliosis needs to be prevented to maintain stable recording parameters, especially in the presence of multiple implants.

FUTURE DIRECTIONS

Although the results of this initial study are promising, further testing is needed to corroborate the effectiveness of the sinusoidal probe as a chronic implant. Testing is needed in larger animals (e.g., non-human primates) where the problem of micromotion is far greater due to different patterns of animal behavior and skull sizes. We have verified that our insertion technique is suitable for non-human primates (data not shown), so this translational step beyond rodents and lagomorphs is a possibility.

CONCLUSION

To our knowledge this is the first study to show the usefulness of addressing micromotion-induced trauma with flexible electrodes more than 6 months after implant. We have shown that the sinusoidal probe appeared to be more stable in recording parameters over a 6–24 month chronic indwelling period in terms of LFP and HVS, especially in terms of LFP power and SNR. Further, we show that it is possible to register neuronal activity beyond 2-years post-implant with the sinusoidal probe. Gliosis was reduced at the recording tip of the sinusoidal compared to the rigid microwire electrodes at 6, 12, and 24-month time points, and there was better neuronal integration at 12 and 24 months. However, further studies are needed to corroborate these initial promising results. This initial study shows that the sinusoidal probe is a potential alternative to silicon, microwire and other polymeric probes for chronic neuronal recording.

ACKNOWLEDGMENTS

This work was supported by the Wellcome Trust, EPSRC, and MRC.

REFERENCES

Allen, J. S., Bruss, J., Brown, C. K., and Damasio, H. (2005). Normal neuroanatomical variation due to age: the major lobes and a parcellation of the temporal region. *Neurobiol. Aging* 26, 1245–1260. doi: 10.1016/j.neurobiolaging.2005.05.023

Azevedo, F. A. C., Carvalho, L. R. B., Grinberg, L. T., Farfel, J. M., Ferretti, R. E. L., Leite, R. E. P., et al. (2009). Equal numbers of neuronal and nonneuronal cells make the human brain an isometrically scaled-up primate brain. *J. Comp. Neurol.* 513, 532–541. doi: 10.1002/cne.21974

Bartels, J., Andreasen, D., Ehirim, P., Mao, H., Seibert, S., Wright, E. J., et al. (2008). Neurotrophic electrode: method of assembly and implantation into human motor speech cortex. *J. Neurosci. Methods* 174, 168–176. doi: 10.1016/j.jneumeth.2008.06.030

Biran, R., Martin, D. C., and Tresco, P. A. (2005). Neuronal cell loss accompanies the brain tissue response to chronically implanted silicon microelectrode arrays. *Exp. Neurol.* 195, 115–126. doi: 10.1016/j.expneurol.2005.04.020

Biran, R., Martin, D. C., and Tresco, P. A. (2007). The brain tissue response to implanted silicon microelectrode arrays is increased when the device is tethered to the skull. *J. Biomed. Mater. Res. A* 82, 169–178. doi: 10.1002/jbm.a.31138

Bjornsson, C. S., Oh, S. J., Al-Kofahi, Y. A., Lim, Y. J., Smith, K. L., Turner, J. N., et al. (2006). Effects of insertion conditions on tissue strain and vascular damage during neuroprosthetic device insertion. *J. Neural Eng.* 3, 196–207. doi: 10.1088/1741-2560/3/3/002

Buzsáki, G., Bickford, R. G., Ponomareff, G., Thal, L. J., Mandel, R., and Gage, F. H. (1988). Nucleus basalis and thalamic control of neocortical activity in the freely moving rat. *J. Neurosci.* 8, 4007–4026.

Chorover, S. L., and DeLuca, A. M. (1972). A sweet new multiple electrode for chronic single unit recording in moving animals. *Physiol. Behav.* 9, 671–674. doi: 10.1016/0031-9384(72)90030-3

Collinger, J. L., Wodlinger, B., Downey, J. E., Wang, W., Tyler-Kabara, E. C., Weber, D. J., et al. (2012). High-performance neuroprosthetic control by an individual with tetraplegia. *Lancet* 38, 557–564. doi: 10.1016/S0140-6736(12)61816-9

Dickey, A. S., Suminski, A., Amit, Y., and Hatsopoulos, N. G. (2009). Single-unit stability using chronically implanted multielectrode arrays. *J. Neurophysiol.* 102, 1331–1339. doi: 10.1152/jn.90920.2008

Geddes, L. A., and Roeder, R. (2003). Criteria for the selection of materials for implanted electrodes. *Ann. Biomed. Eng.* 31, 879–890. doi: 10.1114/1.1581292

Giaume, C., Koulakoff, A., Roux, L., Holcman, D., and Rouach, N. (2010). Astroglial networks: a step further in neuroglial and gliovascular interactions. *Nat. Rev. Neurosci.* 11, 87–99. doi: 10.1038/nrn2757

Gilletti, A., and Muthuswamy, J. (2006). Brain micromotion around implants in the rodent somatosensory cortex. *J. Neural Eng.* 3, 189–195. doi: 10.1088/1741-2560/3/3/001

Gould, H. J. III. (1986). Body surface maps in the somatosensory cortex of rabbit. *J. Comp. Neurol.* 243, 207–233. doi: 10.1002/cne.902430206

Gourine, A. V., Kasymov, V., Marina, N., Tang, F., Figueiredo, M. F., Lane, S., et al. (2010). Astrocytes control breathing through pH-dependent release of ATP. *Science* 329, 571–575. doi: 10.1126/science.1190721

Gray, C. M., Maldonado, P. E., Wilson, M., and McNaughton, B. (1995). Tetrodes markedly improve the reliability and yield of multiple single-unit isolation from multi-unit recordings in cat striate cortex. *J. Neurosci. Methods* 63, 43–54. doi: 10.1016/0165-0270(95)00085-2

Harris, J. P., Hess, A. E., Rowan, S. J., Weder, C., Zorman, C. A., Tyler, D. J., et al. (2011). In vivo deployment of mechanically adaptive nanocomposites for intracortical microelectrodes. *J. Neural Eng.* 8, 046010. doi: 10.1088/1741-2560/8/4/046010

Harris, K. D., Henze, D. A., Csicsvari, J., Hirase, H., and Buzsáki, G. (2000). Accuracy of tetrode spike separation as determined by simultaneous intracellular and extracellular measurements. *J. Neurophysiol.* 84, 401–414.

Hassler, C., Guy, J., Nietzschmann, M., Staiger, J. F., and Stieglitz, T. (2011). Chronic intracortical implantation of saccharose-coated flexible shaft electrodes into the cortex of rats. *Conf. Proc. IEEE Eng. Med. Biol. Soc.* 2011, 644–647. doi: 10.1109/IEMBS.2011.6090143

Hochberg, L. R., Bacher, D., Jarosiewicz, B., Masse, N. Y., Simeral, J. D., Vogel, J., et al. (2012). Reach and grasp by people with tetraplegia using a neurally controlled robotic arm. *Nature* 485, 372–375. doi: 10.1038/nature11076

Hochberg, L. R., Serruya, M. D., Friehs, G. M., Mukand, J. A., Saleh, M., Caplan, A. H., et al. (2006). Neuronal ensemble control of prosthetic devices by a human with tetraplegia. *Nature* 442, 164–171. doi: 10.1038/nature04970

Hubel, D. H. (1959). Single unit activity in striate cortex of unrestrained cats. *J. Physiol. (Lond.)* 147, 226–238.

Hwang, E. J., and Andersen, R. A. (2013). The utility of multichannel local field potentials for brain-machine interfaces. *J. Neural Eng.* 10, 046005. doi: 10.1088/1741-2560/10/4/046005

Jackson, A., and Fetz, E. E. (2007). Compact movable microwire array for long-term chronic unit recording in cerebral cortex of primates. *J. Neurophysiol.* 98, 3109–3118. doi: 10.1152/jn.00569.2007

Kennedy, P. R. (1989). The cone electrode: a long-term electrode that records from neurites grown onto its recording surface. *J. Neurosci. Methods* 29, 181–193. doi: 10.1016/0165-0270(89)90142-8

Kennedy, P. R., Mirra, S. S., and Bakay, R. A. E. (1992). The cone electrode: ultrastructural studies following long-term recording in rat and monkey cortex. *Neurosci. Lett.* 142, 89–94. doi: 10.1016/0304-3940(92)90627-J

Kim, B. J., Kuo, J. T. W., Hara, S. A., Lee, C. D., Yu, L., Gutierrez, C. A., et al. (2013). 3D Parylene sheath neural probe for chronic recordings. *J. Neural Eng.* 10, 045002. doi: 10.1088/1741-2560/10/4/045002

Kipke, D. R., Vetter, R. J., Williams, J. C., and Hetke, J. F. (2003). Silicon-substrate intracortical microelectrode arrays for long-term recording of neuronal spike activity in cerebral cortex. *IEEE Trans. Neural. Syst. Rehabil. Eng.* 11, 151–155. doi: 10.1109/TNSRE.2003.814443

Kohler, P., Linsmeier, C. E., Thelin, J., Bengtsson, M., Jorntell, H., Garwicz, M., et al. (2009). Flexible multi electrode brain-machine interface for recording in the cerebellum. *Conf. Proc. IEEE Eng. Med. Biol. Soc.* 2009, 536–538. doi: 10.1109/IEMBS.2009.5333498

Kozai, T. D. Y., and Kipke, D. R. (2009). Insertion shuttle with carboxyl terminated self-assembled monolayer coatings for implanting flexible polymer neural probes in the brain. *J. Neurosci. Methods* 184, 199–205. doi: 10.1016/j.jneumeth.2009.08.002

Kozai, T. D. Y., Marzullo, T. C., Hooi, F., Langhals, N. B., Majewska, A. K., Brown, E. B., et al. (2010). Reduction of neurovascular damage resulting from microelectrode insertion into the cerebral cortex using in vivo two-photon mapping. *J. Neural Eng.* 7, 046011. doi: 10.1088/1741-2560/7/4/046011

Kuo, J. T. W., Kim, B. J., Hara, S. A., Lee, C. D., Gutierrez, C. A., Hoang, T. Q., et al. (2013). Novel flexible Parylene neural probe with 3D sheath structure for enhancing tissue integration. *Lab Chip* 13, 554–561. doi: 10.1039/c2lc40935f

LaPlaca, M. C., Cullen, D. K., McLoughlin, J. J., and Cargill, R. S. II. (2005). High rate shear strain of three-dimensional neural cell cultures: a new in vitro traumatic brain injury model. *J. Biomech.* 38, 1093–1105. doi: 10.1016/j.jbiomech.2004.05.032

Lempka, S. F., Johnson, M. D., Barnett, D. W., Moffitt, M. A., Otto, K. J., Kipke, D. R., et al. (2006). Optimization of microelectrode design for cortical recording based on thermal noise considerations. *Conf. Proc. IEEE Eng. Med. Biol. Soc.* 1, 3361–3364. doi: 10.1109/IEMBS.2006.259432

Lind, G., Linsmeier, C. E., Thelin, J., and Schouenborg, J. (2010). Gelatine-embedded electrodes – a novel biocompatible vehicle allowing implantation of highly flexible microelectrodes. *J. Neural Eng.* 7, 046005. doi: 10.1088/1741-2560/7/4/046005

Ludwig, K. A., Langhals, N. B., Joseph, M. D., Richardson-Burns, S. M., Hendricks, J. L., and Kipke, D. R. (2011). Poly(3,4-ethylenedioxythiophene) (PEDOT) polymer coatings facilitate smaller neural recording electrodes. *J. Neural Eng.* 8, 014001. doi: 10.1088/1741-2560/8/1/014001

Ludwig, K. A., Uram, J. D., Yang, J., Martin, D. C., and Kipke, D. R. (2006). Chronic neural recordings using silicon microelectrode arrays electrochemically deposited with a poly(3,4-ethylenedioxythiophene) (PEDOT) film. *J. Neural Eng.* 3, 59–70. doi: 10.1088/1741-2560/3/1/007

Marblestone, A. H., Zamft, B. M., Maguire, Y. G., Shapiro, M. G., Cybulski, T. R., Glaser, J. I., et al. (2013). Physical principles for scalable neural recording. *Front. Comput. Neurosci.* 7:137. doi: 10.3389/fncom.2013.00137

Metzen, R. P. V., and Stieglitz, T. (2012). The influence of annealing on the electrical stability of parylene C structures. *Biomed. Tech. (Berl.)* doi: 10.1515/bmt-2012-4272 [Epub ahead of print].

Miller, K., Chinzei, K., Orssengo, G., and Bednarz, P. (2000). Mechanical properties of brain tissue in vivo: experiment and computer simulation. *J. Biomech.* 33, 1369–1376. doi: 10.1016/S0021-9290(00)00120-2

Nicolelis, M. A. (2001). Actions from thoughts. *Nature* 409, 403–407. doi: 10.1038/35053191

Nicolelis, M. A., Dimitrov, D., Carmena, J. M., Crist, R., Lehew, G., Kralik, J. D., et al. (2003). Chronic, multisite, multielectrode recordings in macaque monkeys. *Proc. Natl. Acad. Sci. U.S.A.* 100, 11041–11046. doi: 10.1073/pnas.1934665100

Pang, C., Cham, J., Nenadic, Z., Musallam, S., Tai, Y. C., Burdick, J., et al. (2005). A new multi-site probe array with monolithically integrated parylene flexible cable for neural prostheses. *Conf. Proc. IEEE Eng. Med. Biol. Soc.* 7, 7114–7117.

Patrick, E., Orazem, M. E., Sanchez, J. C., and Nishida, T. (2011). Corrosion of tungsten microelectrodes used in neural recording applications. *J. Neurosci. Methods* 198, 158–171. doi: 10.1016/j.jneumeth.2011.03.012

Perge, J. A., Homer, M. L., Malik, W. Q., Cash, S., Eskandar, E., Friehs, G., et al. (2013). Intra-day signal instabilities affect decoding performance in an intracortical neural interface system. *J. Neural Eng.* 10, 036004. doi: 10.1088/1741-2560/10/3/036004

Polikov, V. S., Tresco, P. A., and Reichert, W. M. (2005). Response of brain tissue to chronically implanted neural electrodes. *J. Neurosci. Methods* 148, 1–18. doi: 10.1016/j.jneumeth.2005.08.015

Potter, K. A., Buck, A. C., Self, W. K., and Capadona, J. R. (2012). Stab injury and device implantation within the brain results in inversely multiphasic neuroinflammatory and neurodegenerative responses. *J. Neural Eng.* 9, 046020. doi: 10.1088/1741-2560/9/4/046020

Prasad, A., Xue, Q.-S., Sankar, V., Nishida, T., Shaw, G., Streit, W. J., et al. (2012). Comprehensive characterization and failure modes of tungsten microwire arrays in chronic neural implants. *J. Neural Eng.* 9, 056015. doi: 10.1088/1741-2560/9/5/056015

Rousche, P. J., and Normann, R. A. (1998). Chronic recording capability of the Utah intracortical electrode array in cat sensory cortex. *J. Neurosci. Methods* 82, 1–15. doi: 10.1016/S0165-0270(98)00031-4

Sasaki, T., Beppu, K., Tanaka, K. F., Fukazawa, Y., Shigemoto, R., and Matsui, K. (2012). Application of an optogenetic byway for perturbing neuronal activity via glial photostimulation. *Proc. Natl. Acad. Sci. U.S.A.* 109, 20720–20725. doi: 10.1073/pnas.1213458109

Schwartz, A. B. (2004). Cortical neural prosthetics. *Annu. Rev. Neurosci.* 27, 487–507. doi: 10.1146/annurev.neuro.27.070203.144233

Seymour, J. P., and Kipke, D. R. (2006). Fabrication of polymer neural probes with sub-cellular features for reduced tissue encapsulation. *Conf. Proc. IEEE Eng. Med. Biol. Soc.* 1, 4606–4609. doi: 10.1109/IEMBS.2006.260528

Seymour, J. P., Langhals, N. B., Anderson, D. J., and Kipke, D. R. (2011). Novel multi-sided, microelectrode arrays for implantable neural applications. *Biomed. Microdevices* 13, 441–451. doi: 10.1007/s10544-011-9512-z

Simeral, J. D., Kim, S. P., Black, M. J., Donoghue, J. P., and Hochberg, L. R. (2011). Neural control of cursor trajectory and click by a human with tetraplegia 1000 days after implant of an intracortical microelectrode array. *J. Neural Eng.* 8, 025027. doi: 10.1088/1741-2560/8/2/025027

Subbaroyan, J., Martin, D. C., and Kipke, D. R. (2005). A finite-element model of the mechanical effects of implantable microelectrodes in the cerebral cortex. *J. Neural Eng.* 2, 103–113. doi: 10.1088/1741-2560/2/4/006

Suner, S., Fellows, M. R., Vargas-Irwin, C., Nakata, G. K., and Donoghue, J. P. (2005). Reliability of signals from a chronically implanted, silicon-based electrode array in non-human primate primary motor cortex. *IEEE Trans. Neural. Syst. Rehabil. Eng.* 13, 524–541. doi: 10.1109/TNSRE.2005.857687

Suyatin, D. B., Wallman, L., Thelin, J., Prinz, C. N., Jörntell, H., Samuelson, L., et al. (2013). Nanowire-based electrode for acute in vivo neural recordings in the brain. *PLoS ONE* 8:e56673. doi: 10.1371/journal.pone.0056673

Swadlow, H. A. (1989). Efferent neurons and suspected interneurons in S-1 vibrissa cortex of the awake rabbit: receptive fields and axonal properties. *J. Neurophysiol.* 62, 288–308.

Swadlow, H. A. (1990). Efferent neurons and suspected interneurons in S-1 forelimb representation of the awake rabbit: receptive fields and axonal properties. *J. Neurophysiol.* 63, 1477–1498.

Swadlow, H. A. (1994). Efferent neurons and suspected interneurons in motor cortex of the awake rabbit: axonal properties, sensory receptive fields, and subthreshold synaptic inputs. *J. Neurophysiol.* 71, 437–453.

Swadlow, H. A., and Hicks, T. P. (1996). Somatosensory cortical efferent neurons of the awake rabbit: latencies to activation via supra – and subthreshold receptive fields. *J. Neurophysiol.* 75, 1753–1759.

Takeuchi, S., Yoshida, Y., Ziegler, D., Mabuchi, K., and Suzuki, T. (2004). Parylene flexible neural probe with micro fluidic channel. *Lab Chip* 5, 519–523. doi: 10.1039/b417497f

Taylor, D. M., Tillery, S. I. H., and Schwartz, A. B. (2002). Direct cortical control of 3D neuroprosthetic devices. *Science* 296, 1829–1832. doi: 10.1126/science.1070291

Thelin, J., Jörntell, H., Psouni, E., Garwicz, M., Schouenborg, J., Danielsen, N., et al. (2011). Implant size and fixation mode strongly influence tissue reactions in the CNS. *PLoS ONE* 6:e16267. doi: 10.1371/journal.pone.0016267

Tseng, W.-T., Yen, C.-T., and Tsai, M.-L. (2011). A bundled microwire array for long-term chronic single-unit recording in deep brain regions of behaving rats. *J. Neurosci. Methods* 201, 368–376. doi: 10.1016/j.jneumeth.2011.08.028

Vetter, R. J., Williams, J. C., Hetke, J. F., Nunamaker, E. A., and Kipke, D. R. (2004). Chronic neural recording using silicon-substrate microelectrode arrays implanted in cerebral cortex. *IEEE Trans. Biomed. Eng.* 51, 896–904. doi: 10.1109/TBME.2004.826680

Ward, M. P., Rajdev, P., Ellison, C., and Irazoqui, P. P. (2009). Toward a comparison of microelectrodes for acute and chronic recordings. *Brain Res.* 1282, 183–200. doi: 10.1016/j.brainres.2009.05.052

Winslow, B. D., and Tresco, P. A. (2010). Quantitative analysis of the tissue response to chronically implanted microwire electrodes in rat cortex. *Biomaterials* 31, 1558–1567. doi: 10.1016/j.biomaterials.2009.11.049

Winslow, B. D., Christensen, M. B., Yang, W.-K., Solzbacher, F., and Tresco, P. A. (2010). A comparison of the tissue response to chronically implanted Parylene-C-coated and uncoated planar silicon microelectrode arrays in rat cortex. *Biomaterials* 31, 9163–9172. doi: 10.1016/j.biomaterials.2010.05.050

Witteveen, J. A., Suyatin, D. B., Gällentoft, L., Schouenborg, J., Danielsen, N., and Prinz, C. N. (2010). Gelatin/glycerol coating to preserve mechanically compliant nanowire electrodes from damage during brain implantation. *J. Vacuum Sci. Technol. B* 28, C6K13–C6K16. doi: 10.1116/1.3498764

Wu, F., Im, M., and Yoon, E. (2011). "A flexible fish-bone-shaped neural probe strengthened by biodegradable silk coating for enhanced biocompatibility," in *Proceedings of 16th International Solid-State Sensors, Actuators and Microsystems Conference (TRANSDUCERS)*, Beijing, 966–969.

Yoshida Kozai, T. D., Langhals, N. B., Patel, P. R., Deng, X., Zhang, H., Smith, K. L., et al. (2012). Ultrasmall implantable composite microelectrodes with bioactive surfaces for chronic neural interfaces. *Nat. Mater.* 11, 1065–1073. doi: 10.1038/nmat3468

Zimmermann, J. B., Seki, K., and Jackson, A. (2011). Reanimating the arm and hand with intraspinal microstimulation. *J. Neural Eng.* 8, 054001. doi: 10.1088/1741-2560/8/5/054001

21

Paying attention to smell: cholinergic signaling in the olfactory bulb

Rinaldo D. D'Souza[†] and Sukumar Vijayaraghavan*

Department of Physiology and Biophysics and the Neuroscience Program, School of Medicine, University of Colorado, Aurora, CO, USA

Edited by:
Darwin K. Berg, University of California, San Diego, USA

Reviewed by:
Joseph F. Margiotta, University of Toledo College of Medicine, USA
Jie Wu, Barrow Neurological Institute, USA

Correspondence:
Sukumar Vijayaraghavan, Department of Physiology and Biophysics and the Neuroscience Program, School of Medicine, University of Colorado, MS 8307, P18-7121, 12800 East 19th Avenue, Aurora, CO 80045, USA
e-mail: sukumar.v@ucdenver.edu

†Present address:
Rinaldo D. D'Souza, Department of Anatomy and Neurobiology, Washington University School of Medicine, St. Louis, MO, USA

The tractable, layered architecture of the olfactory bulb (OB), and its function as a relay between odor input and higher cortical processing, makes it an attractive model to study how sensory information is processed at a synaptic and circuit level. The OB is also the recipient of strong neuromodulatory inputs, chief among them being the central cholinergic system. Cholinergic axons from the basal forebrain modulate the activity of various cells and synapses within the OB, particularly the numerous dendrodendritic synapses, resulting in highly variable responses of OB neurons to odor input that is dependent upon the behavioral state of the animal. Behavioral, electrophysiological, anatomical, and computational studies examining the function of muscarinic and nicotinic cholinergic receptors expressed in the OB have provided valuable insights into the role of acetylcholine (ACh) in regulating its function. We here review various studies examining the modulation of OB function by cholinergic fibers and their target receptors, and provide putative models describing the role that cholinergic receptor activation might play in the encoding of odor information.

Keywords: muscarinic, nicotinic, glomerular, GABAergic, filter

INTRODUCTION

The network of cholinergic fibers acts as a major neuromodulatory system in the brain. It is not only implicated in the pathophysiology of neurodegenerative disorders like Alzheimer's disease, but it also plays a central role in the functioning of the healthy brain. The release of ACh by these fibers is involved in the enhancement of sensory perception during wakefulness, particularly during periods of sustained attention (Himmelheber et al., 2000; Jones, 2005). Studying how ACh controls various brain systems at the level of circuits and synaptic transmission is critical for the understanding of how ACh affects brain function, both in health and in disease. The mammalian main OB provides for a convenient model system to study the modulatory control of sensory circuits. It is located centrally in the olfactory pathway (only one synapse away from odor input into the nose and one synapse away from higher cortical processing), and its excitatory and inhibitory neurons are relatively well-segregated. Importantly, its circuits and function are strongly modulated by ACh. Cholinergic input to the OB is provided primarily by axons of neurons whose cell bodies reside in the HDB in the basal forebrain (Wenk et al., 1980; Senut et al., 1989). While a more recent study has demonstrated the presence of choline acetyltransferase (ChAT)-expressing neurons within the OB itself (Krosnowski et al., 2012), a functional role has yet to be ascribed to these cholinergic interneurons. ACh released by HDB cholinergic neurons acts on both, nicotinic and muscarinic receptors (nAChR and mAChR, respectively) resulting in the control of olfactory function that is dependent upon the brain state of the animal – whether it is sleeping, performing a task, or simply awake and immobile. In this review, we focus on studies that have helped us gain better insights into how the release of ACh in the OB affects olfaction at the cellular, circuit, and behavioral level, and discuss how it might modulate odor coding during attentional control of OB circuits.

MULTIPLE, COMPLEX MECHANISMS INVOLVED IN OLFACTORY CODING

The OB represents a convergence point for incoming odor signals and contains the synapse transferring odor information between the ORNs and higher cortical regions. ORNs send their axons (which form the ON) into defined structures called glomeruli (**Figure 1**). Projections from ORNs that recognize the same odor epitope converge onto about two (of about two thousand) glomeruli in the ipsilateral bulb (Vassar et al., 1994). Within the glomerular neuropil, these neurons provide direct (Najac et al., 2011) and indirect (Najac et al., 2011; Gire et al., 2012) synaptic inputs onto the MCs, the principal output neurons of the OB. Modulation of odor information provided by these inputs occurs in the glomerulus as well as in the other layers of the bulb by a number of bulbar interneurons. Two key neuronal cell types that modulate glomerular output are the GABAergic PG cells and the glutamatergic external tufted (ET) cells, both of which are

---

Abbreviations: ACh, acetylcholine; ET cell, external tufted cell; HDB, horizontal limb of the diagonal band of Broca; M/T cells, mitral and/or tufted cells; mAChR, muscarinic acetylcholine receptor; MC, mitral cell; nAChR, nicotinic acetylcholine receptor; OB, olfactory bulb; ON, olfactory nerve; ORN, olfactory receptor neuron; PG cell, periglomerular cell; GC, Granule cells.

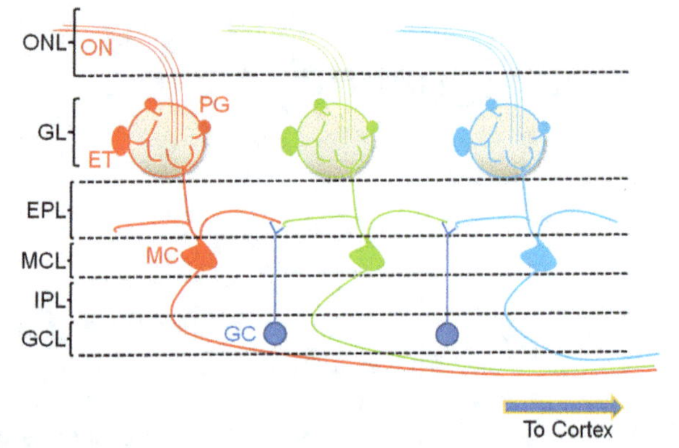

FIGURE 1 | A simplified cartoon of the bulbar circuit. ORNs in the nasal epithelium send their axons ON to the glomerular layer of the OB. Each glomerulus receives convergent ON input from ORNs that recognize the same odor epitope (color coded). Resident interneurons in the juxtaglomerular region receive ON input and modulate glomerular signaling. The two major glomerular interneuron classes are the glutamatergic external tufted (ET) cells and the GABAergic PG cells. Together, these cells regulate the glomerular output resulting in the excitation of MCs, the principal neurons of the OB. A second interneuron type, the granule cell (GC), forms dendrodendritic synapses with the lateral dendrites of the MCs. These neurons exert GABAergic control over multiple MCs resulting in lateral inhibition. The modulated output of the MC is then transmitted to the pyriform cortex. ONL, olfactory nerve layer; GL, glomerular layer; EPL, external plexiform layer; MCL, mitral cell layer; IPL, internal plexiform layer; GCL, granule cell layer.

also directly excited by ON input (Gire and Schoppa, 2009). The lateral dendrites of the MCs receive a second set of GABAergic inputs from granule cells (GCs) within another distinct layer called the external plexiform layer (EPL; **Figure 1**). Other interneuron types and subtypes have been described (Batista-Brito et al., 2008) but are not considered here in the context of cholinergic modulation.

Much of the information on odor representations (Xu et al., 2000; Bozza et al., 2004) and MCs responses to odor (Kashiwadani et al., 1999) comes from studies on anesthetized animals. However, recent studies have shown a much more complex scenario in awake animals, requiring re-evaluation of our notions of olfactory processing (Kato et al., 2012; Wachowiak et al., 2013). MCs in awake, behaving animals are spontaneously active (Rinberg and Gelperin, 2006; Rinberg et al., 2006; Davison and Katz, 2007) with firing that is often locked to the respiration cycle (Cury and Uchida, 2010; Wachowiak, 2011). Odor-evoked responses are not encoded in simple changes in firing frequencies; instead, the OB adopts various sophisticated mechanisms, involving the activity of MCs, to detect and encode odors. For example, upon odor onset, the latency of the first MC spike in response to the odor (Margrie and Schaefer, 2003; Junek et al., 2010), reduction in MC firing frequency (Rinberg and Gelperin, 2006; Rinberg et al., 2006; Davison and Katz, 2007), alterations in the relative temporal phase of individual spikes (Dhawale et al., 2010), relative timing of MC spikes (Haddad et al., 2013), and fine-scale changes in temporal spike patterns (Friedrich and Laurent, 2001; Cury and Uchida, 2010) are all thought to play important roles in odor coding. Each of these mechanisms is a potential target for modulation, thus leading to a multifold increase in the computational power of the OB.

It has now been demonstrated that the OB is not merely an encoder of odor information that is subsequently decoded downstream in the cortex, but that it is itself involved in "higher order" processing. The response of MCs to odors, for example, depends not only on the chemical structure of odorant molecules, but also on more behaviorally relevant properties. *In vivo* recordings have shown that synchrony between MC spiking, in response to an odor, can be altered depending on whether the odor is rewarded in a behavioral task or not (Doucette and Restrepo, 2008; Doucette et al., 2011). Such an associative cortex-like feature (Doucette et al., 2011) suggests an advanced role for the OB in sensory information processing. This is consistent with studies which show that the activity of OB neurons can be profoundly affected by feedback inputs from the cortex (Gao and Strowbridge, 2009; Markopoulos et al., 2012). Task-dependent control of circuits in the OB thus plays a vital role in processing odor information.

THE OLFACTORY BULB AND ITS CHOLINERGIC INPUT

A cluster of cholinergic neurons from the basal forebrain sends diffuse projections to the entire cortical mantle. All cortical areas receive cholinergic innervation, though there appears to be differences in the density of innervation across specific layers (Lysakowski et al., 1989; Mesulam et al., 1992). The lack of consistent topographic precision leads to the idea that cholinergic activation might lead to uniform effects across structures. However, there are different clusters of basal forebrain cholinergic neurons that have been identified and described that might suggest modality-specific control by the transmitter (Zaborszky, 2002).

The cholinergic input from the HDB is a major centrifugal projection into the OB. Cholinergic neurons of the basal forebrain regulate cortical activity in a state-dependent manner. These neurons fire bursts of action potentials during awake and paradoxical sleep states while remaining more or less silent during slow wave sleep (Jones, 2004, 2005). During active periods, the burst discharge of these neurons appears to be synchronized with gamma and theta oscillations (Lee et al., 2005).

Incoming fibers from the HDB show diffuse innervation across different layers of the bulb (Macrides et al., 1981; Zaborszky et al., 1986; Durand et al., 1998). This innervation is complete by postnatal day 12 (Salcedo et al., 2011). However, during further maturation, there is a distinct patterning of the innervation, with the predominant projections being directed to the glomerular layer (**Figures 2** and **3**) and sparser projections to other OB layers (Macrides et al., 1981; Salcedo et al., 2011). Within the glomerular layer, there are variations in projections (**Figure 2**) with some atypical glomeruli showing much denser innervation (Macrides et al., 1981; Gomez et al., 2005; Salcedo et al., 2011). The identity of odor inputs into these glomeruli, or the functional significance of their dense cholinergic innervation is, as yet, unclear. This suggests considerable pruning of cholinergic afferents during maturation (Salcedo et al., 2011).

Occluding sensory input to the bulb from one naris revealed that cholinergic input is modulated by olfactory activity (**Figure 3**). When unilateral naris occlusion was performed on

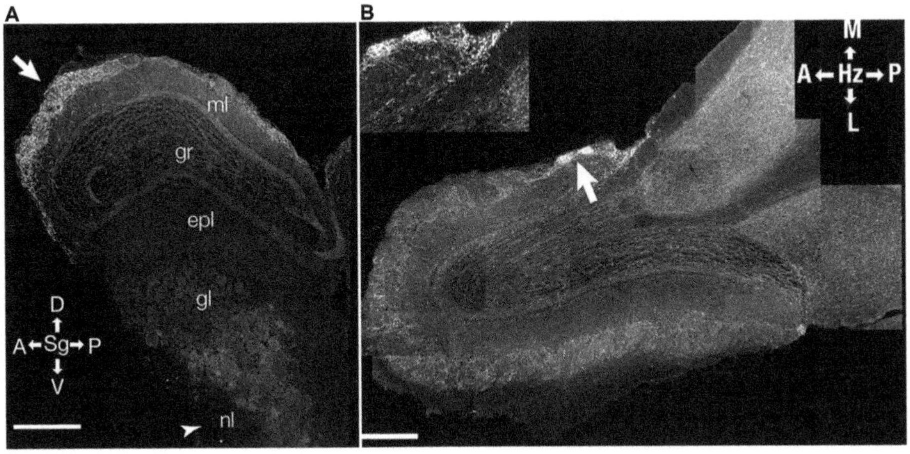

FIGURE 2 | Distribution of cholinergic innervation in the OB. Distribution of incoming cholinergic fibers from the HDB was examined in sections from a 3 month-old mouse expressing a tauGFP fusion protein under a choline acetyltransferase promoter (ChAT-tauGFP mouse). **(A)** Parasagittal section (Sg). *Arrow* points to region of relatively heavy GFP labeling in the anterior glomerular region of the bulb. *Arrow head* indicates the olfactory nerve layer (nl) where relatively little labeling is found. ml- mitral cell layer; gr, granule cell layer; epl, external plexiform layer; gl, glomerular layer; nl, olfactory nerve layer. **(B)** Micrograph of a horizontal (Hz) cross-section of the OB. Arrow points to heavily stained atypical glomeruli shown in inset. **(B inset)** High-resolution micrograph of two atypical glomeruli with a relatively high amount of GFP staining. D, dorsal; V, ventral; A, anterior; P, posterior; L, lateral; M, medial. Data, with permission, from Salcedo et al. (2011).

postnatal day 2, the pattern and intensity remained unchanged up to postnatal day 12. However, significant reductions in intensities were observed in the ipsilateral bulb of the adult (**Figure 3**). In addition, the patterning was lost during this period. These results suggest that odor-induced activity is required for the maintenance and patterning of the cholinergic innervation.

CHOLINERGIC RECEPTOR DISTRIBUTION IN THE OB

The anatomy and function of cholinergic receptor expression in the OB appear to be layer-specific. Quantitative autoradiography in rat OB slices point to the presence of presynaptic cholinergic terminals in the glomerular layer and in the EPL (Le Jeune et al., 1995), suggesting that the glomerulus and the secondary dendrites of MCs are important targets for cholinergic modulation. There is no evidence to suggest that cholinergic terminals form direct synaptic contacts on MCs. On the other hand, asymmetric cholinergic synapses have been described on dendrites of PG cells and GCs (Kasa et al., 1995). The prevalence of synaptic versus non-synaptic cholinergic signaling in the OB, like with other brain areas, remains unresolved to date.

The markers for the cholinergic receptors indicate an age-dependency of cholinergic receptor expression in the OB, with lowest levels of these markers observed at birth, and adult values observed by the end of 4–5 postnatal weeks (Le Jeune et al., 1996). This is consistent with the patterning of cholinergic innervation in the glomerular layer (Salcedo et al., 2011). The postnatal development of cholinergic innervation also extends to the EPL where GC dendrites make GABAergic contacts with the MCs.

Binding of $[^{125}I]$ α-bungarotoxin, a marker for the α7-containing nAChRs, was observed in the glomerular neuropil, suggesting a role for the α7 nAChR subtype in glomerular signaling. On the other hand, $[^{3}H]$ cytisine, which targets heteromeric nAChR subtypes, labeling $\alpha4\beta2^*$- and $\alpha3\beta4^*$-nAChRs (Xiao et al., 1998; Mao et al., 2008), binds to juxtaglomerular neurons and MCs. In addition to the ubiquitous α7 receptor, the rat OB also exhibits the presence of messenger RNA (mRNA) transcripts of nAChR genes that encode the α2, α3, α4, α5, α6, α9, β2, β3, and β4 subunits (Keiger and Walker, 2000), pointing to the possible expression of multiple receptor subtypes and, perhaps, indicating a diverse functional role of for nAChRs in the OB.

M1 and M2 mAChRs were shown to be highly expressed in the EPL indicating that mAChRs might be involved in regulating the dendrodendritic interactions between MCs and GCs. This has been experimentally verified by electrophysiological studies in acute slices (Castillo et al., 1999; Ghatpande et al., 2006; Pressler et al., 2007; Ghatpande and Gelperin, 2009), as well as *in vivo* (Tsuno et al., 2008).

CHOLINERGIC SIGNALING IN THE OB

A major site for nAChR regulation is the glomerulus of the OB. Consistent with autoradiographic studies (Le Jeune and Jourdan, 1993; Le Jeune et al., 1995) functional nAChRs have been described in MCs and ET cells (D'Souza and Vijayaraghavan, 2012; D'Souza et al., 2013). These functional receptors belong to the heteromeric $\alpha3\beta4^*$-nAChR and the $\alpha4\beta2^*$-nAChR subtypes. On MCs, nAChRs appear to be selectively clustered at the primary dendritic tuft within the glomerular neuropil. Removing the primary dendrite drastically attenuates ACh-induced nAChR currents (D'Souza and Vijayaraghavan, 2012). Overall, these results suggest that nAChRs are expressed primarily on excitatory neurons in the glomerular microcircuit. Further, activation of glomerular nAChRs leads to increased glutamate release within the neuropil, resulting in an excitation-dependent feedback inhibition onto the MCs and ET cells. This occurs via increased GABA release from activated juxtaglomerular interneurons, presumably the PG cells (D'Souza

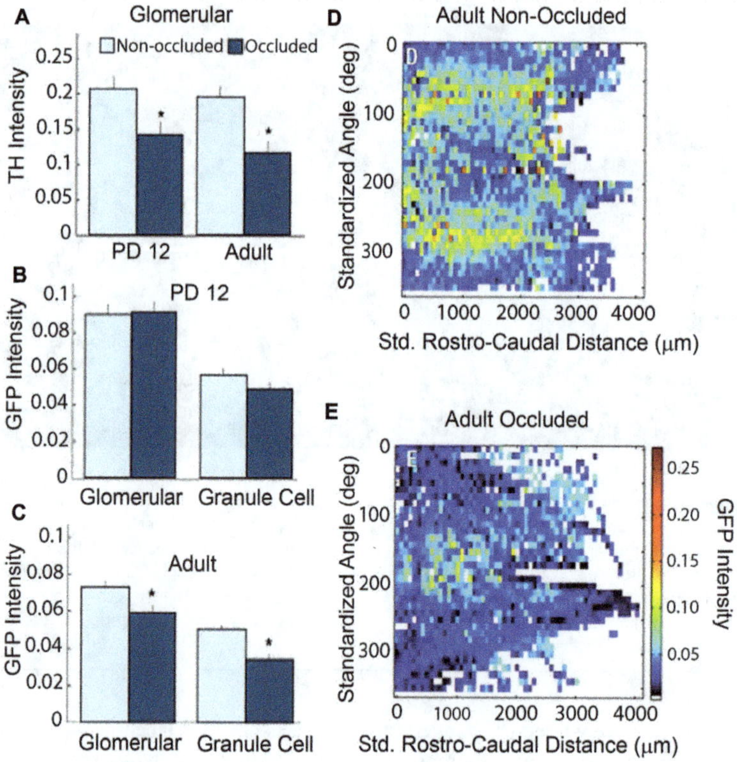

FIGURE 3 | Naris occlusion abolishes differential GFP staining pattern in adult animals. Background subtracted intensities from 12-bit images were converted to a 0–1 scale and plotted. Details of image processing are given in Salcedo et al. (2011). **(A)** Significantly lower tyrosine hydroxylase (TH) intensity in occluded bulbs as compared to non-occluded bulbs confirmed that the occluded bulbs had reduced olfactory activity in both PD12 animals and adult animals (*t*-test, *p*-value $= 1 \times 10^{-2}$ and 3.6×10^{-4}, respectively). **(B)** PD12 animals: mean GFP intensity did not vary significantly between occluded and non-occluded bulbs in either the glomerular or granule cell layers of PD12 bulbs. **(C)** Adult animals: mean GFP intensity fell significantly in both the glomerular and granule cell layers in the occluded bulbs of adult animals (*t*-test, *p*-values: 2.2×10^{-3} and 2.4×10^{-8}, respectively). **(D–E)** Average intensity map in the occluded bulb **(E)** showed a markedly reduced differential patterning of GFP intensity throughout the GL as compared to the non-occluded bulb **(D)**. Data, with permission, from Salcedo et al. (2011).

and Vijayaraghavan, 2012; D'Souza et al., 2013). The predominant effect of nAChR activation appears to be to inhibit incoming signals from the ORNs, leading to a "filtering" mechanism wherein only ORNs excited above a certain intensity threshold transmit their information to cortex (**Figure 4**). A possible mechanism for this inhibition is the shunting of ORN inputs due to the increase in the membrane conductance of MCs upon the opening of a large number of channels, particularly the nAChRs and GABA receptors. Thus, the receptors act as high pass filters that attenuate weak signals while allowing stronger ones to pass, thus setting odor detection thresholds.

Potentially important players in the increased GABA release within the glomerulus upon nAChR activation are the ET cells (D'Souza et al., 2013), a population of OB neurons whose physiological properties have been characterized over the last decade. ET cells are thought to be a major source of excitation for juxtaglomerular neurons (Hayar et al., 2004), as well as drivers of feed-forward MC excitation via glutamate release within the glomerulus (De Saint et al., 2009; Najac et al., 2011; Gire et al., 2012). As targets for neuromodulation by cholinergic (D'Souza et al., 2013), serotonergic (Liu et al., 2012) and endocannabinoid receptor-mediated (Wang et al., 2012) mechanisms, ET cells are well placed to play a vital role in the state-dependent control of OB function. Similar to MCs, glomerular nAChR activation leads to an enhancement of ET cell excitability. This excitation, along with MC excitation, is likely responsible for the increase in the frequency of GABA release within the glomerulus upon nAChR stimulation. There is one report suggesting that a subpopulation of PG cells might, themselves, express nAChRs (Castillo et al., 1999) but their contribution to the glomerular microcircuit is yet to be determined.

mAChRs, on the other hand, appear to mainly control a second inhibitory circuit in the OB, involving GCs and the lateral dendrites of MCs (see **Figure 5A**) within the EPL. Activation of M1-mAChRs, via mobilization of endoplasmic reticulum store calcium, release GABA onto the MCs at the dendrodendritic synapses between GCs and MCs (Castillo et al., 1999; Ghatpande et al., 2006; Ghatpande and Gelperin, 2009). At the same time, M1-mAChRs increase GC excitation thus providing an additional inhibitory drive on to MCs (Pressler et al., 2007). Similar mechanisms of cholinergic modulation were also observed in the accessory OB where M1-like mAChRs control GC-to-MC inhibition, while nAChR activation increases MC excitability (Smith and Araneda, 2010).

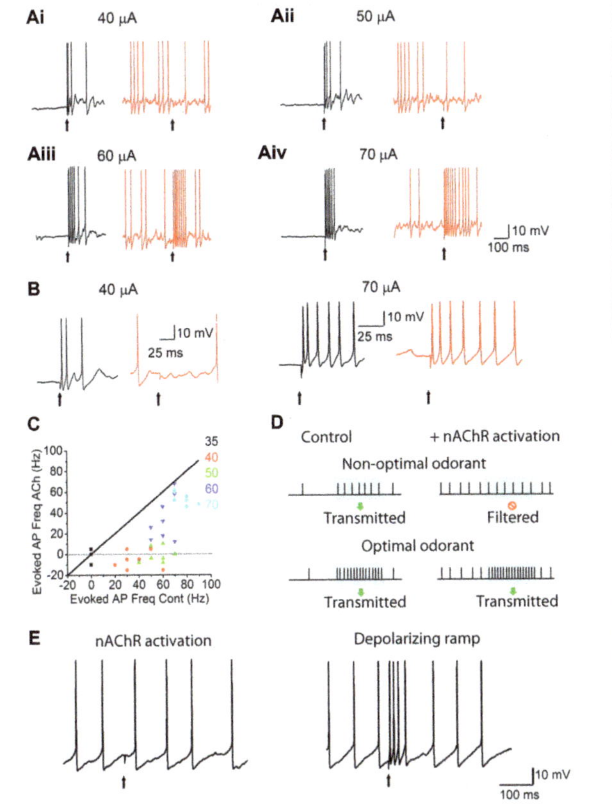

FIGURE 4 | nAChRs act as high-pass filters of glomerular output. **(Ai)**: Responses of MCs to ON stimulation, recorded under current-clamp. Left: **(A)** 40 μA ON stimulus causes an MC to exhibit a burst of spikes. Right: during a ACh/At-mediated depolarization (and enhanced background firing), the 40 μA stimulus fails to evoke a response in the same MC. ACh/At refers to a 1 s focal application of 1 mM ACh in the presence of 2 μM atropine, the latter also added in the bath in order to block mAChRs. **(Aii–iv)**: Similar data for 50, 60, and 70 μA stimuli, respectively. While the 50 μA stimulus also fails to evoke a response during the ACh/At-mediated spiking in the same MC as in Ai, the MC responds to higher stimuli with increased spiking. In all cases, control traces are in black and traces in the presence of ACh/At are in red. **(B)**: Expanded traces from Ai and Aiv. **(C)**: Scatter plot of net increase in spiking upon ON stimulation, during the ACh/At-mediated depolarization, plotted against the same during control conditions. Data is from the same cell as in **(A,B)**. Net increase in spiking was calculated by subtracting the mean firing frequency before ON stimulation from the mean firing frequency during the 100 ms window after ON stimulation. While responses to all stimulus intensities were suppressed during the ACh-mediated depolarization, lower intensity stimuli (up to 50 μA) show a filtering of MC responses (not different from 0). Diagonal line (slope = 1) is where the points would lie if there were no ACh-mediated filtering. **(D)**: Cartoon summarizing the effects of nAChRs on MC responses. Period of odor exposure shown by shaded box. Under non-optimal conditions (weak odor), a MC fires a burst of APs during odor exposure leading to signal transmission. On the other hand, nAChR activation, causes an increase in basal MC firing but shows no net change in firing patterns during the period of odor exposure thus resulting in filtering of the response. Under optimal conditions (i.e., strong odor), there is a net increase in MC firing during odor exposure both under control conditions and when nAChRs are activated. **(E)**: Filtering shown in the presence of ACh/At (left trace) is not seen when the same cell is depolarized via current injection to elicit APs in the absence of ACh/At (right trace, from the same cell). This suggests that optimal excitation-driven feedback inhibition requires the activation of more than one MC, and that the filtering is not merely a result of MC membrane depolarization. Figures **(A–C,E)** adapted, with permission, from D'Souza and Vijayaraghavan (2012).

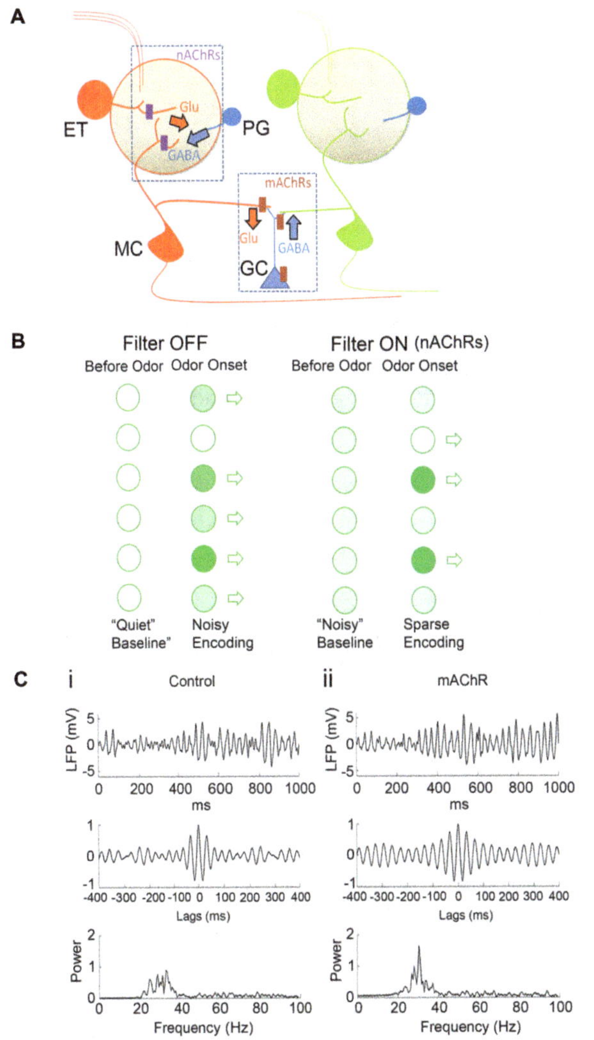

FIGURE 5 | A working model for cholinergic modulation of OB circuitry. **(A)** Cartoon of the OB circuit showing major sites of cholinergic inhibition. In the glomerular microcircuit, nAChRs (purple rectangles) are expressed in the primary dendritic tufts of MCs and on the ET cell (in red). Activation of these receptors depolarizes the neurons resulting in the release of glutamate (Glu). Released glutamate excites nearby PG cells (blue) eliciting a feedback GABA release on to the excitatory neurons. **(A)** Similar feedback circuit exists at the dendrodendritic synapses between GCs and secondary dendrites of MCs allowing for lateral inhibition of adjacent MC dendrites. **(B)** Cartoon showing glomerular output (open arrows). In the absence of receptor activation (Filter OFF) there is less baseline activity ("Quiet baseline.") Odor stimulations at different strengths (light and dark green circles for weak and strong stimulation, respectively) are transmitted through. Upon nAChR activation, (Filter ON), excitation of ET cells and MCs lead to a noisier baseline (i.e., all light green). However, upon odor input, excitation-driven inhibition results in filtering out of weaker inputs, such that only strong ones pass through. Further, increased basal activity also allows for potential "inhibitory readouts" (open circle) where net MC firing rates can be reduced to levels below that prior to odor onset (see **Figure 4C**). The time window of the nAChR-evoked inhibition will determine the efficacy of this filter. Thus determining the temporal patterns of ACh release, in relation to behavioral stages, is necessary in order to predict the direct consequences of this filter mechanism. **(C)** Modeling the activation of mAChRs in the OB (with permission from Li and Cleland, 2013). In this model, mAChR activation does not alter MC firing rates but the receptor

(Continued)

FIGURE 5 | Continued
activation enhances sLFP oscillatory power and imposes more stringent phase locking between MC spikes and sLFP oscillations. **(i)** Control responses: simulated sLFP during odor presentation **(top)** with autocorrelation **(middle)** and power spectrum **(bottom)**. **(ii)** Same as **(i)** but during active mAChR modulation. In response to odor, MC spikes were locked to the gamma frequencies under both control conditions and upon mAChR activation, but the responses were more tightly phase constrained when mAChRs were active. This is consistent with the idea that modulation of lateral inhibition by mAChR signaling at GC-MC synapses imposes a stronger synchronization of MC firing in the OB.

mAChRs AND nAChRs CONTROL OB FUNCTION VIA DISTINCT MECHANISMS

Results from a variety of behavioral and *in vivo* electrophysiological studies point to the importance of cholinergic receptor activation in modulating the detection and discrimination of odors, as well as in olfactory perceptual learning, i.e., learning to distinguish between two or more perceptually similar odors (Fletcher and Wilson, 2002; Wilson and Stevenson, 2003; Wilson et al., 2004; Fletcher and Chen, 2010). For instance, increasing the level of ACh in the OB results in the sharpening of the molecular "receptive field" of individual MCs in response to odors, while the addition of nAChR and mAChR blockers into the OB impairs the ability to distinguish between similar odors, both at the level of MC spike frequency, as well as in behavioral tests (Chaudhury et al., 2009).

In addition to modulating odor detection and discrimination (Chaudhury et al., 2009), nAChRs are also involved in olfactory working memory. Mice that lacked the α7 nAChR showed impairments in working memory when compared to wild type mice (Young et al., 2007a), while acute nicotine administration could fully restore deficits in olfactory working memory in a transgenic mouse model that overexpressed the caspase-3 protein (Young et al., 2007b). Olfactory working memory could also be enhanced in rats via subcutaneous administration of specific agonists for the α4β2 and the α7 receptor subtypes (Rushforth et al., 2010).

mAChRs have been shown to be involved in the behavioral state-dependent control of dendrodendritic synapses between MCs and GCs (Tsuno et al., 2008). Results from this work indicated that inhibition of MCs by GCs was most enhanced during the slow-wave sleep state and successively weaker during light sleep, awake immobility, and awake moving states. Activation of mAChRs were responsible for this inhibition. This supports the observation that ACh levels in the brain are higher in the awake state than when the animal is asleep. Real time monitoring of ACh levels demonstrate that the awake state is characterized by low levels of ACh (Parikh and Sarter, 2008), though relatively higher than that during slow wave sleep, which might signal via mAChRs to maintain a tonic GABAergic control on the basal firing rates of MCs. It appears, therefore, that an important function of cholinergic input to the OB is to inhibit the activity of GCs, thereby disinhibiting the MCs during wakefulness and behavior. *In vivo*, mAChRs have been suggested to play a role in potentiating the firing rates of MCs upon stimulation of the basal forebrain (Zhan et al., 2013), as well in olfactory perception and short-term olfactory memory (Chaudhury et al., 2009; Devore et al., 2012).

Interestingly, optogenetic excitation of cholinergic neurons in the HDB of anesthetized animals inhibits the basal firing rate of (M/T) cells, while also inhibiting the basal firing of the GABAergic granule and PG cells (Ma and Luo, 2012). This observation is quite surprising because, as described above, MCs have been shown to be excited by nAChR activation. Further, work from a number of labs using acute OB slices have demonstrated that mAChRs, in contrast to the optogenetic study, excite GCs, leading to increased GABAergic postsynaptic currents in MCs (Pressler et al., 2007). It is therefore unclear as to how cholinergic input inhibits GCs *in vivo*. It must be pointed out, however, that general anesthetics have effects on nAChR function and might, therefore, confound interpretations when testing cholinergic effects in anesthetized animals (Hara and Harris, 2002; Weber et al., 2005; Liu et al., 2009). Further, a more recent study demonstrated that exciting the cholinergic axons in the OB, instead of exciting the cell bodies in the HDB, leads to an enhancement of M/T cell firing (Rothermel et al., 2014). This observation suggests that activating cholinergic somata in the HDB may lead to indirect inhibition of M/T cells and other bulbar neurons, via pathways that remain to be elucidated (Rothermel et al., 2014).

Activation of basal forebrain cholinergic neurons also results in the sharpening of M/T cell responses so that when these inputs are activated, M/T cell responses to the optimal odorant (i.e., an odorant that elicits the maximal response in the M/T cell under control conditions) are enhanced, while responses to non-optimal odorants are suppressed (Ma and Luo, 2012). It should be noted, however, that direct activation of the cholinergic axons in the OB did not lead to such a suppression for non-optimal odors; instead, excitation of these fibers led to an enhancement of odor-evoked M/T cell responses independent of control response strengths (Rothermel et al., 2014). Thus, there appears to be qualitative differences between activating cholinergic cell bodies within the HDB and activating their fibers in the OB to study the effects of cholinergic input on bulbar function. Regardless of these differences, these results strongly imply that cholinergic input to the OB is responsible for enhanced olfactory function, potentially playing a central role in the detection of weak odors and in the discrimination of chemically similar odorants. Computational models based on experimental observations suggest that mAChRs are likely responsible for the generation of gamma oscillations in the OB while the activation of nAChRs sharpen the tuning curves of MCs in response to odor input (Li and Cleland, 2013), thus pointing to a role of mAChRs (via the modulation GC-MC interactions in the EPL) in controlling MC spike timing, and the role of nAChRs in enhancing contrast between activated glomeruli.

OTHER PLAYERS IN THE CHOLINERGIC MODULATION OF THE OB

Our knowledge of cholinergic modulation of the OB output is far from complete as we are still discovering the extent of receptor distribution and cell types that they can act upon. The functional role that the α7 receptor plays in modulating OB function is still unresolved. Anatomical studies have revealed that α7 nAChRs are highly expressed in the glomerulus (Le Jeune et al., 1995; Hellier et al., 2010), while behavioral studies point to an important role for this receptor subtype in olfactory function (Hellier et al., 2010, 2012). However, electrophysiological studies suggest that α7 nAChRs do not play a significant role in modulating the spontaneous activity of MCs (D'Souza and Vijayaraghavan, 2012). It is possible that glomerular α7 nAChRs are expressed not on the glomerular tufts of MCs, but on the axon terminals of ORNs, which provide the input to the OB. Other possibilities include the expression of these receptors on glomerular astrocytes, or on centrifugal fibers that innervate the glomerulus. The observation that the release of other neuromodulators such as serotonin and noradrenaline can be altered by cholinergic activation (Decker and McGaugh, 1991; Levin and Simon, 1998), and that circuits in the OB are also modulated by these two neuromodulators (Fletcher and Chen, 2010; Devore and Linster, 2012; Liu et al., 2012), point to the possibility of a sophisticated interplay between these three neuromodulatory systems in regulating the output of the OB. While α7 nAChRs do not appear to play a significant role in inducing nicotinic currents in MCs, or altering the frequency of spontaneous postsynaptic currents on them, they might play a role in mediating plasticity in the OB. This is supported by observations that the receptor is important for olfactory learning (Hellier et al., 2010, 2012; Rushforth et al., 2010).

Similarly, we have no information on the role M2-mAChRs play in the cholinergic modulation of the bulbar output. Anatomical evidence suggests that these receptors are localized on GC synapses in the EPL, on second-order GABAergic neurons in the infra-mitral cell layer, and on some juxtaglomerular GABAergic interneurons, suggesting complex inhibition/disinhibition roles for these receptors on MC output (Crespo et al., 2000).

Our knowledge of the function and regulation of various juxtaglomerular interneurons is incomplete as well. For example, the short axon cells, a type of juxtaglomerular cells that mediates interglomerular inhibition (Aungst et al., 2003), have been studied with increased detail only in recent years (Kiyokage et al., 2010; Liu et al., 2013; Whitesell et al., 2013). Their role in cholinergic modulation remains unresolved, although it's possible that this cell type was previously identified as "bipolar PG cells" that exhibited prominent, slow, inward currents upon nicotinic activation (Castillo et al., 1999).

POSSIBLE MECHANISMS FOR CHOLINERGIC CONTROL OF OLFACTORY CODING

The vast repertoire of cholinergic receptor subtypes expressed throughout the brain exhibit a variety of physiological properties. These include the sensitivity of these receptors to ACh, as well as their desensitization rates. A major puzzle in the field of cholinergic function is to understand the roles played by these different receptor subtypes. Cholinergic transmission in the brain can be broadly classified as occurring via two modes, synaptic, and diffusion-based, resulting in the release of ACh with concentrations that vary over orders of magnitude. Varying concentrations of ACh acting on receptor subtypes exhibiting a myriad of sensitivity and desensitizing properties indicate a dynamic control of sensory processing over multiple timescales that is dependent on the behavioral state of the animal.

As we described earlier, behavioral and *in vivo* work have shown that during light sleep or awake immobility, a low, tonic level of ACh primarily activate mAChRs expressed on GCs (Tsuno et al., 2008). This sets a basal cholinergic tone for GABAergic control of OB output. In contrast, during the anticipational/attentional phase of behavior, there is a rapid and transient increase in MC firing, and it has been suggested that this spontaneous activity in the alert animals might be driven by basal forebrain cholinergic activity (Rinberg and Gelperin, 2006). Consistent with this finding, real-time measurements of ACh levels in the brains of rats performing attention-dependent tasks indicate that cholinergic activity acts on three distinct timescales depending on effort: (1) cue-evoked transient increases in ACh levels that act on the scale of seconds, (2) pre-cue cholinergic signals on the scale of tens of seconds when the rat is anticipating or predicting a cue, and (3) a tonic level of activity that lasts for minutes throughout the session (Parikh et al., 2007, 2008). The transient increase in ACh levels during sustained attention would be sufficient to activate the lower affinity nAChRs, especially the slowly desensitizing heteromeric receptor subtypes. This excitation, in conjunction with feedback GABAergic inhibition, could potentially result in the gating of odor input so that only MCs belonging to strongly activated glomeruli are excited. Such a mechanism would potentially filter out "noise" from weakly activated glomeruli, and lead to enhanced contrast between odor maps encoding chemically similar odors. Noise, in this context, refers to the non-optimal activation of glomeruli via weakly excited ORNs (see **Figure 5B**). This model, therefore, predicts a role for both tonic and phasic modulation for cholinergic inputs (Parikh and Sarter, 2008; Sarter et al., 2009a,b).

Direct excitation of MCs by cholinergic activation has important implications for odor processing. First, the depolarization of MCs can drive them to spike with a high basal firing rate (D'Souza and Vijayaraghavan, 2012). If attention-dependent cholinergic input leads to an increase in the basal firing rate of MCs, it would allow an odor input to alter the frequency, as well as the timing, of spikes. For instance, a decrease in spike frequency or changes in the fine temporal structure at the level of individual action potentials, upon odor input, would not be possible if the cells were not already firing in the first place. Having a baseline firing rate before odor input therefore provides a template for the incoming odor input to manipulate and provide more information to process. Second, depolarization of MCs *before* the onset of an odor signal would trigger the PG-cell driven feedback inhibition, such that, only MCs belonging to glomeruli that receive a strong odor input would transmit the information to the cortex. Third, increasing the basal firing frequency of MCs would increase the probability of coincident synaptic excitation of GCs. Since GCs form reciprocal dendrodendritic contacts with the lateral dendrites of MCs, an increase in the excitation of GCs would, in turn, increase lateral inhibition between MCs (Arevian et al., 2008). Slice and computational studies have implicated the role of GC-mediated lateral inhibition in the synchronization of MC action potentials (Galan et al., 2006; Schoppa, 2006). The cause of this synchrony is the near-simultaneous recovery of MCs from synchronized GABAergic inhibition, and is thought to underlie synchronous neuronal oscillations in the gamma frequency (Schoppa, 2006). Computational modeling supports the idea that cholinergic excitation of the OB circuit increases the synchronization, as well as the sparseness, of MC action potentials in response to odor input (de Almeida et al., 2013). The observations that cholinergic influence mediate gamma frequency oscillations within neuronal populations (Dickson et al., 2000; Simon et al., 2011) suggest a possibility for a synchronized activity baseline in the OB prior to odor input that could be altered by a subsequent inhalation of odors, providing for a mechanism for allowing the detection and higher-order processing of olfactory information.

OB CHOLINERGIC MODULATION AND NEURODEGENERATIVE DISEASES

The notion that olfactory dysfunction is one of the early symptoms in neurodegenerative diseases is gaining recognition (Attems et al., 2014). As olfactory deficits have been shown to manifest themselves years prior to onset of characteristic symptoms, they might act as early biomarkers of these diseases (Barresi et al., 2012). Major deficits in odor detection, identification, and discrimination have been described in Parkinson's disease (PD) patients, prior to the onset of motor disturbances (Mesholam et al., 1998; Tissingh et al., 2001; Doty, 2009), even leading to a theory that PD might be a primary olfactory disorder (Hawkes et al., 1999).

Similar evidence exists for patients with Alzheimer's disease (AD) where early loss of olfactory discrimination and anosmia has been reported (Christen-Zaech et al., 2003; Djordjevic et al., 2008). Changes in the number of dopaminergic PG cells and loss of OB volume have been described in AD (Mundinano et al., 2011). In mouse models of AD, early onset of olfactory deficits also corresponds to early depositions of amyloid β protein prior to central pathology (Wesson et al., 2010; Kim et al., 2011).

The cholinergic hypothesis for diseases like AD has had dominance for many decades (Bartus et al., 1982; Coyle et al., 1983; Bartus, 2000) and has led to the development of the only approved drugs for the treatment for early and mild dementia. While cholinergic dysfunction is likely to be one of many causes for neurodegeneration (Craig et al., 2011), these studies nonetheless suggest a dominant role for this neurotransmitter system. Studies with patients suffering from Parkinson's disease have indicated that olfactory deficits, seen early in the disease process, correlates with cholinergic degeneration rather than the nigro-striatal dopaminergic neuron deficits (Bohnen et al., 2010), once again confirming the correlation between olfactory function and the cholinergic system.

Our studies indicate that distribution of cholinergic fibers in the OB is intricately connected to olfactory sensory input (**Figure 3**). Unilateral naris occlusion results in a loss of pruning of incoming cholinergic fibers in the adult and results in diffuse innervation of the OB similar to that seen in young (day 12) animals (Salcedo et al., 2011). Does disruption of axonal pruning in the bulb alter the survival of HDB cholinergic neurons? We do not know this, but if loss of axons results in "die-back" and delayed death of neuronal soma in the basal forebrain, it is possible to conceptualize a mechanism that connects sensory environment to neurodegeneration and memory loss observed in AD or other diseases.

CONCLUSION

In most mammals, the ability to discriminate, effectively, benign odors from those that could signal danger is an essential prerequisite for survival. It is, therefore, logical that systems signaling arousal and attention are brought to bear during tasks of odor discrimination. The key transmitter system invoked in these olfactory tasks involves the cholinergic projections from the basal forebrain, long thought to be involved in attention, arousal, learning, and memory. In the olfactory system, it is well accepted that significant processing of odor information occurs at the OB.

A simple model, based on current state of our knowledge, would postulate that nAChR activity dominates at the glomerular microcircuit, while mAChRs control the GC-driven modulation of MC firing (**Figure 5**). The key process in cholinergic modulation of OB functions, appears to be GABAergic signaling. Activation of nAChRs drives glomerular inhibition via the indirect excitation of PG cells. This allows for normalization of glomerular excitation, setting thresholds for transfer of information. The excitation of MCs and ET cells by nAChRs also increase baseline firing, potentially providing a template for net negative readouts in firing frequencies, as well (see **Figures 4C** and **5B**).

At the same time mAChR-driven excitation of GCs and their modulation of GABAergic signaling at the GC-MC dendrodendritic synapses allows for lateral inhibition. Recovery from inhibition across MCs aids in synchronizing firing which is thought to facilitate the integration of incoming information at a population level (**Figure 5C**). Ongoing efforts at further localizing the relevant receptors and at manipulating cholinergic inputs in awake animals performing olfactory tasks will shed more light on this important modulation of a sensory modality by cholinergic processes.

ACKNOWLEDGMENTS

Funding was provided by NIH Grants R01DC 008855 and R01DA 10266 to Sukumar Vijayaraghavan.

REFERENCES

Arevian, A. C., Kapoor, V., and Urban, N. N. (2008). Activity-dependent gating of lateral inhibition in the mouse olfactory bulb. *Nat. Neurosci.* 11, 80–87. doi: 10.1038/nn2030

Attems, J., Walker, L., and Jellinger, K. A. (2014). Olfactory bulb involvement in neurodegenerative diseases. *Acta Neuropathol.* 127, 459–475. doi: 10.1007/s00401-014-1261-7

Aungst, J. L., Heyward, P. M., Puche, A. C., Karnup, S. V., Hayar, A., Szabo, G., et al. (2003). Centre-surround inhibition among olfactory bulb glomeruli. *Nature* 426, 623–629. doi: 10.1038/nature02185

Barresi, M., Ciurleo, R., Giacoppo, S., Foti, C. V., Celi, D., Bramanti, P., et al. (2012). Evaluation of olfactory dysfunction in neurodegenerative diseases. *J. Neurol. Sci.* 323, 16–24. doi: 10.1016/j.jns.2012.08.028

Bartus, R. T. (2000). On neurodegenerative diseases, models, and treatment strategies: lessons learned and lessons forgotten a generation following the cholinergic hypothesis. *Exp. Neurol.* 163, 495–529. doi: 10.1006/exnr.2000.7397

Bartus, R. T., Dean, R. L. III, Beer, B., and Lippa, A. S. (1982). The cholinergic hypothesis of geriatric memory dysfunction. *Science* 217, 408–414. doi: 10.1126/science.7046051

Batista-Brito, R., Close, J., Machold, R., and Fishell, G. (2008). The distinct temporal origins of olfactory bulb interneuron subtypes. *J. Neurosci.* 28, 3966–3975. doi: 10.1523/JNEUROSCI.5625-07.2008

Bohnen, N. I., Muller, M. L., Kotagal, V., Koeppe, R. A., Kilbourn, M. A., Albin, R. L., et al. (2010). Olfactory dysfunction, central cholinergic integrity and cognitive impairment in Parkinson's disease. *Brain* 133, 1747–1754. doi: 10.1093/brain/awq079

Bozza, T., McGann, J. P., Mombaerts, P., and Wachowiak, M. (2004). In vivo imaging of neuronal activity by targeted expression of a genetically encoded probe in the mouse. *Neuron* 42, 9–21. doi: 10.1016/S0896-6273(04)00144-8

Castillo, P. E., Carleton, A., Vincent, J. D., and Lledo, P. M. (1999). Multiple and opposing roles of cholinergic transmission in the main olfactory bulb. *J. Neurosci.* 19, 9180–9191.

Chaudhury, D., Escanilla, O., and Linster, C. (2009). Bulbar acetylcholine enhances neural and perceptual odor discrimination. *J. Neurosci.* 29, 52–60. doi: 10.1523/JNEUROSCI.4036-08.2009

Christen-Zaech, S., Kraftsik, R., Pillevuit, O., Kiraly, M., Martins, R., Khalili, K., et al. (2003). Early olfactory involvement in Alzheimer's disease. *Can. J. Neurol. Sci.* 30, 20–25.

Coyle, J. T., Price, D. L., and DeLong, M. R. (1983). Alzheimer's disease: a disorder of cortical cholinergic innervation. *Science* 219, 1184–1190. doi: 10.1126/science.6338589

Craig, L. A., Hong, N. S., and McDonald, R. J. (2011). Revisiting the cholinergic hypothesis in the development of Alzheimer's disease. *Neurosci. Biobehav. Rev.* 35, 1397–1409. doi: 10.1016/j.neubiorev.2011.03.001

Crespo, C., Blasco-Ibanez, J. M., Brinon, J. G., Alonso, J. R., Dominguez, M. I., and Martinez-Guijarro, F. J. (2000). Subcellular localization of m2 muscarinic receptors in GABAergic interneurons of the olfactory bulb. *Eur. J. Neurosci.* 12, 3963–3974. doi: 10.1046/j.1460-9568.2000.00289.x

Cury, K. M., and Uchida, N. (2010). Robust odor coding via inhalation-coupled transient activity in the mammalian olfactory bulb. *Neuron* 68, 570–585. doi: 10.1016/j.neuron.2010.09.040

D'Souza, R. D., Parsa, P. V., and Vijayaraghavan, S. (2013). Nicotinic receptors modulate olfactory bulb external tufted cells via an excitation-dependent inhibitory mechanism. *J. Neurophysiol.* 110, 1544–1553. doi: 10.1152/jn.00865.2012

D'Souza, R. D., and Vijayaraghavan, S. (2012). Nicotinic receptor-mediated filtering of mitral cell responses to olfactory nerve inputs involves the alpha3beta4 subtype. *J. Neurosci.* 32, 3261–3266. doi: 10.1523/JNEUROSCI.5024-11.2012

Davison, I. G., and Katz, L. C. (2007). Sparse and selective odor coding by mitral/tufted neurons in the main olfactory bulb. *J. Neurosci.* 27, 2091–2101. doi: 10.1523/JNEUROSCI.3779-06.2007

de Almeida, L. B., Idiart, M. A., and Linster, C. (2013). A model of cholinergic modulation in olfactory bulb and piriform cortex. *J. Neurophysiol.* 109, 1360–1377. doi: 10.1152/jn.00577.2012

De Saint, J. D., Hirnet, D., Westbrook, G. L., and Charpak, S. (2009). External tufted cells drive the output of olfactory bulb glomeruli. *J. Neurosci.* 29, 2043–2052. doi: 10.1523/JNEUROSCI.5317-08.2009

Decker, M. W., and McGaugh, J. L. (1991). The role of interactions between the cholinergic system and other neuromodulatory systems in learning and memory. *Synapse* 7, 151–168. doi: 10.1002/syn.890070209

Devore, S., and Linster, C. (2012). Noradrenergic and cholinergic modulation of olfactory bulb sensory processing. *Front. Behav. Neurosci.* 6:52. doi: 10.3389/fnbeh.2012.00052

Devore, S., Manella, L. C., and Linster, C. (2012). Blocking muscarinic receptors in the olfactory bulb impairs performance on an olfactory short-term memory task. *Front. Behav. Neurosci.* 6:59. doi: 10.3389/fnbeh.2012.00059

Dhawale, A. K., Hagiwara, A., Bhalla, U. S., Murthy, V. N., and Albeanu, D. F. (2010). Non-redundant odor coding by sister mitral cells revealed by light addressable glomeruli in the mouse. *Nat. Neurosci.* 13, 1404–1412. doi: 10.1038/nn.2673

Dickson, C. T., Biella, G., and de, C. M. (2000). Evidence for spatial modules mediated by temporal synchronization of carbachol-induced gamma rhythm in medial entorhinal cortex. *J. Neurosci.* 20, 7846–7854.

Djordjevic, J., Jones-Gotman, M., De Sousa, K., and Chertkow, H. (2008). Olfaction in patients with mild cognitive impairment and Alzheimer's disease. *Neurobiol. Aging* 29, 693–706. doi: 10.1016/j.neurobiolaging.2006.11.014

Doty, R. L. (2009). The olfactory system and its disorders. *Semin. Neurol.* 29, 74–81. doi: 10.1055/s-0028-1124025

Doucette, W., Gire, D. H., Whitesell, J., Carmean, V., Lucero, M. T., and Restrepo, D. (2011). Associative cortex features in the first olfactory brain relay station. *Neuron* 69, 1176–1187. doi: 10.1016/j.neuron.2011.02.024

Doucette, W., and Restrepo, D. (2008). Profound context-dependent plasticity of mitral cell responses in olfactory bulb. *PLoS. Biol.* 6:e258. doi: 10.1371/journal.pbio.0060258

Durand, M., Coronas, V., Jourdan, F., and Quirion, R. (1998). Developmental and aging aspects of the cholinergic innervation of the olfactory bulb. *Int. J. Dev. Neurosci.* 16, 777–785. doi: 10.1016/S0736-5748(98)00087-2

Fletcher, M. L., and Chen, W. R. (2010). Neural correlates of olfactory learning: critical role of centrifugal neuromodulation. *Learn. Mem.* 17, 561–570. doi: 10.1101/lm.941510

Fletcher, M. L., and Wilson, D. A. (2002). Experience modifies olfactory acuity: acetylcholine-dependent learning decreases behavioral generalization between similar odorants. *J. Neurosci.* 22, RC201.

Friedrich, R. W., and Laurent, G. (2001). Dynamic optimization of odor representations by slow temporal patterning of mitral cell activity. *Science* 291, 889–894. doi: 10.1126/science.291.5505.889

Galan, R. F., Fourcaud-Trocme, N., Ermentrout, G. B., and Urban, N. N. (2006). Correlation-induced synchronization of oscillations in olfactory bulb neurons. *J. Neurosci.* 26, 3646–3655. doi: 10.1523/JNEUROSCI.4605-05.2006

Gao, Y., and Strowbridge, B. W. (2009). Long-term plasticity of excitatory inputs to granule cells in the rat olfactory bulb. *Nat. Neurosci.* 12, 731–733. doi: 10.1038/nn.2319

Ghatpande, A. S., and Gelperin, A. (2009). Presynaptic muscarinic receptors enhance glutamate release at the mitral/tufted to granule cell dendrodendritic synapse in the rat main olfactory bulb. *J. Neurophysiol.* 101, 2052–2061. doi: 10.1152/jn.90734.2008

Ghatpande, A. S., Sivaraaman, K., and Vijayaraghavan, S. (2006). Store calcium mediates cholinergic effects on mIPSCs in the rat main olfactory bulb. *J. Neurophysiol.* 95, 1345–1355. doi: 10.1152/jn.00757.2005

Gire, D. H., Franks, K. M., Zak, J. D., Tanaka, K. F., Whitesell, J. D., Mulligan, A. A., et al. (2012). Mitral cells in the olfactory bulb are mainly excited through a multistep signaling path. *J. Neurosci.* 32, 2964–2975. doi: 10.1523/JNEUROSCI.5580-11.2012

Gire, D. H., and Schoppa, N. E. (2009). Control of on/off glomerular signaling by a local GABAergic microcircuit in the olfactory bulb. *J. Neurosci.* 29, 13454–13464. doi: 10.1523/JNEUROSCI.2368-09.2009

Gomez, C., Brinon, J. G., Barbado, M. V., Weruaga, E., Valero, J., and Alonso, J. R. (2005). Heterogeneous targeting of centrifugal inputs to the glomerular layer of the main olfactory bulb. *J. Chem. Neuroanat.* 29, 238–254. doi: 10.1016/j.jchemneu.2005.01.005

Haddad, R., Lanjuin, A., Madisen, L., Zeng, H., Murthy, V. N., and Uchida, N. (2013). Olfactory cortical neurons read out a relative time code in the olfactory bulb. *Nat. Neurosci.* 16, 949–957. doi: 10.1038/nn.3407

Hara, K., and Harris, R. A. (2002). The anesthetic mechanism of urethane: the effects on neurotransmitter-gated ion channels. *Anesth. Analg.* 94, 313–318. doi: 10.1097/00000539-200202000-00015

Hawkes, C. H., Shephard, B. C., and Daniel, S. E. (1999). Is Parkinson's disease a primary olfactory disorder? *QJM.* 92, 473–480. doi: 10.1093/qjmed/92.8.473

Hayar, A., Karnup, S., Ennis, M., and Shipley, M. T. (2004). External tufted cells: a major excitatory element that coordinates glomerular activity. *J. Neurosci.* 24, 6676–6685. doi: 10.1523/JNEUROSCI.1367-04.2004

Hellier, J. L., Arevalo, N. L., Blatner, M. J., Dang, A. K., Clevenger, A. C., Adams, C. E., et al. (2010). Olfactory discrimination varies in mice with different levels of alpha7-nicotinic acetylcholine receptor expression. *Brain Res.* 1358, 140–150. doi: 10.1016/j.brainres.2010.08.027

Hellier, J. L., Arevalo, N. L., Smith, L., Xiong, K. N., and Restrepo, D. (2012). Alpha7-Nicotinic acetylcholine receptor: role in early odor learning preference in mice. *PLoS ONE* 7:e35251. doi: 10.1371/journal.pone.0035251

Himmelheber, A. M., Sarter, M., and Bruno, J. P. (2000). Increases in cortical acetylcholine release during sustained attention performance in rats. *Brain Res. Cogn. Brain Res.* 9, 313–325. doi: 10.1016/S0926-6410(00)00012-4

Jones, B. E. (2004). Activity, modulation and role of basal forebrain cholinergic neurons innervating the cerebral cortex. *Prog. Brain Res.* 145, 157–169. doi: 10.1016/S0079-6123(03)45011-5

Jones, B. E. (2005). From waking to sleeping: neuronal and chemical substrates. *Trends Pharmacol. Sci.* 26, 578–586. doi: 10.1016/j.tips.2005.09.009

Junek, S., Kludt, E., Wolf, F., and Schild, D. (2010). Olfactory coding with patterns of response latencies. *Neuron* 67, 872–884. doi: 10.1016/j.neuron.2010.08.005

Kasa, P., Hlavati, I., Dobo, E., Wolff, A., Joo, F., and Wolff, J. R. (1995). Synaptic and non-synaptic cholinergic innervation of the various types of neurons in the main olfactory bulb of adult rat: Immunocytochemistry of choline acetyltransferase. *Neuroscience* 67, 667–677. doi: 10.1016/0306-4522(95)00031-D

Kashiwadani, H., Sasaki, Y. F., Uchida, N., and Mori, K. (1999). Synchronized oscillatory discharges of mitral/tufted cells with different molecular receptive ranges in the rabbit olfactory bulb. *J. Neurophysiol.* 82, 1786–1792.

Kato, H. K., Chu, M. W., Isaacson, J. S., and Komiyama, T. (2012). Dynamic sensory representations in the olfactory bulb: modulation by wakefulness and experience. *Neuron* 76, 962–975. doi: 10.1016/j.neuron.2012.09.037

Keiger, C. J., and Walker, J. C. (2000). Individual variation in the expression profiles of nicotinic receptors in the olfactory bulb and trigeminal ganglion and identification of alpha2, alpha6, alpha9, and beta3 transcripts. *Biochem. Pharmacol.* 59, 233–240. doi: 10.1016/S0006-2952(99)00326-3

Kim, J., Choi, I. Y., Michaelis, M. L., and Lee, P. (2011). Quantitative in vivo measurement of early axonal transport deficits in a triple transgenic mouse model of Alzheimer's disease using manganese-enhanced MRI. *Neuroimage* 56, 1286–1292. doi: 10.1016/j.neuroimage.2011.02.039

Kiyokage, E., Pan, Y. Z., Shao, Z., Kobayashi, K., Szabo, G., Yanagawa, Y., et al. (2010). Molecular identity of periglomerular and short axon cells. *J. Neurosci.* 30, 1185–1196. doi: 10.1523/JNEUROSCI.3497-09.2010

Krosnowski, K., Ashby, S., Sathyanesan, A., Luo, W., Ogura, T., and Lin, W. (2012). Diverse populations of intrinsic cholinergic interneurons in the mouse olfactory bulb. *Neuroscience* 213, 161–178. doi: 10.1016/j.neuroscience.2012.04.024

Le Jeune, H., Aubert, I., Jourdan, F., and Quirion, R. (1995). Comparative laminar distribution of various autoradiographic cholinergic markers in adult rat main olfactory bulb. *J. Chem. Neuroanat.* 9, 99–112. doi: 10.1016/0891-0618(95)00070-N

Le Jeune, H., Aubert, I., Jourdan, F., and Quirion, R. (1996). Developmental profiles of various cholinergic markers in the rat main olfactory bulb using quantitative autoradiography. *J. Comp. Neurol.* 373, 433–450. doi: 10.1002/(SICI)1096-9861(19960923)373:3<433::AID-CNE8>3.0.CO;2-3

Le Jeune, H., and Jourdan, F. (1993). Cholinergic innervation of olfactory glomeruli in the rat: an ultrastructural immunocytochemical study. *J. Comp. Neurol.* 336, 279–292. doi: 10.1002/cne.903360209

Lee, M. G., Hassani, O. K., Alonso, A., and Jones, B. E. (2005). Cholinergic basal forebrain neurons burst with theta during waking and paradoxical sleep. *J. Neurosci.* 25, 4365–4369. doi: 10.1523/JNEUROSCI.0178-05.2005

Levin, E. D., and Simon, B. B. (1998). Nicotinic acetylcholine involvement in cognitive function in animals. *Psychopharmacology (Berl.)* 138, 217–230. doi: 10.1007/s002130050667

Li, G., and Cleland, T. A. (2013). A two-layer biophysical model of cholinergic neuromodulation in olfactory bulb. *J. Neurosci.* 33, 3037–3058. doi: 10.1523/JNEUROSCI.2831-12.2013

Liu, L. T., Willenbring, D., Xu, Y., and Tang, P. (2009). General anesthetic binding to neuronal alpha4beta2 nicotinic acetylcholine receptor and its effects on global dynamics. *J. Phys. Chem. B* 113, 12581–12589. doi: 10.1021/jp9039513

Liu, S., Aungst, J. L., Puche, A. C., and Shipley, M. T. (2012). Serotonin modulates the population activity profile of olfactory bulb external tufted cells. *J. Neurophysiol.* 107, 473–483. doi: 10.1152/jn.00741.2011

Liu, S., Plachez, C., Shao, Z., Puche, A., and Shipley, M. T. (2013). Olfactory bulb short axon cell release of GABA and dopamine produces a temporally biphasic inhibition-excitation response in external tufted cells. *J. Neurosci.* 33, 2916–2926. doi: 10.1523/JNEUROSCI.3607-12.2013

Lysakowski, A., Wainer, B. H., Bruce, G., and Hersh, L. B. (1989). An atlas of the regional and laminar distribution of choline acetyltransferase immunoreactivity in rat cerebral cortex. *Neuroscience* 28, 291–336. doi: 10.1016/0306-4522(89)90180-2

Ma, M., and Luo, M. (2012). Optogenetic activation of Basal forebrain cholinergic neurons modulates neuronal excitability and sensory responses in the main olfactory bulb. *J. Neurosci.* 32, 10105–10116. doi: 10.1523/JNEUROSCI.0058-12.2012

Macrides, F., Davis, B. J., Youngs, W. M., Nadi, N. S., and Margolis, F. L. (1981). Cholinergic and catecholaminergic afferents to the olfactory bulb in the hamster: a neuroanatomical, biochemical, and histochemical investigation. *J. Comp. Neurol.* 203, 495–514. doi: 10.1002/cne.902030311

Mao, D., Perry, D. C., Yasuda, R. P., Wolfe, B. B., and Kellar, K. J. (2008). The alpha4beta2alpha5 nicotinic cholinergic receptor in rat brain is resistant to up-regulation by nicotine in vivo. *J. Neurochem.* 104, 446–456. doi: 10.1111/j.1471-4159.2007.05011.x

Margrie, T. W., and Schaefer, A. T. (2003). Theta oscillation coupled spike latencies yield computational vigour in a mammalian sensory system. *J. Physiol.* 546, 363–374. doi: 10.1113/jphysiol.2002.031245

Markopoulos, F., Rokni, D., Gire, D. H., and Murthy, V. N. (2012). Functional properties of cortical feedback projections to the olfactory bulb. *Neuron* 76, 1175–1188. doi: 10.1016/j.neuron.2012.10.028

Mesholam, R. I., Moberg, P. J., Mahr, R. N., and Doty, R. L. (1998). Olfaction in neurodegenerative disease: a meta-analysis of olfactory functioning in Alzheimer's and Parkinson's diseases. *Arch. Neurol.* 55, 84–90. doi: 10.1001/archneur.55.1.84

Mesulam, M. M., Hersh, L. B., Mash, D. C., and Geula, C. (1992). Differential cholinergic innervation within functional subdivisions of the human cerebral cortex: a choline acetyltransferase study. *J. Comp. Neurol.* 318, 316–328. doi: 10.1002/cne.903180308

Mundinano, I. C., Caballero, M. C., Ordonez, C., Hernandez, M., DiCaudo, C., Marcilla, I., et al. (2011). Increased dopaminergic cells and protein aggregates in the olfactory bulb of patients with neurodegenerative disorders. *Acta Neuropathol.* 122, 61–74. doi: 10.1007/s00401-011-0830-2

Najac, M., De Saint, J. D., Reguero, L., Grandes, P., and Charpak, S. (2011). Monosynaptic and polysynaptic feed-forward inputs to mitral cells from olfactory sensory neurons. *J. Neurosci.* 31, 8722–8729. doi: 10.1523/JNEUROSCI.0527-11.2011

Parikh, V., Kozak, R., Martinez, V., and Sarter, M. (2007). Prefrontal acetylcholine release controls cue detection on multiple timescales. *Neuron* 56, 141–154. doi: 10.1016/j.neuron.2007.08.025

Parikh, V., Man, K., Decker, M. W., and Sarter, M. (2008). Glutamatergic contributions to nicotinic acetylcholine receptor agonist-evoked cholinergic transients in the prefrontal cortex. *J. Neurosci.* 28, 3769–3780. doi: 10.1523/JNEUROSCI.5251-07.2008

Parikh, V., and Sarter, M. (2008). Cholinergic mediation of attention: contributions of phasic and tonic increases in prefrontal cholinergic activity. *Ann. N. Y. Acad. Sci.* 1129, 225–235. doi: 10.1196/annals.1417.021

Pressler, R. T., Inoue, T., and Strowbridge, B. W. (2007). Muscarinic receptor activation modulates granule cell excitability and potentiates inhibition onto mitral cells in the rat olfactory bulb. *J. Neurosci.* 27, 10969–10981. doi: 10.1523/JNEUROSCI.2961-07.2007

Rinberg, D., and Gelperin, A. (2006). Olfactory neuronal dynamics in behaving animals. *Semin. Cell Dev. Biol.* 17, 454–461. doi: 10.1016/j.semcdb.2006.04.009

Rinberg, D., Koulakov, A., and Gelperin, A. (2006). Speed-accuracy tradeoff in olfaction. *Neuron* 51, 351–358. doi: 10.1016/j.neuron.2006.07.013

Rothermel, M., Carey, R. M., Puche, A., Shipley, M. T., and Wachowiak, M. (2014). Cholinergic inputs from Basal forebrain add an excitatory bias to odor coding in the olfactory bulb. *J. Neurosci.* 34, 4654–4664. doi: 10.1523/JNEUROSCI.5026-13.2014

Rushforth, S. L., Allison, C., Wonnacott, S., and Shoaib, M. (2010). Subtype-selective nicotinic agonists enhance olfactory working memory in normal rats: a novel use of the odour span task. *Neurosci. Lett.* 471, 114–118. doi: 10.1016/j.neulet.2010.01.022

Salcedo, E., Tran, T., Ly, X., Lopez, R., Barbica, C., Restrepo, D., et al. (2011). Activity-dependent changes in cholinergic innervation of the mouse olfactory bulb. *PLoS. ONE.* 6:e25441. doi: 10.1371/journal.pone.0025441

Sarter, M., Parikh, V., and Howe, W. M. (2009a). nAChR agonist-induced cognition enhancement: integration of cognitive and neuronal mechanisms. *Biochem. Pharmacol.* 78, 658–667. doi: 10.1016/j.bcp.2009.04.019

Sarter, M., Parikh, V., and Howe, W. M. (2009b). Phasic acetylcholine release and the volume transmission hypothesis: time to move on. *Nat. Rev. Neurosci.* 10, 383–390. doi: 10.1038/nrn2635

Schoppa, N. E. (2006). Synchronization of olfactory bulb mitral cells by precisely timed inhibitory inputs. *Neuron* 49, 271–283. doi: 10.1016/j.neuron.2005.11.038

Senut, M. C., Menetrey, D., and Lamour, Y. (1989). Cholinergic and peptidergic projections from the medial septum and the nucleus of the diagonal band of Broca to dorsal hippocampus, cingulate cortex and olfactory bulb: a combined wheatgerm agglutinin-apohorseradish peroxidase-gold immunohistochemical study. *Neuroscience* 30, 385–403. doi: 10.1016/0306-4522(89)90260-1

Simon, C., Kezunovic, N., Williams, D. K., Urbano, F. J., and Garcia-Rill, E. (2011). Cholinergic and glutamatergic agonists induce gamma frequency activity in dorsal subcoeruleus nucleus neurons. *Am. J. Physiol. Cell Physiol.* 301, C327–C335. doi: 10.1152/ajpcell.00093.2011

Smith, R. S., and Araneda, R. C. (2010). Cholinergic modulation of neuronal excitability in the accessory olfactory bulb. *J. Neurophysiol.* 104, 2963–2974. doi: 10.1152/jn.00446.2010

Tissingh, G., Berendse, H. W., Bergmans, P., DeWaard, R., Drukarch, B., Stoof, J. C., et al. (2001). Loss of olfaction in de novo and treated Parkinson's disease: possible implications for early diagnosis. *Mov. Disord.* 16, 41–46. doi: 10.1002/1531-8257(200101)16:1<41::AID-MDS1017>3.0.CO;2-M

Tsuno, Y., Kashiwadani, H., and Mori, K. (2008). Behavioral state regulation of dendrodendritic synaptic inhibition in the olfactory bulb. *J. Neurosci.* 28, 9227–9238. doi: 10.1523/JNEUROSCI.1576-08.2008

Vassar, R., Chao, S. K., Sitcheran, R., Nunez, J. M., Vosshall, L. B., and Axel, R. (1994). Topographic organization of sensory projections to the olfactory bulb. *Cell* 79, 981–991. doi: 10.1016/0092-8674(94)90029-9

Wachowiak, M. (2011). All in a sniff: olfaction as a model for active sensing. *Neuron* 71, 962–973. doi: 10.1016/j.neuron.2011.08.030

Wachowiak, M., Economo, M. N., Diaz-Quesada, M., Brunert, D., Wesson, D. W., White, J. A., et al. (2013). Optical dissection of odor information processing in vivo using GCaMPs expressed in specified cell types of the olfactory bulb. *J. Neurosci.* 33, 5285–5300. doi: 10.1523/JNEUROSCI.4824-12.2013

Wang, Z. J., Sun, L., and Heinbockel, T. (2012). Cannabinoid receptor-mediated regulation of neuronal activity and signaling in glomeruli of the main olfactory bulb. *J. Neurosci.* 32, 8475–8479. doi: 10.1523/JNEUROSCI.5333-11.2012

Weber, M., Motin, L., Gaul, S., Beker, F., Fink, R. H., and Adams, D. J. (2005). Intravenous anaesthetics inhibit nicotinic acetylcholine receptor-mediated currents and Ca^{2+} transients in rat intracardiac ganglion neurons. *Br. J. Pharmacol.* 144, 98–107. doi: 10.1038/sj.bjp.0705942

Wenk, H., Bigl, V., and Meyer, U. (1980). Cholinergic projections from magnocellular nuclei of the basal forebrain to cortical areas in rats. *Brain Res.* 2, 295–316. doi: 10.1016/0165-0173(80)90011-9

Wesson, D. W., Levy, E., Nixon, R. A., and Wilson, D. A. (2010). Olfactory dysfunction correlates with amyloid-beta burden in an Alzheimer's disease mouse model. *J. Neurosci.* 30, 505–514. doi: 10.1523/JNEUROSCI.4622-09.2010

Whitesell, J. D., Sorensen, K. A., Jarvie, B. C., Hentges, S. T., and Schoppa, N. E. (2013). Interglomerular lateral inhibition targeted on external tufted cells in the olfactory bulb. *J. Neurosci.* 33, 1552–1563. doi: 10.1523/JNEUROSCI.3410-12.2013

Wilson, D. A., Fletcher, M. L., and Sullivan, R. M. (2004). Acetylcholine and olfactory perceptual learning. *Learn. Mem.* 11, 28–34. doi: 10.1101/lm.66404

Wilson, D. A., and Stevenson, R. J. (2003). Olfactory perceptual learning: the critical role of memory in odor discrimination. *Neurosci. Biobehav. Rev.* 27, 307–328. doi: 10.1016/S0149-7634(03)00050-2

Xiao, Y., Meyer, E. L., Thompson, J. M., Surin, A., Wroblewski, J., and Kellar, K. J. (1998). Rat alpha3/beta4 subtype of neuronal nicotinic acetylcholine receptor stably expressed in a transfected cell line: pharmacology of ligand binding and function. *Mol. Pharmacol.* 54, 322–333.

Xu, F., Greer, C. A., and Shepherd, G. M. (2000). Odor maps in the olfactory bulb. *J. Comp. Neurol.* 422, 489–495. doi: 10.1002/1096-9861(20000710)422:4<489::AID-CNE1>3.0.CO;2-#

Young, J. W., Crawford, N., Kelly, J. S., Kerr, L. E., Marston, H. M., Spratt, C., et al. (2007a). Impaired attention is central to the cognitive deficits observed in alpha 7 deficient mice. *Eur. Neuropsychopharmacol.* 17, 145–155. doi: 10.1016/j.euroneuro.2006.03.008

Young, J. W., Kerr, L. E., Kelly, J. S., Marston, H. M., Spratt, C., Finlayson, K., et al. (2007b). The odour span task: a novel paradigm for assessing working memory in mice. *Neuropharmacology* 52, 634–645. doi: 10.1016/j.neuropharm.2006.09.006

Zaborszky, L. (2002). The modular organization of brain systems. Basal forebrain: the last frontier. *Prog. Brain Res.* 136, 359–372. doi: 10.1016/S0079-6123(02)36030-8

Zaborszky, L., Carlsen, J., Brashear, H. R., and Heimer, L. (1986). Cholinergic and GABAergic afferents to the olfactory bulb in the rat with special emphasis on the projection neurons in the nucleus of the horizontal limb of the diagonal band. *J. Comp. Neurol.* 243, 488–509. doi: 10.1002/cne.902430405

Zhan, X., Yin, P., and Heinbockel, T. (2013). The basal forebrain modulates spontaneous activity of principal cells in the main olfactory bulb of anesthetized mice. *Front. Neural. Circuits.* 7:148. doi: 10.3389/fncir.2013.00148

22

In vivo monitoring of glial scar proliferation on chronically implanted neural electrodes by fiber optical coherence tomography

Yijing Xie[1], Nadja Martini[1], Christina Hassler[2], Robert D. Kirch[1], Thomas Stieglitz[2], Andreas Seifert[3] and Ulrich G. Hofmann[1]*

[1] Neuroelectronic Systems, Department of General Neurosurgery, University Medical Center Freiburg, Freiburg, Germany
[2] Laboratory for Biomedical Microtechnology, Department of Microsystems Engineering(IMTEK), University of Freiburg, Freiburg, Germany
[3] Gisela and Erwin Sick Chair of Micro-optics, Department of Microsystems Engineering(IMTEK), University of Freiburg, Freiburg, Germany

Edited by:
Jürgen Krüger, Bernstein Center for Computational Neuroscience, Germany

Reviewed by:
Luca Berdondini, Italian Instittue of Technology, Italy
Pascal Darbon, Université de Strasbourg, France

***Correspondence:**
Ulrich G. Hofmann, Neuroelectronic Systems, Department of General Neurosurgery, University Medical Center Freiburg, Engesser Strasse 4, Freiburg D-79108, Germany
e-mail: ulrich.hofmann@klinikum.uni-freiburg.de

In neural prosthetics and stereotactic neurosurgery, intracortical electrodes are often utilized for delivering therapeutic electrical pulses, and recording neural electrophysiological signals. Unfortunately, neuroinflammation impairs the neuron-electrode-interface by developing a compact glial encapsulation around the implants in long term. At present, analyzing this immune reaction is only feasible with post-mortem histology; currently no means for specific *in vivo* monitoring exist and most applicable imaging modalities can not provide information in deep brain regions. Optical coherence tomography (OCT) is a well established imaging modality for *in vivo* studies, providing cellular resolution and up to 1.2 mm imaging depth in brain tissue. A fiber based spectral domain OCT was shown to be capable of minimally invasive brain imaging. In the present study, we propose to use a fiber based spectral domain OCT to monitor the progression of the tissue's immune response through scar encapsulation progress in a rat animal model. A fine fiber catheter was implanted in rat brain together with a flexible polyimide microelectrode in sight both of which acts as a foreign body and induces the brain tissue immune reaction. OCT signals were collected from animals up to 12 weeks after implantation and thus gliotic scarring *in vivo* monitored for that time. Preliminary data showed a significant enhancement of the OCT backscattering signal during the first 3 weeks after implantation, and increased attenuation factor of the sampled tissue due to the glial scar formation.

Keywords: chronic implants, flexible microelectrodes, foreign body reaction, optical coherence tomography, fiber catheter

1. INTRODUCTION

Intracortical electrodes are often employed in neuroprosthetic applications or in clinical stereotactic surgery, to deliver therapeutic electrical pulses and collect neuronal electrophysiological signals (Tronnier and Fogel, 2000; Stieglitz et al., 2009; Raspopovic et al., 2014). A reliable and dependable electrode-tissue-interface is crucial in this concept since a neuroprosthetic device is supposed to serve functionally over long period in subject's brain. Unfortunately, the lifetime of a such device is always compromised due to electrode corrosion or so called glial scarring around the indwelling electrode (Edell et al., 1992; Schmidt et al., 1993; Turner et al., 1999; Leach et al., 2010).

When an electrode is implanted into the brain, during the acute phase of the immune reaction, microphages settle in on the area and resident microglia cells of the immune system become activated and start proliferating. Then astrocytes are activated to scavenge the leftover large intruders. Unfortunately, any type of the artificial implant is resistant to this bio degradation, which induces a so called frustrated phagocytosis and leads in consequence to a dense glial scar attempting to isolate the implant from the delicate brain tissue (Turner et al., 1999; Biran et al., 2005; Polikov et al., 2005; Winslow et al., 2010; Potter et al., 2012). This isolation performed by glial sheathing not only changes the electrical coupling to the surrounding parenchyma, but may even cause neuronal loss by neurotoxic factors released from glial cells (Block et al., 2007). This leads to a deterioration and loss of electrophysiological signal over time. Electrical characterization of electrode-tissue state over time is attempted by temporally resolved impedance spectroscopy or signal-to-noise ratio analysis (Ludwig et al., 2006; Mcconnell et al., 2009). Immunohistochemical analysis is performed to characterize astrocytes and microglial cells progression over time. However, this requires tissue to be removed for postmortem examination disqualifying for long term *in vivo* process monitoring of the same animal (Szarowski et al., 2003). Lately, Kozai et al. (2012) reported using two-photon microscopy to reveal immediate microglial reaction to electrode insertion *in vivo*. However, this technique is limited to imaging only a shallow part

(~200 μm) of the brain and only in short term (up to 7 h post implantation).

Alternatively, clinically approved Optical Coherence Tomography, displaying the intrinsic optical scattering properties of the tissue, might be used instead (Huang et al., 1991; Hee et al., 1996; Bonin et al., 2010). OCT features a spatial resolution in cellular range of 5–10 μm, up to 1.2 mm imaging depth in brain tissue, and up to 40,000 axial scans (A-scan) per second (Drexler et al., 2001; Rodriguez-Padilla et al., 2007). When integrated with ultra-small single mode fiber catheter, it is competent to visualize deep brain structures with minimum trauma (Tearney et al., 1997; Böhringer et al., 2006; Xie et al., 2013).

In the present study, we propose to use a fiber based spectral domain OCT to monitor the progression of the tissue's immune response through scar encapsulation progress in a rat animal model. We developed an integrated OCT detection probe consisting of an implantable ferrule based fiber catheter and a fiber patch cable. The fiber catheter was implanted in rat brain together with a flexible polyimide microelectrode array in sight, according to the procedure described in Richter et al. (2013), both intended to induce the brain tissue immune reaction. The OCT backscattering intensity of the brain tissue around the fiber increased during the first 3 weeks. The tissue optical attenuation coefficient altered after implantation and reached a maximum at the week 6 implying that a compact dense tissue sheath has developed around the fiber tip. Further more, the 10 μm thick flexible probe which located up to 2.7 mm away from the fiber catheter tip is still visible in the OCT image and A-scan plot.

2. MATERIALS AND METHODS

2.1. OPTICAL COHERENCE TOMOGRAPHY IMAGING SYSTEM

The imaging modality we used to monitor and assess the foreign body reaction is fiber based spectral domain optical coherence tomography (SDOCT) (Fercher et al., 1995). In this imaging modality, the incident light is transmitted into tissue through an implantable fiber catheter and the backscattered light from the illuminated tissue is also collected by the fiber catheter. The incident light and the backscattered light produce an interference pattern encoding the intrinsic optical properties of the sampled tissue. The interference pattern is detected at a spectrometer to construct A-scan (depth-scan) signals providing the backscattered light intensity as a function of depth.

The imaging system employed composes a commercially available fiber-based OCT module ("Callisto," Thorlabs GmbH, Lübeck, Germany) utilizing a superluminescent diode (SLD) with center wavelength at 840 nm as the light source and a single mode fiber based sampling probe providing the feasibility of minimum-invasive imaging (see **Figure 1**). When equipped with a single mode fiber based detecting catheter, the whole system features an axial resolution of 14 μm and transversal resolution of 20 μm in air. The system's look-ahead capability is 3.5 mm from the tip of the fiber catheter to the tissue, enabling us to evaluate the development of the tissue reaction to the indwelling fiber catheter and to the flexible microelectrode underneath. It has been demonstrated that the fiber based OCT system is competent for imaging brain anatomical structures *in vivo* (Xie et al., 2013).

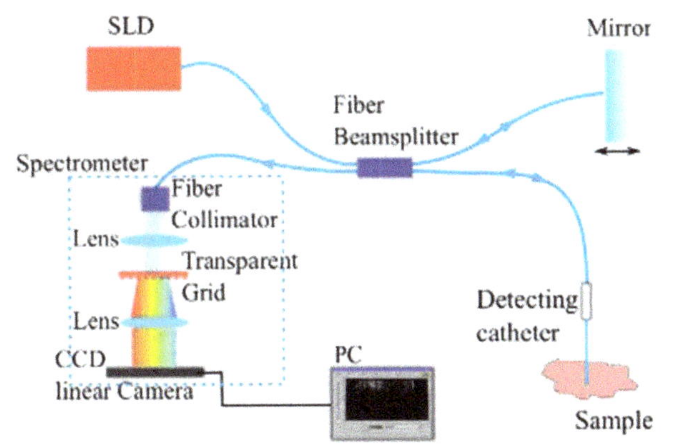

FIGURE 1 | A schematic diagram of the Spectral Domain Optical Coherence Tomography imaging system.

2.2. OPTICAL FIBER DETECTION CATHETER

The aim of this study is to use a chronically implanted OCT fiber cannula to monitor and to assess brain tissue's foreign body reaction to it and to the also chronically implanted flexible microelectrode. The fiber cannula chosen consists of a ceramic FC ferrule (CF126-10, Thorlabs) with 2.5 mm outer diameter and 10.5 mm total length, and a 8 mm long single mode fiber (⌀125 μm, SMF800-5.6-125, Thorlabs) in order to reach deep brain structures (see **Figure 2B** bottom for geometry).

2.3. POLYIMIDE BASED FLEXIBLE MICROELECTRODE

The flexible polyimide microelectrode, which also provokes immune response and which was implanted into the rat brain, is designed and fabricated in-house. The probe shank is 15 mm long, 10 μm thick and 365 μm wide, with a smooth surface. The substrate material of the photolithographically structured probe is a medical grade polyimide type PI2611 (U-Varnish S, UBE, Newyork), with a bulk YoungÕs modulus of around 10 GPa over 20 months in 37°C PBS (Rubehn and Stieglitz, 2010) (**Figure 2B** left). It is exemplifying a "device under test" based on findings (Sohal et al., 2014) that indwelling flexible substrates provoke a less pronounced gliosis compared with rigid micro electrodes presumably due to compliance-matching with brain tissue.

2.4. ANIMAL SURGERY AND DEVICE IMPLANTATION

All animal experiments conducted in this study were performed with approval from the locally responsible Animal Welfare Committe with the Regierungspräsidium Freiburg in accordance with the guidelines of the European Union Directive 2010/63/UE. The animal model chosen consists of adult female Sprague Dawley rats (Charles River, Germany), weighing 280–320 g. The rats were initially anesthetized by administering intraperitoneally a mixture of 100 mg/kg ketamine and 5 mg/kg xylazine. Rats were placed on a the heating pad of a circulating water bath set to 40°C to maintain a body temperature of 35°C. The rat was then fixed into the stereotactic frame with a pair of ear pins and a bite bar. A 15 mm long scalp incision was cut along the midline, the skin was pulled aside to expose the skull surface structure. Bregma was identified and served as coordinate 0.0 mm. A burr hole (0.9 mm

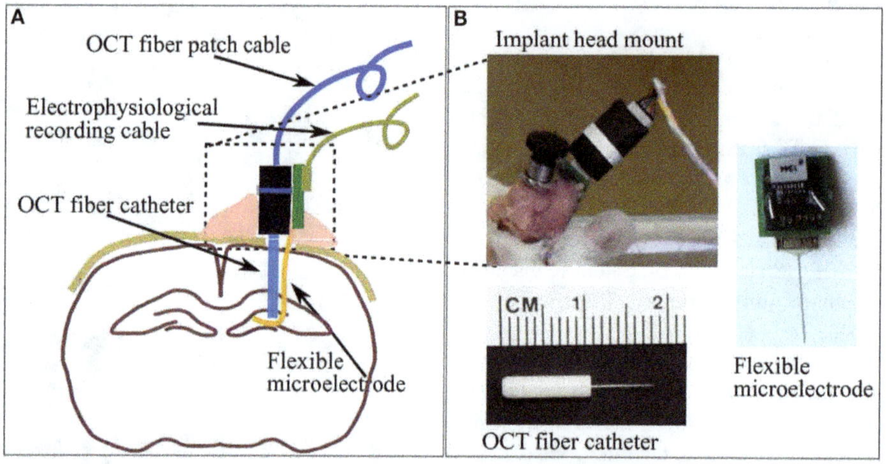

FIGURE 2 | (A) A brief sketch of the implantations including a pair of indwelling probe: the OCT fiber catheter and the flexible polyimide microelectrode. **(B)** The picture on top-left shows the cemented fiber optics connector and PCB for electrophysiology recording taken on the second week after implantation surgery. Pictures on bottom-left and right demonstrate the geometry of the OCT fiber catheter and the flexible microelectrode connected to a PCB, respectively.

in diameter) in the skull at 4.0 mm posterior 2.0 mm lateral from Bregma was drilled. Prior to probe insertion, a small incision was cut on the dura and pia mater underneath the burr hole with a 27 G needle to avoid brain dimpling upon probe penetration.

The flexible microelectrode was inserted in the brain tissue with the OCT fiber catheter, following the protocol prosposed by Richter et al. (2013). The flexible microelectrode was placed on the moist skull surface, with the shank precisely adjusted to overlay the burr hole at the position of 4 mm from the shank distal end. The OCT fiber catheter was firmly clamped to the micro drive equipped stereotaxic frame and positioned on top of the burr hole. The microelectrode shank was placed between the exposed skull and the OCT fiber precisely aligned above the hole (**Figure 3A**). Slowly driving the stereotactic z arm to insert the fiber catheter, the flexible microelectrode was pushed into the brain by the fiber catheter (**Figures 3B,C**). We stopped the insertion when the fiber catheter was at 6 mm under the brain surface (thalamic nucleus area) (**Figure 3D**). In order to avoid electrode displacement while applying dental cement, a small drop of Super Glue (Loctite 4061, Henkel Loctite GmbH) was applied to adhere the rest of the electrode shank to the skull. A small amount of bone wax was plastered to close the skull burr hole. We sealed and tethered the connector part of the fiber catheter and the microelectrode with adequate dental cement (**Figure 2A**). The skin incision was sutured to close and wiped with betaisodona (7.5%, B. Braun Melsungen) to prevent skin infection. Carprofen (4 mg/kg) was then administered subcutaneously for pain management each day for 5 days after surgery. The animals were housed with daily inspection.

2.5. POST SURGERY MEASUREMENT AND OCT SIGNAL ANALYSIS

The OCT signal was collected at week 1, 2, 3, 6, and 12 after the implantation surgery in freely moving rats. During each measurement, the implanted OCT fiber catheter was connected to the OCT sampling cable through FC/FC mating sleeve. Since the FC ferrule features a flat endface, the presence of air at the junction point induces significant signal loss due to the refractive index mismatching between air and fiber material. To achieve the maximum light transmission between the fiber catheter and the sampling cable, we applied a thin layer ($\sim$100 μm thick) of index matching gel (G608N3, Thorlabs) at the junction part. Signal acquisition was performed for about 5 min in each measurement section for analysis.

The OCT signal is presented in gray scale images each of which consists of 1000 A-scan signals aligned in x-axis (see **Figure 4** left panels). Depth-scan profile is plotted by taking an average of 1000 A-scans (see **Figure 4** right panels). For quantification of OCT signals, we calculated the light attenuation factor of the sampled tissue by analysing A-scan signals. The light attenuation factor was defined as the ratio of detected light intensity decline in depth (mm). It is proportional but not equal to the tissue attenuation coefficient which is one of the essential tissue optical properties reflecting the tissue composition and density. A change in attenuation factor implies alterations in tissue properties, such as cell density, cell orientation, predominate cell type and hence backscatter ability. Attenuation factor is calculated as the slope value of the linear fit for the log intensity of the linear portion depth in an A-scan plot (see the red lines on plots in **Figure 4**).

2.6. HISTOLOGY AND IMMUNOSTAINING

Rats were terminated by administering Ketamine and Xylazine mixture intraperitonealy. The brains were removed immediately after decapitation, fixed in 4% paraformaldehyde (PFA) in PBS for 4 days, and then incubated in 30% sucrose in PBS for at least 2 days. During the brain removal procedure, the flexible microelectrode and the OCT fiber probe were carefully cut from their skull-tethered part and were PFA fixed within the brain. Prior to sectioning, the OCT fiber probe was explanted from the brain while the flexible microelectrode was kept *in situ* in the brain. Brains were then embedded in Tissue-Tek O.C.T. (Sakura Finetek,

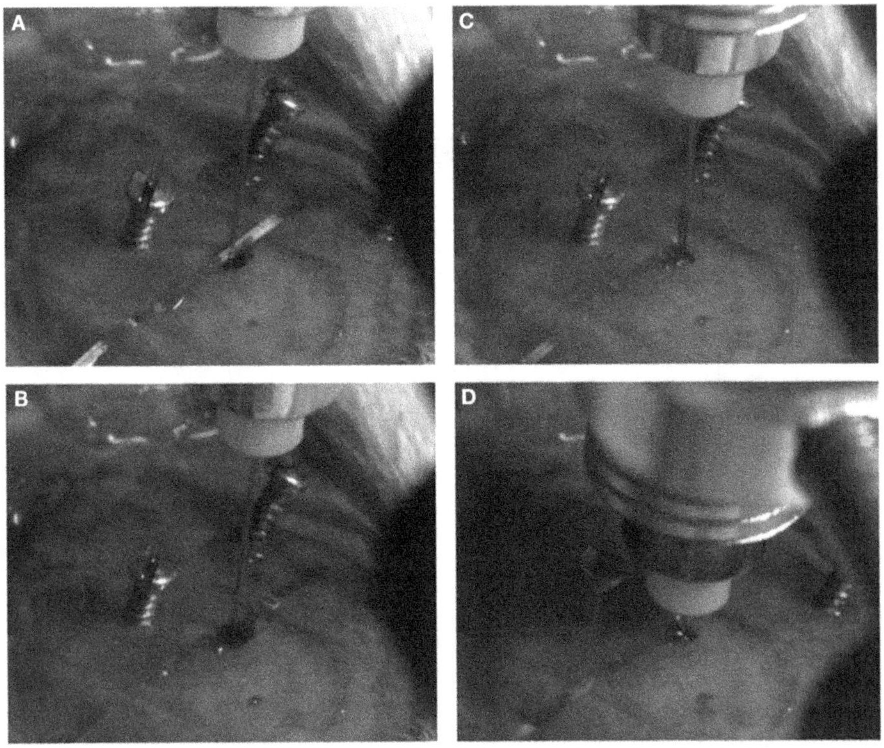

FIGURE 3 | Probe implantation procedures. The flexible microelectrode and fiber catheter are precisely aligned above the burr hole **(A)**. The fiber catheter is slowly and cautiously driven down to push the shank of the flexible mciroelectrode into the brain **(B,C)** until the desired depth is reached **(D)**.

Germany) at −20°C. 20 μm thick transversal or coronal slices were obtained with a cryostat-microtome at −20°C.

Brain slices were double-immunostained for GFAP (glial fibrillary acidic protein) to detect astrocytes and Iba1 (ionized calcium-binding adapter molecule (1) to identify microglia/macrophages. Brain slices were incubated in 10% goat serum to block non-specific binding, then incubated in GFAP antibody (1:1000 dilution, rabbit IgG, Millipore) and Iba1 antibody (1:500 dilution, Goat IgG, Abcam) for 3 h. After 3 rinses in PBS (5 min each), fluorescence-labeled secondary antibodies AlexaFluro 488 anti-rabbit and AlexaFluro 647 anti-goat were applied for 1 h. Both secondary antibodies (Molecular Probes) were used in 1: 1000 dilution. After 3 rinses in PBS (5 min each), brain slices were mounted onto the microscopic slides with Dapi-Fluoromount-G (Southern Biotech) and then covered with a coverslip. Slice images were collected with Jenoptik camera mounted on a Zeiss microscope (Zeiss Imager a1), using the identical exposure time for each immunolabel at each magnification.

3. RESULTS

3.1. OCT SIGNALS FROM THE TISSUE AROUND THE INDWELLING FIBER CATHETER

During 6 weeks after the implantation, the intensity of the OCT signal increased from 60 to 70 dB (**Figures 4A–C**). From week 6 to week 12, the OCT signal intensity didn't demonstrate noticeable change (**Figures 4C,D**). Some sparsely distributed microscopic structures could be identified close to the fiber catheter 1 week post operation, having the shape of as several horizontal stripe patterns and appear in the A-scan signal as multiple peaks (**Figure 4A**). At week 6, a 200 μm thick layer of tissue with high backscattering signal had developed around the fiber catheter (**Figure 4C**). This high reflecting tissue layer developed into a prominent feature in the OCT image at week 12, with a smooth A-scan plot profile (**Figure 4D**). At week 6 and 12, the OCT signal attenuated faster featuring a steep declining slope in the A-scan plot while the backscattering intensity from the tissue surrounding the fiber probe stayed steady at 70 dB (see **Figures 4C,D**). To further characterize the OCT signal, the attenuation factor of 4 animals on each measurement were calculated and presented in **Figure 5**. In general, the attenuation factor evidently raised during the first 3 weeks after the implantation, implying that a compact dense tissue layer was developing during this period. Then the attenuation factor stabilized at 6 weeks and 12 weeks post implantation.

3.2. OCT SIGNALS OF THE INDWELLING FLEXIBLE MICROELECTRODE

At week 1 post implantation, the signal from the flexible probe was evidently visible in the A-scan signal located at 2.3 mm underneath the OCT fiber catheter tip. The maximum backscattering intensity of the OCT signal at week 1 post implantation (p.i.) is about 59 dB, while the backscattering intensity from the flexible electrode is approximately 35 dB presenting a a clearly visible peak (**Figure 6A**). Since before it reached the flexible probe the incident

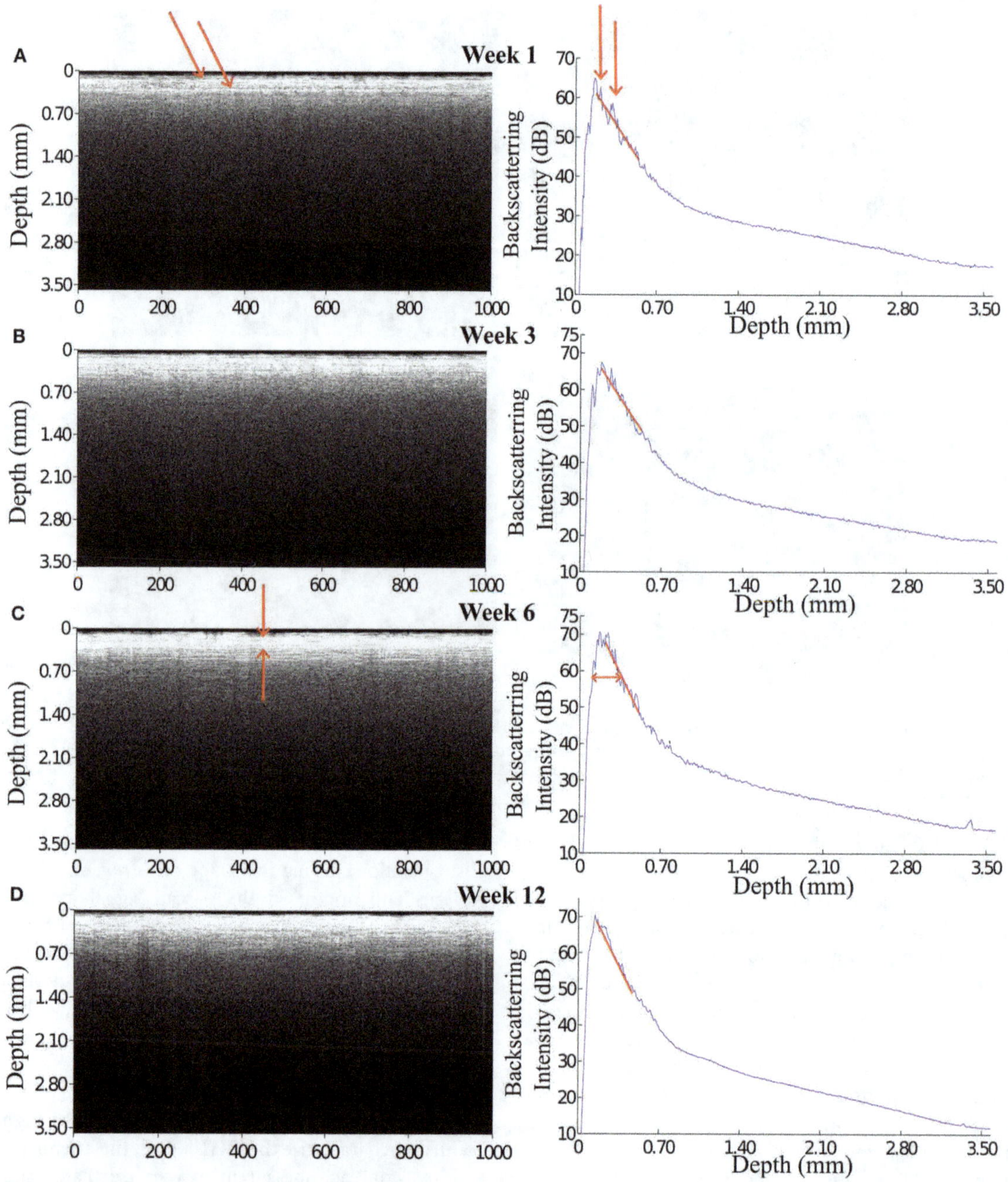

FIGURE 4 | OCT images and the corresponding A-scan profiles acquired at week 1, 3, 6, and 12 after implantation. The intensity of the backscattered light increased during the first 3 weeks post implantation **(A,B)**, while at week 6 and 12 the OCT signal attenuated faster featuring a steep declining slope in the A-scan plot **(C,D)**. Arrows in panel **(A)** indicate the anatomic micro structures viewed by the OCT. Arrows in panel **(C)** indicate a 200 μm thick layer is expressed in the OCT signal.

light was presumably scattered and attenuated by the ongoing scar formation around the glass fiber catheter, the backscattered signal from the flexible electrode dwindled in the following weeks (**Figures 6B,C**). Although the incident light attenuated predominantly in the tissue around the fiber presumably the scar sheath, the flexible electrode was still visible in the OCT scan demonstrating as a noticeable peak in the A-scan plot.

Although the signal of the flexible electrode was expected to diminish due to the strong light scattering in the compact glial sheath around the rigid fiber catheter, we observed in one case that the signal of the flexible electrode reappeared at 6 weeks p.i. (**Figure 7**). This very flexible probe was not visible after the first week, presumably as a result of the incorrect alignment of the flexible electrode and the fiber catheter upon implantation (**Figure 7A**). At week 2 p.i. in addition to the two-layer structure formation at the depth position of around 0.60 mm in the OCT image, a small peak was observed in the A-scan plot at the depth position of 2.70 mm (**Figure 7B**). At week 6 p.i. a pronounced signal at the depth position of 2.70 mm was detected and visible both in the OCT image and the A-scan plot (**Figure 7C**). We assume, that the high intensity signal that reappeared at the image depth of 2.70 mm at 6 weeks p.i. is originating from the flexible electrode. Since this polyimide-based electrode features much lower elastic modulus compared to the conventional metal microelectrode with similar dimensions, the flexible electrode is supposedly able to float with the brain tissue (Jensen et al., 2007). Therefore, during the 6 weeks the flexible electrode's position in the brain might alter and move back to the detection area of the OCT fiber catheter eliciting the high intensity peak in OCT signal.

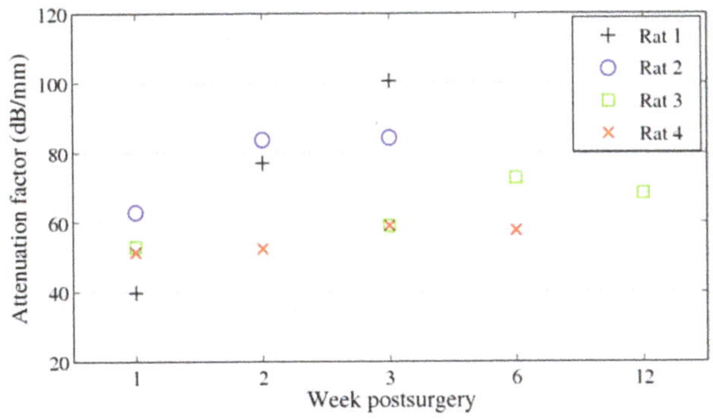

FIGURE 5 | Attenuation factors of the brain tissue around the fiber catheter at week 1, 2, 3, 6, and 12.

3.3. IMMUNOREACTIVITY OF GFAP POSITIVE CELLS AND IBA-1 POSITIVE CELLS AROUND THE INSERTION TRAJECTORY

The reactivity of GFAP-positive cells are widely used to characterize astrocytes star-shaped cell body (Schiffer et al., 1993; Faulkner et al., 2004; Sofroniew, 2005). At week 1, GFAP-positive cells are loosely distributed in an area up to 500 μm from the insertion cavity. A thin layer of the aligned GFAP-positive cells was observed surrounding the insertion channel. At week 3, GFAP-positive cells proliferated and spread to further areas up to 700 μm from the insertion edge with enhanced fluorescence intensity. At week 6, the fluorescence of GFAP-positive cells in the far area appeared reduced. Instead, a layer GFAP-positive cells

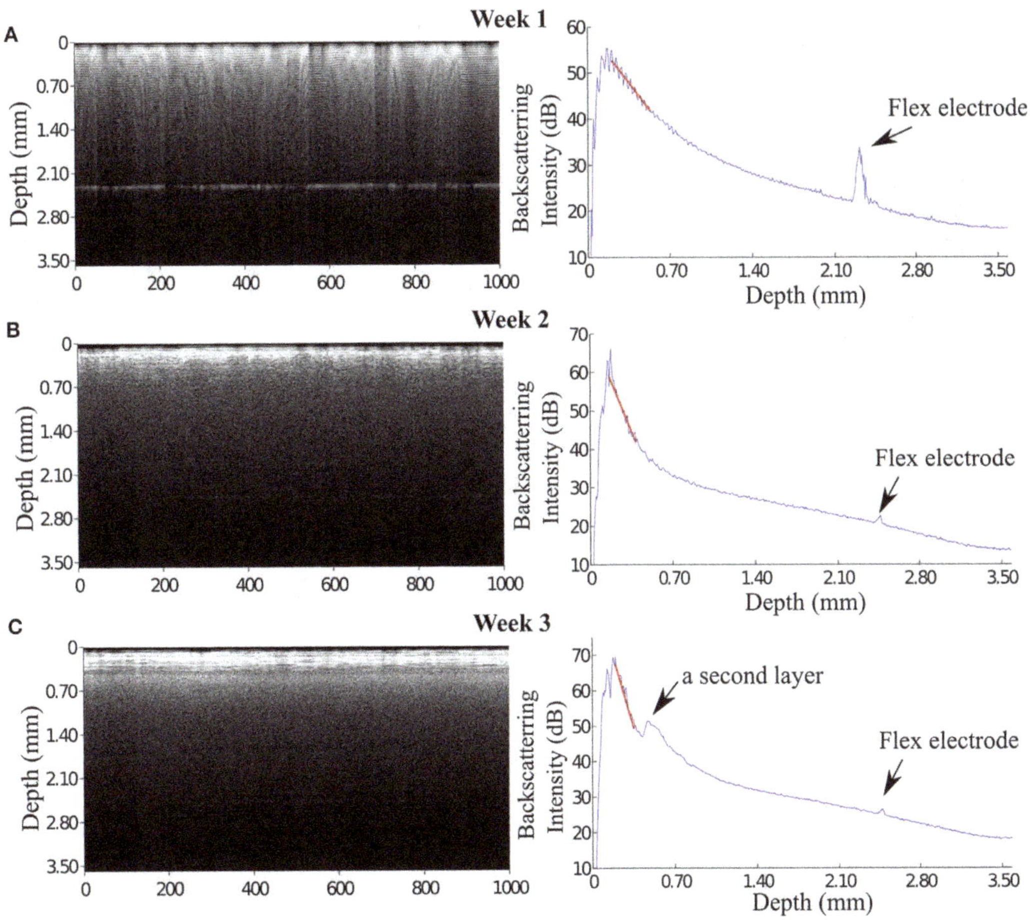

FIGURE 6 | OCT images reveal that the signal of flexible microelectrode underneath the fiber catheter declined. (A) At 1 week, the flexible electrode can be seen distinctly in the OCT image with a approximately 12 dB peak height in the A-scan plot. **(B)** In contrast to the enhanced OCT signal of the brain tissue, the signal of the flexible electrode severely declined. **(C)** Interestingly, at 3 weeks p.i. the OCT image illustrates 2 distinguishable tissue layers. The backscattering intensity of the flexible electrode remains noticeable.

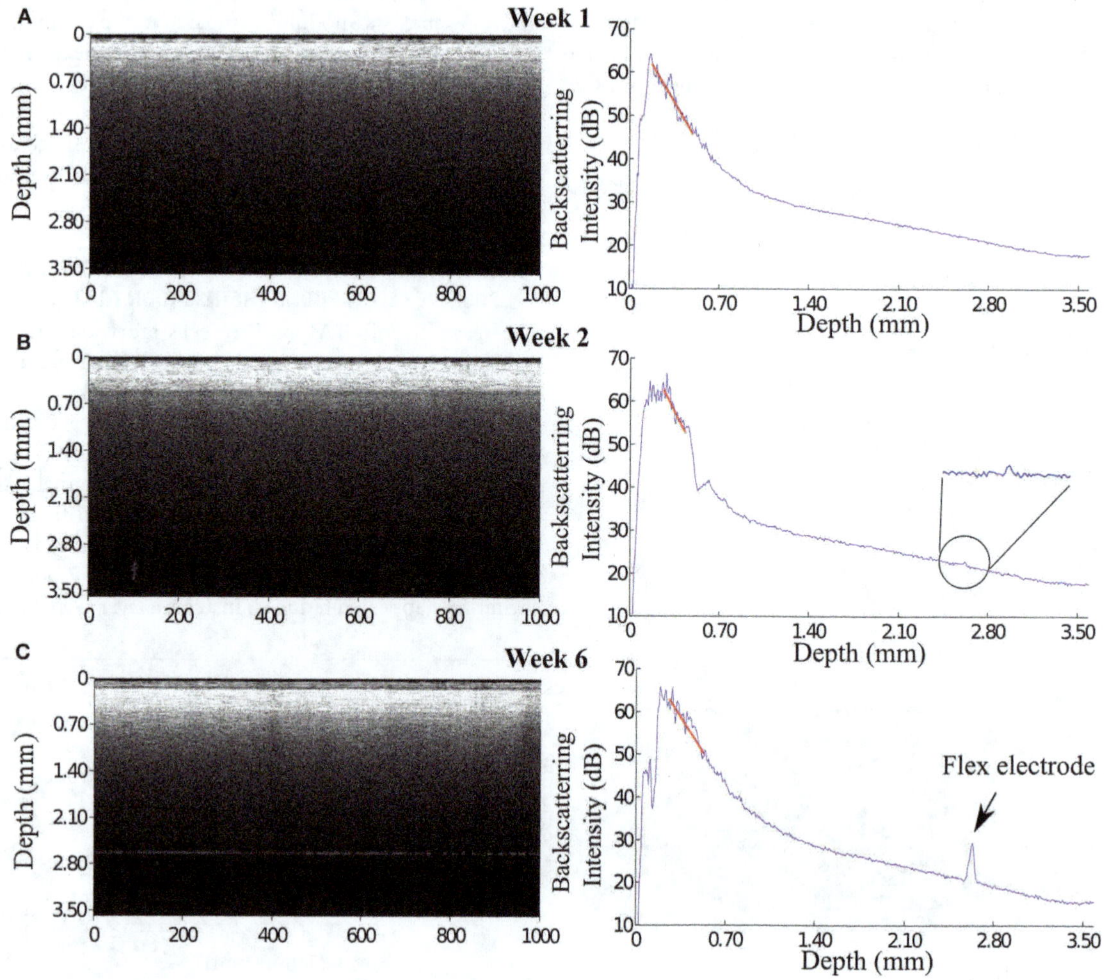

FIGURE 7 | (A) At 1 week, the flexible electrode can not be seen in the OCT image probably because of a misalignment between the flexible electrode and the fiber catheter. **(B)** At 2 weeks, a small but noticeable peak appears in the A-scan plot at the depth position of 2.70 mm. **(C)** At 6 weeks, a pronounced signal is revealed both in the OCT image and in the A-scan plot, presumably, from the flexible electrode.

with high fluorescence intensity encapsulated the insertion site (**Figure 8**).

We assessed the inflammatory process during the experiment by analyzing the expression of the ionized calcium binding adaptor molecule (Iba-1), a marker for both resting and reactive microglia and macrophages (Ito et al., 1998). At 1, 3, 6 weeks, the Iba-1 expression was only found in the close area of the insertion site not in the extended surrounding area (**Figure 8**). The apparent distribution of fluorescence intensity and the number of the Iba-1 positive cells didn't demonstrate any significant changes over time.

4. DISCUSSION

The goal of this study is to introduce a new method to monitor and assess the scarring process around a chronically implanted glass fiber catheter and a synchronously implanted flexible polyimide-based microelectrode by using an OCT imaging system (catheter type, ⌀125 μm). OCT signals were acquired weekly for 12 weeks after implantation even though no technical obstacles prohibit continuous monitoring. The results corroborate that SDOCT with an *in situ* implanted fiber catheter is capable of visualizing the modification in optical properties of the surrounding tissue over time. During the first 3 weeks after implantation, the intensity of the backscattered light, hence the OCT signal of the surrounding tissue increases monotonically. The intensity levels off at 6 weeks after implantation. The increased backscattering intensity from the surrounding tissue is most likely caused by the increased accumulation of astrocytes around the glass fiber itself, which is referred in literature as glial encapsulation (Leach et al., 2010). The analyzed tissue optical property "attenuation factor" demonstrates that a compact dense tissue sheath has been developing during the 6 weeks after implantation. Since we've obtained the attenuation factor of control brain tissue from a previous study, we are able to compare the current result to naive control tissue (**Figure 9**). Besides, it is promising that within the proposed novel monitoring modality (1) the 10 μm thick flexible probe is still visible up to 2.7 mm away from the fiber tip, (2) alteration in tissue anatomical structure is noticeable in OCT A-scans, such as the two-layered structure that developed from week 3 on in (**Figure 6**).

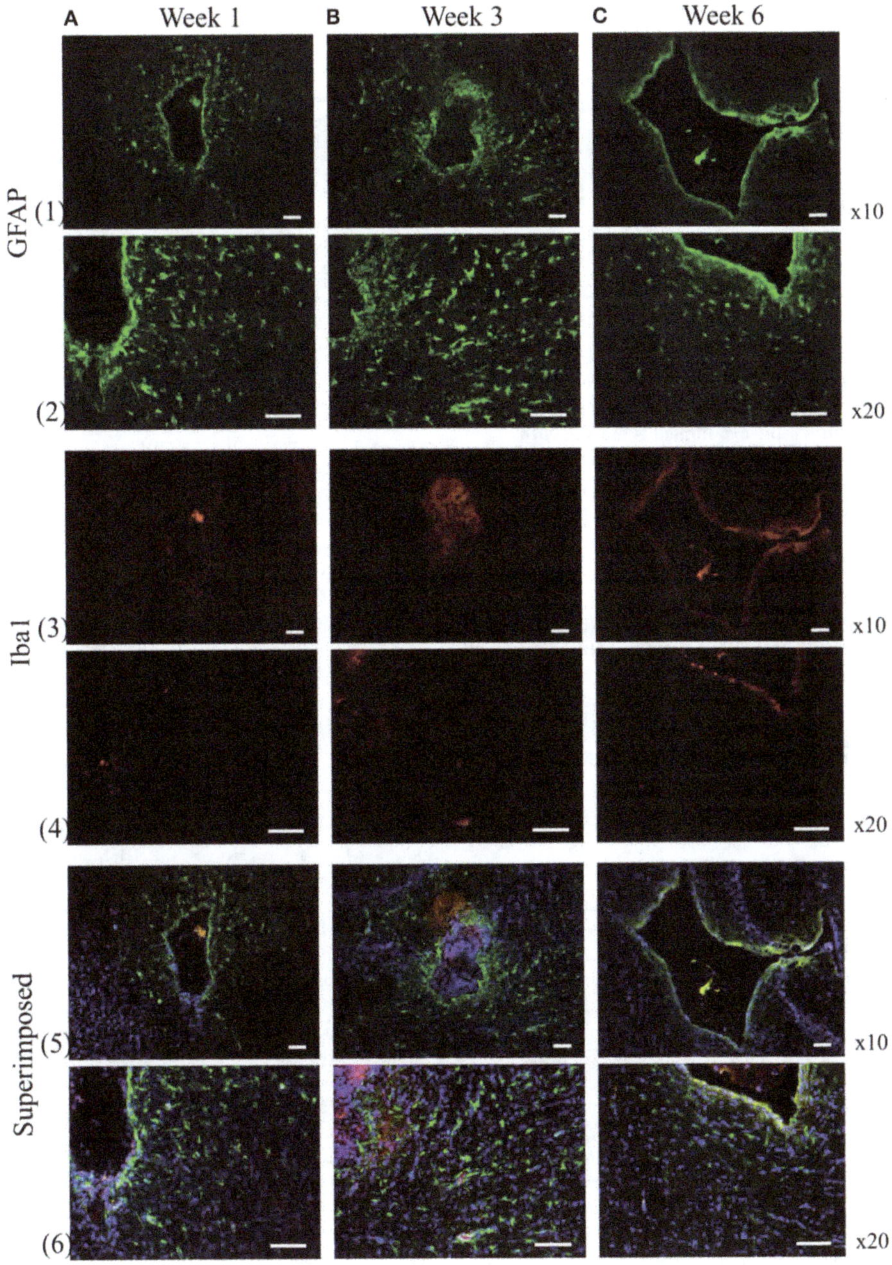

FIGURE 8 | GFAP and Iba-1 reactivity to the chronically implanted fiber catheter and flexible electrode assembly at week 1, 3, and 6, respectively. At week 1 and 3 the GFAP positive cells spread to larger area around the insertion trajectory **(1A,B, 2A,B)**, while at week 6 the GFAP positive cells become less pronounced in the extended surrounding area, instead they construct a compact layer next to the electrode and fiber **(1C, 2C)**. Iba-1 positive cells are much smaller numbers than the GFAP positive cells at all time points **(3A–C, 4A–C)**. No obvious proliferation of the Iba-1 positive cells are observed over time. Row 5 and 6 are the superimposed pictures of GFAP (green), Iba-1 (red) and DAPI (blue) staining. Scale bar = 100 μm.

Since the OCT fiber cannula itself is recognized as a foreign body by the brain tissue, the incident light is scattered and attenuated already at the compact astrocyte sheath around the fiber tip, resulting in a deteriorated detection of the flexible probe, but at the same time providing positive control of immune response. This shortcoming could be overcome by using a probe assembly which consists of a waveguide (for OCT acquisition) that is integrated to a flexible polyimide probe (for electrophysiology acquisition) to gain "inside-out" views of the developing gliosis while maintaining the probe's flexibility.

Still, it must be noted, that the flexible probe remained visible even at distances greater than 1 mm without revealing a change in tissue optical properties. It is a matter for ongoing investigations, whether the flexible probe was indeed not covered by a detectable glial sheath as independent immunocytochemistry results suggest (unpublished data) or whether an existing sheath

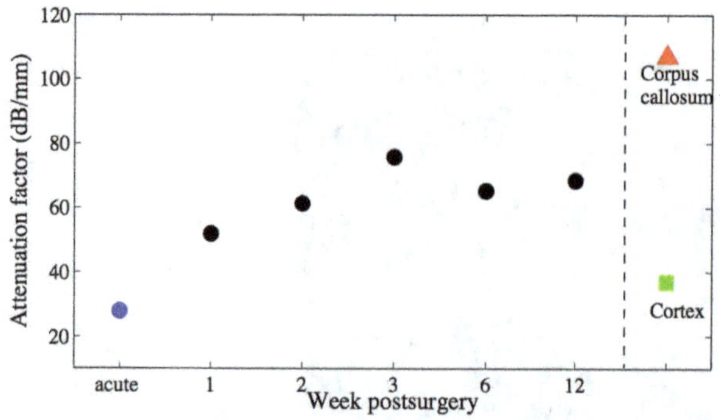

FIGURE 9 | Averaged attenuation factors of the brain tissue around the fiber catheter at week 1, 2, 3, 6, and 12 are marked with black •, attenuation factor obtained from acute experiment is marked with blue •. Attenuation factors of other brain tissue types obtained also in acute experiments (Xie et al., 2013) are marked with △ and □ respectively. No error bars are shown, due to the littel number of animals used.

did not sufficiently backscatter for detection. In any ways, to the best of our knowledge, the presented method appears to be the first optical attempt to monitor brain's immune response on deep implants without prior markers *in vivo*.

ACKNOWLEDGMENT

This work was supported by BrainLinks-BrainTools Cluster of Excellence funded by the German Research Foundation (DFG, grant number EXC 1086).

REFERENCES

Biran, R., Martin, D. C., and Tresco, P. A. (2005). Neuronal cell loss accompanies the brain tissue response to chronically implanted silicon microelectrode arrays. *Exp. Neurol.* 195, 115–126. doi: 10.1016/j.expneurol.2005.04.020

Block, M. L., Zecca, L., and Hong, J.-S. (2007). Microglia-mediated neurotoxicity: uncovering the molecular mechanisms. *Nat. Rev. Neurosci.* 8, 57–69. doi: 10.1038/nrn2038

Böhringer, H., Boller, D., Leppert, J., Knopp, U., Lankenau, E., Reusche, E., et al. (2006). Time-domain and spectral-domain optical coherence tomography in the analysis of brain tumor tissue. *Lasers Surg. Med.* 38, 588–597. doi: 10.1002/lsm.20353

Bonin, T., Franke, G., Hagen-Eggert, M., Koch, P., and Hüttmann, G. (2010). *In vivo* fourier-domain full-field oct of the human retina with 1.5 million a-lines/s. *Opt. Lett.* 35, 3432–3434. doi: 10.1364/OL.35.003432

Drexler, W., Morgner, U., Ghanta, R. K., Kartner, F. X., Schuman, J. S., and Fujimoto, J. G. (2001). Ultrahigh-resolution ophthalmic optical coherence tomography. *Nat. Med.* 7, 502–507. doi: 10.1038/86589

Edell, D., Toi, V., McNeil, V., and Clark, L. (1992). Factors influencing the biocompatibility of insertable silicon microshafts in cerebral cortex. *Biomed. Eng. IEEE Trans.* 39, 635–643. doi: 10.1109/10.141202

Faulkner, J. R., Herrmann, J. E., Woo, M. J., Tansey, K. E., Doan, N. B., and Sofroniew, M. V. (2004). Reactive astrocytes protect tissue and preserve function after spinal cord injury. *J. Neurosci.* 24, 2143–2155. doi: 10.1523/JNEUROSCI.3547-03.2004

Fercher, A., Hitzenberger, C., Kamp, G., and El-Zaiat, S. (1995). Measurement of intraocular distances by backscattering spectral interferometry. *Opt. Commun.* 117, 43–48. doi: 10.1016/0030-4018(95)00119-S

Hee, M. R., Baumal, C. R., Puliafito, C. A., Duker, J. S., Reichel, E., Wilkins, J. R., et al. (1996). Optical coherence tomography of age-related macular degeneration and choroidal neovascularization. *Ophthalmology* 103, 1260–1270. doi: 10.1016/S0161-6420(96)30512-5

Huang, D., Swanson, E., Lin, C., Schuman, J., Stinson, W., Chang, W., et al. (1991). Optical coherence tomography. *Science* 254, 1178–1181. doi: 10.1126/science.1957169

Ito, D., Imai, Y., Ohsawa, K., Nakajima, K., Fukuuchi, Y., and Kohsaka, S. (1998). Microglia-specific localisation of a novel calcium binding protein, Iba1. *Brain Res. Mol. Brain Res.* 57, 1–9. doi: 10.1016/S0169-328X(98)00040-0

Jensen, W., Yoshida, K., and Hofmann, U. (2007). "*In vivo* implant mechanics of single-shaft microelectrodes in peripheral nervous tissue," in *Neural Engineering, 2007. CNE '07. 3rd International IEEE/EMBS Conference on* (Hawaii).

Kozai, T. D. Y., Vazquez, A. L., Weaver, C. L., Kim, S.-G., and Cui, X. T. (2012). *In vivo* two-photon microscopy reveals immediate microglial reaction to implantation of microelectrode through extension of processes. *J. Neural Eng.* 9:066001. doi: 10.1088/1741-2560/9/6/066001

Leach, J. B., Achyuta, A. K. H., and Murthy, S. K. (2010). Bridging the divide between neuroprosthetic design, tissue engineering and neurobiology. *Front. Neuroeng.* 2:18. doi: 10.3389/neuro.16.018.2009

Ludwig, K. A., Uram, J. D., Yang, J., Martin, D. C., and Kipke, D. R. (2006). Chronic neural recordings using silicon microelectrode arrays electrochemically deposited with a poly(3,4-ethylenedioxythiophene) (PEDOT) film. *J. Neural Eng.* 3, 59–70. doi: 10.1088/1741-2560/3/1/007

Mcconnell, G. C., Butera, R. J., and Bellamkonda, R. V. (2009). Bioimpedance modeling to monitor astrocytic response to chronically. *J. Neural Eng.* 6:055005. doi: 10.1088/1741-2560/6/5/055005

Polikov, V. S., Tresco, P. A., and Reichert, W. M. (2005). Response of brain tissue to chronically implanted neural electrodes. *J. Neurosci. Methods* 148, 1–18. doi: 10.1016/j.jneumeth.2005.08.015

Potter, K. A., Buck, A. C., Self, W. K., and Capadona, J. R. (2012). Stab injury and device implantation within the brain results in inversely multiphasic neuroinflammatory and neurodegenerative responses. *J. Neural Eng.* 9:046020. doi: 10.1088/1741-2560/9/4/046020

Raspopovic, S., Capogrosso, M., Petrini, F. M., Bonizzato, M., Rigosa, J., Di Pino, G., et al. (2014). Restoring natural sensory feedback in real-time bidirectional hand prostheses. *Sci. Trans. Med.* 6, 222ra19. doi: 10.1126/scitranslmed.3006820

Richter, A., Xie, Y., Schumacher, A., Loeffler, S., Kirch, R., Al-Hasani, J., et al. (2013). A simple implantation method for flexible, multisite microelectrodes into rat brains. *Front. Neuroeng.* 6:6. doi: 10.3389/fneng.2013.00006

Rodriguez-Padilla, J. A., Hedges, T. R. III, Monson, B., Srinivasan, V., Wojtkowski, M., Reichel, E., et al. (2007). High-speed ultra–high-resolution optical coherence tomography findings in hydroxychloroquine retinopathy. *Arch. Ophthalmol.* 125, 775–780. doi: 10.1001/archopht.125.6.775

Rubehn, B., and Stieglitz, T. (2010). *In vitro* evaluation of the long-term stability of polyimide as a material for neural implants. *Biomaterials* 31, 3449–3458. doi: 10.1016/j.biomaterials.2010.01.053

Schiffer, D., Giordana, M. T., Cavalla, P., Vigliani, M. C., and Attanasio, A. (1993). Immunohistochemistry of glial reaction after injury in the rat: double stainings and markers of cell proliferation. *Int. J. Dev. Neurosci.* 11, 269–280. doi: 10.1016/0736-5748(93)90085-R

Schmidt, S., Horch, K., and Normann, R. (1993). Biocompatibility of silicon-based electrode arrays implanted in feline cortical tissue. *J. Biomed. Mater. Res.* 27, 1393–1399. doi: 10.1002/jbm.820271106

Sofroniew, M. V. (2005). Reactive astrocytes in neural repair and protection. *Neuroscientist* 11, 400–407. doi: 10.1177/1073858405278321

Sohal, H. S., Jackson, A., Jackson, R., Clowry, G. J., Vaisilevskiy, K., O'Neill, A., et al. (2014). The sinusoidal probe: a new approach to improve electrode longevity. *Front. Neuroeng.* 7:10. doi: 10.3389/fneng.2014.00010

Stieglitz, T., Rubehn, B., Henle, C., Kisban, S., Herwik, S., Ruther, P., et al. (2009). "Brain–computer interfaces: an overview of the hardware to record neural signals from the cortex," in *Neurotherapy: Progress in Restorative Neuroscience and Neurology, Vol. 175 of Progress in Brain Research*, eds E. M. H. Joost Verhaagen and D. F. Swaab (Oxford, UK: Elsevier), 297–315.

Szarowski, D. H., Andersen, M. D., Retterer, S., Spence, A. J., Isaacson, M., Craighead, H. G., et al. (2003). Brain responses to micro-machined silicon devices. *Brain Res.* 983, 23–35. doi: 10.1016/S0006-8993(03)03023-3

Tearney, G. J., Brezinski, M. E., Bouma, B. E., Boppart, S. A., Pitris, C., Southern, J. F., et al. (1997). *In vivo* endoscopic optical biopsy with optical coherence tomography. *Science* 276, 2037–2039. doi: 10.1126/science.276.5321.2037

Tronnier, V. M., and Fogel, W. (2000). Pallidal stimulation for generalized dystonia. *J. Neurosurg.* 92, 453–456. doi: 10.3171/jns.2000.92.3.0453

Turner, J., Shain, W., Szarowski, D., Andersen, M., Martins, S., Isaacson, M., et al. (1999). Cerebral astrocyte response to micromachined silicon implants. *Exp. Neurol.* 156, 33–49. doi: 10.1006/exnr.1998.6983

Winslow, B. D., Christensen, M. B., Yang, W.-K., Solzbacher, F., and Tresco, P. A. (2010). A comparison of the tissue response to chronically implanted Parylene-C-coated and uncoated planar silicon microelectrode arrays in rat cortex. *Biomaterials* 31, 9163–9172. doi: 10.1016/j.biomaterials.2010.05.050

Xie, Y., Bonin, T., Löffler, S., Hüttmann, G., Tronnier, V., and Hofmann, U. G. (2013). Coronal *in vivo* forward-imaging of rat brain morphology with an ultra-small optical coherence tomography fiber probe. *Phys. Med. Biol.* 58, 555–568. doi: 10.1088/0031-9155/58/3/555

Permissions

All chapters in this book were first published in ANTYLPFVBR, by Frontiers; hereby published with permission under the Creative Commons Attribution License or equivalent. Every chapter published in this book has been scrutinized by our experts. Their significance has been extensively debated. The topics covered herein carry significant findings which will fuel the growth of the discipline. They may even be implemented as practical applications or may be referred to as a beginning point for another development.

The contributors of this book come from diverse backgrounds, making this book a truly international effort. This book will bring forth new frontiers with its revolutionizing research information and detailed analysis of the nascent developments around the world.

We would like to thank all the contributing authors for lending their expertise to make the book truly unique. They have played a crucial role in the development of this book. Without their invaluable contributions this book wouldn't have been possible. They have made vital efforts to compile up to date information on the varied aspects of this subject to make this book a valuable addition to the collection of many professionals and students.

This book was conceptualized with the vision of imparting up-to-date information and advanced data in this field. To ensure the same, a matchless editorial board was set up. Every individual on the board went through rigorous rounds of assessment to prove their worth. After which they invested a large part of their time researching and compiling the most relevant data for our readers.

The editorial board has been involved in producing this book since its inception. They have spent rigorous hours researching and exploring the diverse topics which have resulted in the successful publishing of this book. They have passed on their knowledge of decades through this book. To expedite this challenging task, the publisher supported the team at every step. A small team of assistant editors was also appointed to further simplify the editing procedure and attain best results for the readers.

Apart from the editorial board, the designing team has also invested a significant amount of their time in understanding the subject and creating the most relevant covers. They scrutinized every image to scout for the most suitable representation of the subject and create an appropriate cover for the book.

The publishing team has been an ardent support to the editorial, designing and production team. Their endless efforts to recruit the best for this project, has resulted in the accomplishment of this book. They are a veteran in the field of academics and their pool of knowledge is as vast as their experience in printing. Their expertise and guidance has proved useful at every step. Their uncompromising quality standards have made this book an exceptional effort. Their encouragement from time to time has been an inspiration for everyone.

The publisher and the editorial board hope that this book will prove to be a valuable piece of knowledge for researchers, students, practitioners and scholars across the globe.

List of Contributors

Sara Bragado Alonso, Max Schulze-Steikow and Federico Calegari
DFG–Research Center and Cluster of Excellence for Regenerative Therapies, Dresden, Germany

András Jakab and Ernst Schwartz
Computational Imaging Research Lab, Department of Biomedical Imaging and Image-guided Therapy, Medical University of Vienna, Vienna, Austria

Gregor Kasprian, Daniela Prayer and Veronika Schöpf
Division for Neuroradiology and Musculoskeletal Radiology, Department of Biomedical Imaging and Image-guided Therapy, Medical University of Vienna, Vienna, Austria

Gerlinde M. Gruber
Department of Systematic Anatomy, Center for Anatomy and Cell Biology, Medical University of Vienna, Vienna, Austria

Georg Langs
Computational Imaging Research Lab, Department of Biomedical Imaging and Image-guided Therapy, Medical University of Vienna, Vienna, Austria
Computer Science and Artificial Intelligence Lab, Massachusetts Institute of Technology, Cambridge, MA, USA

Masayuki Sakamoto
Institute for Virus Research, Kyoto University, Kyoto, Japan
Kyoto University Graduate School of Biostudies, Kyoto, Japan

Ryoichiro Kageyama
Institute for Virus Research, Kyoto University, Kyoto, Japan
World Premier International Research Initiative–Institute for Integrated Cell-Material Sciences, Kyoto University, Kyoto, Japan
Japan Science and Technology Agency, Core Research for Evolutional Science and Technology, Kyoto, Japan

Itaru Imayoshi
Institute for Virus Research, Kyoto University, Kyoto, Japan
World Premier International Research Initiative–Institute for Integrated Cell-Material Sciences, Kyoto University, Kyoto, Japan
The Hakubi Center, Kyoto University, Kyoto, Japan
Japan Science and Technology Agency, Precursory Research for Embryonic Science and Technology, Kyoto, Japan

Salah Sommakia
Weldon School of Biomedical Engineering, Purdue University, West Lafayette, IN, USA
Physiological Sensing Facility at the Bindley Bioscience Center and Birck Nanotechnology Center, Purdue University, West Lafayette, IN, USA

Jenna L. Rickus
Weldon School of Biomedical Engineering, Purdue University, West Lafayette, IN, USA
Physiological Sensing Facility at the Bindley Bioscience Center and Birck Nanotechnology Center, Purdue University, West Lafayette, IN, USA
Department of Agricultural and Biological Engineering, Purdue University, West Lafayette, IN, USA

Kevin J. Otto
Weldon School of Biomedical Engineering, Purdue University, West Lafayette, IN, USA
Department of Biological Sciences, Purdue University, West Lafayette, IN, USA
J. Crayton Pruitt Family Department of Biomedical Engineering, University of Florida, Gainesville, FL, USA

Akiko Nishiyama, Ryusuke Suzuki and Xiaoqin Zhu
Department of Physiology and Neurobiology, University of Connecticut, Storrs, CT, USA

Sara De Faveri
Department of Robotics, Brain and Cognitive Science, Istituto Italiano di Tecnologia, Genova, Italy
Department of Neuroscience and Brain Technologies, Istituto Italiano di Tecnologia, Genova, Italy

Fabrizia Cesca
Department of Neuroscience and Brain Technologies, Istituto Italiano di Tecnologia, Genova, Italy

Emma Maggiolini
1 Department of Robotics, Brain and Cognitive Science, Istituto Italiano di Tecnologia, Genova, Italy

Ermanno Miele and Francesco De Angelis
Department of Nanostructures, Istituto Italiano di Tecnologia, Genova, Italy

Fabio Benfenati
Department of Neuroscience and Brain Technologies, Istituto Italiano di Tecnologia, Genova, Italy
Department of Experimental Medicine, University of Genova, Genova, Italy

Luciano Fadiga
Department of Robotics, Brain and Cognitive Science, Istituto Italiano di Tecnologia, Genova, Italy
Section of Human Physiology, University of Ferrara, Ferrara, Italy

Maria F. Eiriz and Jorge Valero
Center for Neuroscience and Cell Biology of Coimbra, University of Coimbra (CNC-UC), Coimbra, Portugal

João O. Malva
Faculty of Medicine, Institute of Biomedical Imaging and Life Sciences (IBILI), University of Coimbra, Coimbra, Portugal

Liliana Bernardino
Faculty of Health Sciences, Health Sciences Research Center, University of Beira Interior, Covilhã, Portugal

Viswanath Sankar, Erin Patrick, Robert Dieme and Toshikazu Nishida
Electrical and Computer Engineering Department, University of Florida, Gainesville, FL, USA

Justin C. Sanchez and Abhishek Prasad
Biomedical Engineering Department, University of Miami, Coral Gables, FL, USA

Vania Broccoli, Serena G. Giannelli and Pietro G. Mazzara
Stem Cells and Neurogenesis Unit, Division of Neuroscience, San Raffaele Scientific Institute, Milan, Italy

Alexandra Acevedo-Rodriguez and Lifen Zhang
Department of Neuroscience, Baylor College of Medicine, Houston, TX, USA

Fuwen Zhou, Suzhen Gong and Fu-Ming Zhou
Department of Pharmacology, University of Tennessee College of Medicine, Memphis, TN, USA

Howard Gu
Department of Pharmacology, Ohio State University, Columbus, OH, USA

Mariella De Biasi
Departments of Psychiatry, Perelman School of Medicine, University of Pennsylvania, Philadelphia, PA, USA

John A. Dani
Department of Neuroscience, Perelman School of Medicine, University of Pennsylvania, Philadelphia, PA, USA

J. Dudink and K. Pieterman
Department of Neonatology, Pediatric Intensive Care and Pediatric Radiology, Erasmus Medical Center - Sophia Children's Hospital, Rotterdam, Netherlands

A. Leemans
Image Sciences Institute, University Medical Center Utrecht, Utrecht, Netherlands

M. Kleinnijenhuis
Oxford Centre for Functional Magnetic Resonance Imaging of the Brain, University of Oxford, Oxford, UK

A. M. van Cappellen van Walsum
Department of Anatomy, Donders Institute for Brain, Cognition, and Behaviour, Radboud University Medical Center, Nijmegen, Netherlands

F. E. Hoebeek
Department of Neuroscience, Erasmus Medical Center Rotterdam, Rotterdam, Netherlands

Marika Berchicci
BIND - Behavioral Imaging and Neural Dynamics Center, University "G. d'Annunzio" of Chieti-Pescara, Chieti, Italy
Department of Movement, Human and Health Sciences, University of Rome "Foro Italico," Rome, Italy

Gabriella Tamburro
BIND - Behavioral Imaging and Neural Dynamics Center, University "G. d'Annunzio" of Chieti-Pescara, Chieti, Italy
Department of Medicine and Aging Sciences, University "G. d'Annunzio" of Chieti-Pescara, Chieti, Italy

Silvia Comani
BIND - Behavioral Imaging and Neural Dynamics Center, University "G. d'Annunzio" of Chieti-Pescara, Chieti, Italy
Department of Neuroscience, Imaging and Clinical Sciences, University "G. d'Annunzio" of Chieti-Pescara, Chieti, Italy
Casa di Cura Privata Villa Serena, Città Sant'Angelo, Italy

Karl Deisseroth
Department of Bioengineering, Stanford University, Stanford, CA, USA

Feng Yi and Josh Lawrence
COBRE Center for Structural and Functional Neuroscience, The University of Montana, Missoula, MT, USA
Department of Biomedical and Pharmaceutical Sciences, The University of Montana, Missoula, MT, USA

Elizabeth Catudio-Garrett
COBRE Center for Structural and Functional Neuroscience, The University of Montana, Missoula, MT, USA
Department of Biomedical and Pharmaceutical Sciences, The University of Montana, Missoula, MT, USA
Davidson's Honors College, The University of Montana, Missoula, MT, USA

Robert Gábriel
Department of Experimental Zoology and Neurobiology, University of Pécs, Pécs, Hungary
János Szentágothai Research Center, Pécs, Hungary

Marta Wilhelm
Department of Experimental Zoology and Neurobiology, University of Pécs, Pécs, Hungary
Department of Sport Biology, University of Pécs, Pécs, Hungary

Ferenc Erdelyi and Gabor Szabo
Laboratory of Molecular Biology and Genetics, Institute of Experimental Medicine, Hungarian Academy of Sciences, Budapest, Hungary

Eduardo Fernández, Cristina Soto-Sánchez and Arantxa Alfaro
Bioengineering Institute, Miguel Hernández University of Elche, Elche, Spain
CIBER-BBN, Zaragoza, Spain

Bradley Greger
School of Biological and Health Systems Engineering, Arizona State University, Tempe, AZ, USA

Paul A. House
Department of Neurosurgery, University of Utah, Salt Lake City, UT, USA

Ignacio Aranda
Department of Pathology, Hospital General Universitario, Alicante, Spain

Carlos Botella
Department of Neurosurgery, Hospital La Fe, Valencia, Spain

Julio Albisua
Department of Neurosurgery, Fundación Jimenez Díaz and Hospital Rey Juan Carlos, Madrid, Spain

Richard A. Normann
Department of Bioengineering, University of Utah, Salt Lake City, UT, USA

Maria Asplund and Christian Boehler
Biomedical Microtechnology, IMTEK, Albert-Ludwigs Universität, Freiburg, Germany
Freiburg Institute for Advanced Studies FRIAS, Albert-Ludwigs Universität, Freiburg, Germany
BrainLinks-BrainTools Cluster of Excellence, Albert-Ludwigs Universität, Freiburg, Germany

Thomas Stieglitz
Biomedical Microtechnology, IMTEK, Albert-Ludwigs Universität, Freiburg, Germany
BrainLinks-BrainTools Cluster of Excellence, Albert-Ludwigs Universität, Freiburg, Germany

Antonio Luchicchi, John Noel M. Viaña and Huibert D. Mansvelder
Department of Integrative Neurophysiology, Center for Neurogenomics and Cognitive Research, Neuroscience Campus Amsterdam, Vrije Universiteit, Amsterdam, Netherlands

Bernard Bloem
Department of Integrative Neurophysiology, Center for Neurogenomics and Cognitive Research, Neuroscience Campus Amsterdam, Vrije Universiteit, Amsterdam, Netherlands
McGovern Institute for Brain Research, Massachusetts Institute of Technology, Cambridge, MA, USA

Lorna W. Role
Department of Neurobiology and Behavior, Stony Brook University, Stony Brook, NY, USA

Ulises A. Aregueta-Robles, Laura A. Poole-Warren, Nigel H. Lovell and Rylie A. Green
Graduate School of Biomedical Engineering, University of New South Wales, Sydney, NSW, Australia

Andrew J. Woolley
Graduate School of Biomedical Engineering, University of New South Wales, Sydney, NSW, Australia
School of Medicine, University ofWestern Sydney, Sydney, NSW, Australia

Daniel A. Nagode
Department of Biology, University of Maryland College Park, College Park, MD, USA

Bradley E. Alger
Department of Physiology, University of Maryland School of Medicine, Baltimore, MD, USA
Department of Psychiatry, University of Maryland School of Medicine, Baltimore, MD, USA
Program in Neuroscience, Graduate School, University of Maryland Baltimore, Baltimore, MD, USA

Ai-Hui Tang
Department of Physiology, University of Maryland School of Medicine, Baltimore, MD, USA

Anja Richter, Susanne Löffler, Andreas Moser and Volker Tronnier
Neurochemistry Group, Department of Neurology, University of Luebeck, Luebeck, Germany

Yijing Xie
Graduate School for Computing in Medicine and Life Sciences, University of Luebeck, Luebeck, Germany
Neuroelectronic Systems, Department of General Neurosurgery, University Hospital Freiburg, Freiburg, Germany

Anett Schumacher
Department of Psychology, University of Toronto Scarborough, Toronto, ON, Canada

Robert D. Kirch and Ulrich G. Hofmann
Neuroelectronic Systems, Department of General Neurosurgery, University Hospital Freiburg, Freiburg, Germany

Jaafar Al-Hasani, Daniel H. Rapoport, Charli Kruse and Sandra Danner
Fraunhofer Institution for Marine Biotechnology, Fraunhofer Society, Lübeck, Germany

Paolo Peretto
Neuroscience Institute Cavalieri Ottolenghi, Orbassano, Italy
Department of Life Sciences and System Biology, University of Turin, Torino, Italy

Luca Bonfanti
Neuroscience Institute Cavalieri Ottolenghi, Orbassano, Italy
Department of Veterinary Sciences, University of Turin, Torino, Italy

Harbaljit S. Sohal
Newcastle Movement Lab, Institute of Neuroscience, Newcastle University, Newcastle Upon Tyne, UK
School of Electrical and Electronic Engineering, Newcastle University, Newcastle Upon Tyne, UK

Andrew Jackson, Gavin J. Clowry and Stuart N. Baker
Newcastle Movement Lab, Institute of Neuroscience, Newcastle University, Newcastle Upon Tyne, UK

Richard Jackson, Konstantin Vassilevski and Anthony O'Neill
School of Electrical and Electronic Engineering, Newcastle University, Newcastle Upon Tyne, UK

Rinaldo D. D'Souza and Sukumar Vijayaraghavan
Department of Physiology and Biophysics and the Neuroscience Program, School of Medicine, University of Colorado, Aurora, CO, USA

Yijing Xie, Nadja Martini, Robert D. Kirch and Ulrich G. Hofmann
Neuroelectronic Systems, Department of General Neurosurgery, University Medical Center Freiburg, Freiburg, Germany

Christina Hassler and Thomas Stieglitz
Laboratory for Biomedical Microtechnology, Department of Microsystems Engineering(IMTEK), University of Freiburg, Freiburg, Germany

Andreas Seifert
Gisela and Erwin Sick Chair of Micro-optics, Department of Microsystems Engineering(IMTEK), University of Freiburg, Freiburg, Germany

Index

www.ingramcontent.com/pod-product-compliance
Lightning Source LLC
LaVergne TN
LVHW080927210926
848485LV00004B/744